Dr. miriam stoppard's

Family Health Guide

Dr. miriam stoppard's

Family
Health Guide

DK Publishing

For Eden, Violet, Brodie, and Zac

LONDON, NEW YORK, MUNICH, MELBOURNE, DELHI

Senior Managing Art Editor: Lynne Brown
Senior Editors: Julia North, Jennifer Williams
Senior Art Editor: Rosamund Saunders
Art Editor – Life Stages section: Kathryn Gammon
DTP Designer: Karen Constanti
Editors: Jinny Johnson, Kathy Fahey, Jane Perlmutter
Picture Research: Samantha Nunn
Picture Library: Charlotte Oster, Scott Stickland
Production: Heather Hughes

Special Photography: Trish Gant
Photographic Coordination: Sally Smallwood
Illustrations: Richard Tibbitts

This book is not intended to be a substitute for medical diagnosis and you are advised to consult your doctor for specific information concerning your health.

All photography in this book uses models.

First American Edition, 2003
00 01 02 03 04 05 10 9 8 7 6 5 4 3 2 1

Published in the United States by DK Publishing, Inc.
375 Hudson Street, New York, New York 10014

First published in Great Britain in 2002
By Dorling Kindersley Limited

A Cataloging-in-Publication record for this book is available from the Library of Congress ISBN 0-7894-9699-2

Reproduced by GRB
Jacket reproduced by Colourscan
Printed and bound by
Toppan Printing Co (HK) Ltd, Hong Kong

Discover more at
www.dk.com

Contents

How to use this book

The Family Health Guide is about how you can stay well as much as it is about what to do if you are ill. It has been planned so that you can find topics that interest you quickly and easily, with boxed text to highlight areas of special interest, such as tests and treatments, information on what you can do to help yourself, and important points to note. The book is also easy to browse with related topics listed in section openers, overview articles at the beginning of each section, and cross-references between articles.

Section Opener

Throughout the book, the main topics that are covered in each section are listed in section openers, making it easy to find a subject that interests you and enabling you to see other topics at a glance that are related to it.

Sections include
- Golden Rules
- Life Stages
- Symptom Guides
- Directory
- Reference
- Useful Addresses
- Index

SECTION OPENER

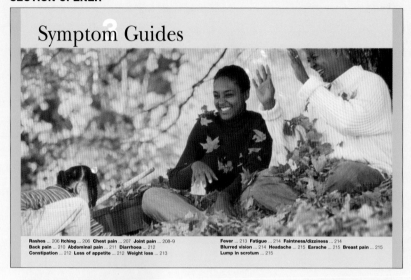

Symptom Guides

Rashes ... 206 Itching ... 206 Chest pain ... 207 Joint pain ... 208-9
Back pain ... 210 Abdominal pain ... 211 Diarrhoea ... 212
Constipation ... 212 Loss of appetite ... 212 Weight loss ... 213

Fever ... 213 Fatigue ... 214 Faintness/dizziness ... 214
Blurred vision ... 214 Headache ... 215 Earache ... 215 Breast pain ... 215
Lump in scrotum ... 215

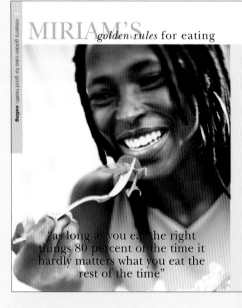

MIRIAM'S *golden rules* for eating

"as long as you eat the right things 80 percent of the time it hardly matters what you eat the rest of the time"

"drink plenty of fluids"

✻ Our bodies don't need balanced meals every time we eat, but **eating a variety of different foods each day promotes good health.** Don't get too worried about picky children who go through food fads – their diet usually balances out over a week.

✻ As long as you **eat the right things 80 percent of the time** it hardly matters what you eat the rest of the time.

✻ **Eat an orange fruit or vegetable every day** for the carotenoids, which help to protect against cancer.

• Drink at least 6–8 large glasses of fluid a day – any liquid will do. Vary water with fruit juice and low-fat milk. A few cups of tea can count too.

✻ No healthy person who **eats a balanced diet** needs vitamin supplements.

✻ For children of two and up, start to moderate fatty foods. Use semi-skimmed milk, **cut the fat off meat**, don't fry – grill.

✻ Always eat some breakfast. Research shows that **breakfast eaters tend to be slimmer** and have healthier diets. Don't eat a heavy meal too late in the evening – it will stop you sleeping.

✻ **Small changes in eating habits reap great rewards,** so there's no need to go overboard and make dietary changes you can't stick to. **Make one or two small adjustments a week** – change from white to wholemeal bread, full cream to semi-skimmed milk, butter to an olive-oil spread.

✻ We really do all need at least **five helpings of fruit and vegetables a day** – fresh, frozen, canned, dried or juiced. There's no alternative.

✻ **Eat oily fish at least once a week.** It is very good for you because it helps to maintain a healthy heart. Have a little olive oil on your salad too.

✻ Drink tea for the flavonoids, which **seem to help reduce the risk of heart disease** and stroke and may even slow ageing.

✻ Around half of our calories **should come from unrefined carbohydrates** – that is, wholemeal bread, oats in any form, rice in any form, pasta, wholegrain cereals, potatoes (in jackets especially good), peas, beans and fruit.

✻ Treat protein like a condiment – a little goes a long way. **Eat some lean red meat a few times a week.** Remember that red meat is an excellent source of protein, easily absorbed iron and zinc, and B vitamins.

✻ Start reading labels for food values, especially fat and sugar. **Sugar adds variety, but is a non-essential food** – don't give your children sugar-coated cereals as this may encourage a sweet tooth for life.

✻ Stop adding salt to food and keep your blood pressure at a healthy level. **The healthy limit for salt is 6g (⅕oz) per day** (equivalent to 2.4g (⅒oz) sodium – salt is usually listed as "sodium" on food labels). But your doctor may advise you to reduce it even further.

✻ Read labels for salt content, too, and **never give foods with a high salt content to babies and** young children; their kidneys can't handle it.

Use fresh fruits as your snack food and try a greater variety – have you tasted mango, papaya, passion fruit, ugli fruit or kiwi fruit? Eat whole fruits as well as drinking fruit juices, and avoid squashes and cordials, many of which contain only fruit flavours.

Choose a variety of yellow vegetables, beans and pulses, and green leafy vegetables each week. Don't add salt to your vegetables and steam or reduce the boiling time for green vegetables.

Eat fresh, unprocessed nuts as snack and give them in salads. Nuts contain essential fatty acids not found in many other foods, and therefore are a vital part of your diet. They are also high in calories so don't eat too many, and limit the roasted, dry-roasted and salted ones.

Potatoes, cereals and grains
As well as potatoes, this group includes wheat, oats, barley, rye and rice and the foods made of them, such as bread, pasta, biscuits and breakfast cereals. Wholegrain products are the most nutritious and contain a lot of dietary fibre. Increase the amount of wholegrain foods you eat.

✻ Choose wholemeal pasta and brown or basmati rice.
✻ Eat at least four slices of wholemeal bread a day.
✻ Buy unsweetened breakfast cereals.
✻ Use wholemeal flour for making pastry (or use half white and half wholemeal).

✻ Eat more potatoes. Try them thinly sliced and steamed, or boiled or baked in their skins, and eat them with low-fat yogurt and herbs rather than butter. Mashed potatoes are tasty made with skimmed milk or low-fat yogurt, parsley and pepper.

✻ Eat fewer cakes and biscuits, even when they are made with wholemeal flour because of their high fat and sugar content. Choose scones, currant buns, fruit and nut cakes and malt loaves, which are lower in sugar and fat than cream-filled and iced cakes.

The only other comment I'd make is that unrefined carbohydrates such as whole grains should provide a solid base to our diet. High-protein diets have absolutely nothing to recommend them. Protein should be taken as a condiment – for example, in pasta sauce. We should take very few of our calories in the form of saturated fats, such as butter and cheese, or sugar.

"Eat whole fruit as well as drinking fruit juices"

◀ **Golden Rules** Guidelines to a healthy lifstyle are easy to understand and easy to follow.

▲ **Explanation** Supporting information explains the whys and hows of the rules.

protect against cataracts and age-related macular degeneration.

grapefruit - One half contains half your daily requirement of vitamin C. Eat the pith – the soluble fibre lowers cholesterol and contains folic acid and bioflavonoids to keep cancer at bay.

protect against cancer, as do all orange foods. Eat at least one every day.

prunes - Contain iron, fibre, potassium, vitamin A.

cranberries - Juice stops bacteria clinging to the lining of the bladder. Ace for women who are cystitis-prone.

Golden Rules

The Golden Rules section of the book gives Dr. Stoppard's concise, essential guidelines for maintaining a lifetime of good health. Each rule is supported by facts that explain why it is important and precise instructions on what you need to do to stay on track.

Topics include:
- Eating • Exercise • Safe drinking limits • Giving up smoking • Safe sex • Restful sleep • Avoiding stress

Life Stages

The Life Stages section offers advice and information on issues affecting health and well-being at each stage of life.

Stages covered
• 0–1 years • 1–4 years • 4–11 years
• 11–18 years • 18–40 years • 40–60 years • 60+ years

MINI CONTENTS

Body — **Happy mealtimes**...96 **Veggie child**...84 **Sweets**...85 **Junk foods**...85 **Importance of physical activity**...86 **Healthy feet**...86 **Adventurousness**...87 **Teeth**...87 **Guiding principles**...88

"children can't survive, let alone thrive, without close parental interest"

Social — **Holidays away from home**...92 **Pocket money**...91 **Self-confidence**...91 **Road safety**...90 **Knowing where to draw the line**...92 **Children and the too-friendly stranger**...92 **Being considerate**...90 **Changing patterns of friendship**...90 **Bullying**...91 **Problem behaviour**...91 **A healthy attitude to nudity**...90 **Masturbation is normal**...90

tell your children the facts of life as soon as they begin to ask

Mind — **Preparing your child for school**...96 **Project work**...96 **How parents can help with reading**...97 **Helping with numbers**...97 **Why does a child cheat?**...98 **Why does a child lie?**...98 **Hyperactivity**...99 **Why does a child steal?**...99 **Sex play is normal**...100 **Answering questions about sex**...101 **Television?**...101

CHAPTER OPENER

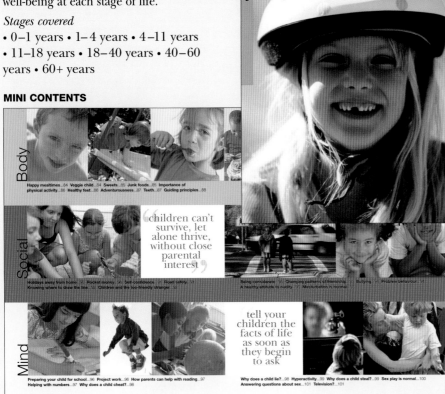

"a child needs self-belief if she is to fulfil her potential"

life stages: 4 to 11 years

Between the ages of 4 and 11 your energetic, loving, mischievous pre-schooler is going to grow and develop into a reflective, kind, industrious, cooperative adolescent whom everyone enjoys. That's a tough assignment for any 4-year-old and there are many complex skills to acquire along the way, not the least of which are self-control and self-discipline.

Most important, milestones can only be achieved if parents show loving care to their children. Children can't survive let alone thrive without close parental interest. They can get by of course and most do, even if parental care isn't forthcoming.

Achieving self-belief

But there are some milestones that are exceedingly difficult for a child to master alone and they can go astray without feedback and guidance. Let me give you just one example of a milestone that involves an important step in personal development – achieving **self-belief**.

Call it self-confidence, call it self-assurance, but without it a child will not only fail to fulfil her potential, she could get into all kinds of trouble because she won't know how to control her emotions or how to rechannel her frustrations and anger to gainful purpose.

You may think, well, she'll grow into a shy child, unsure of herself. That would be bad enough, but it's worse than that.
● She grows into a child who becomes a loner without friends, which is heartbreaking for any parent to see.
● She may seek attention and affection to bolster her waning ego with all kinds of inappropriate behaviour, sometimes being labelled as **hyperactive**.
● And then, if no one helps her to build belief in herself, she resorts to lying, stealing, bullying, even to drinking and taking drugs to feel good about herself.

You can see that without achieving **self-belief**, there are problems ahead. So important is this milestone, and several other crucial milestones, that I call them **islands of development**. If a child doesn't reach the haven of these islands, there can be disastrous fallout later.

Think of your child as bobbing along on a river of development trying to negotiate the equivalent of white water, the flow sometimes fast as she goes through a spurt of skill acquisition, or slower and more placid as she consolidates her achievements.

These islands make the river navigable. They're places where your child can rest up, so to speak, take stock and move on to the next milestone – with lots of encouragement and praise from you of course. The islands are also an insurance policy. If you can help your child to reach one she'll tackle the next stretch of white water with determination, courage and good sense. And, having enjoyed the security of reaching one of these islands, your child can safely be given responsibilities of increasing gravitas both for herself and others.

In the pages that follow, I offer guidelines where appropriate, advice where I feel there may be a need and strategies for dealing with difficult situations.

The right age to...

● A child is ready to learn to tie her own shoelaces at about 4 years old.
● A child may be able to cope with moving into a proper bed at about 5 years old.
● A 6-year-old is probably ready to receive pocket money and decide how to spend it.
● At 7 a child can learn to cross the street alone.
● A child of 8 can sleep over at a friend's house.
● A 9-year-old is ready to learn about puberty.
● A child of 10 may enjoy the responsibility of looking after a pet.
● An 11-year-old can be left at home alone for short periods.

▲ **Life Stages** Dr. Stoppard outlines and gives her views on the most significant health-related issues that arise at each stage of life.

◄ **Contents** Picture time lines help you to pick out the subjects that interest you most.

▶ **Category** For each life stage Dr. Stoppard discusses health implications related to mind, body, and social development. Life stages are color-coded so that you can find the one that interests you at a glance.

BODY **SOCIAL** **MIND**

feeding children

The best way to make sure that your children eat a healthy, balanced diet for the rest of their lives is to help them develop good habits from the beginning.

Happy mealtimes

do
✓ Make mealtimes an important family ritual so your child can learn how to be part of a group.
✓ Set up some basic ground rules for meals so that everyone knows they can't throw tantrums or just grab and run.
✓ Have meals at regular times so that you set up a rhythm for family life – children love this.
✓ Encourage thoughtfulness for others – never take the last portion without offering it to everyone else.
✓ Foster chat and discussion and make sure each child is listened to, including the youngest.
✓ Trivialize accidents and spillage so that the conviviality isn't broken.

don't
✗ Let meals become battlegrounds. You can't force a child to eat. Let them refuse food, they'll ask for it soon enough if you don't insist.
✗ Let a child spoil family calm and harmony at the table for everyone else, remove them to another room.
✗ Exclude children from your conversation – they become naughty to attract your attention.
✗ Let meals tail off without a formal ending. Each child should say they've had enough and ask to go and play.
✗ Let the youngest be last to get her food. Give it to her first – her patience is shortest.
✗ Have the television on or music playing during meals.

Veggie foods

It's quite safe for a child to be a vegetarian from the age of eating solid food, but think about the following points.
● Their diet should contain dairy products and eggs and be carefully planned to contain all essential ingredients.
● With supplements, and ingenuity on the parents' part, even a vegan diet excluding dairy, eggs, and meat can be okay.
● Children can on a vegan diet tend to be smaller and lighter than average. While their height does "catch up," vegan children usually remain lighter and leaner.
● The slow growth is because a typical vegetarian diet contains fewer of the high-energy foods needed for growth.
● Children need high-energy foods for growth and play so nut products, cheese, and avocado are useful. Vegetarian children should be given whole milk to provide crucial calories. Go easy on bulky foods such as a lot of fruit and vegetables and high-fiber cereals, which reduce absorption of iron and zinc.
● Variety is key. All four food groups should be included in these daily ratios. Cereals and grains 4–5 servings; fruit 1–3 servings; vegetables 2 servings; legumes, nuts, and seeds 1–2 servings; animal protein (milk, cheese, and eggs) 3 servings.
● Vegetarian children should have some vegetable oil/butter/yeast extract.
● Good sources of vegetable protein are nuts, legumes, tofu, and soy in any form. Milk and dairy products and eggs are "complete" proteins.
● To keep up intake of calcium, iron, and vitamin C, children need to eat plenty of fortified foods – for example, breakfast cereals and whole grain bread – diced fruit, dark green vegetables, and dairy.
● Vitamin C promotes iron absorption so food containing these nutrients should be eaten together.

Junk foods

■ How many times a week does your family eat fast food?
Rarely (1)   Once (2)
Twice (3)   More (4)

■ Do you serve french fries with food?
Never (0)   Occasionally (1)
Frequently (3)   Very frequently (5)

■ Do you give in if your child whines for a Big Mac?
Never (0)   Sometimes (1)
Often (2)   Always (4)

■ How often do you use junk food as a bribe?
Never (0)   Now and then (2)
Quite often (5) All the time (7)

■ Do you put hamburgers and fish sticks on your weekly shopping list?
Never (0)   Once a month (1)
Every two weeks (3) Every week (5)

■ Do you have sweet carbonated drinks in the fridge?
Never (0)   Sometimes (1)
Often (3)   All the time (5)

■ Do you finish off meals with a sweet dessert, e.g. ice cream?
Never (0)   Now and then (1)
Every day (5)   Every meal (7)

■ Is there ketchup on the table?
Never (0)   Occasionally (1)
Often (2)   Always (3)

■ How often does your family eat take-out?
Never (0)   Now and then (1)
Weekly (2)
Often (3)   Very frequently (7)

■ Do you serve much fried food?
Never (0)   Sometimes (1)
Often (3)   Very frequently (7)

Now add up your score.
Up to 15: Okay – your family's diet slips occasionally but it is generally good.
Up to 25: Too much – the junk food level is creeping up. Try to cut it down.
More than 35: STOP! Your family is eating far too much junk food and it will damage their health.

Candy

I don't believe in giving candy freely nor in placing a total ban on candy – that only encourages children to be secretive and dishonest. What I do believe in is rationing candy, and this always worked with my own children. If you let your child have a little candy after a meal and encourage him to brush his teeth afterward, you'll be helping him develop good eating habits, self-control, and good oral hygiene. Candy might seem like an appropriate reward for children and it is, but not all the time. There is no hard and fast rule on this, and no reason why you shouldn't occasionally reward your child with candy as long as you make it clear that this is a one-time treat. It's worth making an effort, though, to devise other forms of reward, such as a favorite yogurt flavor or a small toy.

Symptom Guides

These guides help you make sense of the most common symptoms you and your family are likely to experience and direct you to the right information.

Charts include:
• Fatigue • Faintness • Fever
• Headache • Weight loss • Blurred vision • Earache • Chest pain
• Back pain • Joint pain • Abdominal pain • Loss of appetite • Diarrhea
• Constipation • Rash • Itching
• Breast pain • Lump in scrotum

SELF-HELP SYMPTOM GUIDES

Chapter openers These list all conditions covered.

Directory

With a strong emphasis on prevention and cure, the Directory covers over 280 of the most common medical conditions. These are grouped by body system and are explained in friendly, nonspecialized language.

Chapters include:
• Heart, Blood, & Circulation • Sexuality & Fertility • Threats to Mental

Well-being • Allergies & the Immune System • Infections • Digestion
• Kidneys & Bladder • Chest & Air Passages • Brain & Nervous System
• Bones, Joints, & Muscles • Skin, Hair, & Nails • Eyes & Vision • Ears, Nose, & Throat • Teeth & Gums • Hormones

Plus:
A special section on children's conditions

ESSAY   ANATOMY

DIRECTORY

FOCUS ON

▶ **Essay & Anatomy**
These pages give Dr. Stoppard's personal view of each medical area, with a guide to the basic anatomy of the body system dealt with in the chapter.

▶ **Directory**
Each entry gives an explanation of the condition, how and why it occurs, how a doctor might treat it, and what you can do to help yourself.

▶ **Focus On**
Focus On pages give Dr. Stoppard's personal view of a topic of special concern, helping you to understand it in greater depth.

CHILDREN'S CONDITIONS

Special section on children's conditions

▶ **Children's conditions**
This section gives advice on what to do when your child is ill and includes over 50 common medical conditions and developmental problems that occur in childhood.

▶ **Development**
Key aspects of behavior and development that may cause concern include dyslexia and dyspraxia, developmental delay, and attention deficit hyperactivity disorder.

FIRST AID

Reference

This section includes first aid for common emergencies, how to keep healthy when traveling abroad, and a list of useful addresses and websites relating to topics covered in the book.

Features
• First aid • Travel health • Useful addresses, telephone numbers, and websites • Index • Acknowledgments

▶ **Step-by-step** The first aid section gives step-by-step instructions to help you deal with minor and more serious medical emergencies.

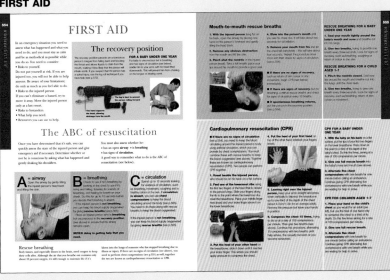

Index
The index is designed to help you find the information you want with the minimum of effort.

Page numbers for main entries are in bold; page numbers for topics covered in boxes are in italics.

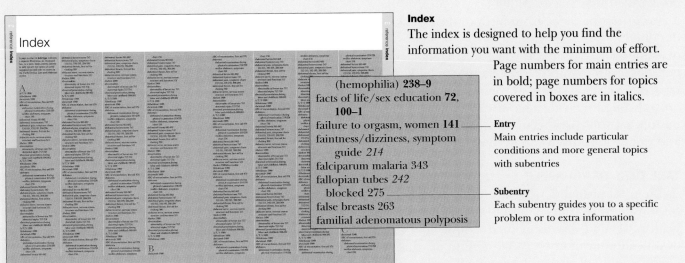

Entry
Main entries include particular conditions and more general topics with subentries

Subentry
Each subentry guides you to a specific problem or to extra information

MIRIAM'S introduction

Why another health book you may ask. There are many answers, the first being that my goal is to inform parents and through them promote healthy families. So while you'll find many topics and issues that affect you yourself, there are many others that are important to you because they affect your children and your parents.

When I wrote this book I had you in mind: the mom or dad who has growing children at one end of the spectrum and aging parents at the other. You are the person who has the most need of good, accurate, usable information that will clarify, reassure, and inform you about the health and well-being of all your family on a day-to-day basis.

Toward this end I've included a section in the book called Life Stages, which takes a look at the major issues that arise from birth to death. It's designed to give you warning of the sorts of questions you may face as you go through each decade. It offers you the opportunity to look back, say from your 40s or 50s, at your children as they grow through their teenage years and beyond, and on to what your parents may be experiencing now and what you yourself will in the future.

TAKE CARE OF YOURSELF

As the most pivotal person in your family you have a responsibility to yourself and to them to stay fit and healthy. When I was disinclined to look after my own health, my mother would remind me that the family would fall apart if I became ill. "Who will take "your lifestyle can easily give you ten more years of life"

"improve the health and well-being of the whole family"

"those tough workouts in the gym aren't life expanding at all"

care of your four little boys?" she'd ask, and that was usually a good enough corrective to make me pay attention to what I was eating and to get exercise.

"healthy eating doesn't have to be a chore"

SMALL CHANGES – HUGE DIFFERENCES

These days healthy eating shouldn't be a chore. Quite the opposite in fact. There are a few very simple tips (what I've called Golden Rules) about eating which, if followed even approximately, will improve the health and well-being of the whole family. Small changes in eating make huge differences, especially since a list of what can truly be called power foods has emerged in the last few years and no person should go without them. No one would claim that

simply by eating a plentiful supply of these power foods that we can live longer. Food alone won't do that, but evidence is emerging that your lifestyle can easily give you ten more years of life – or take ten away.

CLUES TO A LONG LIFE

Long-term studies on the Okinawan people, the longest-living race on the planet, give us plenty of clues about how to increase our lifespan and defy the biological markers of age. The Okinawans, who live on an island off the coast of Japan, are, decade for decade, biologically younger than we are in the West. Many of the beneficial aspects of Okinawan life are the direct opposite of what we pursue here.

They don't smoke, for instance, and they drink very little. They don't eat just five portions of fruit and vegetables as we're exhorted to do, but anything from 9 to 19. They are the opposite of sedentary – our most life-shortening habit is sitting down – and they putter all day long; walking, gardening, dancing, and engaging in gentle martial arts.

In fact we now know that those tough workouts in the gym aren't life expanding at all. Keeping active, even gently, is. If I had to recommend just one life change to instantly improve your health and life expectancy it would be to get more exercise in the way the Okinawans do. Nothing onerous, three or four sessions a week of gentle cycling or brisk walking will do. The payoffs are quite surprising.

First, you won't be fat. Second, you won't be in danger of developing type II diabetes and you'll lower your chances of a heart attack or stroke. Osteoporosis and fractures will probably pass you by. If, in addition, you follow my Golden Rules for your lifestyle, you could find you've avoided many cancers.

KEEP INFORMED

Despite our best efforts we are prey to illness and you'll find most of the common ones in the ready-reference disease directory. I hope you'll dip in and out of it to make sure you're well enough informed to know a potentially serious symptom when it arises, what to do in a household emergency, and how to be an equal negotiator with your doctors and carergivers.

"our most life-shortening habit is sitting down"

Golden Rules

for Good Health

MIRIAM'S *golden rules* for eating

"as long as you eat the right things 80 percent of the time it hardly matters what you eat the rest of the time"

✳ Our bodies don't need balanced meals every time we eat, but **eating a variety of different foods each day promotes good health**. Don't get too worried about fussy children who go through picky phases – their diet usually balances out over a week.

✳ As long as you **eat the right things 80 percent of the time** it hardly matters what you eat the rest of the time.

✳ **Eat an orange fruit or vegetable every day** for the carotenoids, which help to protect against cancer.

✳ **Drink at least 6–8 large glasses of fluid a day**. Vary water with fruit juice and low-fat milk. A few cups of tea can count too.

✳ No healthy person who **eats a balanced diet** needs vitamin supplements.

✳ For children of two and up, start to moderate fatty foods. Use low-fat milk, **cut the fat off meat**, don't fry – broil.

✳ Always eat some breakfast. Research shows that **breakfast eaters tend to be slimmer** and have healthier diets. Don't eat a heavy meal too late in the evening – it will stop you from sleeping.

✳ **Small changes in eating habits reap great rewards**, so there's no need to go

"drink plenty of fluids"

overboard and make dietary changes you can't stick to. **Make one or two small adjustments a week** – change from white to whole grain bread, whole milk to low-fat milk, butter to an olive oil spread.

✳ We all really do need at least **five helpings of fruit and vegetables a day** – fresh, frozen, or juiced is best. There's no alternative.

✳ **Eat oily fish at least twice a week**. It is very good for you because it helps maintain a healthy heart. Have a little olive oil on your salad too.

✳ Drink tea for the flavonoids, which **seem to help reduce the risk of heart disease** and stroke and may even slow aging.

✳ Around **half of our calories should come from unrefined carbohydrates** – that is, whole grain bread, oats in any form, brown rice, whole wheat pasta, whole grain cereals, potatoes (with skins are especially good), peas, beans, and fruit.

✳ Treat protein like a condiment or a side dish – a little goes a long way. **Eat some lean red meat, fish, or poultry a few times a week.** Remember that red meat is an excellent source of protein, easily absorbed iron and zinc, and B vitamins.

✳ Start reading labels for food values, especially fat and sugar. **Sugar is a nonessential food** – don't give your children sugary cereals since this may encourage a sweet tooth for life.

✳ To help keep your blood pressure at a healthy level, stop adding salt to food. **The healthy limit for salt is ⅕oz (6g) per day** (equivalent to ⅒oz (2.4g) sodium – salt is usually listed as "sodium" on food labels). Your doctor may advise you to reduce it even more.

✳ Read labels for salt content, too, and **never give foods with a high salt content to babies** and young children; their kidneys can't handle it.

"eating a healthy diet helps you control your weight"

How to eat healthily

Changing from an unhealthy to a healthy diet is not difficult; it simply involves making some different choices and emphasizing certain foods. It does require a little effort and determination, but once you start following the golden rules, you'll really enjoy it, feel marvelous, and be encouraged to continue.

Most of the foods you should eat are easily available and, contrary to what you might have thought, you can eat more of some of them. You will soon find that a healthy diet can be delicious and satisfying. It doesn't involve hunger pangs, which would

only lead to excessive snacking and overeating later. In fact, you'll find that your desire to snack will gradually decrease and that eating a healthy diet helps you to control your weight without effort.

There are very few foods we need to eat every day. I'd narrow them down to:

✳ at least two fruits, more if possible; one should be orange in color
✳ at least two veggies, more if possible
✳ a large bowl of leafy vegetables.

Otherwise, eat a variety of foods each day from the other three main food groups: meat, fish, or legumes; breads,

potatoes, and cereals; and milk and dairy foods. Most of us eat enough meat and dairy products but need to increase the amount of fruit and vegetables as well as cereals and grains.

Fruit and vegetables

Fresh fruits and vegetables provide a lot of vitamins, minerals, and fiber. Eat more of them and a greater variety – aim for at least five portions each day.

Eat more salads of all kinds: try beans, corn, potato, celery, apple, carrot, bean sprouts, beets, rice, watercress, and chickpeas as delicious alternatives to the familiar lettuce, cucumber, and tomato.

Superfoods

avocados · Contain vitamins B1, B6, and E, potassium, magnesium, and healthy fatty acids that help regulate cholesterol levels. Make a great first food for babies. Beware, though, they are high in calories.

broccoli · Contains vitamins C, A, and E, calcium, folic acid, and sulforaphane.

tomatoes · Good source of vitamin C and flavonoids. Contain the antioxidant lycopene, which helps protect against prostate cancer and heart disease.

corn · Contains fiber, potassium, and lutein, which may help protect against cataracts and macular degeneration (deterioration in vision).

grapefruit · One half contains half your daily requirement of vitamin C. Eat the pith – the soluble fiber lowers cholesterol and contains folic acid and bioflavonoids to keep cancer at bay.

red onions · Contain folic acid, B6, and potassium as well as flavonoids to help reduce risk of heart disease. May help raise HDL ("good" cholesterol).

beets · Fresh, not pickled, beets contains folic acid.

strawberries · Rich in vitamin C and ellagic acid, a compound with cancer fighting effects.

black currants · Very rich in vitamin C, vitamin K, and body-protecting flavonoids.

carrots · Contain carotenoids, which protect against cancer, as do all orange foods. Eat at least one every day.

prunes · Contain iron, fiber, potassium, vitamin A.

cranberries · Juice stops bacteria from clinging to the lining of the bladder. Good for women who are cystitis-prone.

Use fresh fruits as your snack food and try a greater variety – have you tasted mango, papaya, passion fruit, ugli fruit, or kiwi? Eat whole fruits, drink fruit juices, and avoid fruit "drinks" and sodas, many of which contain only fruit flavors.

Choose a variety of yellow and orange vegetables, beans and legumes, and green leafy vegetables each week. Don't add salt to your vegetables, and steam or reduce the boiling time for green vegetables.

Eat fresh, unprocessed nuts as snacks and put them in salads. Nuts contain essential fatty acids not found in many other foods, and therefore are a vital part of your diet. But they are also high in calories so don't eat too many, and limit the roasted, dry-roasted, and salted ones.

Potatoes, cereals, and grains

In addition to potatoes, this group includes wheat, oats, barley, rye, and rice and the foods made from them, such as bread, pasta, muffins, and breakfast cereals. Whole grain products are the most nutritious and contain a lot of dietary fiber. Increase the amount of whole grain foods you eat.

✻ Choose whole wheat pasta and brown or basmati rice.
✻ Eat at least four slices of whole grain bread a day.
✻ Buy unsweetened breakfast cereals.
✻ Use whole grain flour for making pastries (or use half white and half whole grain).
✻ Eat fewer cakes and cookies, even when they are made with whole wheat flour, because of their high fat and sugar content. Choose scones, biscuts, fruit and nut cakes, and muffins, which are lower in sugar and fat than cream-filled and iced cakes.

"eat whole fruit as well as drinking fruit juices"

✻ Eat more potatoes. Try them thinly sliced and steamed, or boiled or baked in their skins, and eat them with low-fat yogurt and herbs rather than butter. Mashed potatoes are tasty made with skim milk or low-fat yogurt, parsley, and pepper.

The only other comment I'd make is that unrefined carbohydrates such as whole grains should provide a solid base to our diet. High-protein diets have absolutely nothing to recommend them. Protein should be eaten as a side dish – for example, in pasta sauce. We should get very few of our calories in the form of saturated fats, such as butter and cheese, or in the form of simple sugars.

MIRIAM'S *golden rules* for exercise

"always exercise to the
point where you have
to breathe deeply to fill every
corner of your lungs"

* **Do some physical activity for 30 minutes** at least five days a week. Brisk walking will do.

* If you're over 40, take any medication, or have a chest or heart condition, **never start an exercise program without a medical checkup.**

* If you want, wear a heart rate recorder and **never exceed the maximum heart rate for your age.**

* **Always do warm-up exercises before you start** – 5–6 minutes. Cold muscles injure easily. The older you are, the longer you should spend warming up – 10–15 minutes if you're over 50.

* **Always spend five minutes "warming down"** after exercise. Do a few stretches to prevent stiffness and aching.

* **Swimming is excellent as we get older** because it supports stiff joints and exercises the whole body.

* **The most important muscles to keep fit are the quads on the front of the thighs** – without them you'll become tied to a chair because you won't be able to get out of it. Cycling is good for the quads.

* **If anything hurts, stop** – the saying "no pain, no gain" is nonsense – sharp pain is bad.

"take up an activity or sport that you adore"

* You should always **exercise to the point where you have to breathe deeply** to fill every corner of your lungs – this helps protects your lungs from infection.

* **Increase the time and vigor of your exercise program gradually**, say a week at a time.

* **Weight-bearing exercise is best** because it protects against osteoporosis (brittle bones).

* Exercises aren't just for strength and stamina, they **promote balance, agility, and mobility** – very important as you get older.

* **Yoga is superb exercise** because it exercises muscles through stretching. **Only some forms benefit heart and lungs**

* To ensure the success of your exercise program **take up an activity or sport you adore**, so it's never a chore.

Here's my list of the good things resulting from exercise. It:

* keeps your heart and lungs healthy
* promotes endorphins which give you an eight-hour high
* helps relieve headaches, irritable bowel syndrome, and migraines
* controls appetite
* can change your eating habits to healthy ones
* makes you want more exercise
* burns calories
* helps insomnia
* relieves anxiety
* helps relieve panic attacks
* treats depression
* reshapes your body
* alleviates jet lag
* reduces cholesterol
* lowers blood pressure.

In addition to these benefits, we now know that exercise also improves self-esteem, self-confidence, performance, and mental health.

Benefits of exercise

Physical activity can boost mental as well as physical well-being and change your outlook on life. It could even prevent problems from starting. As I know from personal experience, regular activity can lift your mood, help you deal with negative emotions like anger, and bring you a general sense of mental well-being.

I've noticed that if I wake feeling a bit down, 30 minutes on my exercise bike cures the blues. That's because exercise floods my body with hormones that reduce tension levels and feelings of stress or fatigue. These changes happen right after a session, particularly since I do six hill programs. No wonder I'm addicted to it and can't miss a day. This kind of exercise can make a difference to anyone suffering from anxiety, depression, or low self-esteem – and it has no side effects.

Self-image

Studies have shown that people feel better about themselves once they start an exercise program. Changes to body shape – as you begin to lose weight and feel your muscle tone getting better – improve your self-image, which can boost mental well-being.

Exercise helps you to see just what you're capable of, giving you a sense of achievement. Learning a new skill or achieving a goal, however minor, boosts self-esteem and motivation.

Social life

Joining a local group, going to classes at a gym or health club, or bicycling with a friend or relative, for example, can give you a way to meet people and socialize. It gives you something

"regular exercise can lift your mood"

in common and helps break the ice. If you'd prefer not to join in with others, there are many activities you can enjoy on your own, such as swimming or walking.

Health benefits

People who are active have half the risk of developing coronary heart disease of those who aren't. Regular exercise ameliorates common risk factors for heart disease such as high blood pressure, obesity, and high cholesterol levels.

Keeping up an active lifestyle is good for bones, joints, and muscles and it can help delay the onset of osteoporosis and arthritis. It can significantly improve and maintain the strength and flexibility of your muscles, helping to prevent injury and reducing the risk of falling,

allowing you to enjoy life to the fullest as you get older.

It can also help control conditions such as diabetes and may reduce the risk of some cancers – in particular bowel cancer.

Staying active

Recent research on the longest-living people in the world, the Okinawans living on islands between Japan and Taiwan, suggests that beneficial physical activity can simply mean everyday puttering – gardening, cleaning, and walking to catch a bus, as well as exercise such as bicycling, swimming, or working out, or playing sports such as soccer, golf, or volleyball. It doesn't necessarily mean an intensive workout in the gym, but it does mean being active for 30 minutes at least five days a week.

MIRIAM'S *golden rules* for not smoking

* **Giving up smoking is one of the best things you can do for your body.**

* **Stop smoking three months before trying for a baby** – men and women.

* **Don't smoke during pregnancy.**

* **Tobacco is the gateway drug to other drugs,** including marijuana.

* **No one who smokes should hold a baby** (to lessen the risk of crib death).

* **Don't smoke high-tar cigarettes.**

* **Never smoke right down to the filter,** this is where cancer chemicals are concentrated.

* **If possible smoke only five cigarettes a day.**

* **Don't smoke while drinking alcohol** – you'll find you can't have one without the other.

* **Most people find quitting much easier than they first thought** and wish they had done it earlier.

* **Smokers with a young family must smoke outside.**

* **Inflicting your smoke on other people is antisocial.**

Giving up smoking

Addiction to cigarettes is the most common and vicious of all the addictions, worse than heroin and more difficult to kick – and it's legal! Quitting smoking brings both short-term and important long-term health benefits.

Here are some of the dangers:

There are 3,000 dangerous chemicals in cigarette smoke.

Up to 5 percent is carbon monoxide – the same deadly gas that's in car exhaust fumes – and it stops your blood from absorbing oxygen properly.

The same tars that are used to surface roads are in tobacco smoke, and can cause cancer.

The most dangerous tar is a powerful nitroso chemical, one part per billion in food is a hazard: in tobacco smoke there are 5,000 parts per billion.

The other chemicals inhaled include ammonia, a chemical found in explosives, bleach, and bathroom cleaners; cyanide, a deadly poison; and phenols, chemicals used in paint stripper.

Here are some of the reasons why people smoke:

When nicotine reaches the brain, it makes the head spin and people feel stimulated and alert.

Nicotine makes the heart beat faster, so more blood circulates

"giving up smoking is one of the best things you can do"

"within 5 years of quitting, the lung cancer risk decreases by half"

around the body per minute; people say they feel ready to get up and go.

Nicotine reduces tension in muscles, which makes people feel relaxed and seems to relieve stress.

Nicotine seems to help people work by improving concentration: it can stave off boredom and fatigue.

Effects on your health

Lung cancer: Smoking causes lung cancer, which can be less than six months from diagnosis to death.

Fatal heart disease: Nicotine makes your heart beat faster and raises your blood pressure – the end result can be a heart attack.

Stroke: Smoking makes your blood thick and more likely to clot. A clot in the brain can mean permanent brain damage, paralysis, even death.

Gangrene: Your blood gets so sticky it can block the arteries in your legs, leading to gangrene and amputation.

Emphysema and bronchitis: Air passages become clogged, narrow, and damaged until you're crippled by breathlessness.

Cancers of the mouth, throat, esophagus, bladder, pancreas, kidney, cervix, and breast are all more common in smokers.

Ulcers: You are more likely to get stomach and duodenal ulcers if you smoke.

Why quit?

Cigarette smokers look older than their age because smoking speeds up aging of the skin.

The risk of premature death is double that of nonsmokers.

Smoking-related diseases kill 40 percent of smokers before they reach retirement.

Nonsmokers live at least six years longer than smokers.

What are the benefits of quitting?

Giving up smoking has instant benefits.
✻ Within 20 minutes blood pressure and pulse fall.
✻ Within 2 hours lung airways relax, making it easier to breathe, and the volume of air our lungs can hold increases.
✻ Within 8 hours carbon monoxide levels drop to normal and the oxygen level goes back up to normal.
✻ Within 24 hours the risk of a heart attack decreases.
✻ Within 48 hours damaged nerve endings start to regrow, so smell and taste become stronger.
✻ Within 1 to 3 months circulation improves; lung function improves by up to a third.
✻ Within 5 years the risk of lung cancer decreases by half.
✻ Within 10 years the risk of lung cancer is normal.

Helping yourself quit

Many people wonder if aids to quit smoking work and if they should try them. Most smoking experts agree, and I am with them, that there's no substitute for willpower, but you could try nicotine gum or skin patches, hypnosis, acupuncture, and going to smoking support groups.

Here are 20 tips for helping you to quit smoking:

Don't try to do them all at once. Choose three or four, never more, to begin with, then add one or two more each day. Good luck!

1 Never smoke in the car.
2 Refuse every cigarette that's offered to you.
3 Don't have a cigarette before breakfast.
4 Buy only one pack at a time.
5 Keep only 10 cigarettes in a pack.
6 Buy a different brand of cigarettes every time, not just your favorite.
7 Before you light up, count to 10.
8 Every time you get a cigarette, put the pack away in another room.
9 When you run out of cigarettes, never take one from someone else.
10 After each puff, put the cigarette down.
11 Never smoke outdoors.
12 Never smoke in bed.
13 Stop smoking at work.
14 Don't smoke in the house.
15 Stop carrying your lighter or matches with you.
16 Stop smoking a cigarette more than halfway down.
17 After a meal, don't smoke until you've left the table.
18 Don't smoke while you're relaxing with a drink.
19 Only smoke if you're sitting in an uncomfortable chair.
20 Keep a rubber band around your cigarette pack as a reminder.

Smoking and pregnancy

✻ **Mothers:** Don't smoke when pregnant or you risk harming your unborn baby, having a miscarriage, or giving birth to an underweight baby, vulnerable to infections.

✻ **Fathers:** The children of fathers who smoke 20 or more cigarettes a day have a higher risk of cancer than children of nonsmoking fathers. Smoking damages sperm, so men should quit smoking at least three months before trying for a baby.

Smoking increases the likelihood of crib death (SIDS).

MIRIAM'S *golden rules* for safe drinking

✳ Drink twice as much flat water as alcohol, and **a big glass of water before bed to avoid dehydration**.

✳ Avoid carbonated drinks. The **bubbles get the alcohol to your brain faster**.

✳ Remember that **alcohol has a greater effect on women than on men**.

✳ **Don't mix drinks and drugs**, you won't be able to handle an emergency.

✳ **Make a note of how much alcohol you go through in a week**. A diary can be a real eye opener!

✳ **No one should drink every day.** Have some alcohol-free days every week.

✳ **Stay off alcohol for a few days** after a party to let your liver recover.

"no one should drink every day"

✳ **Keep below recommended limits**. These are no more than 3–4 units a day for men and 2–3 for women. One unit = 10 ounces of beer, medium glass of wine, or one shot of spirits.

✳ **Don't binge on the weekend** and drink a week's allowance in a short time; **it's bad for your liver**.

✳ Don't mix the grain (beer) with the grape (wine) if you want to avoid a hangover.

✳ **Always sip alcohol rather than gulp it.**

✳ Eat first if you plan to drink: **even a glass of milk can help prevent a hangover**.

✳ **Don't drink and drive** and never ride in a car driven by someone who has been drinking.

✳ **Don't mix drink and sex** – you're more careless and could catch an STD or get pregnant.

✳ **Eat food as you drink** to soak up the alcohol.

✳ Plan how you'll get home after drinking – **call a taxi**.

✳ **Don't keep pace with your friends** – drinking isn't a competition.

✳ For teenagers – **don't think that drinking alcohol means you're grown up**. It doesn't.

✳ **Being drunk at sports events could invite trouble.**

"vitamins C and E can help accelerate alcohol detoxification"

Dangers of heavy drinking

Alcohol is intoxicating, and although it gives you an initial lift, it's a depressant drug. It slows down responses (affecting coordination) and the way the brain works (affecting judgment), so it makes people clumsy and dopey. It's one of the most widely used drugs, above and below the legal age limit. In large quantities over a short time, alcohol is a poison and will kill.

What happens to alcohol in your body?

Although it takes minutes for alcohol to reach the brain, it takes the liver an hour to break down the alcohol in a glass of wine or beer. The less you weigh, the more alcohol affects you, so there's a good reason for alcohol being illegal below a certain age. A slim teenage boy will get drunk far more quickly than a large adult male. A woman will feel the effects of alcohol faster and for longer than a

man because women don't have enough body fluid to dilute alcohol the way men do.

Drinking too much always has horrible effects

Drinking too much can make you aggressive and violent. You're more likely to start arguments and pick fights.

You become uncoordinated and clumsy and you shouldn't try to use sharp instruments or machinery.

Too much alcohol gives you double vision and slurred speech.

Drinking when you're feeling down can make you more depressed.

Alcohol is loaded with calories. It can make you fat, and is bad for your skin.

A bad hangover makes you feel really fragile. Your head pounds and you have an upset stomach. You can't work or study.

Alcohol can damage a man's fertility and potency (lowers sperm count and affects an errection).

It's difficult to get and maintain an erection if you've been drinking.

Avoid alcohol if you're:

✱ taking any over-the-counter medicines – even cold medications – without first checking the labels
✱ taking any prescribed or illegal drugs
✱ going to drive a car, ride a bike, or operate machinery.

Check the dangers of drinking

If you drive after you've had only one drink, you're still five times more likely to have a car accident than a nondrinker.

Accidents are more common with alcohol because your reflexes slow down and you lose coordination.

You're more likely to be careless and have unprotected sex if you're drunk, thereby risking a pregnancy or a sexually transmitted disease.

You can black out or forget what you did for whole periods. If you wander off alone you could pass out and choke on your own vomit.

Serious binge-drinking can cause you to fall, injure yourself, and even lose consciousness or have seizures.

Alcohol has a high sugar content, so anyone with diabetes is advised to avoid it entirely.

Drinking during pregnancy can cause fetal alcohol syndrome in your developing baby. The baby could develop abnormally in your womb and behave abnormally as he or she grows up. Keep to one or two units a week or don't drink at all.

Long-term heavy alcohol use leads to physical dependence – which means you can't do without it – and seriously damages the heart, liver, stomach, and brain.

Final stages of alcoholic dependence aren't pretty – DTs or delirium tremens (a state of confusion accompanied by trembling and hallucinations), swollen abdomen, cirrhosis of the liver, weak heart, coma, and death.

Drinking and sex

Because alcohol lowers inhibitions, more than half of all teenagers have sex for the first time when drunk. This may have disastrous results.

Both sexes get careless about contraception and this can lead not only to unwanted pregnancy but also to HIV/AIDS, herpes, and other sexually transmitted diseases (STDs).

It's harder to maintain an erection when you're drunk. Girls think boys' lovemaking is fumbling and confused when they're drunk.

Stages in alcohol dependence

The first stage is when the heavy social drinker finds that he or she is able to drink more and more alcohol without noticing its effects.

Then come periods of memory loss, followed by the realization that they are no longer in control of their drinking. They can't be certain they can stop whenever they want.

The next and final step is characterized by prolonged binges and by serious physical and mental problems.

Treatment

Different methods of treatment – psychological, social, and physical – are appropriate for different people and may be combined.

Psychological treatments involve psychotherapy and are commonly carried out in groups. There are various types of group therapy.

Social treatments, like Alcoholics Anonymous, may help with problems at work and some will include family members in the treatment process.

Physical treatment is needed only by some alcoholics. It generally includes the use of disulfiram, a drug that sensitizes the drinker to alcohol so that he or she is afraid to drink because of the unpleasant side effects.

Detox

Many alcoholics require medical help in getting over the physical symptoms when they stop drinking, and this may mean staying at a detox clinic for a few days or maybe longer. This must be followed up by long-term treatment, which depends on individual needs. For example, some people benefit from psychotherapy, which is often carried out in grou

"alcohol is loaded with calories. It can make you fat"

Alcoholics can also suffer from nutritional deficiencies. Studies have shown that supplements of zinc and vitamins C, E, and Thiamine can help accelerate alcohol detoxification and prevent liver damage.

Naxtrexone

A new and revolutionary alcohol treatment, naxtrexone, has been introduced that allows patients to continue drinking during and after treatment. Trials have shown it to be a powerful technique for patients who have not descended too far into alcoholism and who are sufficiently motivated to get well. In Finland, 78 percent of patients had still not relapsed after three years.

Naxtrexone recently won FDA approval for its use in the US. It is prescribed for the treatment of alcoholism and available by doctor's prescription only.

Alcohol and children

Although the legal drinking age in the US is 21, the majority of young people have taken their first drink as a teenager – without knowing the facts about the dangers of drinking. Here are some disturbing statistics.

Alcohol use is the number one drug problem among young people.

Young people who begin drinking before age 15 are four times more likely to develop alcohol dependence than those who begin at age 21.

During a typical weekend, an average of one teenager dies each hour in a car crash – nearly half involve alcohol.

Teens who drink are four times more likely to have sex.

Alcohol is a factor in the three leading causes of death among 15–24 year olds: accidents, homicides, and suicides.

MIRIAM'S *golden rules* on drugs

My goal is to inform and educate children about the dangers of drugs, and certainly not to advocate their use. But I don't believe in scare tactics or moral indignation. I find it as unrealistic to imagine a society without drugs as one without alcohol or sex.

✱ **Don't mix alcohol and drugs**, the effects are addictive and dangerous.

✱ **Keep sipping water if you take drugs** – you need 10oz (300ml) every half hour.

✱ **Keep your salt levels up** by eating salted chips or nuts.

✱ **Learn CPR and basic first aid for emergencies.**

✱ **High-energy drinks are best**, then fruit juice.

✱ **Never wear a hat**, you need to stay cool.

✱ At a club or rave take frequent rests so you **don't overheat**.

✱ Memorize the **poison control telephone number**.

✱ Never take drugs from someone you don't know.

✱ Always stay with friends.

✱ **Don't mix drugs**, all side effects are much worse, especially dehydration.

✱ ...now where to go for help.

"always stay with friends"

My main concern is the welfare of children and, although we may never eliminate drug use completely, I believe we can minimize the dangers by giving young people sound, honest, realistic information. Then the consequences for them and the community at large will be the least damaging.

What you need to know about drugs

The mere mention of drugs is enough to strike fear into almost every parent's heart. Parents fear that their child might want to experiment and ultimately pay with their life, especially when there seems to be no end to the tragic cases of young people who die after taking drugs.

But most young people today see occasional drug use in the same way as their parents see alcohol – as part of normal life. Most describe it as something that makes them feel good and gets rid of their inhibitions. Mainly, I think they're as responsible about drugs as most of us are about alcohol.

The "just say no" approach to drug taking is based on the belief that our sons and daughters are incapable of making decisions about drugs. And it implies that adults aren't interested in their opinions and experiences. Well, I do respect young people's ability to reason, and feel they should have reliable, accurate information about drugs. I discuss drugs in honest terms of harm to mind and body, without relying on the law to separate what's dangerous from what isn't.

My goal is to be scientific and even-handed, separating real from imagined dangers. I've been lecturing, making television

documentaries, and researching drugs for more than 20 years. As a mother myself, I felt it was important to speak directly to concerned parents as well as to potential drug users as part of that research. It's not surprising that many teenagers reject all advice – good and bad – from adults on the subject of drugs.

The messages are often exaggerated or false, sometimes ridiculous, but nearly always inconsistent with their own observations and experience. I have tried to avoid exaggeration and judgment and I have re-examined the assumptions that are too often made about drugs.

A realistic examination has to consider the following:

✱ Despite possible dangers, most drugs induce some pleasurable feelings.
✱ Total abstinence may not always be a realistic goal.
✱ The use of illegal substances doesn't necessarily mean abuse.
✱ One form of drug use doesn't

inevitably lead to other, more harmful forms.
✱ Understanding the risks of drug use will not necessarily deter young people from experimentation.

Heroin (street names: H, Smack, Junk)

A depressant drug that numbs the brain and body and kills pain. It's highly addictive. Comes in three forms, all of which can cause overdose: brown (which should never be injected), China white, and pharmaceutical heroin, which can easily cause overdose. Brown is sometimes dissolved in vinegar or lemon juice and can cause vision problems if injected. Sores and open wounds can develop with heavy heroin use. On withdrawal, addicts suffer craving, panic attacks, cramps, nausea, and diarrhea.

Cocaine (street names: Coke, Blow, Snort)

A powerful stimulant that brings on feelings of euphoria and well-being. It's highly addictive. Long-term users

"users can become psychotic, delusional, and violent"

may become psychotic. Snorting can burn a hole in your nostrils. Injecting cocaine is highly dangerous because there is a real risk of overdosing. Mixing it with heroin (speedballing) is also very dangerous. Most street cocaine comes as a powder that is "cut" with glucose, lactose, or even anesthetics. Cocaine content may be as low as 30 percent.

Marijuana (street names: Grass, Pot, Weed)

Often exaggerates the way a person already feels. Users become talkative and think they have a greater "insight" into the world. They often find everything hilarious. Some long-term, heavy users may get panic attacks, exaggerated mood swings, and feelings of persecution. Mixing marijuana with speed or ecstasy can make you seriously dehydrated and cause other severe problems such as heart attacks. There are three forms: herbal, resin, and hash oil.

Acid (LSD) (street names: Trip, Blotter, Dot)

An extraordinarily powerful, mind-altering drug, causing hallucinations. Acid is unpredictable and should never be taken on the spur of the moment. If you are feeling down, you are more likely to have a "bad trip." There's virtually no risk of physical side effects and it's not addictive, but the mental effects can be very serious. It can unlock a mental illness of which you weren't aware, which can lead you to become depressed, paranoid, or even needing psychiatric treatment. Bad trips can cause terrifying, uncontrollable flashbacks. Acid is almost always soaked in small squares of blotting paper. The average amount in an acid tab is

around 50 micrograms – enough to induce a fairly mild trip – but could contain as much as 250 micrograms, enough to cause the equivalent of a nervous breakdown.

Ecstasy (street names: X, E, Adam)

Releases mood-altering chemicals, such as serotonin and L-dopa, which generate feelings of love and friendliness. It's also hallucinogenic. Ecstasy can cause the body to overheat, resulting in potentially fatal heatstroke. It can also interrupt blood flow in the brain, leading to a stroke, and cause fatal kidney and liver failure. Pills come in different designs, often with logos on them. Ecstasy may be "cut" with talcum powder or ketamine (a horse tranquilizer), producing horrible side effects.

Amphetamine (street names: Speed, Meth, Crank)

A stimulant that makes you more energetic and alert. Users become very talkative and can stay awake for

hours. You can still be "wired" 12 hours after taking the drug. It can cause heatstroke and may also lead to a heart attack. Liver and kidney failure can occur if you mix it with alcohol. Injecting it is highly dangerous since the heart can't take the shock. Speed is least dangerous when it is swallowed.

Crack (street names: Rock, Wash, Cloud)

According to users the intensity of the hit can't be exaggerated. It comes within seconds but is short-lived. It can give an intense euphoria and an energy surge with an incredible sense of well-being and power. It's highly addictive. After the hit, users will often feel weak, tired, paranoid, and depressed. The comedown can last for days. Crack use can lead to severe psychological problems. Users can become psychotic, delusional, and violent. Combining crack with any other drug is potentially lethal. Crack is cocaine that has been processed and can be 80–100 percent pure, which makes it much more dangerous. It is generally smoked.

The penalties

Remember, above all, that if you get caught in possession of illegal drugs, or intend to supply them, the penalties are harsh and vary from state to state. Here are some of the minimum federal penalties for possession of certain amounts.

Drug	Amount	Penalty	Sentence
Heroin	100 grams	Prison	Minimum of 5 years
Speed	5-49 grams	Prison	Minimum of 5 years
Marijuana	Less than 50kg	Prison	Up to 5 years

MIRIAM'S *golden rules* for good sex

✳ Be open, **talk about what does and doesn't turn you on** and show reciprocity by asking for feedback.

✳ **Low, medium, and high sex drives are all normal** so be generous when your partner's libido is different from yours.

✳ **Don't hold back sexual grudges**, get them off your chest – the longer you leave it the more difficult they become to discuss.

✳ **Anything is okay** between consenting adults.

✳ **Find out what pleases you** by masturbating, then show your partner how to please you.

✳ **Simultaneous orgasms aren't the holy grail of sex** so stop chasing them.

✳ **Multiple orgasms aren't either, one is fine**, so is one a night.

✳ **When a woman says NO, that means no sex**. Anything else means rape.

✳ **The G spot is fiction**.

✳ **Sex isn't an athletic competition**.

✳ **Smoking, drugs, and alcohol impair erection**, arousal, and orgasm.

✳ **The female orgasm resides in the clitoris**. The penis is therefore not the best kind of stimulation, the tongue, finger, or a vibrator are often superior.

"be open, talk about what turns you on"

MIRIAM'S *golden rules* for restful sleep

✱ Do whatever you have to do to sleep more – **have a hot milky drink, read a book or the paper,** watch television, or do all three.

✱ Just as a bedtime routine helps children, so the body and brain of adults respond to bedtime cues and rituals, **so have a wind-down routine that you follow most nights**.

✱ Alcohol doesn't help you to sleep, it does the opposite, so if it's sound sleep you want, **avoid alcohol late in the evening**. You may fall asleep but you'll wake a few hours later and be unable to go back to sleep.

✱ Two drops of oil of clary sage or **lavender on the pillow can aid sleep**.

✱ Being either too hot or too cold can prevent sleep, so **spend some effort on keeping your bedroom temperature steady**.

✱ If you have a tendency to insomnia, anything will keep you awake, so **turn off dripping faucets, close squeaking doors, and batten down anything that can flap in a draft**.

✱ **Learn some kind of self-hypnosis that induces sleep very quickly** when you can't drop off – mine is counting backward from ten, repeating "I'm falling asleep" with each number – I've never gotten beyond five.

✱ **Wear loose-fitting cotton sleepwear** or none at all.

✱ **Change your mattress every seven years or so**.

✱ If your partner likes music or television before bed, don't get upset – **snuggle down with ear plugs and eyeshades**.

✱ If you wake up in the early hours and can't get back to sleep, **don't lie there and fume; get up**, do a chore, make a cup of warm milk, do a crossword, read, and when you're feeling sleepy go back to bed.

✱ **Only take sleeping pills in the short term to get you over a bad patch**.

✱ **Sex is the best prelude to sleep**.

"sex is the best prelude to sleep"

MIRIAM'S *golden rules* for managing stress

✱ Some stress is good for us. It increases productivity, so don't rule it out altogether – find your optimum level.

✱ The body *loves* the stress of exercise and releases hundreds of beneficial hormones as a result.

✱ Desensitize yourself to excessive levels of stress with instant relaxation, imagery training, activity of any kind, and writing out an action plan.

✱ Instant relaxation is a quick, simple exercise that you can do whenever you can to **conquer stress in a few minutes**:

1 close your eyes
2 lower your shoulders
3 halve your breathing rate
4 count to five breathing in and to five breathing out
5 think of black velvet.

✱ Simple breathing techniques can relieve stress. Learn yoga breathing.

✱ Exercise itself relieves stress but it also increases your *resistance* to stress, so walk briskly when you can, climb stairs, and incorporate some formal exercise into your life every day if you can. It doesn't have to be excessive – 30 minutes of walking is enough.

"desensitize yourself to excessive levels of stress"

✱ Stress-relieving aromatherapy includes oil of clary sage and lavender – a couple of drops on a handkerchief or pillow and in the bath.

✱ Learn biofeedback to keep your heart rate and blood pressure down when you feel stress taking its toll.

✱ Learn deep muscle and deep mental relaxation techniques. Then you can control stress.

✱ Massage will relieve the muscle tension, aches, and pains that result from stress, so incorporate sessions into your life.

Life Stages

"your baby is a lot more robust than you think and has a strong instinct to survive"

life stages: 0 to 1 years

You're thrilled by the arrival of your new baby, and like most new parents you'll probably feel nervous about handling this tiny scrap of humanity who seems so weak and vulnerable. But, in fact, from the moment of birth your baby is a lot more robust than you think and has a strong instinct to survive.

The importance of bonding

A newborn baby sleeps for most of her first days, so try to spend all of her waking time together. Research has shown that physical contact with you, the sound of your voice, and the smell of your body are very important during the first few days of life. During this time your baby forms a bond with you which, if encouraged, is unique and unbreakable.

To help the bonding process, make sure your baby has frequent contact with your skin since this is critical for establishing bonding. Make feeding a time of physical intimacy; hold her close and talk gently.

Growth and development

In your baby's first year, growth and development cover three main areas:
- **Brain** – she will be using her brain to think and to develop language
- **Mobility** – she will be learning to stand upright and walk, starting with attempts to control her head as early as her first week
- **Dexterity** – she will be acquiring fine control of her fingers so that by around 10 months she can pick up a pea between thumb and index finger.

All that you have to do to help a skill develop is take your lead from your baby. This is the golden and unbreakable rule of child development. And your baby will always show you with some sign that she wants to and can move on. It's important to follow her lead because if you do you'll hit exactly the right moment when it's essential for her to acquire the skill.

This makes her feel very pleased with herself (especially if you praise her) and you'll be building her self-confidence and self-esteem right from the start. Just think what a confident, balanced, affectionate child she'll grow into. And all the groundwork is laid in the first year.

Emotional continence

It is also vital for your baby to learn "emotional continence" in her first year. Emotional continence means being able to manage emotions, not letting them get out of hand. It involves being able to control strong emotions by turning them to good purpose.
- Babies learn emotional continence from you.
- If emotional continence isn't learned in the first year it's very difficult to acquire later.

Without this skill she finds it very difficult to cope with anything that thwarts her wishes or stands in her way as she grows up – in other words she becomes emotionally incontinent. The classic outcome of emotional incontinence is a preschooler who bullies, is disruptive, even destructive at home and at nursery school.

In the pages that follow I offer guidelines on what happens during your baby's first year and advice where I feel there may be a need.

Building emotional continence

It's not difficult to impart early lessons in emotional continence to your baby. There are three easy steps in any situation.

- *Legitimize* your baby's emotions. Tell her "I know it hurts" if she's fallen over or "That is annoying" if she's frustrated by something and becomes angry.

- *Defuse* your baby's emotions. Say "Mommy will kiss it better" or "Daddy gets annoyed with that too, you know."

- *Move on* from the emotion. Suggest "When it's stopped hurting we'll go out to play" or "Let's forget that and cuddle."

Body

a baby's
bond with
you is
unique and
unbreakable

Mind

Social

"your new baby has a number of amazing innate skills"

"she learns to be loving and friendly by imitating you"

your new baby

Your feelings on the birth of your new baby are likely to be pride, wonder, and exhilaration mixed with exhaustion. Your baby may seem smaller than you imagined and very vulnerable, but don't worry – your baby is equipped with reflexes and behavior that help him survive.

Premature babies

Over 11 percent of babies born in the US today are premature. The medical definition of a premature baby is one that is born at less than 37 weeks. All premature babies need special treatment but not necessarily in a neonatal unit. Premature babies are not well equipped for life outside the womb and may have the following problems:

● **Breathing** Due to the immaturity of their lungs, most premature babies experience difficulty in breathing, known as respiratory distress syndrome (RDS).
● **Immune system** An underdeveloped immune system and a body that is too weak to defend itself properly means there is a greater risk of infection.
● **Digestion** A premature baby's stomach is small and sensitive, which means he is less able to hold food down, and so is more likely to vomit. The immaturity of his digestive system makes it difficult for him to digest essential proteins so they have to be given in a predigested form.

● **Temperature regulation** A premature baby's temperature control is inefficient and he is likely to be too cold or too hot. He has less heat insulation than a full-term baby, since he lacks sufficient body fat.
● **Reflexes** Inadequate development of his reflexes, particularly his sucking reflex, creates difficulties in feeding. Premature babies usually need tube feeding.

Progress

The development of a premature baby can be slow and erratic. It can be a shock to see just how tiny your premature baby is, but he will have a great will to live. For a premature baby, every day can be an uphill battle. Periods of improvement may be followed by setbacks, and this uncertainty makes you and your partner very anxious. It is encouraging to know, however, that most babies born after 32 weeks will develop normally. Of those babies born at 28 weeks, 6 out of 7 will survive.

Baby skills at birth

Although your baby is physically helpless at birth, he has a number of amazing innate skills. Your newborn
● is wired to communicate
● is programmed to imitate the facial expressions and sounds you make when you talk
● loves eye contact and skin contact
● sees everything 8–10in (20–25cm) away clearly and responds eagerly to your face at this distance, looks intensely
● at 8–10in (20–25cm) can "read" emotions and may smile if he sees you smiling
● can hear your voice very clearly and recognize it.

What you can do to help
● Trust, warmth, and sociability are developed in the first few months, and during this time you must teach your baby most of the basic ways to relate to people. So most important, be positive in all you do, and overt in all you express.
● Smiling is your most important tool to show pleasure, approval, love, and joy. Voice comes next. Babies are sensitive to loving, approving, delighted, and joyful tones of voice, pitched light and high.
● Body contact – the warmth, closeness, and smell of your body – is important, too, as are touch and physical demonstrations of affection.

Preventing crib death

Sudden infant death syndrome (SIDS), commonly known as crib death, is the sudden and unexpected death of a baby for no obvious reason.

The exact causes of crib death are still unknown, and there is therefore no advice that can absolutely guarantee its prevention. There are, however, many ways in which parents can vastly reduce the risk. Recent surveys have shown that routine immunizations reduce the risk, as does keeping your baby in your room with you at night for the first six months of her life. Falling asleep with your baby on the sofa greatly increases the risk of crib death.

A mother who smokes during pregnancy increases the risk of SIDS. The risk of crib death in babies born to smokers is twice that for babies born to nonsmokers, and with every 10 cigarettes a day the risk increases threefold.

Reducing the risk

● Always place your baby on her back to sleep.
● Don't smoke, don't allow smoking in your house, and avoid taking your baby into smoky places.
● Don't let your baby get too hot.
● When covering your baby, allow for room temperature – the higher the temperature, the fewer bed covers your baby needs and vice versa.
● Avoid tucking in, so your baby can throw off bed covers if she is hot.
● If you think your baby is unwell, don't hesitate to contact your doctor.
● If your baby has a fever, don't increase her wrappings; reduce them so she can lose heat.

Your new baby's appearance

When you hold your baby for the first time, her appearance will probably surprise you. She's undoubtedly a joy to you, but you may have expected a clean and placid bundle, similar to the babies that appear in baby food commercials. Real life (as you'll now suddenly discover) is a bit different.

Skin

● **Vernix** – a whitish, greasy substance – may cover your baby's skin. This natural emollient cream prevented the skin from becoming waterlogged in the uterus. It may be removed at once, or left to give your baby some natural protection against minor skin irritations such as flaking and peeling.

● **A blotchy red rash** is quite common in the first week. There's no need for treatment; it will disappear very quickly.

● **Milia** are small white spots seen mainly on the bridge of the nose but also elsewhere on the face.

● **Heat rash** – if she's too warm, your baby may get small red spots, particularly on her face.

Head

The soft spots on the top of your baby's skull where the bones are still not joined are called the fontanels. The skull bones won't fuse completely until your baby is about two. Be careful not to press the fontanels.

Eyes

Your baby may not be able to open her eyes right away due to puffiness caused by pressure on her head during birth. This pressure may also have broken some tiny blood vessels in her eyes, causing harmless small, red, triangular marks in the whites

that need no treatment and disappear in a couple of weeks. She may have "sticky eye" – a yellow discharge around the eyelids. This is quite common, and although not serious should always be treated by a doctor.

Hair

Some babies are born with a full head of hair; others are completely bald. The color of your baby's hair at birth may not be the color she will end up with. The fine, downy hair that many babies have on their bodies at birth is called lanugo, and this will fall off soon after birth.

Genitals

The genitals may look swollen and enlarged.

Legs and arms

The baby's legs and arms are still bent, as they were in the uterus.

helping your baby to sleep

Some babies sleep through the night early on, some do not. As a rule, the more active your baby is and the more energy she uses, the more soundly she sleeps – her sleep being divided between daytime naps and nighttime.

Sleep patterns

The way babies fall asleep differs from adults; adults can crash suddenly, whereas babies sleep lightly for about 20 minutes, then go through a transitional stage before reaching deep sleep. **Nothing will wake them, until they've had enough sleep.** This means that babies who are simply "put down" will not necessarily go to sleep peacefully. You may need to nurse your baby to sleep for quite a while, so try to be patient, particularly if you are trying to get him back to sleep at night, when you are longing to go back to bed yourself.

Where should a baby sleep?

Where a baby sleeps isn't important to start with. He won't automatically fall asleep when put into a darkened bedroom; light doesn't bother him at all. He's much more likely to be disturbed by being too hot or too cold. Your baby will be happiest going to sleep hearing your voices and the household noises that he is used to in the background, so from the start, be kind to yourselves and the baby by letting him sleep in an infant seat or Moses basket placed in whichever room you happen to be.

Using a baby monitor

If you leave your baby in another room, set up a baby monitor so you can hear him as soon as he wakes.

Keep in mind that your baby may feel disturbed by the silence when you leave the room, and this could make him more fretful; leave the door open so he can hear you moving around the house – unless you have a cat which may climb into the crib. Avoid going back into the room once your baby is asleep; your smell could wake him, so resist the temptation to check on him too frequently.

Encouraging longer sleep periods at night

A young baby requires nourishment and calories at regular intervals, so he'll wake for a feeding when his body tells him he needs it. The way to encourage your baby to sleep for a stretch (four, then rising to five or six hours) during the night is to make sure he's taken in sufficient calories to last that long. This means feeding him whenever he shows he's hungry during the day. As he steadily gains weight, he can go longer between feedings and by about six weeks he could be sleeping for at least one period of about six hours – hopefully during the night. **When he wakes for a night feeding, make as little fuss as possible:** feed him in bed; if he needs changing, do it gently and quickly in dim light. Don't make this a time for chatting and games and he'll begin to learn that waking at night doesn't bring any special privileges.

Pacifiers

Babies are born with a sucking reflex. Without it, they wouldn't suckle or be able to nourish themselves. **I feel it's important that babies are allowed to indulge their desire to suck.**

Some babies are more "sucky" than others. One of mine wanted to suck all the time, whether he was hungry or not. With all my sons, I used to put their thumb gently into their mouth so they could suck to soothe themselves. **But at the same time, I see nothing wrong with using pacifiers as comforters**, although very young babies will not take to them readily.

There are several types of pacifier. Some are molded to the shape of the baby's mouth; others are designed to move in and out like a human nipple when sucked.

Pacifiers for a very young baby should be sterilized in the same way as bottles and nipples. But once your child is being weaned and starts to use his fingers for feeding himself, it is pointless to sterilize pacifiers. Careful washing and rinsing are all that is needed. Have several pacifiers so that they can be changed for fresh ones when they get damaged.

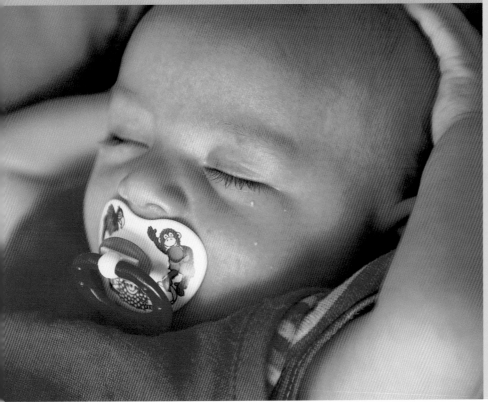

Sleep tips for older babies

● Keep the time just before bed as happy and pleasant as possible.

● Try giving a comfort suck from the breast or the bottle just before putting your baby to bed.

● Develop a routine and stick to it. Don't just put your baby right to bed: work out a routine of play, bath, bed, story, song, and then say goodnight. But don't leave the room; quietly tidy up so that your baby learns that she can drift off to sleep without actually "losing" you.

● Let your baby develop comfort habits such as using a blanket, a stuffed animal, a handkerchief, a doll, or her own thumb. There is nothing wrong with any of these. There's no particular age at which comforters should or shouldn't be used and, like bed-wetting, children grow out of them.

Soothing and settling your baby

There are numerous ways to soothe and console your baby if she's crying. As a general rule, most babies respond to either movement or sound, or both.

● Any movement that rocks her, whether it is you holding and rocking her in your arms, going gently back and forth on a swing, or rocking her in a cradle or rocking chair.

● Walking or dancing with an emphasis on rhythmic movement, since it will remind her of the time when she was being jogged inside your uterus.

● Bouncing her gently in your arms, the crib, or on the bed.

● Putting her in a sling and walking around with her. If you're by yourself, just get on with whatever you want to do and try to ignore the crying.

● Taking her for a ride in the car or in a carriage, or for a walk in a sling, even at night (you may want to take a cell phone with you).

● Any form of music as long as it is calm, rhythmic, and not too loud; special CDs are available.

● A steady household noise, for instance the washing machine.

● Your own soft singing voice, especially if you sing a lullaby.

caring for your baby

Caring for your baby does not require any specialized skills – just some basic knowledge, plenty of common sense, and a willingness to ask for help and advice.

Immunizations

Immunization is vital to every growing child to make sure the immune system is strengthened. **Most parents don't realize that when we vaccinate our babies we don't just protect our own, we protect all other babies.** If the number of babies vaccinated against measles drops below 75 percent, measles can escape into communities. For a community of babies to be protected, 95 percent must be vaccinated.

● Before the introduction of the mumps vaccine in the US, the maximum number of cases in one year was 152,209 in 1968. In 1999, there were 352 reported cases of mumps in the US, a decrease of 99%. Mumps can also cause permanent deafness.

● Measles has nasty complications including encephalitis, ear infections, and pneumonia.

● Fifteen percent of children who suffer from measles encephalitis will die and 20–40 percent of survivors will suffer brain damage.

● I sincerely do not believe there is any scientific evidence to support a connection between the combined MMR vaccine and autism. Nor is there any evidence that giving the vaccine in three separate doses is safer than giving it in a single dose.

How effective is measles vaccine?

Following the introduction of the measles vaccine in 1963, there has been a 99% reduction in the number of cases.

Why immunize if the diseases are so rare?

There are several important reasons.

● The diseases are now rare but will only remain rare because of vaccination.

● These diseases can have serious consequences. Low immunization rates in preschool children led to an increase in cases of measles betweeen 1989 and 1991.

● These highly contagious diseases can be brought into the US by visitors, putting unimmunized children at risk.

● There will always be some susceptible children who cannot be vaccinated, so high immunization rates must be maintained to prevent epidemics.

Breast-feeding

Breast-feeding has to be learned and you should seek support and advice from your family, from friends with babies, and from your doctor or midwife. Above all you will learn from your baby, by understanding his signals and discovering how to respond to them.

Colostrum and breast milk

During the 72 hours after delivery, the breasts produce a thin, yellow fluid called colostrum, made up of water, protein, and minerals. Colostrum contains antibodies that protect the baby against a range of intestinal and respiratory infections. In the first few days, your baby should be put regularly to the breast, both to feed on the colostrum and to get used to latching on to the breast.

Once your breasts start to produce milk, you may be surprised by its watery appearance. When your baby sucks, the first milk that he gets – the foremilk – is thin, watery, and thirst quenching. Then comes the hindmilk, which is richer in fat and protein.

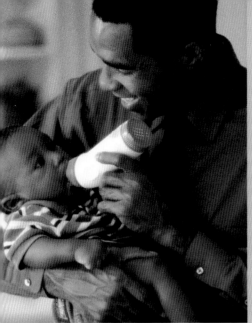

Bottle-feeding tips

Bottle-feeding is straightforward, but you will need to make sure that your baby can swallow properly, and that she is not taking in air with the milk.

● Before you start feeding, test the temperature of the milk by dropping a little onto the inside of your wrist. It should feel neither too hot nor too cold.

● Never leave your baby with the bottle propped up on a pillow or cushion; this can be dangerous. She could become very uncomfortable if she swallows a lot of air with the formula, and could choke. She will also miss the cuddling she should enjoy while she is feeding.

● Tilt your baby on your arm. It is very difficult for your baby to swallow when she is lying flat so don't feed her in this position; she may gag or even be sick.

● If your baby has a stuffed nose she can't swallow and breathe at the same time. Your doctor can give you nose drops to be used before each feeding.

● Don't change your formula without first consulting your doctor or midwife, even if you think your baby doesn't like it. It is very unusual for a brand of formula to be responsible for a baby's not feeding well; very rarely cow's milk causes allergies in babies and your doctor may advise you to use a substitute soy formula.

● Your baby knows when she's had enough, so don't try to force her to go on feeding and finish the bottle after she has stopped sucking.

Vegetarian eating

A growing baby can get all the nutrients necessary for health and vitality from a diet that excludes meat, fish, and poultry, provided a proper balance of the different food groups is maintained.

● Your baby's main source of calories will still be milk, so give this at each feeding.

● Cereals and grains provide carbohydrates and some protein for energy, while vegetables and fruits supply essential vitamins and minerals. Legumes (puréed or mashed beans or lentils), eggs, cheese and cheese sauce provide protein and minerals for growth and development.

Hard cheese, eggs, and gluten should not be given to your baby before he is six months old.

Foods for teethers

When your baby is teething, she will like to chew and suck to soothe her gums. Any piece of raw vegetable or fruit that is large enough to hold easily and can be sucked or chewed makes a good teething food, particularly if it is chilled but not frozen solid. The following are all suitable:

● celery stick
● Italian breadstick
● zwieback
● peeled cucumber
● peeled raw apple
● plain oat biscuit
● teething biscuit
● carrot stick.

Never leave your baby alone while she is eating in case she chokes.

Keeping baby teeth healthy

Make toothbrushing fun for your baby.

● Start brushing your baby's teeth as soon as the first one appears in his mouth.

● Babies are born mimics and one way your baby will learn is by watching you brush your teeth, so make sure he sees you.

● Use a small baby brush and a tiny smear of nonfluoride baby toothpaste.

● Make toothbrushing part of a baby's morning and bedtime routine.

● Baby toothpastes may have a milder taste but do not give as much fluoride protection. Check with your dentist whether they provide enough fluoride for your baby's needs.

● Sing a song as you brush his teeth. Make up a toothbrush song to a favorite nursery rhyme.

Moving to solids

Somewhere toward the end of five or six months, according to her size, is a good time to start your baby on solid foods. By this time she's drinking milk to full capacity at each feeding but still doesn't have enough calories for her needs.

Have a small amount of prepared food to hand. Start by feeding her from one breast or giving half the usual bottle, then give one or two teaspoons of food. The midday meal is ideal because your baby will not be ravenous but will be wide-awake and cooperative.

● Your baby may be reluctant to try new foods, so give her time to get used to each food and don't persist if she seems to dislike something.

● Use unprocessed infant cereals rather than ones that are prepared and make them up in small quantities.

● Don't give foods containing nuts, gluten, whole cow's milk, or egg until at least six months, to minimize the risk of your child developing allergies later.

● Give one new food at a time. Try it once and wait a few days before giving it again to see if there's a reaction.

the baby skill map

	0-1 months	1-2 months	2-3 months	3-4 months	4-5 mon

In developing skills such as language and movement all babies follow the same path, but the time it takes to reach each milestone varies from one baby to another. The ages given below are only a rough guide. All you have to do to help a skill develop is take your lead from your baby.

mind

gets excited at sight of breast or bottle

looks at own hand

spontaneous smile

listens and is alert

moving

supports upper bod

lifts head to 45°

talking

blows raspberries and bubble

squeals

mouths

hands

grasps rattle

holds hands open

grasps your finger tightly

friendliness

cries at disapproving tone of your voice

jerks whole body when sees you

months   6-7 months   7-8 months   8-9 months   9-10 months   10-11 months   11-12 months

shows you things in a book and shakes head for "no"

waves good-bye

holds arms out

understands "no"

stands and cruises

crawls

sits unsupported

"dada" and "mama" with meaning

single syllables "da" and "ma"

stacks blocks

bangs cubes together

points – then thumb/finger grasp

grasps with one hand

eaches out

loves theatrical show of emotions, laughs at "jokes"

plays clapping games

touches your face and touches other babies

how your baby learns to move

Movement begins with head control. Your baby cannot sit up, stand up, or crawl without being able to control the position of her head. Development of any kind goes from head to toe.

Lifts head

By two to three months your baby is really learning how to use and control his body. This means that he

● has stronger neck muscles so there's much less head lag when you pull him into a sitting position. His head is steady for several minutes when he's held in a sitting position or is propped up, but his back is curved

● can raise his head and hold it up when lying on his tummy and he's learned to lift his chest from horizontal by supporting himself a little on his hands, wrists, and arms

● practices bending his knees while lying prone

● enjoys the control that he now has over his movements and kicks and waves his arms around when he's lying down – for this reason, never leave him unattended on a changing table or bed.

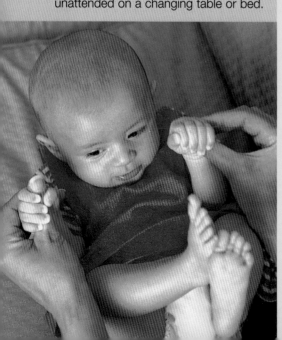

Supports upper body

By four to five months your baby's muscles are developing fast. She's gaining important head control and so she can

● move her head from side to side easily, without it wobbling

● keep her head in line with her body when she's pulled to sitting without it lagging behind – a major milestone in her development

● keep her head steady when sitting up, even if gently rocked to and fro

● raise her chest off the floor when she is lying on her tummy and look forward steadily, supporting herself on her arms.

Now that her upper body is strong and mobile and head control is complete you can play bouncing games on your knee. She may also start to roll from her front to her back, so play floor games and roll around.

Safety tips

Before your baby starts walking make your home childproof.

● Never leave your baby alone.

● Remove all furniture with sharp edges and corners from the room.

● Remove anything breakable from a surface that is less than a yard (3ft) from the floor.

● Make sure there are no electric wires trailing across the floor.

● Make sure all electric sockets are covered with safety plugs.

● Make sure that there are no extension cords less than a yard (3ft) from the floor.

● Make sure that all doorways and staircases have adjustable safety gates.

● Try and keep the floor clear of small, sharp toys.

● Make sure all fires are guarded.

● Don't leave any cloths hanging from tables that a baby could reach and pull.

● Make sure that all furniture and fixtures are sturdy and safely attached.

● Never leave anything hot on a table in the same room as your baby.

● Make sure that stair railings are too narrow for a small child to squeeze through.

● Make sure that all cabinet doors are closed firmly and that the handles are out of a crawling baby's reach; if they aren't, lock them or seal them up with masking tape.

● Make sure there are no containers of poisonous substances on the floor or within reach.

Sits unsupported

At six to seven months he'll make great strides in the way he moves. Now he
- can lift one hand off the floor in the push-up position and take all his weight on one arm
- can sit quite safely without support
- is strong enough to lift his head to look around when he's lying on his back
- can roll over from his back to his tummy (much harder than the other way around)
- can use his muscles to straighten his legs without wobbling so that he can take his whole weight steadily when you stand him on your lap
- bounces by bending and stretching his ankles, knees, and hips.

Now he can roll over from his back to his tummy, try some floor games. Don't be afraid to be a bit silly – he's developing a great sense of humor and it's good for you too. On his tummy he can rest on one hand so give him things to reach when in this position to improve his balance and strength.

Starting to move

By eight to nine months your baby is discovering that sitting up isn't enough – she wants to propel her body and to try to bring herself upright. Encourage her to pull herself up by placing furniture that will give support and hold her upright yourself. Her muscles have developed to the extent that she
- can sit for up to 10 minutes before she gets tired
- can lean forward without falling, although she can't lean sideways or swivel at the waist
- won't give up if she wants to reach an object, she'll try various ways of moving to reach it, but she is still unsteady
- may roll over to get to a sitting position and may move around this way
- may try crawling movements if you put her on her tummy and ask her to come toward you; don't be surprised if she goes backward though – her brain can't yet sort out the correct muscles for forward and backward
- may pull herself to standing in her crib or by holding on to furniture, but she flops down because she hasn't got the balance or coordination to sit down in a controlled way.

Crawls

By nine to ten months your baby may really be on the move and he
- can pull himself up to standing with ease, confidence, and good balance
- crawls or shuffles on his bottom, pulling himself forward with his hands, but his tummy may still not be completely off the floor when crawling
- may miss crawling or shuffling altogether, but however he moves, he's confidently mobile and moves forward on to his hands and knees when he's sitting
- loves his movement skills – he'll roll over and over, get himself into a sitting position, pull himself to standing, then sit down again
- can nearly control the movement from standing to sitting without toppling over.

He's learning to balance his body now because he
- is beginning to twist his trunk around in an attempt to swivel, but is still unsure
- can move from his tummy to sitting up and from sitting up to lying on his tummy
- has perfect balance when seated.

He's so good at crawling you'll be worn out if you try to crawl at the same rate! Create play tunnels and play crawling chase games on the floor or out on the grass in the yard.

Stands and cruises

By ten to eleven months, your baby is striving to get upright most of the time and she
- tentatively practices lots of pre-walking movements, so when she's standing holding on to the furniture or your hands, she'll lift her foot off the ground in a stepping movement and may stamp her foot a few times
- can scamper about swiftly on all fours if she's a crawler, with her tummy well clear of the floor

- can lean over sideways when sitting without toppling over
- can twist her trunk right around to reach something behind her and still keep her balance
- will cruise around the furniture to reach something she particularly wants. Now she'll start to pull herself up and cruise around the furniture, so help her with a treasure trail or an obstacle course or hold her hands to encourage her to walk. Be adventurous!

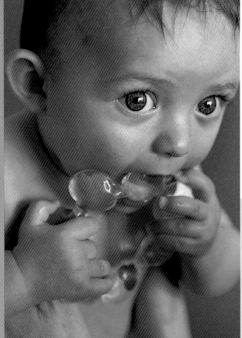

learning how to use her hands

Your baby was born with the reflex to grasp anything that is placed in her palm – such as your finger – and not let go. At first your baby has little interest in her hands, but as she becomes more aware of her body they'll begin to fascinate her more and more, and she gets more dextrous.

Grasps your finger tightly

It will be awhile before your baby realizes his hands are a part of him or that he has any control over them. His fingers remain tightly curled for at least the first three weeks of his life.

Once the grasp reflex that he was born with is lost, his hands relax and they will begin to open. Meanwhile your baby will hang on to your finger even when he's asleep. Play with his hands and fingers to encourage him to open his fists.

Grasps rattle

At four to five months your baby is beginning to realize that his hands are great tools and he
● has found his toes and discovered he can pull them into his mouth
● puts everything, including his fists, into his mouth since it's his most sensitive area
● tries to grasp his toys for the first time with his hand wide open, palm down, and mainly by curling his little finger in to his palm – he can only do this with large objects because he hasn't any fine finger movements yet
● reaches out for everything, grabbing and hitting, but beware – he loves to grab hold of long hair!
● loves crumpling paper, clothing, or blankets.

Holds hands open

At one to two months your baby will soon be fascinated by her hands. In preparation for this, she
● has completely lost the grasp reflex she was born with by the end of the second month – her fingers are hardly ever curled in a fist now, they remain wide open most of the time, ready for clasping things she wants in her palm
● is becoming aware of her fingers and she'll begin to study them intently by the end of the second month
● has very sensitive fingertips and

enjoys having them held, tickled, and massaged by you
● may take a swipe at a toy which is held out to her. She'll miss at this stage – even though her arm movements are becoming more purposeful, her ability to judge the distance between the object and her hand (known as her hand-eye coordination) is still quite poor, as is her muscle control.
Increase her awareness of her hands by using all kinds of tactile stimulation.
Open her hands and tickle her palms.

Grasps with one hand

By six to seven months your baby's grasp is becoming more and more precise – it's the key to so much future learning and independence. He's also putting things expertly in his mouth to explore so don't let him hold very small objects that he can swallow. He has so much more control over his hands and arms now and he

- can easily pass a toy from one hand to another
- reaches for a toy with one hand and not two as previously
- reaches for a block with his fingers

instead of palming it with an open hand
- holds on to one block in one hand and takes another block offered to him in the other.

Help your baby practice his grasping and improve his coordination by giving him finger foods and his bottle to hold, and introduce him to a two-handled cup for drinking. Give him small objects to hold between his fingers (but not so small that he can swallow and choke on them). He loves to make a noise so show him how to bang with the flat of his hand and play "Patty-cake."

Fine grasp

By nine to ten months, your baby will be able to do a lot more with her toys now that she

- reaches out for small objects with her index finger guiding her hand accurately to them
- has entirely mastered her fine grasp between finger and thumb
- has excellent hand-eye coordination so she can pick up a small object with ease (but be careful what you leave lying around)
- loves dropping and picking up games now that she can release her grip – she'll drop toys endlessly from her high chair and she'll watch them fall, she knows exactly where they've gone even if they roll out of sight and she'll shout and point for you to pick them up again
- loves rummaging in bags and boxes and will repeatedly take things out and put them back.

The finest movement she'll ever learn – the pincer grip between thumb and forefinger – is perfected at this time, so give her small, safe objects to pick up on her high chair tray or give her a treasure basket to sort through.

Points – then thumb/finger grasp

At eight to nine months your baby's grasp is getting finer. His ability to handle small objects is improving and he demonstrates this perfectly when he

- tries to turn the pages of a book, although he often turns several at a time
- holds a block in each hand and can bang them together
- holds an object between his thumb and fingers
- "rakes up" small pieces of food, like raisins, with his fingers and thumb.

Pointing is an important milestone in his development. Control of the index finger is the first step toward mastering the

very fine skill of bringing together the thumb and forefinger to nip or pinch small objects, which happens between 10 and 12 months. Give him small objects such as raisins and cooked peas to pick up to practice his grip and hand-eye coordination.

Encourage him to point at things by asking, "What do you want?" and "Show daddy." Point at the pictures as you look at books together to encourage him to copy.

Show him how to stack blocks one on top of the other because he can release his grasp now.

Stacks blocks

By eleven to twelve months her wrist bones have grown so her hands are more maneuverable and she

- is much more accurate at getting food into her mouth with a spoon
- has stopped mouthing everything she picks up – how an object feels in her hands is more important now
- is quite good at throwing
- can hold two blocks in one hand
- is able to build a tower of two blocks, thanks to her improved hand-eye coordination and steadiness
- will hold a crayon and may try to scribble if you show her how.

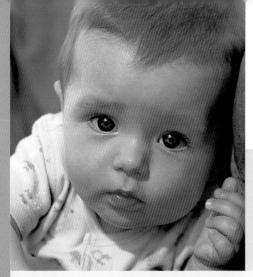

your baby's mind

Your baby's world is a confused blur of sights and sounds at first, and in the early weeks he is fully occupied with figuring out the things that have significance. Your face and voice will be among the first things he recognizes.

Listens and is alert

Your baby "understands" from the moment of birth – he's not inanimate. You can chart his progress in the first month. For example:

Day 1 He "stills" when he hears your voice – he becomes quiet and alert, his body stops moving, and he concentrates on listening.

Day 3 He responds when spoken to and his gaze becomes intense.

Day 5 At 8–10in (20–25cm) he's attracted to things that move and will watch your moving lips or your gently fluttering fingers with interest.

Day 9 His eyes will "dart" at the sound of a high-pitched voice, indicating that he can hear you.

Day 14 He can tell you apart from other people.

Day 18 He turns his head to sounds.

Day 28 He's learning how to express and control his emotions and will adjust his behavior to the sound of your voice: he'll get upset if you speak roughly or loudly and quiet down if your voice is soothing.

Play your baby some classical music. In addition to soothing him it will encourage him to listen, make sounds, and, believe it or not, add up numbers later.

Spontaneous smile

By one to two months your baby is taking more of an interest in her surroundings and soon she

● knows who you are and recognizes you, she's very interested to see you and shows her excitement by jerking her whole body with pleasure, kicking and waving her legs and arms

● smiles readily as soon as her eyes can focus at any distance, usually around six weeks

● watches what's going on around her; if she's propped up on cushions or in a bouncing chair, she will look in the direction of any sounds and movements

● stares steadily at things that interest her as though she's "grasping" them with her eyes.

When she smiles, smile back and tell her she's clever. Smiling means she's happy so let her know you're happy too. She loves looking at things so make sure she has plenty to look at – frequently change pictures or mobiles hanging over her crib to give a lot of interest.

Looks at own hand

Even at two to three months she's a keen thinker and she

● is fascinated by her own body and is beginning to understand that she can make it move – the first step in understanding the concept of cause and effect

● enjoys looking intently at her hands and fingers while she moves them in front of her face

● is attracted by moving objects and has sufficient control over her head to follow a slow-moving object with her eyes – if you hold a brightly colored toy in front of her, she'll take a moment to focus on it and then her eyes will follow it to either side as you move it (in a week or two she'll be able to focus instantly and follow the movement easily)

● is very curious about what goes on around her and watches everything with interest – sit her propped up so she can see better.

Gets excited at the sight of breast or bottle

At four to five months he is asserting his personality and relating more to other people. He

- loves the breast or bottle and shows this by patting it when feeding
- has a repertoire of emotions such as fear, anger, disgust, frustration, sadness, and pleasure to which he wants you to respond sympathetically – and you should because it makes him feel comfortable with his emotions
- loves all games because this is the way he learns and as he wants to learn he'll join in anything you suggest. He'll even make up simple games like splashing the bath water and he studies intently the effect of his hands and feet in the water
- is learning to concentrate, and spends a long time just looking at something he holds in his hands, although he often drops it
- smiles at his reflection in a mirror, although he doesn't yet realize it's actually himself
- moves his arms and legs to attract your attention and makes noises to call you to him
- is desperate to learn and to imitate, so try new games with rhymes and actions.

Understands "no"

By seven to eight months you'll notice signs that your baby understands what you say even though she can't speak words with meaning. At this time she

- can remember opposites through touch (hot and cold; hard and soft)
- understands some differences – for example,"mommy's coat," "baby's coat"
- can begin to judge the size of objects up to a yard (3ft) away
- understands phrases if they're part of routines so when you go into the bathroom she understands, "It's time for a bath"
- understands that "no!" means stop, don't do it, or don't touch
- shows determination and reaches for a toy she really wants – she's persistent and may cry with frustration if she's unsuccessful
- plays for a long time with her toys, examining and concentrating on them
- is becoming very assertive about showing she wants to feed herself. Now that she understands the words "yes" and "no," use them all the time. Be extra positive about "yes" and be careful about saying "no."

Try not to make "no" an automatic reaction because she'll soon figure out you're just pulling rank. Always make "yes!" a celebration.

Waves goodbye

By nine to ten months your baby enjoys showing off her understanding. See how she

- is becoming very familiar with routines and enjoys them
- puts her foot up when you hold out her sock and holds her hand up to go into the sleeve of her coat
- waves "bye-bye" when you say it
- knows her favorite soft toys and pats and strokes them when you say, "nice teddy bear."

Shows you things in a book and shakes head for "no"

By ten to eleven months his recognition skills and his understanding of concepts are sharpening so that he

- points to familiar things in a book that he likes
- understands that the cat and kitten in his book, his toy kitten, and grandma's cat are all cats, even though they're so different
- enjoys playing games that involve opposites – hot/cold, rough/smooth, round/square, big/little – especially if you act them out
- still has a short attention span when looking at books and will want to turn the pages quickly
- is learning about cause and effect – drop the block and you pick it up, bang the drum and it makes a noise, shake the rattle and it rings a bell
- enjoys putting things into a container and taking them out and pouring water into and out of containers in the bath
- nods or shakes his head to indicate "yes" and "no" to simple questions like "Do you want a drink?"

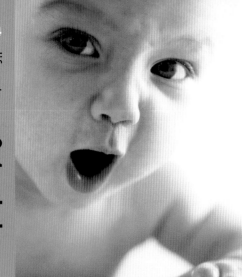

how your baby learns to talk

Babies need and want to communicate from their very earliest days, and even before they begin to talk to you they will listen and try to imitate sounds.

Mouthing

Your baby was born wired for sound and is longing to talk. He's a natural conversationalist.

● From birth he'll respond if you speak animatedly to him with your face 8–10in (20–25cm) from his by "mouthing" with his lips and tongue, like a fish.

● From two weeks he makes his own nonspecific sounds.

● From three weeks he has a baby sound vocabulary.

● From four weeks he understands the interchange of conversation and knows how to respond when you talk to him. From early on he leads the conversation and *you* follow *him*.

The more your baby is talked to and encouraged to respond, the earlier he will learn to speak and the better the quality of his speech will be. Start talking to your baby the instant he's born and never stop. Say his name over and over (and watch his eyes dart in response).

Squeals

By two to three months he's found his voice and takes every opportunity to practice his full range. In doing so he

● makes all kinds of noises to indicate pleasure – you'll hear squeals, gurgles, shouts, and cooing sounds

● may be starting to add consonants to his vowel sounds, the first normally being "m," then the explosives – you can help him by showing him how to blow raspberries

● tends to use "p" and "b" when unhappy, and then by three months he'll use more guttural sounds, "j" and "k," when happy.

Speak rhythmically in a sing-song voice and laugh a lot; jog him in time to your rhythmic speech. Respond to the many different kinds of noises your baby is now beginning to make by talking as much as possible to him while making full eye contact. Repeat every sound your baby makes.

"Dada" and "mama" with meaning

At nine or ten months your baby understands language as more than just vocal patterns. As proof of this new skill she

● understands the precise meaning of quite a few words, although she can't say any yet

● may say one word with meaning by about this age, but don't worry if she doesn't do this, just

understanding the meaning is more important for now

● develops the word "mama" soon after "dada," which she says more often when mommy is present than when she's not

● might begin to sound the beginning of words like "do" for "dog" – help her hear the "g" on the end of the word by emphasizing it with another

syllable, as in "doggie," "horsey," "mommy," "daddy."

She's babbling away so babble with her. Ask a lot of simple questions and recite nursery rhymes to promote her understanding of words. Repeat her words, such as "dada" for daddy, "doe-doe" for dog, but with meaning – say, "Yes, there's daddy" or "Look at this picture of a dog."

Single syllables

At five to six months she's getting the hang of taking turns in conversation and trying new sounds. Listen as she

- attempts to converse with her mirror image and has a "conversation" of gurgles with herself
- has a growing repertoire of speech sounds, especially the blowing and raspberry sounds that she practices all the time
- makes special sounds to attract your attention, even trying a cough
- starts to join real vowels and real consonants together in a simple way, saying "ka," "da," "ma," and "ergh"
- is intent on imitating your conversation and uses her tongue a lot, poking it out and playing with it between her lips
- begins to respond to her name – use it at every opportunity so she'll achieve a sense of self and feel important
- understands bits of what you say, such as, "Here's your bottle," "Daddy's coming," "yes" and "no"
- begins to babble – repeats sounds over and over, listens, then tries them out again.

Talk to her all the time – tell her what you're doing all the time, point out interesting things, especially animals, when you're out and about. Repeat phrases and praise her when she appears to understand you. Sing songs and say rhymes to her. Play clapping games together. Read books together, pointing, naming, and making the sounds of animals.

Blows bubbles

At three to four months your baby will start trying to hold a "conversation" with you now that he

- makes more than simple vowel and consonant sounds
- tries to imitate sentences like yours by stringing sounds together or coming out with "words" like "gaga" or "ahgoo"
- can blow through his lips – he shows off his new skill by blowing bubbles
- uses quite a repertoire of sounds, and by 16 weeks he'll express his feelings, many of which signify delight, by chuckling, laughing, and squealing. All babies love to make someone laugh – it's instant feedback.

Starting to talk

At eleven to twelve months her speech is really taking off and she

- can say two or three words with meaning and make animal noises
- starts "jargoning" – an imitation of what she hears you say to other people or an attempt to copy the running commentary you keep up when you're with her – you'll notice long ramblings of sound and, here and there, the odd intelligible word
- has completely mastered "yes" and "no" while nodding and shaking her head
- understands simple questions like "Where's your shoe?" or "Where's your book?" and will search for them
- doesn't drool much any more, a sign that she's gaining control over her tongue, mouth, and lips ready for speech. Encourage those first words she uses with meaning by repeating stories with her, repeating nursery rhymes, call and response games, clapping games, music, and puppet play.

your friendly baby

Your baby needs to exchange love and friendliness, especially with you, her parents. She learns to be loving and friendly by imitating you, first with facial expressions, then with gestures and movements, and finally with a whole range of friendly behavior.

Jerks whole body when he sees you

From the moment of birth your baby is a highly developed person with many accomplishments. He is born friendly and longs for company so he
● wants to respond to you and listens and looks intently even at birth
● demonstrates this with whole body jerks, mouthing, sticking out his tongue, nods, bobs, throwing out his hands, and spreading his fingers
● smiles from birth if he can see you talking and smiling at him from a distance of 8–10in (20–25cm)
● loves to have eye contact and skin contact, especially when he's feeding
● can show emotions by using the correct face muscles to smile and grimace – he'll be upset if he hears a harsh-sounding voice.
Cuddle him when he's awake. Try to give him skin-to-skin contact with both parents whenever possible. By stroking, caressing, and massaging him you'll make him feel loved and secure.

Cries at disapproving tone of your voice

By four to five months your baby is learning how to express his feelings in a variety of ways. By the end of the fifth month he
● knows your voice and its modulations very well and doesn't like the different tone of voice you use when you say "no," although he doesn't yet know what it means
● eagerly smiles at people he knows
● uses body movements, facial expressions, and sounds as well as crying, to show his different moods.

Tone of voice

Because your baby is disturbed by an angry tone of voice he'll stop when you sound displeased to see if you really disapprove of him. This response is the basis of all future discipline – all that's needed is a change in the tone of your voice. He loves a friendly voice and will do almost anything to hear one, even refraining from doing what he wants.

Touches your face

By five to six months she's showing love for the first time. Get her to touch your face and say "hello" as she does so. Put a mirror in a position where she can see herself and help her to pat her image. There are many games you can play with reflections. Teach her to show love with lots of patting and stroking of pets and cuddly toys and show her books with pictures of mother animals and their babies. You'll notice that she
● makes a lot of advances to you and wants to touch you, but because she hasn't developed refined movement, she tends to pat you roughly
● loves your face – she'll nuzzle and stroke it and she may also grab a handful of hair!
● may begin to be shy with strangers toward the end of the sixth month – she'll bury her head on your chest if someone she doesn't know speaks to her or to you, and may cry if a stranger picks her up.

Naturally outgoing

At three to four months she's naturally outgoing and at this stage not at all shy. This is clearly seen in the way she
- looks, smiles, grunts, and coos at anyone who speaks to her or pays her attention
- knows you and the rest of the family and recognizes family pets
- gets lonely and lets you know she doesn't like being alone for too long when she's awake
- stops crying when you go to her, showing pleasure at your presence
- jerks her body when she sees you
- uses laughter to charm you.

Pats other babies

At six to seven months your baby may like company but he's becoming more self-contained and happy with his own company too. He
- recognizes other babies as being like himself and reaches out to them in friendship
- pats other babies or his own reflection, just as he pats you
- vocalizes to himself and other babies, just as he does to you
- joins in games like "Patty-cake" and "This little piggy"
- is very sociable and wants you to understand him so he laughs, coughs, cries, squeals, blows bubbles, smiles, and frowns to converse with you.

Plays clapping games

By eight to nine months your baby's personality is emerging – he may be serene, a fusspot, noisy, determined, irritable, sensitive. Whatever he's like, he
- loves to join in everything that you do, although he's quite good at playing on his own
- enjoys playing with you – batting balloons or playing clapping games like "Patty-cake" – and anticipates actions involved
- understands when someone is going and may start to wave "bye-bye"
- enjoys a joke and teasing games.

Try some cooperative games like rolling a ball backward and forward, Itsy-bitsy spider and Peekaboo.

Friendliness

By eleven to twelve months your baby knows the power of her affections and will give them or withhold them for effect. For example she
- kisses on request, but won't if she doesn't feel like it
- shows many emotions, especially affection, and will pat the dog, kiss mommy, or hug daddy
- is apt to be shy with strangers but loves family gatherings and outings in the car or in her stroller
- loves being in a crowd, especially with other children, but she'll hold on to you until she's confident enough to join in – even then she'll keep checking that you're close by and may cry if you leave the room unexpectedly.

She loves babies of her own age so invite little friends to play at your house and go to parent-and-toddler groups where she can meet other babies.

"your child will see himself as a separate entity than you; he'll be aware of self"

life stages: 1 to 4 years

During the first year of your baby's life the accent is on learning physical things: he learns to crawl, to stand up, and possibly even to take a few steps. The ability to do these things brings with it a sense of physical achievement and a sense of independence. He is able to go and explore the world without having to wait for you to bring it to him.

During the next few years he'll not only consolidate all the physical skills he acquired in his first year, but he'll also master one of the most difficult intellectual ones – speech. Your child will be struggling to express his thoughts and desires through speech and with his increasingly able brain he'll now see himself as a separate entity than you; he'll be aware of "self." He'll probably be quite frustrated at times and you may notice more tantrums. He'll need a lot of affection, much encouragement, and constant support.

Learning spurts

Your child doesn't grow, develop, and learn at a constant rate. Learning spurts are well known and every child has them. During a learning spurt, your child will gobble up new ideas, acquire new skills, and put them into practice immediately. However, while he's going through these learning spurts some activities, and possibly certain skills that he's already learned, may appear to slip. Don't worry. They won't be gone for good. It is just that your child is using all his concentration to learn something new, but once it is learned he'll regain all the other skills he'd mastered previously.

During a learning spurt try to make your child's life as interesting as possible. Of course if he shows that certain things are enjoyable then you should do them as often as you can, but don't hesitate to introduce him to new things; he is ready to learn and absorb information very fast. And don't be too discriminating about the kind of entertainment you give. Young children simply screen out what they prefer and understand and let the rest go by.

Such spurts are invariably followed by periods when development appears to slow down. Treat them as recovery periods during which your child can consolidate newly learned skills and prepare himself for the next spurt. Don't get anxious about this – just let him practice the skills that he has already learned. You can help during these slower learning times by playing and practicing with him, saying something like "let's sing that song again," or "why don't we try to push the peg through the hole again."

Let your child guide you

All the way through life, teachers who succeed do so by helping us to develop and reach our full potential. They maximize our strengths and minimize our weaknesses. As your baby's teacher you should try to make the best of his good points and play down his bad ones.

You also have to give your child the kind of help he needs when he needs it. Giving help is worthless if the person who is being helped doesn't really require it or like it, so while you have to be an active helper, you shouldn't be an interfering one. Your baby should not be learning what *you* want him to learn, he should be learning what *he* wants to learn, and this should be your first priority.

You have to suppress any ideas of what you think a child of his age ought to be doing and respond to what he wants to do. This means that you have to be guided by your child and respond to his needs. While it is your job as a good parent to introduce him to as wide a range of interesting things as possible, it isn't your job to decide which of those things he should find interesting. In other words, having presented the menu, you must let him choose the dishes.

In the pages that follow, I offer guidelines where appropriate, advice where I feel there may be a need, and strategies for dealing with potentially difficult situations.

Body

Social

" be guided by
your child
and respond
to his needs "

Mind

"toddlers
need almost
constant
activity
to develop
normally"

she is ready
to learn
and absorb
information
very fast

your growing child

Watching your child grow and develop is one of the most exciting aspects of being a parent, and during the early years you'll be astounded by how quickly he changes.

Why your child should exercise

Human beings were born to be active, not sedentary. Toddlers are so named because they toddle almost ceaselessly. And so they should. Their bodies need almost constant activity in order to develop normally. Woe befalls the toddler who isn't encouraged to run around or, even worse, is left parked with a snack to be baby-sat by the Teletubbies. This toddler will be fat because he isn't burning off enough calories with natural exercise. And a fat toddler means a fat child. A fat child may develop diabetes in his teens and be a candidate for heart disease by the time he is in his 20s.

The human race has evolved very efficiently to survive without food for a period. It has never had to accommodate a sedentary life. A sedentary life that starts in infancy can be fatal, so exercise is crucial for your baby and child. Encourage it whenever you can. Join in. Play a family sport even if it's only tossing a ball around.

Encouraging your child to eat

As with all feeding, the key word is flexibility. You and your child should enjoy yourselves, so give a little thought to making mealtimes entertaining.

● If she wants to use a knife, give your child a plastic or blunt-ended one.
● Let her use a straw for drinking sometimes. So that she won't tip the drink over, cut the end of the straw so that there is not too much projecting above the cup.
● Ice-cream cones don't have to be used just for ice cream. Fill one with cheese and tomato chopped together or with tuna salad and give your three-year-old a snack on the move.
● Be open to innovation and occasionally serve your child's meal on a doll's plate or on a flat toy.
● Fill a cake pan with a lot of different finger foods such as cheese cut into cubes, bits of cold meat, raw vegetables, fruit, potato chips, and tiny peanut butter sandwiches and let your child pick out what she wants.
● Let your child "build" her meal from sandwiches, cubes of cheese, and vegetables. She could make a house or a car, and eat it when it's finished.

Physical milestones

Remember that every child develops at his own rate. Don't force your child to go more quickly than he wants to – it will serve no purpose. Let him go at his own pace, while still providing all the help and encouragement you can.

13 months

Let him practice standing alone. If you place furniture close together, he'll "cruise" around and may even take his first independent step. Stable toys or pieces of furniture with rounded edges are ideal for holding on to and help independent stepping and cruising. Once he is mobile, keep an eye on him at all times.

15 months

Provide him with a sturdy chair so that he can kneel and lower his body to sit without support and enjoy getting in and out of the chair. You'll be helping him to practice bending and flexing his hips and knees. Make sure the chair will not tip over if he uses it to hold on to when he stands up. His steps are high, unsteady, and of unequal length and direction. Use stairguards – he can creep upstairs now.

18 months

Show him how to squat to accelerate his muscle development. Encourage him to imitate you. Climb the stairs with him until he can do so unaided, both feet on each step, though he'll need to hold on. He walks with a steadier, lower-stepping gait, runs, walks backward, and rarely falls.

21 months

Let him join in your daily activities because he's fascinated by everything you do and he'll want to imitate your every move. He can pick up objects without falling over now. Encourage games such as soccer so he can show you how fluent his movements are – he walks backward easily; he can also walk up stairs, both feet on each step, but without holding on, and can stop quickly and turn corners.

2 years

Encourage dancing and singing because your child is starting to get rhythm, and making movements to rhythmical music is something he'll enjoy. Dance with him – it will also give

him practice in making a wide range of movements. He can run, but not slow down, and can squat with ease so get down on the floor with him.

2½ years

Provide him with a moving toy with wheels that he can sit on and use his feet to propel. He is probably too young for a tricycle, but there are many simpler, suitable moving toys you can get. He'll love to jump with his feet off the ground and walk on tiptoe. He's steady enough on his feet to carry a breakable object and he can sit and hold a baby brother or sister on his knee for a few moments.

3 years

Play hopping games. He's much more nimble so show him jumping games, such as hopscotch, which are also good for working off excess energy. Include hopping in other games such as "Simon says." He can walk up stairs with one foot on each step, stand on one foot for a second, swing his arms like an adult when walking, and ride a tricycle.

4 years

Show him how to use a jump rope because he's now very active and should be well coordinated. All his muscles are working together and play such as this gives him a workout for a wide range of movements. Make sure he has access to outdoor apparatus. He races around, hopping, jumping, climbing, and goes downstairs rapidly one foot per step. He can even carry a cup of liquid without spilling any.

Visiting the dentist

Take your child for her first dental checkup around her third birthday, and make sure this visit is as pleasant as possible. Get your child used to the sight of instruments and the smell of the surroundings by taking her with you when you go for your own checkup. If she can be trusted, and your dentist has no objections, let your child sit on

your lap while the dentist examines you. She'll watch with fascination and will be delighted to copy your example. Just before your child's first visit, play a game of going to the dentist and look into each other's mouths. Then, when you get to the office, arrange for the dentist to look at your mouth just before he looks at your child's.

learning hand skills

Between the ages of 1 and 4 hand and finger skills really flower. Given how crucial they are for writing, encourage your child all you can.

Hand-eye coordination

Your child's first attempt at hand-eye coordination is feeding herself. She learns how to steer food to her mouth with her hand and eye very quickly and from then on her skills develop rapidly. You can start a one-year-old with stacking blocks and fingerpaints, and go on to materials like Legos and games with a bat and ball.

13 months

Offer food to eat with a spoon. If you give her more solid food that sticks to the spoon, and doesn't slide off easily, she'll be encouraged to feed herself. As she learns to rotate her hand to get the food to her mouth she will become more and more accurate. Throwing things is a favorite game and she can also make lines with a pencil and hold two blocks in her hand. Having mastered relaxing her grip to release objects, she can build a tower of two blocks.

15 months

Help her build towers to increase her hand skills. She can now manage putting three blocks on top of one another. She also tries to turn over the pages of a book, so read with her often. Let her try to put on some of her clothes herself, too. Feeding herself with a spoon, and getting it

to her mouth before anything runs off, is very easy now.

18 months

Give her an activity board or similar toy to practice turning, twisting, spinning, dialing, and sliding movements. She's good with zippers and other fasteners and they fascinate her. Her fingers are dextrous, so provide the materials for fingerpainting and drawing. She'll read a book with you, turning over two or three pages of a book at a time. Give her the chance and she'll feed herself completely and use a cup without spilling anything.

2 years

Encourage her to dress and undress herself and put on her own socks, shoes and gloves as much as she can – plenty of scope for fine finger movements. As she's mastered a screwing movement, she can turn a door knob and unscrew loose lids from jars, and undo and do up a zipper, so get her to show you. She can use a pencil more deliberately, so draw together. Let her show you how she can build a tower four blocks high.

2½ years

Give her blocks and toys to build models that require pressing and

fitting pieces together and use the small muscles of the hand. Let her thread beads and show you how she can fasten an easily placed button into a loose buttonhole. Drawings are more representational; she may also build a tower that is eight blocks high.

3 years

Ask her to help with simple tasks that involve a number of coordinated movements, like setting the table. Encourage her to fasten and unfasten buttons by herself, so she can dress and undress herself completely, if she wishes. She'll draw a recognizable image and her towers may now be nine blocks high. Help her start to try to use scissors – a huge step forward in brain/muscle coordination, and in manual dexterity.

4 years

Give her lots of practice with small movements, such as arranging small toys. She's getting much better at fine tasks, so ask her to set the table properly, wash her own face and hands, make her bed, and put her clothes away tidily. Show your four-year-old how to draw a circle and she will. She can also copy two straight lines crossing at right angles, though imperfectly.

Suitable toys

Give your child toys to help her develop coordination and manipulative skills. Toys that make use of both of these will provide the most enjoyment, but be prepared for your child to be a bit clumsy at first and give her quite large, straightforward items. Household objects are popular, but other toys may stretch both coordination and mental processes further:

- shape sorter
- stacking blocks
- building blocks
- hammering table
- push/pull toys
- dolls
- cars
- frame
- crayons and markers
- paints and brushes
- blackboard
- books
- playdough
- sand box
- slide
- wading pool
- cart
- swing.

Right- or left-handed?

If both you and your partner are left-handed, 1 in 3 of your children will be too; the chance of this happening with two right-handed parents is 1 in 10. **There is no natural law that states that one hand is superior to the other** so it should never bother you if your child is left-handed.

Your child has no control over which of his hands is dominant; dominance is decided by the developing brain. Think of the brain as two linked halves, each of which controls different activities. One of these sides becomes dominant as your child's brain develops. If it is the left side of the brain that dominates, the child is right-handed. If it is the right side, the child is left-handed. In the first few months your baby may seem to have no preferences but in fact most newborns turn their heads more to the right than to the left.

As your child's coordination improves and he starts to acquire manual skills, you may find that he starts to use one hand more than the other. Don't be worried if he doesn't do this. Your child will develop at his own speed. Never, ever, try to dissuade your child from being left-handed. You may think that by "encouraging" your child to use his right hand instead of his left you're doing him a favor for later life. You are not. And, what's more, you could well risk causing psychological side effects like stuttering, as well as reading and writing difficulties, by altering what his brain naturally wants to do.

Is my child stimulated enough?

If you provide the right environment and the right equipment, you shouldn't worry about whether your child is being stimulated enough. At this stage your child is developing his thinking about playing, and what he needs is freedom to allow his thought processes to expand so that he can follow new ideas as they occur to him, and see play though to its conclusions. It is your job to provide the floor space, the tools, and uninterrupted time.

You can't teach your child to use his imagination, but you can encourage his natural gift for fantasy by doing the following.
- Play make-believe games with your toddler.
- When you tell a story, act out the character's parts and make up all the various characters' voices.
- Play "What's this?" games. Get your child to shut his eyes then gently stroke an object across his skin. Ask him to guess what it is.
- Help your child in his imaginary world by giving him some hand puppets – either store-bought ones or brown paper bags with faces drawn on them.
- Start to stock a dress-up box. Put in old shoes, shirts, skirts, dresses, hats, and scarves. Add some special cheap jewelry as well. Make a wrap from a length of fabric and attach a clasp at one end.

Bedtime routines

Bedtimes should be happy times and even if you're worn out, try your best to be calm and relaxed. If you're not, your child will pick up your anxiety and be fretful, and you may have to spend twice as long trying to get him to go to sleep than if you had given him an extra five minutes of your undivided attention in a quiet, direct way.

Helping your toddler to sleep

● Don't put your child to bed immediately after an exciting game or rough-and-tumble play – he will have great difficulty settling which will be frustrating for you. Give him time to quiet down, sitting with you watching television or looking at a book.
● Even a small child likes looking at a book in bed, so if yours is happy, leave him with a favorite nonscary book.
● Put a dab of your perfume or aftershave on your child's pillow and suggest that he breathes it in deeply. Deep breathing is relaxing and calming and will help your child drift off to sleep.
● Give your child a bath before bedtime and follow this with a warm drink and a story in bed.
● There is nothing magical about bedrooms. Let your child go to sleep where he is most comfortable: at your feet on the floor, on a couch, in your lap.
● Be flexible about bedtimes. Left to themselves, most children go to sleep at around seven or eight o'clock in the evening, whether you put them to bed or not. Why should they be unhappy in a room on their own, instead of happy in your company?

1-4 daily care

Keep your child healthy by looking after her hygiene and sleep needs and making sure she has a safe environment.

Safety

Once your child starts to move around the house easily, your main concern will be to keep her safe. Here are some guidelines:

Indoors

● Block open stairways and other unsafe areas with gates. These should be made of a rigid mesh with a straight top edge and should be swung open from a stationary surround.
● The bathroom and kitchen may contain poisonous and dangerous substances, and children should never be allowed to roam free in either room. Many houseplants are also dangerous to young children.

Outdoors

● Keep garden gates locked with child-resistant locks.
● Install swings, slides, and climbing toys on grass or sand, never on concrete or pavement. Check equipment regularly for strength, stability, and signs of corrosion.
● Check all play equipment to ensure that there is no risk of scissoring, shearing, or pinching injuries and that surfaces are free from snags and splinters.
● Instruct children carefully on what they can and can't do on play equipment.

Toilet teaching

I am whole-heartedly against anything that resembles toilet training. For me there are no arguments in favor of it, only against. I believe that toilet training and the attitudes that advocate "training" a child's bowel movements and bladder function should be expunged from child care and child development.

There are good reasons to feel this way: it is impossible to train children to do anything unless their bodies have developed to a point where they are anatomically and physiologically able to perform the tasks that you demand. Applied to bowel and bladder control this means that it is impossible for your child to control either of these functions unless the bowel and the bladder muscles are strong enough to hold urine and feces, and that at a given order from the brain the nerves to the bowel and bladder are mature enough to obey the order and evacuate.

If this level of development has not been reached, there is nothing that your child can do to meet your expectations. You can see immediately what a dreadful position this puts your child in. She is aware of what you want, but her body is unable to perform the task. Your child's desire to please you overrides almost all other desires and in this she is frustrated. She becomes unhappy at not being able to do what you want and may then feel inadequate, ashamed, guilty, and finally resentful.

If you insist on a toilet program when your child is not ready for it, the end can only be sadness. Your relationship with your child will deteriorate. You will become a source of unhappiness, and bowel movements and potty training will become a battle ground of your child's will against your nerves – and you will always be the loser. You cannot make your child pass a stool, or keep a diaper dry, and if you try to do either of these things you'll make her suffer every time the inevitable accident occurs.

Toilet teaching tips

● Let your child develop at her own pace. There is no way that you can speed up the process, you can only be there to help your child along.

● Let your child decide whether or not to sit on the potty. You can suggest that she does but you should never force the issue.

● Do treat your child's feces in a sensible manner, and never show any disgust or dislike for them. They're a natural part of your child and initially she'll be very proud of them.

● Do not delay once your child has signaled that she wants the potty since control is only possible for a short time.

● Praise your child and treat her control as an accomplishment.

● Whenever you travel, make sure that you have a potty with you so that your child can go under any circumstances without having to wait.

● Tell your child very firmly and sympathetically that accidents will always be ignored and forgiven and that she's not to worry about them.

● Some children acquire bowel and bladder control much later than others and in nearly all cases it is wrong to blame the child. Most doctors feel that there is no need to investigate this difficulty before your child is three years old, and if she is only wet at night your doctor may feel that these investigations can be put off until she is five.

a loving child

To help our children grow up into generous, loving adults we must respond to their social demands from the very outset. In doing so, we make them responsive, friendly, outgoing, and affectionate.

Social milestones

12–15 months

Include your child in as many activities as possible, and make certain she has a ringside seat. Social gatherings are fun and she will follow conversations, making noises in the gaps. She can say one or two words with meaning, ask for things, indicate thank you, and will stop doing something at the word "no." But she's not so independent that she doesn't want to hold your hand for security.

15–18 months

Encourage your child to express love. Praise her when she shows affection and care toward others – siblings, relatives, pets, or toys.

Encourage helpfulness, both with chores and dressing and undressing. Keep her with you because she loves being with adults and wants to imitate them, but don't expect too much. At social gatherings, she'll play next to, but not with, another child.

18 months–2 years

Help her to understand sharing. Invite her friends to the house so that she can start to play group games and share play materials. Attention-seeking devices such as grabbing your arm, hitting you, and doing forbidden things are common and she will often refuse to obey. But there is much less fighting and more cooperation with other children so she'll modify selfish behavior to accommodate a playmate.

2–2½ years

Make sharing a game. Initiate games that involve giving things to others and she will learn to share with them. Sharing is hard for her and she'll show feelings of rivalry and will try to force her will on other children. She wants to be independent but also seeks your approval, so give it often. She may react to frustration by having tantrums, which are best ignored.

3 years

Encourage her to play with others. Sharing leads to social acceptance, and this leads to generosity. Have her friends play and stay at your house. Independence is flourishing and she's more outgoing toward other children. Unselfishness starts to blossom, and firm friendships with other adults and children form. She will show signs of sympathy when someone is distressed and be more generous – share that with her.

4 years

Talk to her about her feelings as much as you can. By the age of four your child is showing signs of being a fledgling adult in terms of her emotional development. She loves animals, may cry if they're hurt, and rushes to help and heal them. She's very fond, too, of her family and friends who are clearly special to her.

How to help a shy child

Shyness is something that affects many children. Common types of shy behavior include disliking new experiences, reluctance to join in social gatherings, unwillingness to talk to unknown people, and difficulty in making new friends. Don't think of shyness as something wrong with your child; many well-adjusted adults are quite shy. The best way of dealing with it is not by criticism or forcing change but by preparing your child for any situation he's likely to find difficult, perhaps with stories or role playing. In most cases, time and patience are all that is needed.

If your child has poor social skills there are various ways that you or your child's preschool teacher can help:

Opposite pairing Pairing a neglected or unsocial child with a child who is outgoing and social. By being seen as the friend of a popular child, the shy child will gain a significantly higher level of social acceptance in a short time – in some cases as little as three weeks.

Younger pairing Pairing a child with poor social skills with a younger child can be another way of conferring status. A study done in the 1980s showed that when unpopular children between the ages of four and five played with children younger than themselves, their level of popularity increased by at least 50 percent. Younger playmates offer friendship which helps build self-esteem and assertiveness.

Clique activities Although it might seem bad for children to form small, exclusive groups within a large group, allowing them to mix in their preferred clique motivates them to get along with their peers outside the clique. Clique-based activities give children a sense of security and confidence about all social relationships.

Small groups It is sometimes mistakenly assumed that an unsocial child will become social when surrounded by a big group. In fact, small groupings are better at facilitating friendships because in a large group the unsocial child can remain very much in the background; in a small group he can't be ignored. A preschool teacher can help by placing an unsocial child in a small group – of say three or four children – then gradually extending the size of the group.

Star responsibility Establishing definite roles, such as giving the most popular children responsible tasks to do, appears to have a settling effect on all children of preschool age. Tasks could include giving out the straws for milk or arranging tidying up. Unsocial children appear to benefit from this strategy as much as other children.

Leaving your child

Children in this age group dislike being separated from their parents, even if you are only going to spend the evening out of the house. It is quite usual for a child to shed a few tears until she is reassured about some of the details of the evening. These might include what time you are leaving; how far away you will be going; who you will be with; what you will be doing; and what time you will return.

● Start getting dressed 15 minutes early so that you can spend a few moments with your child quietly doing something nice before you leave. Never rush off without enough warning.

● If you make a promise that you will be back by a certain time, keep this promise and, as you are going, remind your child that you will always come back.

● Have a goodbye ritual – tell a story or play a game, give a hug or blow a kiss as you get into the car.

● Think up a few games – kiss her palm, fold her fingers around it and say that if she needs a kiss while you are away there is one for her to have.

● Never keep the fact that you are going to go out a secret from your child. In fact, talk about it well ahead of your absence. Try to do it very casually the day before and once or twice during the day.

● When your child is very small, don't use time frames that she can't grasp; instead, compare the time with some of her favorite activities. For example, say, "I'll be gone half an hour – that's four cartoons' worth."

● If you are going to have a baby-sitter, ask her to come a good half hour before you leave so that she can get involved in a game with your child before you go.

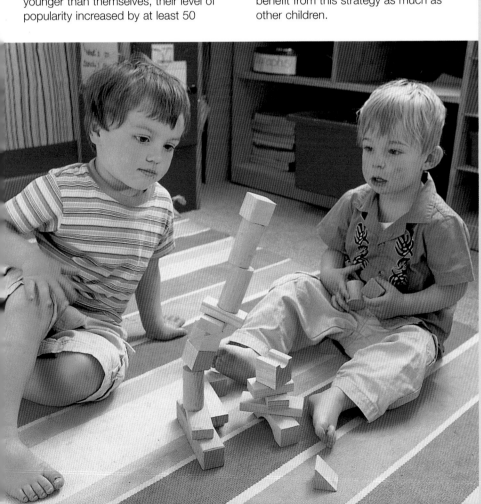

learning to fit in

One- to four-year-olds face many changes as they mature and may feel "hurried." Be patient with problems and allow your child to develop in her own good time.

Right and wrong

Your child will only learn the difference between right and wrong if it's clearly pointed out. If your child understands why you want her to do or not do something she is much more likely to do it willingly, so try to explain and then ask her opinion.

But there are situations that are non-negotiable: when your child's safety is threatened, when the thoughts and feelings of others should be considered, and when your child is tempted to tamper with the truth. You should be very firm on these points and she will gradually learn a sense of responsibility for disciplining herself as she grows up.

Boldness can often be mistaken for impertinence, but unless your child is imposing on the feelings of others, she may be displaying nothing more than a healthy resistance to authority which can be useful, if sensibly directed.

A spoiled or overindulged child will behave in a self-centered way and this may be the result of the over-protectiveness, favoritism, or the high expectations of her parents. The best cure is to let her go to playgroup or preschool at two-and-a-half to three as a leveler. She will get used to mixing with other children and start learning how to get along with them.

Tantrums

Toddlers between the ages of 2 and 3 may often have temper tantrums as a means of venting frustration when they can't do or get what they want.

This is quite normal behavior. At this age your child will not have sufficient judgment to control his strength of will or the language to express himself clearly, but as his knowledge and experience of the world broadens, the occasions when his will is pitted directly against yours become less likely.

A tantrum may be brought on by such feelings as frustration, anger, jealousy, and dislike. Anger is brought on by not getting his own way and frustration by his not being sufficiently strong or well coordinated to do what he wants. A tantrum usually involves your child throwing himself on the floor, kicking, and screaming.

The best thing you can do during a tantrum is to stay calm, since any attention on your part will only prolong the attack. If he has a tantrum in public, take him away from too much attention, without making a fuss.

At home an effective technique is simply to leave the room. Explain to your child that, while you still love him, you have to leave the room because you are getting upset. Never confine him in another room because this denies him the option of coming back and saying sorry.

Your child's position in the family

No position in the family can be regarded as best. Firstborn children grow up in a more child-centered environment where the family activities concentrate on the child more than is possible for later-born children. Firstborn children have more guidance and help in their development, receive more complex language from their parents during infancy, and because of parental pressures on them, they usually achieve more than later-born siblings. Firstborn children tend to be better accepted by adults and are more likely to take up leadership roles because they conform more closely to social expectations.

On the other hand, parents are less skilled at parenting with the first child and tend to intervene, intrude, restrict, and use more coercive discipline and more punishments of all kinds than they do with later children. This can lead to first children receiving more feelings of anxiety from their parents, in other words, "am I doing right?" However, there is little doubt that if children born later in the family were given the same guidance and attention as first-

borns, they would probably achieve as much and be as well accepted socially.

The effects of family position become persistent very quickly and greatly influence the personal and social adjustments children make as they grow up. For example, there is evidence that firstborn children are more health conscious than their younger siblings and as adults consult doctors more often. They also tend to be more cautious and take fewer risks.

The number of small children in the family greatly affects a child's development. Children with several younger brothers and sisters must share their parents' attention. If one child is needy, he is likely to get the lion's share of parental attention, leading to sensitivity about favoritism in the others. Rivalry between siblings, competition, bad feelings, and resentment will be heightened. In addition, a needy child is likely to develop a "follower" personality pattern, and feelings of inadequacy and martyrdom, while the stronger may feel discriminated against and learns to play the leader.

Fantasy and reality

In order for a child to tell a lie he must have reached a stage in his psychological development where he can distinguish fantasy from reality. For example, if a 15-month-old baby is chastised by his mother for smearing finger paint on a wall, and he shakes his head vigorously in denial, he is not lying – it may be that he has genuinely forgotten the action, wishes that he hadn't done it, or simply cannot recognize the difference between fantasy and reality. Only when a child reaches the age of 3 or 4 years is he capable of lying, and most children will lie if they find a situation sufficiently threatening. So to encourage a truthful child, avoid a threatening atmosphere and reward the truth.

How serious is lying?

Children lie for many different reasons and some types of lying are more serious than others. For instance, a make-believe lie is a natural part of a child's fantasy life, whereas a cover-up lie is a conscious attempt to avoid punishment. Because children lie for different reasons, every child and every lie must be treated individually.

do

✔ Act calmly – your child may simply be confusing reality and fantasy.

✔ Try to understand the motive for a lie. Your child is not lying because he wants to be malicious, but because he is afraid of punishment.

✔ Explain why it is wrong to lie. Use examples that he can understand.

✔ Make your child aware that, although you are upset by the lie, you still love him.

don't

✘ Ridicule the child who persists with bragging lies. Bragging indicates low self-esteem and you should work to increase your child's self-confidence with praise and affection.

✘ Use physical punishment on a child who lies. Research shows that constant hitting for lies only encourages children to lie more, because they are afraid of being hit again.

open attitudes

Children who grow up in a secure, loving home, able to discuss anything with their parents, are likely to become well-adjusted, responsible adults, but most will have a few worries along the way.

Answering children's awkward questions

Parents whose responses are shifty or furtive when faced with controversial questions not only make it difficult to raise subjects like race, sex, religion, or drugs within the family, but also encourage their children to be furtive themselves. Parents who are open, responsive and frank encourage self-esteem, balance, and fairness in their children and give them the space to think, weigh up options, make decisions, and act responsibly. This

healthy dialogue between parents and children has to begin early – from the very first question – and should continue throughout the time they are at home.

● Treat your child's questions seriously and always try to give the most accurate, truthful answer you can.

● Think about the point of questions. If a child asks what a ruler is, for example, he may want to know more than just the name. Explain what it is used for and try measuring something together.

● If you don't know an answer to a question, be truthful and say that you don't know but suggest that you look it up or ask someone else together.

● Don't shy away from giving truthful and accurate answers to children on difficult topics. Always answer questions on matters such as death and sex truthfully. But don't feel you have to give the whole truth. Supply as much as you feel your child can cope with and understand at that time.

Make her proud of her body

A child's sex education begins with the first cuddle. All children take pleasure in physical contact and joy in their parents' reciprocity. They grow up realizing that people touch one another as an act of friendship as well as an act of love.

As your child gets older she will become pleasantly aware of her body, without being at all self-conscious about it. **You can encourage this by having an open attitude to nudity within the family.** Like everything else, a child learns patterns of behavior and attitudes from you. The child who sees her parents unclothed and unembarrassed will take nudity as a matter of course and is unlikely to grow up concerned about nakedness. But if you are worried about it she will almost certainly worry too; if you're embarrassed she is likely to be too.

Childhood emotions

Your toddler's emotions develop very rapidly. She can feel guilt, shame, jealousy, and dislike, and be so upset that these emotions make her cry. Even in the most loved, secure child, fear, too, is quite near the surface and will provoke tears.

Dealing with fears

The most common childhood fears are of the dark and thunder. One of the best ways to dispel fears is to talk about them, so encourage your child to be open and frank about what frightens her. Give her your full attention and ask questions, so that she knows that you are taking her seriously. Very often fears are difficult to put into words, but hear your child out. Help her to explain by supplying a few examples and confess that you have similar fears too. Never scold or ridicule your child about her fears. Do something simple and reassuring, like demonstrating to your child that it is fun in the swimming pool and the water is nothing to fear. Your child will trust you and her fear will gradually diminish. When she's old enough, try to explain how things work: for instance, that lightning is just like a giant spark of light, like striking a match.

A new baby in the family

Your child is bound to feel pretty distressed at the thought of a new baby brother or sister and the "dethronement" that she thinks will follow. Take all the precautions you can to make her feel good about the baby. When you talk about the baby, refer to it as her new sister or brother, and let your child feel your tummy as the baby grows and kicks. Show her where the baby is going to sleep, and teach her all kinds of helpful things she can do to look after it. If you are having the baby in a hospital, make sure your child is at ease with the person who is going to take care of her while you're there. When you come home, have someone else carry the baby; you should have your arms free to scoop up your child and cuddle her. Don't turn to the new baby until she asks to see her. Make sure that you bring home a present from the baby for her. If you have to stay in the hospital, let her visit you as often as she likes and when she does, make sure that the baby is not in your arms but in a crib, so you're free to hold your child.

Over-tiredness

A child of this age very often becomes overexcited and overtired toward bedtime. She'll try to put off going to bed for as long as she possibly can and simply become more and more distressed. Your child might become so fragile that the slightest discomfort or frustration will make her cry inconsolably.

If you are expecting your child to have a late evening or a special treat such as a birthday party or a school play, make sure she has a nap during the day so that her energy will last. If she does become overexcited and overtired, it is especially important that you remain calm and quiet. Talk to her gently, cuddle her, be infinitely patient, and take her gently to her bedroom. Sing her a song or read her soothing story until she has become calm and quieted down, ready for sleep.

1-4

learning to talk

During these years your child's language will progress rapidly. She'll be able to talk to you and ask for what she wants and, equally important, understand what you are saying to her.

Talk to your child

If you want your teenager to feel free to talk to you about anything, then you have to set this up early in your child's life and talk about anything to him. **So talk endlessly to your toddler, and go on introducing new words and making your meaning clear with gestures and facial expressions.** It is just as important, however, that you give him space to respond so that he learns that conversation works two ways. If he initiates a conversation by showing you something or asking you a question, always make eye contact and give him your full attention. If you are impatient, or just respond with "that's nice" without even looking at him, he'll become discouraged and give up trying to talk to you.

Talk about everything you are doing in detail. When you are dressing him, give a running commentary: "now we'll do up your buttons… one, two, three." Describe objects you are using: "let's put the apples in the glass bowl." "Would you like a yellow candy or a red candy?"

While you shouldn't correct your child when he makes mistakes, there is no reason why you should talk to him in his own baby language. If he makes a mistake in grammar or pronunciation – "grandma goed" – just repeat his words giving the correct form: "Yes, grandma went home."

Developing language

Your toddler learns new words all the time and she starts to put them together, even if it's only two at a time, "teddy fall." Her pronunciation will be indistinct, but this is no cause for worry; if she is using words with meaning and putting them together, then her language is developing. Mild speech defects, such as lisping, are very common in children, and usually disappear without any intervention.

Language in girls
● Right from the moment of birth, girls are more responsive to the human voice than boys, and they have better verbal skills throughout childhood.
● Girls talk earlier than boys, and begin to string words into sentences earlier. They have better articulation, pronunciation, and grammar, and are better at verbal reasoning. They also learn to read earlier than boys.
● The structure of the female brain is believed to be the reason for girls' superior verbal skills: the speech centers are more tightly organized in the female brain than in the male brain and have more and better connections with other parts of the brain.

Language in boys
● Boys are almost always slower than girls at developing language skills and this discrepancy lasts right through childhood.
● Boys are later in talking than girls, are slower to put words together in sentences, and take longer to learn to read. Speech disorders such as stuttering are far more common in boys than in girls, and boys outnumber girls in remedial reading classes by four to one.
● Although this difference in linguistic ability levels out somewhat during the teenage years, you can help your son's language skills in the preschool years by reading aloud to him and playing a lot of word games.

Speech and language milestones

There is great variation in the speed at which children learn to talk, so don't feel the need to compare your child with others of his age and don't worry if his development doesn't match the timetable given here: I give these dates merely as average guidelines, and no child corresponds to the average.

12–18 months

● Your toddler's comprehension is miles ahead of his ability to express himself, e.g. "mama" can mean lots of things, including "mommy, give me a drink." When you discover what he means, say "mommy will get you a drink" and say the word "drink" again. Soon he'll say, "mommy, dink."
● Introduce your toddler to all kinds of noises, such as those made by animals, vehicles, and music. He is very switched on to sounds, so point them out: doors squeak, faucets drip, paper rustles.
● Read books as often as you can, going over and over favorite ones, repeating names and objects. Point to familiar objects. Give their names. Ask him to repeat the names. Show pleasure when he remembers.
● Name everything, everywhere. Name colors, textures, and other properties.
● Start counting and use numbers whenever the opportunity arises.

18 months–2 years

● Start to use adjectives whenever you can. The first are usually "good," "bad,"

"nice," "nasty," "hot," "cold," Couple them with nouns ("cold milk," "nice girl," "good teddy bear") especially when you are describing food, people, and toys – your toddler's favorite subjects.
● Use adverbs, too, such as "here" and "where." Emphasize all verbs and add actions to promote understanding.
● Prepositions are understood long before your toddler uses them, but always stress them and show what you mean. Always indicate where "under," "on top of," and "behind" are.

2–3 years

● Your child will talk more to children of his own age than to adults, so exposing him as often as possible to the company of other children will help develop his linguistic abilities. This is one of the reasons why preschool becomes important. At this age, speech ceases to be egocentric and becomes more social, so contact with other children is essential if your child is to develop social language.
● Repeat favorite stories, so that your child can figure out his feelings about the world around him.
● Read more complex stories and introduce new words, explaining them by using them over and over in your speech.

3–4 years

● Never overtly correct your child's mistakes; just repeat what he has just said, but correctly. If he hesitates over a

word, supply it instantly, to maintain his momentum and interest.
● Your child responds well to reasoning, so include him in simple problem-solving, with questions, options, and solutions – openly discussing each step. Ask his opinion about something you know you can agree with, so that he feels he has made a decision.
● Make sentences longer and more complex. When your child speaks to you, turn to him and listen attentively. Nod, and incline your head to show you are listening.
● Always answer questions. There is no need to tell the whole truth, just the amount that he can handle, but never lie or dissemble. Your child will find you out and distrust you. Your child will ask the same question over and over; just give the answer again, never become impatient.
● Children like whispering, so play whispering games to aid expression.
● In your child's list of reading include fairy tales, because they help your child to come to terms with his own world without it hurting him, and because they improve his concepts of real and unreal; past, present, and future; fairness and injustice; good and evil; kindness and brutality, and so on.
● Language acquisition is not smooth, it stops and starts, so follow your child's lead and don't push. Don't compare your child with anyone else; language is learned at different rates by different children.

a growing mind

Sharing your child's pleasure in new skills and achievements is one of the great joys of parenthood. Help your child by giving a lot of praise and encouragement.

Television

Some parents see television as a built-in baby-sitter because it keeps children amused when there is no one who wants to watch them. For quite a lot of children, television is more popular and consumes more of their playtime than all other play activities put together.

Television is at its least useful when a child is left to watch alone. Even if she's watching a highly educational program she'll get less out of it if she watches it in an entirely passive way. If she watches it with other children who comment on it, or with an adult who asks questions and makes observations, the program acts as a springboard for ideas and discussion rather than one-way, non-participatory communication.

Television prevents your child from:

- scanning, sifting, and analyzing information and then applying it to everyday situations
- practicing motor skills
- using more than two senses at a time to expand the appreciation of her environment
- asking questions and receiving helpful educational answers
- exploring and using her curiosity
- exercising initiative or motivation
- being challenged and solving problems
- thinking analytically
- using her imagination
- having conversations with the rest of the family and improving verbal skills
- writing and reading
- being either creative or constructive
- developing the ability to concentrate for long periods because of the flicker of the television screen
- developing logical, sequential thinking because the action in programs constantly shifts backward, forward and laterally in time.

Mental development milestones

Many brain and body skills advance on a tide of growth and expansion as general understanding increases. The determining factors are your child's sociability and personality, and the environment you create for him.

15 months

Let him help you as much as he can with simple tasks like tidying up that are well within his abilities and encourage feelings of pride. Get him to point to parts of his body, make animal sounds and help take off his clothes – he loves it. He understands the concept of "cattiness" – he knows that a picture of a cat, a toy cat, and a real cat are all cats, even though very different, so keep pointing out to him the defining features of things.

18 months

Use repetition for learning. Whenever you do something, repeat certain key phrases over and over. "Jack has an apple. Yes, Jack has an apple." Help him recognize a few items on a page and ask him to point to them if you say their names. Give him a few chores – he's dying to try and will try to imitate your actions. He'll carry out a request that requires assessment and memory: "go and bring me your teddy bear."

21 months

Describe the character of things. When showing something to your child, point out whether it is hard or soft, its color, if it makes a noise, and so on. Introduce opposites such as rough and smooth. Encourage him to ask for food, drink, toys, and about going to the potty. He's beginning to understand more complicated requests: "please get your hairbrush from the bathroom." He may grab your arm or use other gestures to get your attention.

2 years

Stimulate his spatial sense by helping place the various cubes, rectangles, and squares into their correct receptacles in a shape-sorting toy or box. Use names all the time to stimulate a rapidly increasing vocabulary of names and objects and so that he can describe the properties of familiar items and identify them. Give him complicated orders, and ask him to find an object played with previously to encourage a good memory. Stimulate him to talk nonstop by answering his questions and asking him questions too.

2½ years

Play a lot of number games. Incorporate numbers into everything you do. Count items when you shop, get dressed, or say what you have to do. A toy farmyard is a good toy at this age – use it to count cows, sheep, pigs, and chickens. He's starting to add detail to broad concepts – a horse has a long tail – and he knows one or two nursery rhymes, so ask him to find them in his book. He's starting to ask "why" and says "no," "won't," "can't" in answer to everything.

3–4 years

Add to his sense of self. Encourage independence and self-reliance by involving your child in simple decisions: ask him to choose his clothes and food. Your child asks questions incessantly – "what?", "where?", "how?", "why?" Always answer them. Encourage a good memory by referring to the past and reminding him what you did the day before. He knows his own gender now so point out differences with girls.

Books and reading

If I had to choose a single way in which a parent could enrich their children's environment and help them to develop well, I would suggest having books in the house. If you enjoy reading, make it obvious and talk about it, your child will too. Words are crucial to the way our brains function: reading is therefore very important and there is a correlation between how many books you have in the house and how much your child will read as he grows up and later in life.

Books are one of the great pleasures of life and are vital in providing your child with the words to express feelings, ideas, and thoughts. Moreover, books can help to explain the world he lives in – describing relationships, depicting situations, and introducing personalities.

Books provide the impetus for imaginative play, they introduce ideas, and they are fun. In our house, books were given to the children as soon as they were born, and reading was a shared experience up to the age of 10.

Bad dreams and nightmares

Nightmares Three- and four-year-olds very often have bad dreams. Your child may walk or talk in her sleep, or have night terrors. They're normal because while her understanding of the world is growing, she cannot make sense of it, and so she goes to sleep with unresolved questions. She's also getting more in touch with her feelings and she knows what it is to be afraid or feel something is not quite right. These feelings come out at night.

Often a child cannot explain her dreams and has difficulty in going back to sleep. Animals, especially wolves and bears, may chase your child during a nightmare, or she may dream of strange, bad, or odd-looking people, fires, and deep water. Only if your child wakes up should you try to console her and take her in your arms. If she remains asleep, don't do anything to wake her; simply stay by her. If you find that she is sleepwalking periodically, put a gate across the stairs to prevent falls.

Night terrors Sometimes you will find your child in bed, apparently awake, terrified, and possibly thrashing around and screaming. She may be angry or desperately upset. This is a night terror rather than a nightmare, and it can be very alarming. You will feel quite anguished at your child's fear and pain, but all you can do is stay close and wait for the terror to pass. There is no point in trying to reassure your child specifically, because she is beyond reason. Don't leave or scold her; that would simply make the terror worse. She won't remember anything in the morning.

learning by play

Play is crucial to your preschool child's development. Once she has practiced her creative talents during play, she can apply them to the real world.

Parent as teacher

A child starts to absorb information from the moment she is born, and it is from her parents that she gets most of this information. A parent is responsible for encouraging a child's imagination and teaching helpfulness and self control, among other things, and there are simple ways to approach all these lessons.

Set appropriate goals

Never pursue perfection since this will lead to frustration and you will end up with an unhappy, demoralized child who simply cannot thrive and develop well. Never fall into the trap of expecting too much too soon, but be aware of the small successes that your child achieves every day. Try not to focus on deficiencies; concentrate instead on noticing and praising every single positive act or achievement.

Always join in

One of the jobs of being a teacher to your child is that you actually have to DO THINGS. Your child learns through example and imitation until she is over eight years old, so get up and do something in front of her or with her. This means that you do not rely on just giving your child orders or directions. Instead of telling her to "go and tidy up your toys," you need to get down on your knees with her,

and make a game of tidying up the toys together.

Repeat, repeat, repeat

With all children, but especially young children, it is frustrating but necessary to tell them over and over again to do the same thing. For example, a young child will not sit calmly while she is eating lunch or waiting for anything. So you may have to repeat certain messages like "we don't swing our legs and kick the chair while we are eating" for months

Know when to forbid

I found only three situations in which it was absolutely necessary to say "no" to a child:

● When my child might harm himself; for instance, reaching for a pot on the stove.

● When my child's actions could have been harmful to others; for example, something as simple as playing noisily or banging toys near a sleeping baby.

● When my child's action would result in real damage; for example, trying to use crayons on the living room wall. Even when you say "no" it does not have to be a head-on confrontation. The best way to do it is to distract your child with something interesting.

and months until your child's body gets the message as well as her mind.

Give positive examples

Remember, whenever possible, to state something in a positive way. Say, "yes that is a nice little dog; let's pat the dog" and show your child how to do it. Don't shriek, "don't hurt the little puppy." Sentences that begin with "do not" communicate displeasure from the moment you start to speak. An infant's brain does not necessarily process every word, so in the case above, your message may come out as "… hurt … puppy!" – your opposite intention.

Don't interrupt

A lot of children have difficulty with concentration span, and it is hard to foster because a small child simply cannot concentrate as well as an adult. One of the major things you can do to help your child sustain attention is not to interrupt when she is clearly absorbed in something.

Give attention

A child only feels that she is being listened to if you make eye contact and stop what you are doing in order to listen. If you do this from a very early age, your child will know that she has a voice, and that you respect her as an individual.

Drawing can help him understand his ...

...Emotions You can help your child to become in touch with his feelings and to recognize emotions in others by getting him to draw happy faces and sad faces, first with a guiding hand from you. Then move your child on to looking at photos of people he knows and deciding how they are feeling in the picture. This not only helps your child to recognize emotions but to empathize, and to relate closely to them. Later, you can show your child pictures in newspapers and magazines. When your child is a little older, you can draw stick figures and ask what the various postures mean in terms of feelings. Then get your child to draw stick figures and to express the various emotions that they feel.

...World You can also use drawings to expand your child's view of the world. A very simple idea would be what happens when you spill water. You and your child could do a drawing of knocking over a pitcher of water and it spilling onto the floor and making a puddle, perhaps running off the edge of the table onto the floor in big drops and splashes. This kind of exercise reinforces your child's memory and provides him with his own experience.

Whenever you are telling or writing a story, or when your child is old enough to do either of these things, always ask if there is any part of the story that could be illustrated. At first, help your child draw some kind of picture, so that he can visualize what is in his imagination and express it in pictures, not only words, then ask him to do one by himself.

Even in conversation you can introduce the idea of mind pictures and get your child to describe the picture in his mind's eye in words, not just in drawings.

Ideas for play

Sometimes your child will be absorbed in a make-believe world of her own and won't need your involvement. At other times you can add to her enjoyment by suggesting new games, or new ways to play with her toys.

Make-believe play Your child will create a little world of her own as part of her imitation of adults. An instant tent or playhouse can be made from a couple of chairs or a small table draped with a blanket. Children love playing with cardboard boxes as long as they are big enough to climb into. Small ones become boats and cars; piles of them turn into castles and houses. Dressing up is a favorite game at this age: a few simple props can transform your child into a doctor or firefighter and, in her fantasy world, she is the adult, and a teddy bear or doll serves as a child.

Messy play Any play involving water, sand, mud, or dough will stretch your child's intellect. To make your supervision easier, set aside a time when messy play is allowed and a place where the mess can be contained, and encourage your child to look forward to it.

Domestic play Helping you around the house is play rather than work because she's so eager to copy you. She helps in the kitchen by tearing salad leaves or arranging bread on a plate, and will enjoy setting the table, so improving manipulative and counting skills as well as independence and self-worth.

Musical play All children are born with perfect pitch so any child with normal hearing adores musical sounds. She probably won't be able to play melodies, but she may be able to hum them and will enjoy banging out a rhythm. Rattles, wooden clappers, trumpets, and drums are all very good for this purpose, as are old pans or baking dishes and wooden spoons. A xylophone will enable her to identify musical sounds and experiment with high and low notes.

"a child needs self-belief
if she is to fulfil her potential"

life stages: 4 to 11 years

Between the ages of 4 and 11 your energetic, loving, mischievous preschooler is going to grow and develop into a reflective, kind, industrious, cooperative adolescent with whom you can have a serious conversation, on whom you can rely, and whose company everyone enjoys. That's a tough assignment for any 4-year-old and there are many complex skills to acquire along the way, not the least of which are self-control and self-discipline.

Most important, milestones can only be achieved if parents show loving care to their children. Children can't survive let alone thrive without close parental interest. They can get by of course and most do, even if parental care isn't forthcoming.

Achieving self-belief

But there are some milestones that are exceedingly difficult for a child to master alone and they can go astray without feedback and guidance. Let me give you just one example of a milestone that involves an important step in personal development – achieving **self-belief**.

Call it self-confidence, call it self-assurance, but without it a child will not only fail to fulfill her potential, she could get into all kinds of trouble because she won't know how to control her emotions or how to rechannel her frustrations and anger to gainful purpose.

You may think, well, she'll grow into a shy child, unsure of herself. That would be bad enough, but you're wrong, it's worse than that.
● She grows into a child who becomes a loner without friends, which is heartbreaking for any parent to see.
● She may seek attention and affection to bolster her waning ego with all kinds of inappropriate behavior, sometimes being labeled **hyperactive**.
● And then, if no one helps her to build belief in herself, she resorts to lying, stealing, bullying, even to drinking and taking drugs to feel good about herself.

You can see that without achieving **self-belief**, there are problems ahead. So important is this

milestone, and several other crucial milestones, that I call them **islands of development**. If a child doesn't reach the haven of these islands, there can be disastrous fallout later.

Think of your child as bobbing along on a river of development trying to negotiate the equivalent of white water, the flow sometimes fast as she goes through a spurt of skill acquisition, or slower and more placid as she consolidates her achievements.

These islands make the river navigable. They're places where your child can rest up, so to speak, take stock and move on to the next milestone – with a lot of encouragement and praise from you of course.

The islands are also an insurance policy. If you can help your child to reach one she'll tackle the next stretch of white water with determination, courage, and good sense. And, having enjoyed the security of reaching one of these islands, your child can safely be given responsibilities of increasing gravitas both for herself and others.

In the pages that follow, I offer guidelines where appropriate, advice where I feel there may be a need, and strategies for dealing with difficult situations.

The right age to…

● A child is ready to learn to tie her own shoelaces at about 4 years old.

● A child may be able to cope with moving into a real bed at about 5 years old.

● A 6-year-old is probably ready to receive pocket money and decide how to spend it.

● At 7 a child can learn to cross the street alone.

● A child of 8 can sleep over at a friend's house.

● A 9-year-old is ready to learn about puberty.

● A child of 10 may enjoy the responsibility of caring for a pet.

● An 11-year-old can be left at home alone for short periods.

Social

> "children can't survive, let alone thrive, without close parental interest"

Mind

"encourage physical activity in your child as early as possible"

tell your children the facts of life as soon as they begin to ask

feeding children

The best way to make sure that your children eat a healthy, balanced diet for the rest of their lives is to help them develop good habits from the beginning.

Happy mealtimes

do

✔ Make mealtimes an important family ritual so your child can learn how to be part of a group.

✔ Set up some basic ground rules for meals so that everyone knows they can't throw tantrums or just grab and run.

✔ Have meals at regular times so that you set up a rhythm for family life – children love this.

✔ Encourage thoughtfulness for others – never take the last portion without offering it to everyone else.

✔ Foster chat and discussion and make sure each child is listened to, including the youngest.

✔ Trivialize accidents and spillage so that the conviviality isn't broken.

don't

✗ Let meals become battlegrounds. You can't force a child to eat. Let them refuse food, they'll ask for it soon enough if you don't insist.

✗ Let a child spoil family calm and harmony at the table for everyone else; remove them to another room.

✗ Exclude children from your conversation – they become naughty to attract your attention.

✗ Let meals tail off without a formal ending. Each child should say they've had enough and ask to go and play.

✗ Let the youngest be last to get her food. Give it to her first – her patience is shortest.

✗ Have the television on or music playing during meals.

Veggie foods

It's quite safe for a child to be a vegetarian from the age of eating solid food, but think about the following points.

● Their diet should contain dairy products and eggs and be carefully planned to contain all essential ingredients.

● With supplements, and ingenuity on the parents' part, even a vegan diet excluding dairy, eggs, and meat can be okay.

● Children put on a vegan diet tend to be smaller and lighter than average. While their height does "catch up," vegan children usually remain lighter and leaner.

● The slow growth is because a typical vegetarian diet contains fewer of the high-energy foods needed for growth.

● Children need high-energy foods for growth and play so nut products, cheese, and avocado are useful. Vegetarian children should be given whole milk to provide crucial calories. Go easy on bulky foods such as a lot of fruit and vegetables and high-fiber cereals, which reduce absorption of iron and zinc.

● Variety is key. All four food groups should be included in these daily ratios. Cereals and grains: 4–5 servings; fruit: 1–3 servings; vegetables: 2 servings; legumes, nuts, and seeds: 1–2 servings; animal protein (milk, cheese, and eggs): 3 servings.

● Vegetarian children should have some vegetable oil/butter/yeast extract.

● Good sources of vegetable protein are nuts, legumes, tofu, and soy in any form. Milk and dairy products and eggs are "complete" proteins.

● To keep up intake of calcium, iron, and vitamin C, children need to eat plenty of fortified foods – for example, breakfast cereals and whole grain bread – diced fruit, dark green vegetables, and dairy.

● Vitamin C promotes iron absorption so food containing these nutrients should be eaten together.

Junk foods

■ **How many times a week does your family eat fast food?**
Rarely (0)   Once (2)
Twice (3)   More (4)

■ **Do you serve french fries with food?**
Never (0)   Occasionally (1)
Frequently (3)   Very frequently (5)

■ **Do you give in if your child whines for a Big Mac?**
Never (0)   Sometimes (1)
Often (3)   Always (4)

■ **How often do you use junk food as a bribe?**
Never (0)   Now and then (2)
Quite often (5)   All the time (7)

■ **Do you put hamburgers and fish sticks on your weekly shopping list?**
Never (0)   Once a month (1)
Every two weeks (3)   Every week (5)

■ **Do you have sweet carbonated drinks in the fridge?**
Never (0)   Sometimes (1)
Often (3)   All the time (5)

■ **Do you finish off meals with a sweet dessert, e.g. ice cream?**
Never (0)   Now and then (1)
Every day (5)   Every meal (7)

■ **Is there ketchup on the table?**
Never (0)   Occasionally (1)
Often (2)   Always (3)

■ **How often does your family eat take-out?**
Never (–5)   Now and then (1)
Weekly (2)
More than once a week (4)

■ **Do you serve much fried food?**
Never (0)   Sometimes (1)
Often (5)   Very frequently (7)

Now add up your score.
Up to 15: Okay – your family's diet slips occasionally but is generally good.
Up to 25: Too much – the junk food level is creeping up. Try to cut it down.
More than 35: STOP! Your family is eating far too much junk food and it will damage their health.

Candy

I don't believe in giving candy freely nor in placing a total ban on candy – that only encourages children to be secretive and dishonest. What I do believe in is rationing candy, and this always worked with my own children. If you let your child have a little candy after a meal and encourage him to brush his teeth afterward, you'll be helping him develop good eating habits, self-control, and good oral hygiene. Candy might seem like an appropriate reward for children and it is, but not all the time. There is no hard and fast rule on this, and no reason why you shouldn't occasionally reward your child with candy as long as you make it clear that this is a one-time treat. It's worth making an effort, though, to devise other forms of reward, such as a favorite yogurt flavor or a small toy.

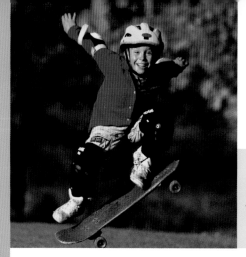

active children

Healthy, happy children have boundless energy. Encourage their adventurousness and allow them to be independent.

Importance of physical activity

There is a great deal of medical evidence to show that physical activity in children favorably affects efficient action of the muscles and the heart and lungs, a tendency to leanness rather than to fatness, and the strength and growth of bones. Since the benefits of physical activity depend on its intensity and duration, it follows that children who play hard and exercise hard are likely to be healthier adults. Active children are generally leaner and show greater physical capacity at all ages than their less active contemporaries.

Just how much exercise is necessary during the growing years is not known and individual variation is great, but it is a good idea to encourage physical activity in your child as early as possible. Promote taking up hobbies and sporting activities that involve strenuous exercise and do not be overprotective, preventing your child from being physically active and adventurous. The more the whole family can join in, the better – and it won't do couch potato parents any harm either.

A sedentary child is nearly always a fat child and a fat child is in danger of developing diabetes, simply as a result of being overweight. Obese children are also in danger of developing conditions of "old age," like heart disease, in their 20s. Another persuasive reason for encouraging your child to be active.

Healthy feet

Children are born with soft, pliable feet. As their feet grow, the toe bones are the last to harden so they are easily bent out of shape. Let small children go barefoot around the house so that toes have room to move.

When you buy shoes for your child it is important to have his feet properly measured for width and length by a trained fitter, so go to a shop that specializes in children's shoes. There should be plenty of room for the child's toes in the front of the shoe when he is standing up: half your thumbnail between the top of the shoe and his toes is a rough guide. Choose shoes with an adjustable strap across the instep and with supple uppers which give support but bend easily during walking. Remember that your child's feet will probably increase by at least two sizes a year until he is 6 or so, so keep an eye on how his toes are growing.

Teeth

The first of your child's 32 permanent teeth will probably come in around the age of 5½. These are the first molars, one on each side at the back of the upper and lower jaw. They appear before any of the baby teeth are lost. Around the same time come the incisors, the sharp teeth at the front of the mouth, which we use for cutting food. After that come the premolars or bicuspids, the square back teeth we use for gripping or tearing food.

Your child will usually have her new set of permanent teeth by about 12 or 14 years of age, with the wisdom teeth coming through several years later. There is no difference between the time teeth come through on the right and left sides of the mouth but there is a marked difference between boys and girls: every tooth appears earlier in girls, by two months for the first molars and as much as 11 months for the canines. Do not worry if your child's teeth seem to be slow in coming through. The timetable for dental development varies from child to child, just as the timetables for height and weight vary.

Brushing teeth

Until your child is about 8, you will probably have to help her to brush her teeth efficiently. Some children can manage earlier than this, but you will need to keep a check on how well they are brushing their teeth until you are sure they can be trusted to do it properly.

Adventurousness

Encouraging your child to be adventurous has countless pay offs, not least that you'll help her to push herself to the limit and develop her full potential. It's the quickest way to self-confidence.

● Good parents separate their fears from their children's. Her own fears are sufficient to make her sensible and circumspect. Your fears cripple her curiosity and spirit.

● Overprotective parents don't allow their children to test their abilities, master new skills, and move on to new feats. They hold children back so that they lack the coordination and confidence that gives them pride and trust in their own bodies and their own abilities.

● By the age of four your child has a clear sense of self and her abilities and can experiment to find out what's feasible and safe on her own without danger. Play equipment such as a jungle gym allows such experiments, and research shows that children, left to their own devices, rarely overstep the limits.

● Your child has boundless energy and can tackle demanding activities like climbing, pedaling, and skating. Your role is to provide the tools within sight of the house for easy supervision.

● If necessary, guide her through the most difficult tasks or add training wheels to her bike, but don't stop her. This way you'll lay the foundations for a lifetime of enjoyment and give her the desire to further her skills and the confidence to venture into the unknown. And you'll help her to become a well-balanced, confident person.

Encourage girls to be adventurous

● Never fuss about her getting dirty.
● Encourage games with energetic movements.
● Think of her as a boy; encourage all "boy's" games – climbing, swinging, balancing, kicking a ball.
● Get her physical toys like a bike early rather than late.

Encourage boys to be adventurous:

● Start physical games on large soft floor cushions early.
● Introduce "spatial" toys like Legos early to stimulate adventurous thinking.
● Help his imagination by giving him items like toilet paper tubes and old egg cartons to make anything he can think of.
● Provide him with physical apparatus – rope ladder, swing, bike, skates, ball.

growing up

Children in this age group grow fast. Parents should make sure that their children are prepared for the changes in their bodies and what they mean.

Guiding principles

There are certain well-established guiding principles about the growth and development of children which are useful for parents to keep in mind:

● Each child is an individual. His growth and development will be different from other children and will differ at different times of his life. These variations are partly due to the tendencies he inherits from his family and partly to the environment in which he is brought up – for example, how well nourished he is. Parents should never expect the same growth and development, or behavior for that matter, in each of their children.

● A child's happiness varies and this can affect development. Happy children are normally healthy and energetic, whereas unhappiness tends to sap strength and energy and reduce well-being. Happy children use their energy purposefully, while unhappy children tend to dissipate their energy in brooding and self-pity.

● There is no point in parents trying to plot their child's size and weight on a complicated graph to see if he is "correct" for his age. Averages in the physical growth of children mean very little in relation to your child. The most important index of your child's normal development is his health and happiness, rather than his size.

Height

In the first year after birth children increase their length by about half. During the third, fourth, and fifth years height gain falls off but is relatively steady at about 2½–3in (6–8cm) per year. Between then and the growth spurt at about 11 years in girls and 13 years in boys, weight remains fairly constant with a height gain of about ½in (1cm) per year.

Weight

During the second and third years of life a child gains from 3-5lb (1.4–2.3kg) a year. After this, weight gain tends to slow down. During the third, fourth, and fifth years weight gain is fairly steady at about 4½lb (2kg) a year. In addition, most children become relatively lean in comparison with their early body shape.

The early school years are a period of relatively slow but steady gain in weight, on average about 7lb (3.2kg) a year. By the time a child is five years old he typically weighs about five times his birth weight and by adolescence he is between 80 and 90lb (36 and 40kg).

Toward sexual maturity

The age for the onset of puberty varies but is quite often around 10 or 11 for girls and around 12 years for boys. Besides growing faster, children will notice changes in their bodies. For a girl, this begins with the dark area around the nipple (the areola) growing larger or puffing up slightly. Then the breasts begin to develop, becoming slightly conical in shape at first, then rounding out as her menstrual periods start.

For a boy, puberty means that, besides growing taller, his penis and

testicles enlarge and pubic hair begins to grow. Later his voice will crack and deepen. Though puberty comes later in boys than girls, in some early developers it can begin as early as 10 years of age.

An explanation before the event of what will happen, in a calm and reassuring manner, is the best way of preparing your son and daughter. If a girl's first period comes without warning it can be a frightening experience, particularly as at this stage the discharge will not be bright red, as

she might expect, but brownish black. Girls are menstruating, on average, nine months earlier than their mothers did. An increasing number of girls begin their period at 10 or 11, which may be before they begin middle school. And 1 in 6 girls now begins her periods at 8 years old, and 1 in 14 boys of 8 years old has pubic hair. For the first time, we have 8-year-old children who are sexually aware. They must have good sex education, and parents are the adults who must give it.

Menstruation

Periods start because hormones from a gland in the brain (the pituitary gland) tell the ovaries to manufacture the female sex hormones, estrogen and progesterone. The ovaries begin producing a monthly egg and you begin to menstruate (have periods). Although 12 is the average age for periods to begin, anything between 8 and 16 is normal.

The start of menstruation is called menarche. Even before your first period you may be fertile, which means that you can get pregnant if you have unprotected sex. Menstruation ends at menopause, when you're about 50 years old. Some pain during a period is common but if you have very painful periods, see your doctor.

Calculated from the first day of bleeding, the cycle is about 28 days.

Hormones make the ovaries produce an egg, and the lining of the womb grows. The egg travels to the womb through the fallopian tubes. If the egg isn't fertilized, it is shed with the womb lining.

Days 1–5 Menstruation: the lining of the womb is shed and flows out through the vagina.

Days 1–12 Pituitary hormones stimulate growth of an egg follicle; estrogen from the ovaries causes womb lining to thicken.

Days 12–16 Ovulation: an egg is released. Ovary starts to produce progesterone.

Days 17–24 Egg travels along the fallopian tube to womb.

Days 24–28 If conception does not occur, your ovary stops producing progesterone, triggering menstruation.

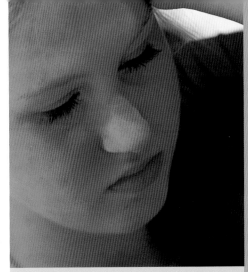

Coping with periods

Your choice of pads and tampons

Ordinary pad Bulky pad that fits inside underwear, usually with self-stick panel.

Shaped pad Fits inside underwear. Held in place by self-stick panel.

Pad with wings Self-stick "wings" anchor the pad more securely within underwear.

Panty liner For light bleeding. Has self-stick panel.

Tampon Small, convenient, but requires manual insertion.

Tampon with applicator Applicator pushes tampon into vagina.

How pads and tampons work

Ordinary pad Worn externally inside the the underwear.

Tampon Worn internally in the vagina. String through vaginal opening allows removal.

Sanitary hygiene during your period

● Change a pad or tampon 3–4 times a day.

● Wash your hands before and after changing pads and tampons.

● Wash your vulva daily from front to back, using baby soap and water. Don't use talc or deodorants.

● To minimize risk of infection, don't use tampons overnight. Use a pad.

● There is a very rare infection called toxic shock syndrome (TSS), which is thought to be linked with using tampons. To avoid this, always use the least absorbent type of tampon to meet your needs and never leave a tampon in for longer than eight hours.

gaining confidence

More than anything, children need caring, interested parents who will help them learn to make their way in the world and build self-confidence.

Vacations away from home

Your child can gain a good deal of confidence and independence from being away from home, helping with the chores, and taking responsibility for keeping his own things neat and tidy. For many children, their first experience of going away with people their own age, instead of their parents, is a short camping trip with the Boy or Girl Scouts. The cost is quite low and the camp leaders are trained and experienced in taking care of children. Any early homesickness usually disappears as soon as the fun starts, but only you can judge whether your child is ready, at the age of nine or so, to take the step toward independence. It is probably best to be guided by the child's enthusiasm; don't push him into it because you think it will do him good.

Camps often have open days for parents, when it is important to go along if you possibly can. A child can feel let down and isolated if all the other parents are there and his are not.

Pocket money

The ability to manage money is not something that comes naturally, it has to be learned. Most of us have less money than we need, or would like, so we are always having to choose between different kinds of spending. For a child, pocket money is the first chance to learn how to manage money.

● For children under six, give a small amount to spend when you are out shopping together, so that she gets used to handling money and realizes that she can choose between buying herself a lollipop or a comic book.

● When you are deciding on the amount of her weekly allowance, ask other parents to get an idea of the going rate so your child has about the same as her friends.

● By the time she is seven or so, sit down with your child and draw up a "balance sheet," so that you can figure out how much she will need and she will know what her pocket money is supposed to cover: for example, is she only expected to buy candy and ice cream or does it also cover her Girl Scout dues and her bus fares?

● Encourage your child to put something in her piggybank each week to save up for special extras or vacation money.

● When relatives who are visiting hand out cash presents, it is reasonable to allow the child to spend them as she wants, as a treat. If large sums are involved, then she could spend some and have the rest put into a savings account in her name.

● Most children enjoy earning a little extra for jobs around the house. This does not mean that they should be paid any time they lend a hand, or they could soon become mercenary, but if they undertake a real job – like cleaning the inside of the car – then small payments can be put toward something they really want.

Self-confidence

A child is not born with a sense of "self-awareness." He develops it gradually through his dealings with other people – parents, brothers and sisters, friends, and teachers. His self-image is moulded by the way they see him and the way he wants them to see him. If his immediate circle of family and friends is a happy, relaxed, and outgoing one, which loves and accepts him as he is, he will have a good self-image, adjust well to the world around him, develop his independence, and get along well with others. If, however, they are always tense and critical, so that he feels he is constantly letting them down, he will have a poor view of himself, be anxious and defensive, and find it far more difficult to form relationships.

As he grows he has to master all sorts of skills, from getting dressed and learning to read to social skills, the making of friends, and talking easily with members of the opposite sex. He needs sufficient confidence to know that he can cope. If he has never developed that confidence, he may feel inferior and inadequate. The more inadequate he feels, the more likely he is to fail.

If your child sees that you notice and care when he makes the effort to master a new skill, or when he tries hard with his schoolwork, he will want to step up his efforts. Make sure you encourage any progress he makes, even if he happens to be slower at learning to read than your friends' children or has difficulty keeping up with the rest of his class. You can easily destroy a child's confidence if you only seem to notice when he makes mistakes or does badly and go on nagging or criticizing about it. Of course, you are only trying to spur him on, but it doesn't look like that from his angle.

Parental interest is vital in helping a child develop his abilities to the full – providing it is not too intense or demanding. Then it can do more harm than good. If parents have unrealistically high expectations, so that the child can never quite meet them, his self-esteem will suffer. Then he may opt out and stop trying altogether. A confident child may be spurred on to try harder by a failure. A child who already feared he was "no good" may see the failure as confirming his worst fears and simply give up. There are children who never reach their full potential because they are so afraid of failing that they avoid any situation where they might be tested.

Road safety

It is never too early to start a road safety drill. Every time you are out with your child, holding her hand so that you stay close together, give a running commentary on what you see, so she learns to judge the speed of an oncoming car, knows that she should never run across the road but always walk at a steady pace, and so on. Children under the age of 6 should never be allowed on the road alone, and children between the ages of 6 and 10 are not mature enough to be completely safe on the road. Once your child is old enough to be out on her own, teach her several unbreakable rules:

● Never dart into the road after a ball or a pet.
● Never walk or play along the curb, particularly near a blind corner.
● Stop, look, and listen for traffic before crossing a road, or even crossing a gateway whose opening may be obscured by walls.
● Never cross the road between parked cars if you can avoid it.
● Whenever you have to cross the road, choose a place where you have a good view of the traffic in both directions. Always use a marked crossing if you can.
● Treat a marked crossing as if it were not there – approach the curb, stop, look, and listen. Always walk across, never run.

4–11

learning to live with others

Parents have the daunting task of turning infants into sensible, social children and eventually into responsible, loving adults who relate well to others.

Knowing where to draw the line

At some time, most parents are filled with doubt about when and how to discipline their children. Naturally they want to strike a balance between constantly nagging them and being too lax. We all like to think of ourselves as positive encouragers, not punishing dictators. The last thing we want is for our children to fear us and we'll do anything to keep channels of communication open. However, day in, day out, there are times when we don't know quite where to draw the line.

The goal of teaching children discipline should be to help them exercise self-discipline. It isn't about exerting control over them or pulling rank. Most harm is done by being too rigid. A classic study from Berkeley in California examined three disciplinary styles and how they affected kids.
● Authoritarian parents (controlling, cold, and detached) had children who were

discontented, withdrawn, and distrustful.
● Permissive parents (warm but non-demanding) at the other end of the spectrum, had the least self-reliant, inquisitive, and self-controlled children.
● Authoritative parents (setting firm limits but warm, rational, and receptive), however, were the most likely to have self-reliant, self-controlled, and contented children.

Strike a balance
Your child begs to stay up past her bedtime to watch television. What's your response?
● Too hard: "Bed! Now! Or I'll ban television for a month."
● Too soft: "Oh, all right, but just this once."
● About right: "Come on now. You know the rules. You can watch television late Friday and Saturday nights only."

Your child wants to wear tattered jeans to her grandmother's birthday party.
● Too hard: "Put on your best pants. That's final!"
● Too soft: "Well, all right, but put on a nice sweater."
● About right: "I don't want to upset grandma and you should look nice for her. I'll help you choose some nice clothes if you want."

As a parent, I wanted to keep rules for my children to a minimum, but those that were important weren't negotiable. For instance:
● activities that were dangerous to my children or others were banned
● respect for, and kindness to, others were the order of the day
● cruelty in life and on television had no place in our family
● the truth would always be rewarded (no matter what was confessed).

Children and the too-friendly stranger

When children are out alone, it is possible that they will meet an undesirable stranger and, because most children are trusting, they may put themselves in danger. It is every parent's duty to inform their children of the risks of being out in public places. There is no need for this explanation to be alarming, but all children should be on the alert for friendly strangers who talk to them, offer them candy or a treat, or a ride in their car when they are in

parks or in playgrounds, on playing fields, in public bathrooms, or even walking down the street.

It is always better to be as honest as you can with children, and your warning words in this instance may be lifesaving. Be perfectly frank and tell your children that adults who are mentally sick may do more than just try to speak to them, but may touch them, invite them to look at pictures, try to undress them, or handle their

genitals. These adults may also undress or touch themselves.

Be very clear in giving instructions about what your child must do if this ever happens. The priority is to get help. They should not worry about where they get it from – they should go into a store, stop a passer-by, or knock on someone's door. Also warn your child that he should never go off to play with another child without asking your permission first.

Being considerate

Good manners and consideration for others – saying "please" and "thank you," offering a helping hand, giving a seat to an elderly or infirm person, waiting our turn in line – are the outward signs that we feel that other people and their rights matter. The actions themselves may be trivial but what they show about our concern for others, whether they are friends or strangers, is very important. Without a generally accepted code of manners, life would become thoroughly brutish and unpleasant, so parents need to pass them on to their children.

The best way to teach your child good manners is by consistent example. If you see a mother yelling at her child: "hey you – get in here!" you won't be surprised to find the child has obnoxious manners. A father who elbows his way to the front of the line, dragging his young son behind him, is likely to produce the sort of child who pushes others out of the way to grab the best piece of cake for himself.

If you treat other people, including your child, with consideration, you will need very little in the way of formal manners teaching. Of course, you will have to prompt, remind, and explain occasionally. A child starts off as a self-centered little being and he does not naturally think of the other person. As he gets older and identifies with you, he will want to copy your style of behavior and if you are considerate to others, so will he be.

Changing patterns of friendship

Friendship patterns change dramatically with age and the factors which govern friendship in young children are quite different from those which apply among teenagers or adults.

The relationships of preschool children are normally friendly and cooperative rather than hostile or competitive, even among the most aggressive youngsters. They tend to have a number of friends, none favored over the others. Don't worry too much if your child is not very popular at this stage. Friendships among this age group are casual and unstable, here today gone tomorrow, so they are not likely to have important or lasting effects on the child's personality.

Studies of preschool children show that it is the girls who seek to make friendships, spending more of their time playing with friends, while boys prefer some sort of physical activity like running and chasing.

Once they are established at school, around the age of 5 or 6, individual friendships are more likely to develop and they attach themselves to a few special pals. They choose friends of the same age, perhaps the child who sits next to them in class or at meals or is in their group when they take turns at playing in a playhouse. It is unusual for a child of this age to be playing alone most of the time.

Sex differences seem unimportant in small children's play but by the age of 8 or 9, they are playing in single-sex groups. Boys of 9 to 13 probably belong to a group, though they may have one particular friend in the group. Girls usually have a best friend – though not always the same best friend – and if they belong to a group or "club" it is less tightly knit and less important to them. Both boys and girls are now forming friendships on the basis of interests rather than proximity.

Children's temperaments vary and so do their social needs. You may have one child who sticks to the same close friend for years and takes little interest in other children – another who has such a wide and changing circle of friends that you can hardly remember their names. As long as your child is content with the way things are, there is no reason for you to interfere.

4-11 sensitive issues

At some stage in nearly every child's life, problems and questions arise that need careful handling from parents.

Bullying

Bullying is one of the most insidious problems within schools – and it can exist in any school, no matter what the system or age of the children. Vigilant teachers in a school with a positive policy on bullying will be eager to nip it in the bud, so if your child's questions hint at bullying, see your school's principal immediately.

● Bullying is always wrong and must be stopped. Convince your child of this fact in whatever way you can. She will find it easier to tell you about bullying if she is clear about this basic belief.

● Boys are particularly conscious of the ridiculous code that they mustn't tell on bullies, even if they are the victims. Convince your children that this code is wrong and that they must seek help if they are being bullied.

● You may wonder whether your child should retaliate if faced with bullying. Under the age of nine, I used to tell my son to give the bully one warning and then hit back, but a child shouldn't do this if faced with several others. A child can ask a trusted older child to help deal with bullies, but you should always report bullying to the school, even if it is happening outside school premises. Ask for the staff's help to bring bullies to book, but in a discreet way to protect your child.

● Girls are just as capable of bullying as boys, and very often it takes the form of a cruel, whispering campaign, or excluding a child from a group of friends. If prolonged, this can be just as wounding as physical violence and should be taken seriously.

● Children aren't born bullies but they often learn a pattern of selfishness, victimization, and bullying from adults in their own homes. This may be due to excessive strictness from an authoritarian parent or arise in a home which is disorganized, where a child is neglected.

● Bullying is a child's response to pain and lack of love. While bullying can never be condoned, these children need help to change their pattern of behavior.

Problem behavior

When should we begin to worry that problem behavior goes beyond bounds and becomes abnormal? There is no simple answer. The point about real "problem" behavior and emotions is that they are too intense and too frequent, so that they lead to unhappy consequences for the child and the people around him. It is one thing to wet the bed at two and half, but think what a terrible time an 11-year-old who could not control his bladder at night would have.

Several criteria are helpful when considering whether problem behavior has stepped outside bounds. The first three concern the frequency, persistence, and intensity of a particular symptom. Many children have fears, tell lies, and steal, but for most of them it is simply a bad patch and they soon leave it behind. But occasionally a child may be so full of fears that as soon as one disappears, another takes its place, or he may go on making up fantastic stories which seem totally real to him long after most children have learned to distinguish fact from fiction. Then he could be having psychological difficulties in adjusting to the world he lives in and may need help.

Most children bite their nails at some time or other. However, few do it so fiercely they draw blood. Such intensity suggests emotional disturbance rather than just a bad habit. Another example is the child who seems unable to tell the truth, even when it would be better for him if he did.

The fourth criterion is age. We need to measure the child's behavior by the norm for his stage of development. It is common for a four-year-old to have a lot of temper tantrums, but they are so rare in an 11-year-old that they are likely to be a sign of emotional disturbance.

A healthy attitude to nudity

The subject of nudity is unfortunately often surrounded by taboos, but there doesn't have to be be any inhibition within a family with children under 11.

● Try not to program your children with your own hang-ups about nudity, if you have them. Your younger children will be naturally unembarrassed; take your lead from them.

● At around eight or nine, however, some children (particularly girls) may give you very clear signals that they are no longer comfortable about exposing their bodies. You may find that your daughter starts to bolt the bathroom door for the first time, and cover herself up when changing for swimming or sports. When this happens, respect her need for privacy.

● The fewer limits set, the better. My own children followed me into the bathroom until they were five or six years old and felt free to come into the bedroom at any time while I was dressing. Some parents may well feel shy about this, but my primary concern was to make myself available to my children at all times, as well as to make them feel comfortable with nakedness and therefore with their own bodies.

● Of course, your child also will have to learn that outside your home others may not be so open about nudity and some, particularly older people such as grandparents, may see things differently; you may need to explain that it's good manners not to embarrass other people. What is perfectly acceptable at home may not be possible or advisable elsewhere.

Masturbation is normal

Masturbation can be a difficult question for parents to face – not because the subject is in itself complicated, but because of their own attitudes to it. Your child has the right to be relaxed about masturbation. Being clear in your own mind that masturbation is normal and beneficial will help to dispel the myths that surround it.

● Many parents feel very confused about masturbation because of misunderstandings starting in their own childhood. Masturbation is not bad in itself; treat it as a normal part of growing up and don't plant the seeds of shame.

● Tolerate or ignore masturbation; if questions arise, answer them; agree that "It feels nice to touch your penis," but set limits: "This is something we do in private." If your child masturbates in public, treat it as you would bad manners or lack of thoughtfulness.

● Up to the age of 5, one child touching another is nearly always innocent. Make sure that one child is not an unwilling victim and that they are not trying to put things into themselves. The exception to this would be a child who has been abused when very young.

● If a child talks about someone who is significantly older and more developed touching him, you should treat this as a danger signal. Calmly ascertain exactly what has happened (if anything) and be vigilant when he's with that person.

● Masturbation is a healthy and natural way to release tension. The only time I would be concerned is if a child were masturbating habitually to escape from a horrible world, because he was being emotionally deprived. A child like this needs help; the way to correct it is to give love, not punishment.

4.11

starting school

If you prepare your child gently and carefully, she should take starting school and learning to read and count in stride.

Preparing your child for school

It will help your child to cope with her first few weeks at school if she can
● say both her names and her address clearly
● handle a knife and fork to cut up her food
● ask for the bathroom without using special "family" names for it
● deal with buttons and zippers
● use faucets, towels, and flush toilets.
It is natural enough for parents to feel anxious as the day approaches for their child to take her first big step into the outside world, especially if she is the first or only child. Parents who have been cementing a close relationship with a child

for four or five years sometimes see school as taking their baby away and destroying something of that precious relationship.

If your child has been to preschool or a playgroup, she is already used to the idea of school and being away from home for part of the day, so she should settle in without problems. If she is the second or third child in the family, she may already be quite envious of her older brother or sister, who seems so much more sophisticated.

If your child has not spent any time at preschool, particularly if she is an only child, then make sure she is used to being parted from you for short periods, perhaps spending an afternoon playing with a

neighbor's children, knowing you will collect her at a set time. A regular walk past the school at playtime can help, too. This gives her an opportunity to look in and see what is going on. She will see other parents near the railings, perhaps waving to their children and you might promise that you will come and wave to her from time to time, when she is one of the children in the playground. Most schools encourage new parents to visit the school with their child at least once before the actual starting date, so that she can see the other children working happily and know there is nothing frightening awaiting her.

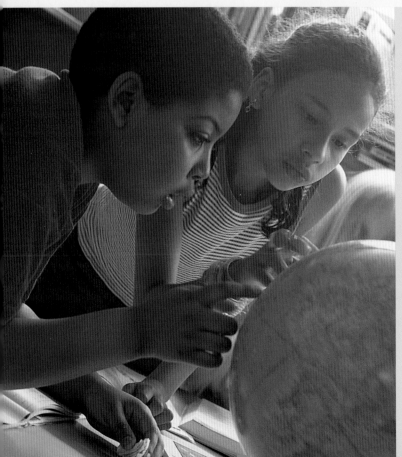

Project work

Project work has been devised to use children's natural curiosity to explore a wide range of subjects. Instead of learning to recite lists of dates or capital cities, they develop a real feeling and understanding for history, geography, and the other subjects that make up the formal curriculum.

If they are working on a project about Native Americans, for example, they might make a map of Native American settlements in America, discuss the reasons behind the choice of site, and study how they traveled. They could figure out how they hunted or gathered food, investigate their religious beliefs, make a model of a teepee, write and act in a play about Pocahontas, and visit a museum to see objects made by Native Americans. By the end of the project, each child should have a personal folder of written work, pictures, and charts and will have learned a good deal about collecting, recording, and presenting information.

How parents can help with reading

If your child seems to be making little progress with the first stages of reading it may be that his whole approach is wrong and he is relying too much on his eyes, instead of using his brain. Settle down with him one evening and ask him to read a little from his school reading book. If, as he reads, he struggles from one word to another and comes out with a sentence which is a nonsensical jumble, it is because he is trying to interpret a string of shapes, instead of thinking about the meaning of the words. Without taking the meaning into account, he cannot check whether he has it right or not. Yet when his mother talks to him, he understands without needing to identify every word or syllable. For some reason he is not applying the same technique in reading. He is not using his knowledge of language to guess what is coming next, so that interpreting the symbols becomes much easier.

You can use a simple reading game to help him. When you read him a story, move your finger along the line of words, so that he follows it with his eyes. After two or three sentences, suddenly stop and let the child guess the next word. If the sentence was: "mom said Jenny could go out and play but she had to be home by…", the child might guess five o'clock. He might be wrong, but he knows it must be a time that is missing and he knows children have to come in from play around dinner time. Soon he will realize that he only needs to identify the first one or two letters of the unknown word to get the answer right. If you repeat the game over and over again he should eventually get into the habit of using his brain as well as his eyes as he tries to read.

Reading for information

If children can be encouraged to see reading as a useful and necessary part of life in dozens of different ways every day, then they will accept the written word easily and naturally instead of being slightly nervous of it all their lives, like many adults. Help your child by putting him in charge of the grocery list, for example, and asking him to read out the items one by one as you go around the supermarket. Or ask him to read out a recipe as you cook or to look up the time of a movie in the paper.

Helping with numbers

Many parents still teach their child to count to 10 by heart or by pointing to her fingers one at a time, but it will be far more useful to her if she learns by moving raisins or pennies into groups. Then she won't begin with the idea that four means the fourth in a series, rather than all four in a set of objects.

Once she has grasped the idea, you can practice by spotting men with umbrellas or dogs on leashes when you are out walking: this helps concentration as well as counting. Instead of threading big wooden beads on the laces just as they come, she can try threading two red ones together, then three green ones, and so on.

Sorting games can be an excellent path to learning. You could ask your child to sort out household items, such as different types of nuts from one large bowl into four smaller ones.

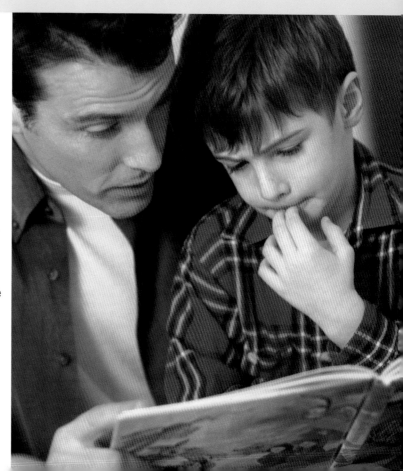

problems of growing up

All children go through phases of "problem behavior" that worry their parents. Most are solved in time, but children may meanwhile need understanding and sensitivity.

Why does a child cheat?

Parents are usually horrified if their child, who has been brought up to think that honesty is very important, is found to be cheating at school.

A normal child cheats when he wants to cover up a real or imagined weakness. If he is self-confident and secure, he will seldom feel the need to cheat. If you find your child is persistently cheating, ask yourself why he feels he cannot stand on his own ability. Often

the trouble comes from putting children in fiercely competitive situations and only praising those who come out on top. Perhaps your child feels he cannot keep up with the rest of the class, in which case his teacher may be able to suggest a way around the problem. It may be that you are pushing him too hard and expecting too much, so that he cheats in a misguided attempt not to disappoint you.

Why does a child lie?

Children often try to boost their prestige in a world where they feel small and insignificant by telling their friends tall tales about the family's gleaming new sports car, which is really a battered old sedan, or father's important jet-setting lifestyle, when he actually has a routine office job. They only do this because they have learned from the adults around them that these are the things that will bring them admiration and esteem.

But sometimes children who "lie" simply are not seeing things the way you do and feel thoroughly misjudged if you call them untruthful. When two brothers fight, it is always the other one who started it. It is always the other sister who suggested climbing onto the toolshed roof or picking all the flowers in the garden.

When you judge whether or not a child is lying, take into account the way she sees the world. Childhood is a period of vivid imagination, make-believe, and

fantasy. For a child with an active imagination, the borderline between fact and fantasy is not clearly defined. What she has wished and dreamed may sometimes be more real to her than mere fact. So if she comes and tells you she has been talking to a little green man in the garden – "he was there, honestly mommy, I'm not making it up" – why not join in the fun, at the same time making it clear that you know it is all a fantasy.

As a child gets older and gains more confidence she normally finds she no longer needs all the little lies that bolstered her self-esteem. But of course some children go on lying into adulthood and, in the end, have trouble distinguishing truth from untruth.

Persistent lying is a danger signal. Parents need to make sure they are not aggravating the problem by being too strict. If the punishment for breaking the rules is too severe, the child will go to

great lengths never to admit she has broken them. If a child accidentally breaks a treasured ornament and owns up, only to find you lose your temper and hit her, she is far more likely to blame it on the cat next time. The main step in teaching a child not to lie is to reassure her sufficiently, so that she does not feel she has to lie.

If she feels that lying is the only way to keep up with her playmates – perhaps they come from a more expensive part of town, so she pretends her home is as grand as theirs – teach her that possessions are not all-important and that people will like her for what she is, not what she brags about.

Finally, make sure you set her a good example. You may tell her fibs for the best possible motives, saying that there is no candy left when there is plenty hidden away, but she will have trouble seeing why her lies are wrong and yours are not.

Hyperactivity

For want of a label, some difficult but completely normal children are said to be hyperactive. To my mind this is unjustified. The word "hyperactive" is the broad term formerly used to describe children who have Attention Deficit Disorder (ADD) and Attention Deficit Hyperactivity Disorder (ADHD) – behavioral conditions that include disruptive behavior, poor attention span, sleeplessness, and excitability (see p.529). Contrary to parental belief, certain food colorings and flavorings have never been proven to contribute to hyperactivity, and sympathetic handling by parents can improve the behavior of most children. There are only a few degrees of hyperactivity in children that are abnormal, serious, or need medical treatment. I, personally, am against the use of drugs such as Ritalin without very careful assessment by several doctors, especially since so many children respond to kinder cognitive and behavioral therapies.

Genuinely hyperactive children will probably need specialized help in retraining their habits, known as "behavior therapy." However if your child's boundless energy leaves you limp and exhausted by the end of the day the chances are that he is simply overactive, **not** hyperactive. If your child is always "on the go" and never wants to go to bed, make sure that he has plenty of opportunity to work off his energy through boisterous outdoor play, then use the basic training rules which work with a toddler who is testing the limits you have set for him. Ignore "bad" behavior as much as possible, provided he is not likely to injure himself or others. But never overlook "good" behavior and always praise him when he is calm and cooperative. Instead of telling him off when he knocks things flying as he charges into the room, make him feel he has done well when he walks in normally. It will take plenty of patience, but it will gradually get results.

Why does a child steal?

A child of four or so takes things because she has no clear idea of what is rightfully hers and what belongs to someone else. She is always being urged to share her toys, so if the little girl next door has something she likes, she sees no reason why she shouldn't take it home with her.

She soon begins to learn that it is wrong to steal or use other people's possessions without their permission. But the way children see stealing varies at different ages. Younger children tend to see stealing as a bad thing to do because they fear the punishment that follows. Older children are more likely to see stealing as undesirable because it injures others.

How to deal with stealing

Most parents are alarmed when a child steals because, as adults, we have learned to look on theft as a serious crime. Yet research shows that stealing is common among older children. Punishment is not a very effective way of stamping it out. Try to avoid sermons and melodramatics, making your child feel she has done something unforgivable so that you will never love her in the same way again. Talk to her calmly and firmly, making her see that she is hurting someone else by taking their property. If she has stolen from friends, see that she pays them back. If she has taken goods from a store, take her back there and explain to the shopkeeper that she took something without paying and wants to apologize and return it.

A child may steal from her mother if she feels she is not getting enough love and attention from her – perhaps she thinks that, once the toddler stage with all its cuddling has passed, you do not love her so much, so you need to show her that she is mistaken. Sometimes a child steals objects she does not need, or even want, to prove herself in some way – perhaps the discipline at home is overly strict or her mother is too fussy and protective, so she needs to break out.

Children who go on stealing do need professional help, but if they are seriously disturbed, stealing will not be the only symptom. They are often playing hooky from school and showing other problems.

keep talking together

Stay in touch with your child on everything – from the facts of life to what he sees on television.

Sex play is normal

The way you deal with sex play is important because it can influence the way your child feels about sex later. Sex play becomes far more common once children start pre-school. By the age of 13 as many as two-thirds of boys have taken part, though sexual activity among girls of this age is less common.

Homosexual play

Homosexual play, with youngsters handling each other's genitals, is also more common as children get older. It is far more likely to happen in single-sex boarding schools than in day schools, for obvious reasons, but there is no hard evidence to show that this passing phase of homosexual activity has any bearing on long-term adult homosexuality.

Sexual interest and behavior in children is intermittent, casual, and not at all intense. So why not treat it in the same way? Don't get excited and tell children they are being "naughty" or "dirty." The child may begin to feel guilty and furtive about his sexual feelings

or he may become far more interested and excited because he feels it is forbidden. If you make a great issue of it, you are implying that sex is unnatural. Treat sexual curiosity as normal and natural, but gently insist that there are conventions of behavior that must be followed.

Many problems can be avoided by an open attitude towards sexual subjects from the time children become aware of the difference between the sexes. If your small son wants to compare the size of his penis with his father's, then there is nothing more likely to allay his curiosity than a good look. It will do a lot to prevent him from being neurotic about his own body.

The facts of life

You can also encourage a sensible outlook on sex by telling your children the facts of life as soon as they begin to ask, so that they know there is nothing to be furtive about. So explain clearly to your children about how a baby grows

in the mother's uterus. Once you have dealt with this point, it is important to go on to say how the baby is actually born, so that children do not grow up thinking that the abdomen simply splits open and delivers the baby like a pea from a pod.

Be guided by your child

If possible, separate the account of the growing embryo from a discussion on intercourse. Parents can be guided by a child's questions, so that they give him all the information he wants at the time without launching into a full lecture on sex before he is ready to understand fully.

Try to use simple accurate language, so that words like penis, vagina, and sperm are never something to giggle over. If you are worried about putting the information over properly, there are plenty of simple books in the library that will help – but don't just hand over the book to your child to look at by himself, sit and read it together.

Answering questions about sex

Answering questions such as "What is making love?", "What is a penis?", etc., provides an opportunity to emphasize to children that sex should come from love and that with love comes responsibility: the responsibility to put the other person before themselves, never to coerce, pressure, or force, and to have respect for others and for themselves.

● Don't shrink from telling your child the truth. You owe your child an honest and open answer without any fear of being embarrassed.

● Don't feel that you have to give every single detail to a young child: it's neither necessary nor good for your child, who may be frightened by what she can't grasp. Remember there's rarely need for detailed information about the mechanics of sex for a child under 8.

● Think of each question your child asks as an opportunity to convey your standards and values and to help your child feel loved and well-informed.

● Try to anticipate your child's concerns. Remember that sex is also about self-control and abstinence and you should school your child about these qualities.

● Don't ever scold your child for being sexually curious about people of the opposite sex; satisfy that curiosity by answering questions frankly and honestly.

● Talk to sons and daughters together. Boys need to know about girls because knowledge and understanding will help to instill in them a sense of responsibility and understanding of girls' and women's needs from an early age.

Television?

Most of us have our own firm opinions about whether the overall influence of television is good or bad. But, like it or not, television is here to stay. Many parents find it difficult or impossible to cut down their children's viewing but they worry what effect the frequent scenes of violence will have on their children and about the amount of time being "wasted" when it could be used for reading, hobbies, music, and so on.

Violence on television

Research evidence shows that the effect of television violence on young children is likely to be rather small. This is probably because much of the violence they see is in cartoons or action films, full of characters who are part of a fantasy world quite different from their own. Children imitate people like themselves – other children, brothers and sisters, or their parents and teachers. They are well aware of the difference between real people and Tom and Jerry or a character in *Star Wars*.

"Cops and robbers" films may have slightly more influence, but even then many children, perhaps most, realize that there is a strong element of fantasy. They know that their fathers and brothers do not drive fast cars and spend their time in expensive nightclubs and they know that when someone punches you, it hurts. The evidence shows that it is young adults, rather than children under 12, who are most likely to be affected by the violence in films, because it is often committed by people from their own age group whom they may be tempted to copy.

Surprisingly, it is the real-life news film or documentary that is most likely to affect a child, because there he can see children throwing stones at soldiers in Ireland or youngsters just like his brother fighting at sports events. These are real people behaving violently in real situations. Whether we own a television set or not, our children are likely to be influenced by the attitudes and actions of the society around them. Parents cannot protect them from all that is ugly in life.

Probably one of the most useful things parents can do is to watch news programs with their children, so that they can talk about what is going on and the way they feel about it. Discussion after programs meant purely for entertainment can be useful too, helping children to form and put across their thoughts about the "good guys" and the "bad guys" and the way the characters treat one another.

You can be reassured that the behavior of family and friends, seeing them treating one another with gentleness and consideration, will exert a much more powerful influence on your child than anything he may see on television.

"teenagers need
to experiment
and test limits –
their own and
other people's"

life stages: 11 to 18 years

Until a child is about 10, most parents can confidently say they know them well, as young children mirror what they're taught. This changes when youngsters reach adolescence. Those years of adolescence are often described as "normal insanity" because, in most cases, things do eventually settle down.

Rebellion is normal

Teenagers are natural risk-takers. They need to experiment and test limits – their own and other people's. Rebellion is a normal part of dealing with the emotional changes of adolescence. Teenagers may feel rebellious about the rules and regulations that society tries to impose on them or that their parents expect them to live by.

Much of the natural rebelliousness of adolescents stems from their need to be different from their parents and to establish their own separate identity. This rebelliousness may not be particularly comfortable for the adolescents themselves, and they may make decisions or act in a particular way precisely because they know their parents won't want them to do it.

But remember, most bad behavior is a sign that your child is finding life difficult. In my experience, it makes things easier for everyone if parents:
- **overlook** what they can
- **avoid** too much confrontation and look for ways to compromise
- are **tolerant**.

I'd very strongly advise against fighting fire with fire. It only makes things worse and heightens a teenager's resentment against everyone. That's why it is so important to try to understand the cause of problem behavior, not just concentrate on the fallout from it.

For instance, if your children are having trouble at school, encourage them to explain what their motivation is for behaving badly. Are there any teachers or classes that cause them particular difficulties? Low self-esteem often lies at the root

of problem behavior, so give your teenagers praise when they do something well to give their confidence a boost.

No problem should be too serious for them to share with you. If it seems impossible to talk to your teenage children because you meet a blank wall or tempers flare on both sides, it's worth asking a third party like a friend or relative to talk to them.

The teenager's point of view

Your teenage years are a very precious part of your life; your horizons broaden in a unique way and new choices constantly present themselves. This time is also unique because of how much you grow mentally. You enter the teenage years feeling awkward, clumsy, shy, and bewildered and you emerge from them with clear opinions and ideas about your career, the kind of relationships that you're looking for and possibly the sort of life that's going to make you happy. Probably at no other time in your life will you grow at such a fast rate, both emotionally and intellectually.

Do try to talk to your parents – you need them and their support, and you're unlikely to find anyone else who's as interested in you as they are. What's essential is to persuade them that you have important things to talk about while you're growing up and you need their help. Few parents can resist such a request.

There are few periods in our lives that seem as difficult as our teenage years, and when they're over, you'll probably look back and feel that you did very well in negotiating them. If you manage this, your achievement will be enormous. If you come to the end of this time feeling fairly contented with a positive outlook on life, it's a triumph and you can be very proud of yourself.

In the pages that follow, I offer guidelines where appropriate, advice where I feel there may be a need, and strategies for dealing with potentially difficult situations.

" the key to
a smooth
passage
through
adolescence
is self-esteem "

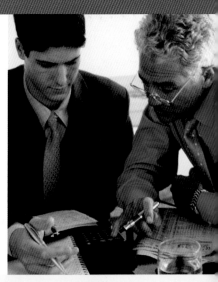

your
teens are
a very
precious
part of
your life

" the only
reason to
have sex
is because
you
want to "

a girl's body

Between the ages of about 8 and 18 a girl's body changes, under the influence of the female hormone estrogen, from that of a child to a woman.

Physical growth

At around the age of 8, a year or so before puberty for most girls, the pelvic bones begin to grow and fat is deposited on the breasts, hips, and thighs. In the adolescent phase, which generally starts between 10 and 16 years, your nipples start to bud, and pubic and underarm hair appears. At this stage, the genital organs develop and your period starts. More fat is deposited on your hips, breasts, and thighs. By the time you are 18 or so, bone growth will be complete and you'll have reached your adult height.

The speed at which your body changes depends on many factors and it varies enormously from individual to individual, so don't worry if your friends are developing more quickly or more slowly than you.

Armpit hair At about 14 years, hair starts to grow in the armpits and the sweat glands become active.

Skin The hormone androgen affects the skin, causing more oil to be secreted. Pimples may appear.

Waist In contrast to broadening hips and breasts, the waist begins to look much more slender and defined.

Pubic hair Hair first appears when you are about 12 years old and then gradually becomes thicker and curlier, spreading up to form a triangle shape. It may not match the color of the hair on your head at first.

Thighs The inner and outer thighs develop pads of fat from about the age of 14, giving the body a more curvaceous, womanly outline.

Hips As the pelvic bones grow, the hips begin to broaden. Fat is then laid down on the hips, helping to give the body its characteristic female shape.

Take good care of your skin

Really great looking skin is a big plus and one of your most important assets. So whether you were born with a perfect complexion, or one that is not so good, you should make an effort to take care of it properly. When you are going through adolescence, your body is trying to adjust to a change in hormone balance, and this affects your skin.

Pimples Never squeeze pimples because this spreads the infection into the deeper layers of the skin. You can squeeze uninflamed blackheads after a hot bath or shower, when all the pores are open, but afterward apply a small dab of antiseptic cream to keep the skin clear. Try using over-the-counter acne cream, and if

your skin is very oily, refrain from using an abrasive cleanser – this simply spreads the bacteria.

Acne Nearly every teenager has acne at some stage. During adolescence, high levels of sex hormones are produced, which lead to the production of large quantities of sebum in the skin. Sebum is an irritant that may block the pores, causing a purplish lump which may become infected and form a pustule. An occasional pimple is normal at this age, but severe acne does tend to scar, so ask your doctor for advice on how to clear it up. There are many good acne preparations available, but the best need a prescription.

Breast development

Breasts come in every shape and size. Remember that it's not true that boys prefer girls with big breasts or that small breasts mean you can't feed a baby.

It's normal for your breasts to feel tender as they grow during puberty, and in the week before your period. You may find that wearing a bra helps to relieve any tenderness. A good bra will support heavy breasts and stop them from wobbling.

Buying a bra

There's no need to wear stiff, heavy bras with underwiring. Today there are plenty on the market specially designed for girls who lead active lives, who need support, and who want to look as natural as possible. Cotton is the best fabric to choose if you can, particularly if you play a lot of sports. But there are good bras made of synthetic fabrics, too.

Measuring for a bra

Measure yourself under the bust and around up to the nearest size. For example, if your measurement is 33in (84cm), you'll need a 34in (86cm) bra. For your cup size, measure around the largest part of your breasts and take the first measurement away from this. If the difference is less than 5in (12.5cm), you are an A cup, less than 6in (15cm) you need a B cup, 6–8½in (15–22cm) a C cup, 9in (23cm) or more, a D cup.

Many stores offer a fitting service with trained assistants and the chance to try on different bras before you buy. This will help you establish what kind of bra works for you.

Problem periods

Girls often experience actual physical distress during their periods, the causes of which have been investigated and treatment is available. Painful periods (dysmenorrhea – see p. 247) can be quite disabling, needing time off school and work.

Dysmenorrhea means menstrual cramps, which can range from very mild to completely disabling. Once thought to be a neurotic condition, it is now known that it's all in our hormones – not in our heads. A girl who has very painful periods either makes too much of the hormone prostaglandin, or her uterus is more sensitive than usual to normal amounts of it.

Drugs containing antiprostaglandins such as ibuprofen, which get to the root of the problem and bring relief in more than 80 percent of cases, are on the market in the United States, Britain, and most European countries. The use of antiprostaglandin has proved to be enormously helpful to many girls. It can shorten the time during which you feel pain and this can reduce how long you have to stay in bed, so that you can continue your studies or your job. Start taking medication the day before your period.

Sharing worries

Many girls worry about how their bodies look and feel, and find their growing sexual awareness disturbing. The "supermodels" used in fashion magazines promote an unrealistic "ideal" image of how girls should look, and it can be hard if you think that you don't match this ideal. Girls may feel that they lack control over their bodies. From time to time they also feel out of tune with their families, schoolmates, friends, and especially their boyfriends. A lot of girls (and increasingly boys) blame the way they look for their low self-esteem, which in turn may lead to more serious problems. If you feel bad about yourself, have the courage to ask for help before things get worse.

Talking about it

● Your mother is the best person for advice but if you can't talk to her, ask another older female relative who is sympathetic.
● Talk to a biology teacher, school nurse, or counselor or see your doctor, and read as many books as you can.
● Compare notes with your best friend. Nearly everyone wonders if other girls are like them and the answer is often a reassuring "yes." Most girls experience the same anxieties.

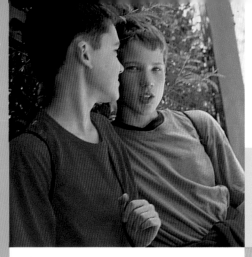

a boy's body

Boys' bodies start to change at 11 to 12 years. Their voices "break" and they begin to grow body hair at 14 to 15. Most boys will have to start shaving at 16 or 17.

Talking over problems

● Like many boys, you may find it difficult to talk about the problems of adolescence with friends or family for fear of losing face. But try to overcome this.
● Read books on the subject or ask your doctor for information.
● A teacher or school counselor will help on matters of fact, and can advise you where to go for help.
● If possible, talk to your dad, an older brother, or a male relative. Ask him about his adolescence, and how he dealt with any problems he had.

How your body changes

● Shoulders and chest grow wider.
● Muscles develop.
● Soft hair, which becomes coarse and curly, grows around the penis.
● Penis grows larger and longer and skin of scrotum darkens.
● Arms, hands, legs, and feet grow bigger and longer.
● Larynx enlarges and becomes an "Adam's apple."
● Voice breaks.
● Hair grows in armpits, on chest, and on arms and legs.

● Testicles grow larger and fuller and become sensitive.
● Wet dreams and erections start to occur.
● Sperm are produced.
● Weight and height increase.
● Body sweats more.
● Face matures as the bones in your face grow.
● Skin becomes oily and pimply.
Be aware of how your body is changing. Boys are affected by hormones just as much as girls.

Worries and questions

The speed at which your body changes at puberty may take you by surprise. The changes take place when your testicles begin making the male sex hormone testosterone. Testosterone also triggers sperm production and makes you sexually aware. You'll begin to get erections because your penis is more sensitive to touch, or because you become excited by something you think about or someone you see.

Penis size
Most boys worry about the size of their penis, but the size of a person's body parts has nothing

to do with how well they work. Also, size when soft has no relation to size when erect. In fact, it is often the opposite: small penises seem to get bigger when erect than large penises. The most important thing to remember is that girls aren't really interested in size, because a big penis doesn't make you a better lover. Just remember – once you start to produce sperm, you are fertile, which means you could father a child if you have unprotected sex.

Wet dreams
When sperm production begins, sperm collect in the seminal

vesicles. Wet dreams act as a safety valve; the pressure builds up to the extent that you may ejaculate in your sleep – that's why it's called a "wet dream." You may be embarrassed when you have a wet dream, but it's totally normal – all boys have them – and they usually stop as you mature physically.

Circumcision
Removal of the foreskin, the protective layer of flexible skin on the penis, is called circumcision. It is a simple operation and may be done for religious or medical reasons, but it doesn't affect the way the penis works.

New feelings

Hormonal changes can affect your mood. All young people experience these changes and you feel miserable and confused, but it's normal.

As your body changes, you'll also start to experience new feelings. Your moods swing up and down like a yo-yo – you're laughing one minute and crying the next. **Sexual desire makes such an untimely entrance in a teenager's life**. Just as you begin to feel attracted to the opposite sex, you find that your emotions are all over the place, and you're feeling really anxious about your body. Your mixed emotions are not the end of the world, even though they feel like it at times. You're learning to handle life's ups and downs, and this is a valuable lesson. It helps to compare notes with a close friend; someone you can confide in.

do

 Be positive
Think about the times when you've triumphed.

 Be active
Try to take the initiative.

 Take care
Make sure your actions don't hurt anyone along the way.

 Be cautious
Don't expect everyone to return your feelings.

Going it alone

Touching yourself "down below" is a perfectly normal habit, no matter what age, gender, or sexual orientation you happen to be. **Everyone masturbates, boys and girls, men and women, and for most of us, it is our first experience of sex**. Masturbation never does any harm, unless it turns into an obsessive occupation, when it may indicate problems to do with poor self-esteem.

Although it's common for boys to masturbate more frequently than girls, masturbation is more important to girls because it allows them to explore and experiment with their bodies long before they have sex with another person. A girl can stimulate her own body to find out what her responses are and what she likes and prefers.

Although they may not often admit it, a lot of boys and girls achieve their best orgasms by masturbating. Nowadays, I am pleased to say, most young people believe that it is acceptable and harmless to do this, and of course they are right.

Masturbation will not make you go blind. Nor will it give you acne, insanity, or hairy palms – these are all myths. It is also quite normal to fantasize about somebody while you are masturbating and these fantasies are almost always innocent. Most people have no difficulty in drawing a line between fantasy and reality, and do not want to act out their fantasies.

teenage troubles

A key factor influencing how teenagers feel about themselves is the way they look. Worries about weight, for example, can affect self-esteem.

Maintaining a healthy weight

Many teenagers go through phases of being very worried about their weight. They may feel that they're too fat all over, or that they're too fat in some places.

Also, at your stage of life, your weight may fluctuate – you may well still be growing, for one thing – and a girl may also weigh more when she is premenstrual. So it's not a good idea just to focus on your weight, but to look at your overall shape and the fact that it does change as you mature and develop breasts and hips. If you are at all concerned about your weight, talk to your school nurse or doctor so they can assess it properly for you.

Some fat is good!
We all need some body fat to stay healthy. Females need more than males – especially once periods start – to make enough of the female hormone estrogen, to be fertile, and to build strong bones. So some fat is good!

When, for whatever reason, your food intake is higher than your energy output, you have an excess that is stored as extra fat. The reverse happens when output outstrips intake; fat becomes a source of energy, it is burned up and weight is lost. If you want to stay a healthy

weight, then the best way to do that is to stay active and to enjoy a healthy diet. No need for drastic diets or to be "model" thin – these are unhealthy and unrealistic measures.

The energy balance
The goal is to stay in energy balance. There are certain influences that can affect the balance of the energy equation. One of these is your basal metabolic rate (BMR), the measurement of the amount of food energy that your body uses to fuel all the functions essential for life and health, such as breathing and

digestion. This accounts for about two-thirds of the body's energy needs and is linked to your height and weight and how much muscle you have. The heavier you are the higher your BMR.

When planning to lose weight, most people opt for cutting down the amount of food they eat because they think they can lose weight quickly this way. In fact, it's more beneficial to change the type of food you eat and increase the amount of exercise you do, because this can affect the energy equation just as quickly, and more effectively, in the long term.

Crash dieting

Crash dieting is a very bad way of losing weight in the long run. Although the amount of weight you lose right away is likely to be impressive, and may be as much as 8½lb (4kg) in the first week, less than half of this will be fat, which is what you're trying to lose. The rest is simply water loss.

Cutting down your food like this is really low-grade starvation; all you'll do is gradually put your body into a state of hibernation – it will turn down the fuel burners to conserve energy and to stay alive. You will also feel hungry, bored, irritable, and likely to binge, which just makes you more miserable, especially as the pounds go back on.

Crash dieting does nothing to retrain your eating habits. If you want to lose weight and keep it off permanently, you must revamp your whole style of eating and adjust your activity levels.

Exercising to stay slim

Exercise not only affects the energy equation in a more subtle way than through direct expenditure of energy, but it is also the only way we know to alter our BMR. If you exercise enough to become fit – that is, four times a week for 30 minutes or longer, over a period of months – muscles become stronger and body fat is better regulated. Exercising muscle has about twice the BMR of fat and resting muscle, so the body adapts and prepares for the increased work done by the heart, lungs, and muscles by working, or metabolizing, at a slightly higher rate, thereby using more energy even on days when you don't exercise.

This makes exercise one of the most valuable of all weight control aids. Research shows that regular activity is the most effective way to control weight in the long term.

Your weight loss depends on how many calories you go without or burn off. If your average calorie needs are 2000 per day, even a fairly generous diet of 1500 calories creates an energy deficit of 500 calories per day or 3500 per week, which is the equivalent in energy terms of 1lb (0.5kg) of body fat. You can double this by getting a moderate amount of exercise.

Self-esteem

The key to a child's smooth passage through adolescence is high self-esteem. Without it, teenagers can run afoul of eating disorders, get into bad company, or even injure themselves. Most people will not have just one idea about their self-worth, but will have a number of views depending on the arena they find themselves in.

An adolescent may report high self-worth around friends, who think he is "awesome"; lower self-worth around parents who think he is "lazy" and "irresponsible"; and the lowest level of self-worth around strangers, who he feels may see him as "a total dork."

Parenting styles contribute to a child's self-worth. But while the behavior of parents continues to be important during the teenage years, the views of peers come to play an increasingly crucial role as young people move towards adulthood.

Another key factor affecting self-esteem, particularly during the early teenage years, is physical appearance. For young people in this age group, it is body image satisfaction that correlates most highly with global self-esteem. In early adolescence girls have much higher levels of dissatisfaction with their bodies than do boys, both during and after puberty. Girls are more dependent on peer approval at this stage in their lives, and more sensitive to the opinions of their friends.

Self-esteem doesn't remain constant during childhood and adolescence. A range of factors will operate to determine the way in which self-esteem varies, depending on things such as success at school, family circumstances, the behavior of friends, and so on.

Research in this area has provided some important new insights into the way adolescent self-esteem alters. Researchers identified four different groups: one with consistently high self-esteem; another showing rising levels of self-esteem between the ages of 12 and 16; a third group showing consistently low self-esteem; and a fourth whose self-worth actually declined during the adolescent stage.

Young people in the third group might be helped by exercises that encourage them to feel better about themselves (for example, write a list of all your good points or write down every positive thing that's happened to you today). In the fourth, the goal might be to identify skills – whether academic, social, or sporting – and then work to improve them in the expectation that better performance in some important areas will lead to a greater sense of self-worth in others.

relationships

11-18

Friends become more important in your teens; they help you broaden your interests and give you loyalty and support. Some friendships may even blossom into deeper relationships.

Deeper relationships

As you grow older and start thinking about having deeper relationships (which may eventually involve sex), you have to start paying attention to your responsibilities. Not only to your girlfriends or boyfriends, but to your family, your friends, and yourself. Responsibility involves morality, which doesn't mean you have to be a prude, it means having a clear idea of the boundaries of fairness and kindness in your behavior to others. It's sensible to approach relationships responsibly – irresponsibility leads to trouble in the long run. You'll know when you're being irresponsible, because the consequences are hard to live with. And when you feel shame and guilt, all this does is create unhappiness, because you're bound to take it out on others. Try to be honest and true to yourself. People will respect you for it.

Good relationships

A good relationship is personally enriching; it provides you with comfort, understanding, and support. You'll feel that you are being loved – you'll get pleasure from giving, too. While your values may be similar to your partner's, any differences are exciting, and you should be able to respect each other's views without any real friction. Good relationships aren't too "exclusive." They don't block off your involvement in other things that are still important.

Thinking about sex

Sex, particularly good sex, is fun and it gives a great deal of pleasure in many contexts. It can be thrilling, exciting, moving, comforting, even consoling. All of these are positive reasons for having sex.

But then there are the questions of safe sex and contraception. Sex is a minefield and you must reflect deeply before stepping onto it.

How old should you be?

For all teenagers, this is the ultimate question. Does age matter anyway, you may ask? I think it does.

For purely medical reasons, I'm against very young girls having sex, because as a doctor I know that if you begin sexual activity, especially with several partners, early during your teenage years, it can make you more vulnerable to cancer of the cervix. I am also against any

teenagers having sexual relationships before they are emotionally mature and have established their sexual feelings and sexual values. For most of us, this is quite a problem and it takes years to do; even adults find it difficult.

In addition to these personal issues, I think you would be unwise to ignore the very strong opinions that are held by society in general. Although conventional thinking doesn't matter as much as the opinions of your parents, teachers, friends, and relatives, it does matter a little and you can't ignore it. Everyone has strong opinions about teenage sexuality and you're almost sure to find that your opinions conflict with those of someone who matters to you. Don't ignore this situation completely because your relationship with that person can only deteriorate if you go against their views.

No one can tell you when sex is okay, but there are a few things you should bear in mind. The first is the law. The law varies on the age of consent (the age under which it is a crime to have sexual intercourse) in different parts of the world, but it usually ranges between the ages of 16 and 18. Therefore you would be breaking the law if you had sex before the age of consent. In any case, coping with sex is difficult under the age of 16.

Another basic requirement when thinking about having sex for the first time is to make sure that there is no risk of an unplanned pregnancy. In other words, both of you should investigate, decide on, and use a method of contraception with the lowest possible failure rate (see p.118). Finally, it is vital that you feel confident that you will not expose yourself to a sexually transmitted disease, including AIDS.

Friendships

Friends of your own age matter a lot and you want to spend as much time as possible with them. You may begin to feel there's a growing rift between you and your parents and that they often cannot see your point of view. You turn to your friends instead – they know what you're experiencing, they're sympathetic with your views, and they make you feel you belong.

Straightforward friendships with other people of your own age are just as important as those that involve sexual attraction. In fact a relationship that isn't also a friendship won't work. But making friends is difficult for a lot of people. Joining a club or group is a great way to meet friends, but you may find you haven't got the self-confidence to take the first step. It helps to know that others are having the same problems.

● Don't judge people too hastily; appearances can be deceptive.
● Do be yourself rather than trying to imitate others or be top dog.
● Do ask others about their interests, such as music or sport.
● Do compliment someone on doing something well.

Friendship means giving and taking. Concentrate on your contribution to a friendship, not what it gives you, and you'll get more out of it.

Remember that each partner in a relationship has the right:

● to have opinions
● to respect
● to see family
● to be trusted
● to show feelings
● to time alone
● to support
● to talk
● to religious beliefs
● to faithfulness
● to make mistakes
● to see friends
● to affection
● to tolerance
● to be listened to
● to security
● to ask for help
● to say "no"
● to have fun
● to be cared for
● to patience.

Use the following as a starting point for your own lists, then, once you have established a relationship, look back at your list of "likes," and see just how close you've come to your ideal.

What I can offer

Fun	Understanding
Support	Respect
Happiness	Togetherness
Love	Company
Trust	Patience
Help with problems	Sense of humor

What I would like

Someone I can laugh with
Someone to go out dancing with
Someone I can really talk to
Someone to lean on
Someone to care for
Someone who won't mind me crying
Someone who really understands me
Someone who won't get jealous

The risks of promiscuity

By far the majority of people decide to have one lover at a time. A few decide to have several at the same time, and if they do, they are behaving in a way that some people would call promiscuous. This may be your choice, but there are certain issues you should consider because, besides any moral and religious judgment of what is right and wrong, there are problems and quite a few risks attached to having sex with more than one person.

● The chances that you could catch a sexually transmitted disease (STD) and, for girls, the risk that you will develop cancer of the cervix, are greatly increased.

● If you or your lover have had other partners, there is a risk of contracting HIV, leading to AIDS. It is therefore crucial for all young couples to use condoms and spermicides every time they have intercourse to reduce the risk, regardless of what other contraceptive they use.

● By squandering time and emotional energy on more than one relationship you may find that you don't have enough time or energy to make any one of them work.

● You are greatly increasing the risk of hurting other people who don't approve of what you're doing.

● You may not think so at the time, but you are running the risk of losing your self-respect if you have even the slightest suspicion that what you're doing isn't right.

● People who disagree with your values are quite likely to label you, and you may get a bad reputation.

11-18

deciding about sex

Girls and boys need courage to withstand the pressure of the moment: to realize they can say "no" without losing face. There are many reasons why you may feel unsure or uncomfortable about sex.

Saying "no" to sex

The only reason to have sex is because you want to. Deciding to have sex should never be taken lightly. No one should ever make you have sex. Young people are presented with many difficult choices and pressures to do things that they feel uncomfortable about – taking drugs, drinking alcohol, smoking, and sex.

For your own sense of self-respect, don't be pressured into having sex because you think your boyfriend or girlfriend will leave you or be disappointed. You and nobody else decides whether you want to enter a sexual relationship. If you haven't managed to figure out your sexual values yet, then you really should say no.

No means no

People can come up with lots of apparently plausible reasons for persuading their partners to have sex when they don't really want to.

Typical ploys include saying things like "if you don't, I'll tell everyone you're a tease" or "you know you want to really" or "I'll leave you if you don't." It's not acceptable to trick your partner in this way – if a person says "no" then you should respect his or her wishes.

Why girls find it hard to say "no"

Almost every girl has difficulty in saying "no" at some time and finds herself on a date having sexual contact when she doesn't really want it.

There are lots of reasons why girls find it difficult to come out and say "no" firmly, the most common is that they don't want to hurt the boy's feelings, or they're afraid of being thought a prude.

Some girls worry that they're not going along with what other girls appear to be doing. With all these pressures, it takes a

brave girl to say "no," but you must say it if that's what you feel. If your boyfriend really cares for you, he'll agree. On the other hand, you'll lose a lot of self-respect if you say "yes" when you really mean "no."

Ways to say no

If you're really concerned about refusing sex, you can practice these replies:
- No, I hate being forced to do anything.
- No, I don't feel ready for it.
- No, I'm really too scared.
- No, I don't think I know you well enough yet.
- No, do you really want to have sex with someone who doesn't want to?
- No, I want to have time just being friends. Then I can decide if I want to have sex with you.
- No, you're hassling me. I'll know when I'm ready.
- No, I don't feel I trust you enough yet.
- No, I believe I should wait until marriage.
- No, I only want to have sex as part of a long-term relationship.
- No, not until we've discussed contraception.
- No, not until we know there are no risks at all.
- No, I don't want to and if you make me that's rape.
- No, you're giving the impression you don't really care about me.
- No, you're making me think that you'll leave me if I don't.
- No, you're moving too fast for me.
- No, you're making me feel really frightened of you.
- No, you're acting like a person I don't really want to know.
A question that will really bring things to a screeching halt is: "Are you ready to be a father yet? "

The risks – STDs

While sex is one of the ways of showing affection, if you don't wear a condom it is also a way of spreading certain sexually transmitted diseases, most of which are very unpleasant and some of which are incurable. They are nearly always infectious and are contracted only by having sex with another person. Here are some of them:

● Genital warts and genital herpes are viral infections; warts are curable, herpes is not, but the symptoms can be treated. The warts virus can also lead to cervical cancer.

● Gonorrhea, syphilis, and chlamydia are bacterial infections, which are treatable with antibiotics. However, chlamydia is difficult to diagnose since it's often symptomless. It can also cause pelvic inflammatory disease (PID) and an inability to become pregnant.

● HIV/AIDS and hepatitis B are incurable viral infections; AIDS can be fatal and hepatitis B can be also.

● Pubic lice ("crabs") and scabies are parasites, which are treatable with insecticides.

● Candidiasis ("thrush") is a yeast infection, which is treatable with a fungicide.

● Trichomonas is a single cell parasite, which is treatable with antiparasitic agents.

How to tell if you have an STD

Some STDs are symptomless in the early stages or have very vague symptoms, but if you suspect that you may have contracted an STD and have any or all of the following symptoms, you should seek medical advice immediately:

● pain when urinating or moving your bowels

● a smelly, discolored vaginal discharge that is greater in quantity and with a worse odor than usual

● any vaginal discharge accompanied by a rash or that makes you sore and itchy

● lower back pain or pain in the pelvis or in the groin

● pain when having sex

● a sore lump or spot on any part of the genital area, including around the anus

● a fever combined with any of these symptoms

● oral sex may lead to symptoms around the mouth, including a sore throat

● anal sex may result in symptoms around the anus.

Where to get help Most people who think that they've got an STD are too embarrassed to visit their own doctor. This need not cause you any delay. There are public health clinics in every major city that are well advertised and guarantee confidential treatment. If you want to find the clinic nearest to you, ask at a local health center, call the hospital, or look in your phone book.

Satisfaction without sex

In a good sexual relationship, there are loads of ways to explore each other's bodies without having actual sexual intercourse. Sex is the iceberg of which intercourse is only the tip – the one-eighth that's showing above the surface. Foreplay is the seven-eighths beneath the surface and can help you to overcome any anxieties that you may have about sex. It can often lead to orgasm and may even be more fulfilling than full sexual intercourse, particularly for girls who may find it easier to have an orgasm with foreplay than with penetrative sex, because foreplay concentrates on the clitoris.

Different kinds of stimulation

● Mutual masturbation is when you stroke and rub each other's genital organs. A girl strokes or rubs her boyfriend's penis while a boy strokes his girlfriend's clitoris.

● Oral sex is when you kiss, lick, nuzzle, and suck each other's genital organs; girls do it to the penis (called fellatio); boys do it to the clitoris (called cunnilingus).

● "69" is when a boy and girl perform fellatio and cunnilingus for each other at the same time (stimulates orgasm).

● Simultaneous orgasm is possible if a boy rubs a girl's clitoris with his penis; he should still wear a condom since semen can enter the vagina even without penetration.

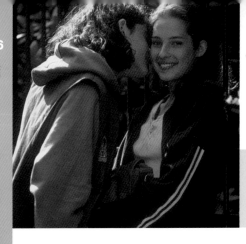

11-18

your sexuality

Whether you're heterosexual or gay, practice safe sex. That means always using a condom.

Making sure sex is safe

In order to be safe from HIV and gonorrhea, you should use a condom for all forms of penetrative sex – anal and oral as well as vaginal. Condoms may be less effective in preventing tranmission of other STDs. Make sure that you know how to use one properly, and never use condoms from expired packages. Practice safe sex; think carefully about your sexual behavior and don't rely on condoms alone to prevent pregnancy. Semen can leak if you haven't managed to use the condom correctly, or if you've used an expired one. It's best for girls to either be on the pill, or to also use a diaphragm.

Getting help

● Your doctor or family planning clinic will gladly give you information on condoms.
● A whole variety of condoms are available, and some of them have been designed to make sex a little more interesting! Condoms are available from retail outlets, supermarkets, pharmacies, and even public bathrooms.
● Safe sex also means that you must report a suspected STD immediately to a clinic where you can get confidential treatment and also say who your suspected contacts are. If you contract a contagious STD such as genital herpes, you must always be honest with subsequent partners.

Safe sex guidelines

Carry a condom
Carry a condom with you at all times, girls as well as boys.

Practice first
Make sure you know how to use a condom before you have sex with someone.

Condoms every time
Use a condom until you're absolutely sure there's no risk of sexual infections to or from your partner.

Once only
Don't ever try to use a condom more than once.

Be frank
Be open about previous sexual experiences when you start a relationship, and tell your partner about any chronic infections, such as herpes.

No casual sex
Don't have sex with someone at a party, or on vacation, whom you hardly know and may never meet again. Be especially careful after drinking a lot.

Accepting that you're gay

Feeling fundamentally different from one's family and friends can be an extremely isolating and unhappy experience. What can make matters even worse is hearing friends and family make disparaging or abusive remarks about gays. Experiences like this can lead many young gay people to feel guilty and ashamed and, as a result, forced to keep this secret about themselves for a very long time. A great many have no idea that there are an enormous number of people who are sexually attracted to members of their own sex just as they are. **In fact, a significant number of the population are gay.** Nobody knows the exact figure because there is a wide gulf between being exclusively heterosexual and exclusively homosexual. Many young people have homosexual feelings or experiences but this does not necessarily reflect their adult sexuality.

A gay person can't help the way they are any more than a blond person can help having fair hair. Medical evidence suggests that a person's sexual orientation is formed before the age of five. So it's highly unlikely that an adolescent could be "turned" homosexual or lesbian simply by contact with another gay person – although such a contact could bring to the fore an orientation which was previously unrecognized.

Be proud of who you are
Accepting the fact that you are gay is the first and most important step in the process of coming to terms with your identity as a gay person. You can't, and shouldn't, live in the shadows, and have every right to be proud of who you are. However, it's important that you shouldn't feel

pressurized into announcing yourself to the world at large. Sexuality is a private matter and if you'd prefer to keep yours under wraps for the time being, that is your choice. The point is that you feel comfortable about yourself – "confessing" to friends and family won't necessarily make this so.

Knowing you are not alone
Meeting other members of the homosexual community should be your next step. Talking to young people who are or have been in a situation similar to your own will help build your confidence and reduce feelings of alienation. You may, at first, prefer not to meet anybody face to face. If so, you should telephone a gay hotline (see p. 567), which is run by gay people to give help, support, and counseling to other gay people. Knowing you are not alone will help you feel stronger and help you to cope with the challenges that lie ahead.

The last and probably most crucial step is sharing what has been a secret part of your life with those whom you love most in the world – your family. This last stage can be especially daunting because the parents of most

gay people are heterosexual with entrenched ideas and expectations for their offspring usually revolving around marriage and a family of their own. You may believe your family and friends will hate you if and when they discover that you're gay. But this need not necessarily be true. **Many people now realize that being attracted to a member of the same sex is absolutely normal for a gay person.**

But it must be accepted that some people are still homophobic. These people usually have never met a gay person in their lives and are content to agree with what their friends say because they don't want to be thought of as different. They haven't had the chance to realize that people are people and should be liked or disliked for their personality, not for their sexuality.

It would be wonderful to say with confidence that your family and friends won't desert you once they discover you are gay, but this is impossible to predict. But it's highly unlikely that they will turn against you. Once they've allowed the news to sink in, I'm sure they will realize that you are still the same person they have loved all these years. That's what you must try to remember. **If they love you now, why shouldn't they love you once they know that you're gay?** After all, nothing will have changed except their false impression of the truth.

As I said, there's no rule which says when you should tell your parents or if you have to tell your parents. It's entirely up to you. Once the news is out, nothing can hide it so it's not something you should do unless you feel completely ready. Good luck!

11–18
preventing pregnancy

Once you decide you want to have full sexual intercourse, it is crucial that you don't have an unplanned pregnancy. If you do get pregnant, never keep it a secret. Tell your parents or your doctor immediately.

Contraception

If you are thinking of starting a sexual relationship, first make absolutely sure that you want it. Talk over your doubts together and make your own decision. Once you decide you want to have full sexual intercourse, it is crucial that you don't have an unplanned pregnancy. Before you start having sex, the most responsible thing to do is to seek advice on contraception from a family planning clinic or your doctor.

The laws vary state to state, but in many a girl under the age of 16 can seek contraceptive advice and receive it without the doctor telling her parents. This is one of the rights of many teenage girls.

Natural methods

These methods include the oldest forms of contraception.

Periodic abstinence Abstinence from intercourse during the time of ovulation. This method is based on calculations using the calendar, plus the rise and fall of the woman's body temperature and an ovulation-prediction kit. Using these indicators, you can decide to abstain from penetrative sex during ovulation. Failure rate is high because ovulation is difficult to be certain of.

Withdrawal Another ancient method with a very high failure rate. The penis is withdrawn just before ejaculation. It doesn't require discussion about methods at clinics and there's no financial cost, but the failure rate is very high because sperm-rich semen comes out before

orgasm and because men often wait too long to withdraw.

Barrier methods

These methods physically block the sperm from reaching the ovum.

Male condom A latex rubber or plastic sheath placed over the erect penis before penetration. It should be lubricated with a water-based lubricant – never use anything oily or greasy – and freed from air so that it doesn't burst inside the vagina. It prevents transmission of sexually transmitted diseases, especially AIDS.

Female condom As effective as the male condom, it's designed to line the inside of the vagina. Consists of a lubricated plastic sheath with an anchoring ring to keep it in place within the vagina and an outer ring that holds the sheath open to allow insertion of the penis. Cumbersome.

Diaphragm and cervical cap A diaphragm is a dome of rubber with a coiled metal spring in its rim. It fits diagonally across the vagina and is used with a spermicidal agent. It must be left in place for six hours after intercourse. The cervical cap is smaller and more rigid and fits over the cervix, where it is held in place by suction. Very efficient.

Hormonal methods

These use hormones (synthetic estrogen and progesterone) to suppress ovulation; they are practically 100 percent effective used properly. They interfere with the

cervical mucus, making it thick and impenetrable to sperm, and thin the uterine lining so that conception cannot occur.

Pill forms include the combined pill, low-dose minipill (no estrogen, only progestogen), hormonal injections, and implants and the post-coital pill. The combined pill must be taken for the full course of 21 or 28 days to be effective. The low-dose minipill is taken continuously.

Injectable contraceptives, ideal for women who have difficulty remembering to take the pill regularly, contain only progestogens and are administered every two or three months.

What are the risks?

A pill containing estrogen may not be appropriate for you if you are overweight, if you smoke, or suffer from diabetes, high blood pressure, a heart condition, deep vein thrombosis, or migraines.

After-sex methods

There are two means of preventing conception after unprotected sex and they must be started within one to five days of intercourse, but they are not recommended as a routine form of birth control.

The hormonal method involves a short high-dose course of the combined "morning after pill" which must be taken within 72 hours. For women who cannot take this pill, a copper-bearing IUD an be inserted within five days of unprotected intercourse; this prevents a possible pregnancy.

Teenage pregnancy

Once you've begun a sexual relationship, there is always a chance of you becoming pregnant, even if you use contraception.

How to tell if you're pregnant

If you have any of the symptoms below, go right to your doctor or family planning clinic and ask for a pregnancy test. You'll need to give them a small sample of your urine. For quicker results, home pregnancy testing kits can be bought from any pharmacy.
● A missed period, if your periods are regular.
● A short, light period at the correct time.
● Swollen tingling breasts and darkening nipples.
● Wanting to pass urine more often.
● More vaginal discharge than usual.
● Feeling really tired.
● Disliking food you liked before.
● A strange taste in your mouth.
● Nausea, vomiting, particularly after a long time without food, such as in the morning.

Telling your parents

● If you find it easier to talk to your mom, tell her first, and ask her to tell your dad.
● It can help if you tell a close relative – someone your parents trust – and take the person along.
● Consider your options before talking to your parents; let them see how responsible you can be.

Girls: telling your partner

If the father wants to be involved but disagrees about the course of action, listen, but explain that the final decision is

yours. If he won't support you, try to get by without him for now; you have enough to worry about.

Boys: getting the news

Try to remember that while you're equally responsible, your girlfriend's burden is infinitely greater. Ultimately you cannot control events, but you'll never have a better opportunity to give your partner your full support.

If you're still in school

If you haven't completed your education but decide to have the baby, you need to consider carefully what your options are.
● Are you above or below the legal age for compulsory schooling? Your school or education authority can advise you on how to continue your education throughout your pregnancy and after the birth.
● You may feel tempted to leave school right away, but try to think of your long-term future before making any rash decisions. You still need qualifications for your career and your self-esteem.

If you're a father

If your girlfriend's pregnant, you'll certainly have views about what your partner should do, even if they're negative.

In most countries you have no legal right to a say in whether she goes ahead with the pregnancy or not. However, this doesn't mean you should be excluded from the discussions. Your attitude and support will count for a lot in helping your

partner to make up her mind. Fathers have rights once the baby's born, and with those rights come all the responsibilities of having a family.

Girls: some of your options

● Getting married: get married to the father and have the baby.
● Live together: live with the father and raise the child together.
● Be a single mom: bring up the child on your own as a single parent.
● Start over: sometimes an abortion is the only answer.
● Family affair: have the baby and stay with your parents, who may be only too glad to help you care for the child.
● Another home: get the baby adopted by a loving family. It's a relief to know your baby will be well cared for.

The right choice for you

Along with your partner, parents, and a close relative, try to talk to a doctor, or a clergyman if you have a religious background.

But in the end, whatever anyone else says, you have to weigh up your future, your strengths, your weaknesses, your ambitions, and the strength of your maternal drive. Only you know how you want your life to be, so only you can make the right decision.

Warning

Don't allow yourself to be forced into a decision you're unhappy with because it seems to be the easiest. You'll always regret it.

Pap smears

Pap smears are important for girls who start having sex in their early teens because the young cervix seems vulnerable to cancerous changes when exposed to semen early in fertile life. The test is simple and quick and results should be available within six weeks.

Cancerous change is even more likely if you have several partners. Promiscuous sex also increases the chance of being infected with genital warts, the virus that also promotes cervical cancers.

alcohol and drugs

More teenagers are drinking and experimenting with drugs, and more and more are battling with alcohol and drug problems. Never be afraid to admit that you need help.

Drugs

When parents ask their children if they take drugs, they're looking for one answer – NO. Some parents don't even get as far as asking. They're not prepared to have any kind of discussion about drugs, except possibly to condemn them out of hand. This is a pity because there could well be a time when you need to talk about drugs to your parents, and not just because they've found out that you've been taking them. It may be that a friend has been taking drugs and you're worried about her health; or another friend may have been caught with drugs and you're frightened about what may happen to him.

The strict approach doesn't work. Being really strict simply means people go to greater lengths to conceal what they're doing. It's human nature – anything that's forbidden is immediately attractive.

Take the initiative

Drugs may be the last thing you want to talk about with your parents, especially if

it means admitting that you've taken them yourself. But for your sake and theirs, it's a good idea to try to take the initiative in starting a dialogue with them about drugs before there's a crisis. Your parents are concerned about your welfare so tell them what you know. Many parents only know scare stories about widely publicized drug-related deaths and jump to the conclusion that so-called soft drugs inevitably lead to hard drugs or believe that all illicit drugs are more harmful than tobacco and alcohol. If your parents are very rigid in their thinking, you may feel inclined to abandon attempts at reasonable discussion and honest behavior. Try to resist this because you'll both lose out in the long run.

Parents and drugs

Some adults are probably as confused and ill-informed as some young people.
● Show your parents the drugs education material you get from school.
● Show them books about drugs.
● Give them leaflets about drugs from nationally recognized agencies such as the National Institutes of Health.

What parents can do

Rather than being judgmental and heavy-handed, there are practical things you can do to help your children:
● Learn about drugs and help your child to learn about them too.
● Think carefully about your views on drugs, and be honest with yourself and your child about your own drug use past and present – be it alcohol, nicotine, tranquilizers, or marijuana.
● Don't be authoritarian; you'll lose your child.
● Know where to get help if it's ever needed.
● Keep drugs in perspective.

Teenage drinking

Alcohol is an intoxicating substance made from fermented starches, and although it gives you an initial lift, it is actually a depressant drug. It slows down responses (affecting coordination) and the way the brain works (affecting judgment), so it makes people clumsy and dopey. It's one of the most widely used drugs, above and below the legal age limit.

The alcohol effect

Drinking alcohol makes people:
● feel like they're having more fun
● feel confident
● feel relaxed and calms their nerves
● feel able to open up and talk more
● let go and lose their inhibitions
● feel they fit socially
● feel really happy and laugh more
● think they have the courage to overcome their fears.

The downside

Drinking too much alcohol always has horrible effects.
● Drinking can make you aggressive and violent. You're more likely to start arguments and pick fights.
● You become uncoordinated and clumsy.
● Too much alcohol gives you double vision and slurred speech.
● Drinking when you're down can make you feel even more depressed.
● Alcohol is loaded with calories. It can make you fat, and it's bad for your skin.
● A bad hangover makes you feel really fragile. Your head pounds and you have an upset stomach.
● Alcohol can damage a man's fertility and potency.

Warning!

Alcohol is responsible for many, many more deaths than hard drugs.

Drug emergencies

Drugs are unpredictable – the same drug can affect different people in different ways. In an extreme case a friend may collapse unconscious after taking a drug. But a drug can also cause a person to become dangerously hot or very drowsy or to have terrifying hallucinations or even a seizure.

Take action

If a friend suffers adverse side effects from taking drugs, it may be frightening for you, but it could be life-threatening for your friend. It's vital to be able to recognize that something is going wrong as well as to know what to do in an emergency – quick action can save lives.
● If you see someone you think has had a bad reaction to a drug, don't hesitate to get help and don't panic.
● If you're in a club, shout for the security staff and ask for someone qualified in first aid.
● If you're not in a club, call an ambulance or, better still, get someone else to make the call while you care for your friend.

Calling an ambulance

Call emergency services, ask for an ambulance, and give the following information as clearly as you can:
● the telephone number you are calling from
● where you are – the name of the club, for example
● what's wrong with your friend: she's very hot or she's collapsed; she's unconscious. Don't be afraid to say that your friend has taken drugs, and preferably name the drug; the information could save her life.

If someone else makes the call, ask him to come back and confirm that it's been done.

Kicking a drug habit

Getting off drugs is difficult and you shouldn't attempt to do it by yourself, but as long as you want to get off you can. Many people before you have gotten off drugs and if you go about it the right way and with the right help you'll succeed too.

Getting help

Find out from a drug help hotline (see p. 567) what services are available in your area; they can advise you on what type of help would be most appropriate. Alternatively, ask your GP to refer you to an appropriate organization. Whatever you choose, remember that all drug agencies and medical services are duty bound to treat your case in complete confidence.

Getting off

Clearing your system can take anything from a few days to a few months, and for safety's sake it must be done under medical supervision. Some drugs can be stopped right away; others, such as barbiturates and tranquilizers, have to be cut down gradually – to stop them suddenly is very dangerous. The first few days are the hardest, so once you're through them hang in there – it will get better, but it takes time.

Staying off

Withdrawal is only half the battle: the toughest part is staying off the drug. Give yourself the best chance:
● Keep yourself busy.
● Stay away from all drugs, and that includes alcohol.
● Avoid situations where there are drugs, and places where you used to go to take drugs and avoid people who take drugs.
● Get support when you feel you might slip back.

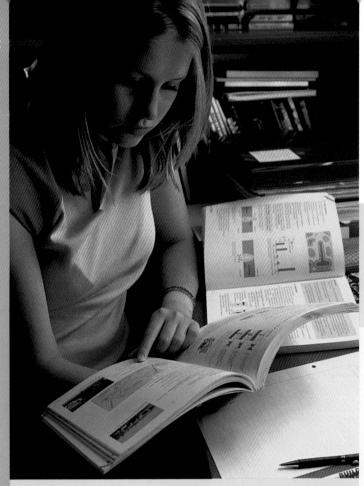

a good education

Education should be a priority in life – it is the best tool a person can have to help them manage their lives, achieve happiness, and enjoy some freedom.

Schoolwork away from school

Most people have to do a great deal of hard work and study for many hours to prepare for exams. You often have several subjects to study, and this work can seem like a real chore. If you don't love information for its own sake, then the most practical way of looking at this work is that it has to be done to give you the freedom to do what you want later on. It's a grind that you just have to go through.

It's good for you to learn determination and develop staying power early in your educational career because you will need a great deal of these qualities later on if you're going to hold down a job successfully in a competitive world. Life beyond school is perhaps not as straightforward as it used to be – even some college graduates with good degrees have difficulty finding jobs.

Fitting it in There's no doubt that while you're having to study in the evenings, you'll sometimes feel jealous and resentful of those of your friends who may have left school, have jobs and money, and go out every night apparently without a care in the world. You're not unique; everyone who studies has experienced this, and many before you have ignored it, continued to study, and become successful.

The right amount of homework Most young people are expected to do about two hours of homework an evening during the week, plus three to four hours on weekends in addition to some extra credit work during vacation periods. Your school should guide you as to the amount of homework you are supposed to do. If very little homework is being given to you, or you're finding that you can do what you're given on your trip home, it's not going to do you much good in the long run. However, if you suddenly realize that you're doing three or four hours a night and more on weekends, you may be overloading yourself or working too slowly. Talk to your parents and teachers about maintaining a balance or possibly learning how to work faster.

Why homework helps

When you do homework, you are understanding and consolidating what you have been taught during the day. Although you may think homework is a chore, it can be the road to great achievements because, in addition to providing the information to do well on exams, it teaches you many personal skills.

● Homework teaches you how to study independently without guidance and how to use your own judgment.

● It teaches you discipline – not only the discipline of routine, but also discipline in the way you have to tackle your work, plan it, present it, and write it out.

● When you have a difficult or long assignment to complete on a deadline, it teaches you persistence and determination – qualities that you need in ample supply if you are to follow a demanding career.

● Learning to manage your schoolwork alongside outside interests and the normal social life that all teenagers need and enjoy actually prepares you for the world of work later. It instills such skills as time management and the ability to handle pressure.

● All of these achievements will bring you a sense of self-respect and confidence, not to mention the pride that your parents and teachers will feel in your successes.

What an education can offer

It wasn't until I was through my adolescent years that I realized that continuing my education offered me the kind of freedom that nothing else in my life possibly could. With qualifications, it was possible to apply for jobs that paid enough so that I didn't have to worry about paying for basic needs like a roof over my head, food, and clothing. **My education made me strong and independent, not just financially, but also emotionally and intellectually**. With it, I had the ability to follow my preferences and exercise my options.

Having an education also means that you will always have interests to fall back on during low or lonely points in your life because it will give you a vast fund of inner resources. It should also mean that you will be able to analyze problems, figure out solutions, and expedite actions at work, in the community, and in your social life.

Making space for home study

Your studies are important and if domestic arrangements allow, you should make sure that the rest of the family understands that keeping up with your schoolwork is one of your main priorities.

You will need:

● **A quiet space**. If you're going to study for long hours alone, it's only fair that you have a room, or at least a space, in your home where you can study, that is quiet, comfortable, and well-heated. This room will probably be your bedroom, but wherever it is, it should be a calm place that is recognized by everyone as being yours and where disturbances from the rest of the family are minimal.
● **Adequate furniture**. You need a minimum of furniture such as a desk, a few drawers or shelves for your files and equipment, and some shelves for your schoolbooks and reference texts.
● A good **reading light** and a **comfortable chair** that gives you good support.

11-18

school pressures

Coping with the demands of school and resisting other temptations is not always easy, but if you persevere you will find it really worthwhile.

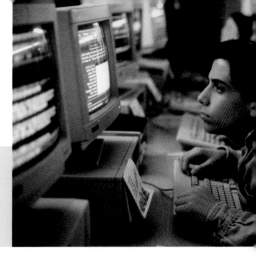

Truancy

Some people play hooky from school because this is their way of rejecting the monotony and the seemingly stupid rules to which they have to conform. But it can also be the case that you're pressured into staying home by one or both of your parents because there's no one else to do the housework or care for small children while they are at work. If you do start to stay at home, you'll fall behind in your schoolwork and going back will become more and more difficult. Once you start, it's an easy step to avoid school and spend your time going out or just staying at home playing music. So if you are getting pressure from your parents, rather than pressure from your own friends, remind your parents that it is actually against the law for them to keep you at home. But if you're staying away from school because you want to, and your parents don't know about it, remember that the school will soon contact your parents and you will be called to account for your absence.

Computers and the Internet – a parent's guide

A research team of psychologists and educators in America found that over-exposure to computers can lead to obesity and long-term emotional damage. Youngsters only really learn through human interaction. Computers simply present them with a huge amount of information they can't properly digest.

The report, which concludes that computers should only be used at middle school level and not by younger children, also warns that there's no real evidence to suggest computers or the Internet help with academic achievement.

Safety and the Internet

Most parents are concerned about the safety of their children using the Internet. Prevention is always better than cure, so parents should look for approved Internet service providers that will carry family friendly safeguards. That way you can ensure your children are logging on in safety. Some, for example, offer a range of censorship levels on the Internet catering for the under-12s, young teens, and older teens. Others automatically filter swear words and sexual references and have an adult to vet messages in the chat room.

Then there are children's e-mail services that come with similar restrictions, including one that only sends e-mails that are first approved by parents.

Everyone knows that teen chat rooms are used by pedophiles. I'm not sure why they are allowed at all.

An educational tool?

Your child may insist that she needs the Internet for school, and there's no denying that it can be a good educational tool. Much is made of the Internet's educational efficacy. She may even claim she can't do her homework without it. But, as one survey found, when children get that much needed computer, a quarter of under-17s log on and head straight to gambling or porn sites. Of the 5 million under-16s who use computers regularly, 1.15 million spend most of their time on-line in chat rooms. So parents are right to be concerned and right to exert some control.

If your child does use a computer at home, make sure that the keyboard and screen are correctly positioned to avoid repetitive strain injury and back strain. Try to limit the hours she spends at the computer and encourage her to take breaks.

Surviving school

Everyone has a few problems at school. There may be teachers you don't get along with and subjects that you don't like. It's possible you may find that certain subjects are beyond you. You may also find that worries about your appearance, social life, and popularity distract you from your schoolwork and sometimes seem more important than your academic abilities.

As you progress through school, and possibly go on to further education, it's sometimes tempting just to give up and have time to enjoy yourself. **Try not to be influenced by friends who've given up studying, who've left school early to get a job**, or feel that marriage and a family at 18 is what's right for them. Remember that they, not you, are the ones who may be narrowing their options for the rest of their lives.

There's no point in saying that it's easy for a young person to survive hard days at school and long hours working at night, especially when the rewards aren't immediately forthcoming or easy to see. It isn't. It takes a lot of staying power, a lot of grit, guts, and determination. It also takes resilience. There will be times when you'll feel depressed and think that it's just not worth the effort. Well, no one can give you the will to keep going and the will to succeed. You're going to have to find that somewhere inside of yourself.

If you feel that your willpower is cracking, have a chat with the teachers you most respect and ask them for tips. Most schools nowadays know that examinations can be especially stressful and will provide review classes and advice on how to manage.

after 18 – what then?

I believe that staying on at school or college after 18 gives you far better career opportunities. But if you do decide to leave, do your best to find a job that interests you.

Continuing your education

Like many other teenagers, I wanted to stop school at 18. I felt a great desire to be independent, to be working, and to be earning money of my own. I wanted to stop studying and start enjoying myself. Fortunately for me, my parents and teachers persuaded me to do otherwise. I went to college after summer break and and then went on to medical school. Thank heavens my parents and teachers won me over.

If you are a teenager who has academic ability, it would be a great shame if you didn't go on to further study, because it's then that you can really start to enjoy complex and more specialized work. Besides

this, your relationships with teachers will become easier, friendlier, and more informal, **you're given responsibility and you're treated as an adult.** In higher education you have more choice – you may go to a community college, a technical school, or a public or private university, where you may study alongside adults. You should be aware that by finishing high school you're preparing for a college career and college life, which will offer independence, living away from home, a new social life, and an open academic curriculum. Don't, therefore, be tempted to leave school on a mere whim.

Thinking about a career

If you know what kind of job or career you want to pursue, get career advice early, and this usually means at around the age of 15 or 16. Schools may begin career guidance at this age, if not earlier, and increasingly there are opportunities for useful work experience with local businesses and professionals arranged through the school.

Career guidance will help you choose the right subjects to study so that a particular career will be open to you. **However, beware of closing off any future options by deciding too early**. You may change your mind later and it will be harder to go back – so

keep your mind open to many possibilities.

The goal of most modern education systems is to provide a well-rounded education for as long as possible and to keep you studying the broadest possible range of subjects. Make sure that your guidance counselors know what kind of career you want to pursue, so that they can put you in touch with the right colleges, universities, or technical schools. They can also provide career information, point you in the direction of relevant internships, and recommend which college prep courses you should take.

Preparing a résumé

If you decide to look for a job, rather than going on to college or a technical training school, get as much help as you can on how to apply for jobs and handle interviews. Some guidance counselors will set up mock interviews, often with professionals or local business people, to help you with the technique. They should also show you how to write good cover letters and fill out application forms. Putting together a lively résumé is an important part of this.

Writing your résumé

Draft your résumé on a computer, if possible, before you even need to think about applying for jobs, and then all you have to do is adapt it to suit your prospective employer.

Obviously, you're not going to have much of a record of employment, although vacation or weekend work is relevant because it shows that you've got some experience with workplace routines. Give the names of two people as references. Most employers ask for this anyway, but line them up beforehand. They need to be people in responsible positions who know you, such as teachers, youth workers, church leaders, or past employers. You should ask their permission first, and let them know that they may be contacted by potential employers.

What goes into a résumé

Your résumé should include the following:
● Your name, address, and telephone number.
● The names of schools and colleges attended and the dates you were there.
● Qualifications – subjects (with grades), plus any other certificates such as music, drama, sports, youth awards.
● If you're looking for a short-term position for a few months before going to college, give details of the course you're going to study and where you'll be studying in addition to the starting date, so that your employer knows exactly how long you're going to be available for work.
● Previous temporary employment, such as weekend, evening, or vacation work, with dates and names of employers.
● Volunteer work, including any community work, fund-raising, or amateur arts involvement, such as membership in a drama or dance group or orchestra.
● All your interests – don't leave any out. Even playing computer games can count because it shows that you're familiar with computers and probably have quick reflexes.
● Future training or education plans. If you're taking a year off before going to college, explain this.

Going to interviews

It's exciting but nerve-racking to go to your first job interview, but you can feel confident by following a few simple rules. (These apply equally to going for an interview at a college.)
● When you get invited for an interview, write as soon as possible to confirm that you can be there on the day and at the time requested. If it's difficult, be open about it, and ask for another appointment. Employers and colleges realize that people may have commitments.
● **Find out as much as you can about the company (or college) beforehand** so that you can tailor your answers. Almost all interviewers will ask why you want to join their organization.
● Go to bed early the night before, and figure out what you're going to wear in advance so that you're not tired or rushed in the morning. Try to look smart, but not flashy.
● Plan how to get to the interview in time, and leave plenty of time so that you're not late – this gives a bad first impression. However, in case you're let down by public transportation, make sure you have the telephone number so you can let them know.
● Don't worry about being nervous; the interviewer will expect it and a good one will try to put you at your ease. Sit down when you're asked. Always refer to your interviewer as Mr. A, Mrs. B, Ms. C, or Miss D unless you're invited to use first names.
● When you answer questions, don't just answer yes or no. Enlarge on what you're asked. Speak clearly and look the interviewer in the eye. Don't forget to smile.
● **Don't be afraid to ask questions** – most interviewers will ask you if there is anything you want to know, usually toward the end of the interview. If it hasn't been made clear or you're not sure, ask the interviewer to confirm the salary, and inform you about possible overtime or weekend work, as well as about vacations.
● You may be offered a job on the spot. If you're undecided, ask for time to think about it, even if it's just overnight. Go home and talk to your parents or teachers so that you can decide calmly.

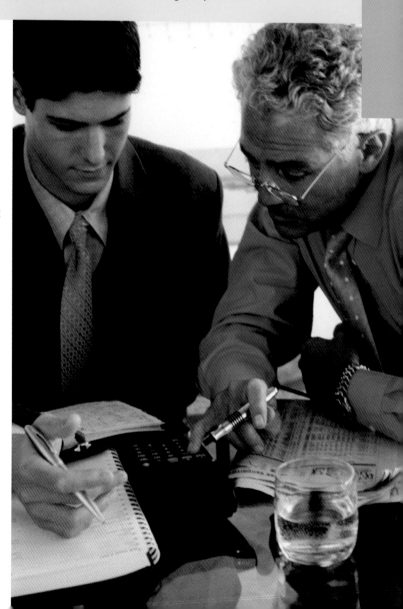

FOCUS
on pregnancy and birth

If you are waiting for everything to be just right before you have your baby, you might as well give up now and take up a hobby instead. It's rare for a couple to feel that the perfect moment has arrived to have a child, but now that men and women have control over their fertility, it gives time for consideration.

WHAT AGE IS BEST FOR HAVING A BABY?

Many women are delaying pregnancy until their 30s and even 40s. This is no more hazardous than being in your 20s as long as you are fit and healthy. Whatever your age, you are likely to have a normal pregnancy and birth, although problems such as infertility and chromosomal defects – for example, Down syndrome – do become more frequent with the increasing age of both parents. Tests for chromosomal abnormalities are always offered to older women.

WHEN DO I STOP CONTRACEPTION?

If you use barrier methods, such as condoms or a diaphragm, you can safely conceive as soon as you stop using them. But most doctors prefer that you have at least one normal period after ceasing other forms of contraception before you start trying to conceive. This allows your

First signs of pregnancy

If you are planning a pregnancy and miss your period, you may suspect that you are pregnant. You may not notice any other changes other than the missed period at first, but an increase in hormonal activity will confirm your pregnancy with one or more of the following physical signs.
• A feeling of nausea at any time.
• A change in taste – you may suddenly be unable to tolerate alcohol or coffee, for example.
• A preference for certain foods, sometimes close to a craving.
• A metallic taste in your mouth.
• Changes in your breasts; they may feel tender and tingly.
• A need to urinate more frequently.
• Fatigue at any time of the day; you may even feel faint or dizzy too.
• Increase in normal vaginal discharge.
• Your emotions swing unpredictably.

metabolic functions to return to normal.

If you've been on the pill, the best plan is for you to stop taking it three months before conception. A month would do, as long as you have a normal period before you conceive.

If you have an intrauterine device (IUD), the same time frame applies – have it removed three months before you intend to get pregnant. Have at least one normal period before stopping all contraception – use a barrier method in the meantime.

DO I NEED GENETIC COUNSELING?

Seek advice and have tests in advance if a genetic disorder runs in your family. Examples of heritable conditions include cystic fibrosis, muscular dystrophy, and hemophilia.

What happens in counseling?

The counselor explains the condition and your family background and shows you the pattern of inheritance through past generations. Not all carriers of a defective gene get the condition: if it's recessive it can be masked by a healthy version, whereas a dominant gene will always show up. With a dominant gene the chances of your baby being affected are one in two, with a recessive gene they are one in four.

HOW DO I PREPARE FOR PREGNANCY?

When you make the decision to become parents, it makes sense to prepare yourselves in advance. To have a healthy baby, research shows that by far the most important factors are your own health and nutrition. As a prospective mother, the healthier you are, the more easily your body will be able to cope with the stresses and strains of pregnancy. But fitness and lifestyle may also change a man's ability to father a child, by affecting sperm production. It's best if you both try to think about your general health and lifestyle at least three months before you're planning to stop contraception.

I'm not in the business of using scare tactics to get a message across, but there are facts you should know for the sake of your baby.

Must I stop smoking?

Smoking is one of the greatest threats to the health of your unborn baby and the major cause of avoidable health problems. The associated risks include miscarriage and stillbirth, damage to the placenta, a low birthweight baby who fails to thrive and an increased chance of fetal abnormalities. Smoking can cause a low sperm count, and a man who continues to smoke while his partner is pregnant risks damaging the health of his unborn baby via passive smoking.

What about alcohol?

Alcohol is a poison that can damage the sperm and ovum (egg) before conception as well as harm the developing embryo. The main risks to the unborn baby are mental retardation, retarded growth, and damage to the brain and nervous system – well documented as fetal alcohol syndrome. Alcohol can also cause stillbirth. Research suggests that the effect of alcohol is variable – the only certainty is that there will be no effect if alcohol is avoided.

And drugs?

Over-the-counter medicines should only be taken when necessary and social drugs should **definitely** be cut out before you conceive. Marijuana interferes with the normal production of male sperm, and the effects take three to nine months to wear off. Hard drugs such as cocaine, heroin, and morphine can damage the chromosomes in the ovum and sperm, leading to abnormalities. It is best to avoid taking anything during pregnancy unless your doctor determines that the benefit to you outweighs any risk to the fetus.

SHOULD I CHANGE MY DIET ONCE I'M PREGNANT?

Your body uses up a lot of energy during pregnancy, and you need to eat well to fuel your requirements and those of your growing baby. Pregnancy is not the time to go on a diet, but you should also forget the myth about "eating for two"; the rule is to eat to satisfy your hunger and no more. Later in pregnancy you may find you simply can't take in much food at any one time, so eat little and often. Keep supplies of healthy snacks such as dried fruit, rice cakes, crispbreads, and hard fruits in your bag, car, or office, and low-fat cheese and yogurt, raw vegetables, fresh fruit, and unsweetened fruit juice in the fridge at home.

What should I eat?
To provide for your baby's needs as well as your own, note the following tips about diet.
● Complex carbohydrates such as pasta, potatoes, or legumes (beans and lentils) are needed for energy.
● Protein is needed for your baby's growth. Eat fish and poultry, dairy products, wholegrain cereals, seeds, and legumes.
● Don't cut out fats altogether, but don't eat too much of them. You'll get enough from dairy products and normal cooking methods.
● Get vitamin C daily from raw fresh fruit and vegetables, and the B complex from whole grains, nuts, and legumes, green vegetables, dairy products, eggs, oily fish, and meat.
● Iron maintains red blood cells; it's found in red meat, fish, egg yolks, apricots, and cereals.

What about morning sickness?
Though called morning sickness, nausea can occur at any time of day. To combat it many women find that small, frequent snacks help

Is it safe to exercise?

Both you and your baby benefit from exercise: your blood starts circulating freely, there's a blast of oxygen to your baby's brain, exercise hormones such as endorphins give you both a wonderful high, and your baby loves the swaying motion. Exercise increases your strength, suppleness, and stamina, which will make pregnancy easier and equip you for the rigors of labor.

But exercise in pregnancy is not just about being physically fit. It helps you to understand your body, to believe in its power, and it gives you the key to relaxation so that you can handle fatigue and prepare yourself for the birth.

Whole body exercise
Try to incorporate some exercise into your day, beginning gradually, at a pace that is comfortable. Always stop if you get out of

breath or feel pain. Whole body exercise is best since it tones your heart and lungs, so walking and swimming are excellent. Dancing is good, too, as long as it's not too energetic. Yoga is ideal because it stretches tight muscles and joints and also relieves tension. Yoga methods can also help with labor and pain relief.

Exercises to avoid
Pregnancy is not a time to start learning an energetic contact sport. However, you can continue sporting activities for a while if you're already fit and play often. Don't engage in sports like skiing, cycling, or horse riding after 20 weeks because balance may become a problem at that time. Take it easy with very energetic sports like tennis or raquetball, and don't do heavy workouts at the gym, especially tough abdominal exercises.

during the difficult weeks. Here are some snack foods that you can prepare at home or have at your workplace to damp down the rising nausea during your working day.
● Raw vegetables such as carrots, celery, tender young beans, peas from the pod, tomatoes.
● Slices of whole grain bread dried in the oven.
● Sandwiches made with whole grain bread and hard cheese.
● Nuts, raisins, and dried apricots.

● Fruit cake (preferably made with whole wheat flour and added wheatgerm).
● Crisp green apples.
● Water crackers and cottage cheese.
● Fresh fruit juices.
● Commercial muesli bars.
● Unflavored natural yogurt with honey.
● Herbal teas.
● Milkshakes made with skim milk.
● Juicy fruits such as peaches, plums, and pears.

Growing bigger

Having a baby growing inside you is like being part of a real life miracle. Sometimes you'll pat your tummy and feel you can hardly believe your child is in there – it seems so amazing and extraordinary. Find out as much as you can about how your baby develops. It will help you both to understand the minor discomforts and ups and downs that a pregnant woman feels.

FOLLOWING YOUR PREGNANCY
No part of a woman's body escapes when she's carrying a baby, and you and your partner need to keep that in mind. For instance, tender breasts that are getting ready for breast-feeding need to be treated gently by a father when he caresses them; the growing uterus pressing on your internal organs means that you must never be too far from a bathroom during the last three months of pregnancy. The guide that follows is a brief outline of the complex changes going on inside your body.

What's happened by three months?
The first three months of pregnancy (the first trimester) are tremendously important in laying the foundations of your baby's healthy development, although there are few visible signs of your baby's phenomenal growth.

You
- You'll really start to gain weight; any morning sickness will soon disappear.
- The uterus is rising out of the pelvis and can be felt.
- The risk of miscarriage is almost zero now.
- Your heart is working flat out and will continue to do so right up to labor.

Your baby
- She has a fully formed body, complete with fingers, toes, and ears.
- Her eyes move, though her eyelids are still closed.
- Her body is covered with fine hair.
- She wriggles if poked – her muscles are growing.

What's happened by six months?
The period from about the third to the sixth month (the second trimester) is when pregnancy sickness ends, your baby really grows, and you begin to feel her move. You're brimming with energy, vitality, and well-being.

You
- You're putting on about 1lb (0.5kg) of weight a week.

Sex in pregnancy

Many women say that sex when they were pregnant was the best they've ever had. There are a lot of reasons for this.

- Physical factors: the blood supply to all the pelvic organs increases and pregnancy hormones make the vulva more erogenous.

- The breasts are more sensitive as they prepare for lactation and become more easily aroused.

- A woman who's relaxed and happy about her pregnancy may feel such a surge of love for her partner that she becomes passionately responsive to him.

You can have sex all the way through pregnancy as long as you're comfortable. However sexual desire varies and there is nothing wrong with you if yyou don't want to have sex. By the way – you might like to know that your baby feels your

orgasm with you and enjoys it just as much. Some women are scared that sex will crush the baby. This is not possible because the baby is suspended in the amniotic sac and surrounded by amniotic fluid, which cushions it from any kind of bumping and bruising.

On the other hand, it is not safe to have sex if you experience either of the following symptoms:

- If bleeding occurs – in such a case, consult your doctor.
- If you have blood-stained vaginal discharge, heralding the onset of labor, or if your water breaks.

Also, if you have had a miscarriage in the past, seek medical advice about having sex. You may be advised to abstain during the early months of pregnancy.

- Your uterus is a good 2in (5cm) above the pelvis.
- You may have bouts of indigestion.
- From 18 weeks or so, you'll feel the baby move.

Your baby
- Her hearing is acute, she can recognize your voice.
- She's becoming better proportioned – her body is catching up with her head.
- She's well muscled but thin.
- Her lungs are maturing fast.

What's happened by nine months (full term)?
The final 12 weeks or so of pregnancy (the third trimester) are when the baby puts on fat in preparation for birth, and the brain and lungs mature in preparation for independent life.

You
- You may feel a "lightening" as your baby's head drops into the pelvis.
- It's more difficult to find a comfortable position for sleep.
- You visit the prenatal clinic every week.
- Your breasts secrete a clear-colored nutritious liquid – colostrum.

Your baby
- She weighs about 6–8lb (2.7–3.5kg) and she measures 14–15in (35–38cm) in length.
- Her head is most likely "engaged," lying just on top of your cervix (although 15% of first babies are not engaged at onset of labor).
- The placenta is 8–10in (20–25cm) across and there are 40oz (1.1 liters) of amniotic fluid.
- Her breasts may be swollen due to the action of your hormones.

COPING WITH FATIGUE
Fatigue is a periodic problem during pregnancy, especially during the first three months and the last six to eight weeks. Its extent may take you by surprise – it's the kind of tiredness that makes you feel you don't even have the energy to blink, but just stare straight ahead. You're sleepy in the early stages of pregnancy because you're sedated by the high levels of progesterone. Your metabolism speeds up to deal with the demands of your baby and the extra work all your organs are called on to do. Later on in pregnancy you're tired because your whole body is working flat out 24 hours a day, and you're carrying extra weight around that puts a strain on your heart, lungs, and muscles. Help yourself by resting when you can, putting your feet up when you sit, and going to bed early at least three times a week.

The birth

These days it's possible to plan exactly the kind of birth experience you want because most doctors, obstetricians, and midwives are well aware that a relaxed, confident, informed mother is more likely to have an enjoyable labor and a successful delivery.

MAKING A BIRTH PLAN

Making a plan for your baby's birth will help to ensure you are actively involved in the way he is born and what happens to you as a family after the birth. By carefully considering all your preferences, and by discussing them with your birth attendant and partner, you will be able to establish a bond of trust and so create a happier and more comfortable birth environment. The following are some of the issues you might want to think about.

BIRTH PARTNERS

Every woman going into labor should have with her someone other than medical and nursing professionals to offer support, comfort, and encouragement. The best assistant is your partner, especially if he has attended your prenatal classes with you, and knows how to help you through each stage of labor, but it doesn't have to be him. Your mother, sister, or best friend would be an excellent choice, particularly if she's had children of her own and can stay calm if things do not go quite as planned. Whoever you choose should be someone that you trust to make decisions on your behalf, if necessary, so make sure they know your views inside out. It can be a help for your birth partner to deal with hospital staff – you may not want your concentration disturbed.

STAYING ACTIVE

The most important thing for a mother in early labor is to keep active. Moving around is a great help in getting and keeping labor established, and most women find it easier to cope with contractions if they're upright. If you have a contraction, just stop and breathe through it. As labor progresses, keeping upright as much as possible helps the contractions work with, not against, gravity.

PAIN RELIEF

For many women, particularly first-time mothers, anticipation of their baby's birth may be overshadowed by worry about pain during labor. Labor invariably involves some level of pain, but you can build up your confidence by preparing for the intensity of contractions, trying to understand your own limits of pain tolerance, and by learning about different methods of pain relief. View the pain as a positive element of labor – each contraction brings the birth of your baby nearer.

Find out as much as you can about the types of pain relief available. Have a discussion with your doctor or midwife and then outline your choices in your birth plan. Be prepared for your plan to change if any complications arise.

Regional anesthetics

These remove sensation from part of your body by blocking the transmission of pain from nerve fibers. The most widely used form of this type of anesthesia is the epidural. This prevents pain from spreading out from your uterus by acting as a "nerve block" in your spine. After an injection of local anesthetic in your back to numb it, the anesthesiologist inserts a fine, hollow needle into the epidural space – the region around the spinal cord – and the anesthetic is injected through this.

A well-managed epidural removes pain from your waist to your knees but does not affect your baby. You will, however, feel pressure and be able to push. An epidural is recommended if you have preeclampsia or severe asthma, or if labor is difficult or a forceps delivery is likely.

Narcotics

The most commonly used is demerol, which is derived from morphine and is given by injection in the first stage of labor. It dulls the sensation of pain but also reduces consciousness and tends to make labor longer. Although demerol is used most often in US hospitals, it is being phased out and replaced with other narcotics such as nubain.

Lamaze

The goal of this widely used method of breathing exercises is to avoid unnecessary medical or technological intervention during

Stages of labor

Labor can start in a variety of ways, but once it's really under way, you will know all about it. If you're unsure, you probably aren't quite in labor.

There are various signs that labor is starting.
• **The bloody show** – brownish/pink discharge that indicates that the mucus plug that has sealed the cervix during pregnancy has come away in readiness for labor.
• **Water breaks** – sometimes the amniotic sac ruptures before labor starts, causing fluid to leak slowly or in a gush from your vagina.
• **Contractions start** – the muscular tightenings of the uterus – contractions – gradually start to pull open the cervix. If they're coming regularly every five minutes, you're in labor.

There are three stages of labor.
• **First stage** – during this stage the cervix opens (dilates) to allow the baby's head to pass through. Before it dilates, the cervix becomes thinned and softened and is gradually pulled up by the contracting uterine muscles. When the cervix is about 4in (10cm) in diameter it is said to be fully dilated. This is the completion of the first stage of labor.

• **Second stage** – this is the expulsive stage, when you push your baby out through the birth canal. It lasts from the full dilation of the cervix until the baby is born. The uterine contractions are 60–90 seconds long at this time and occur at two- to four-minute intervals. As your baby is gradually pushed down your birth canal, you should try to use gravity as much as possible to help, so keep as upright as you can. The first sign that the baby is coming is the bulging of your anus and perineum. With each contraction, more and more of the baby's head appears at your vaginal opening, until the head doesn't slip back at all between contractions. This is known as crowning. If you take your time and let your vagina stretch slowly, you may avoid a tear. As the head emerges, the midwife or doctor will ask you to pant, not push. With the next contractions, she will gently turn the baby so that the shoulders can be born one at a time and the rest of your baby's body can slide out. Now is the moment for which you've waited nine months.
• **Third stage** – once your baby has been born, your uterus will rest for about 15 minutes. It will then start to contract again in order to expel the placenta.

childbirth. The technique uses various patterns of controlled chest breathing, a light massage of the abdomen, and visual concentration on an object. This distraction method is said to decrease the perception of pain or discomfort.

Breathing
Relaxing your body and focusing on your breathing will help alleviate your anxiety and let you ride out your contractions. Practice before the birth with your birth partner.

Massage
This is a wonderful way of getting reassurance from your partner while relieving discomfort, whether you're lying, standing, or squatting. It can be particularly helpful if you have backache during labor, which most women do. Techniques such as firm stroking, rubbing, or

kneading, on your temples, shoulders, neck scalp, feet, hands, or at other tension points are soothing and relaxing during labor. Let your birth partner know what feels good to you.

Acupuncture
I would recommend using acupuncture for pain relief in labor only if you have found it successful in the past. For some women it will undoubtedly work, but the acupuncturist must be practiced at giving pain relief in labor. It is important that you clear acupuncture treatment in labor with your doctor and hospital well before labor. Note that alternative methods of pain relief, such as acupuncture, may not be covered under your insurance.

EPISIOTOMY
This is a surgical cut to enlarge the vaginal outlet

at delivery and is the most commonly performed operation in the West. Episiotomies are used in order to avoid tears, which have ragged edges and are difficult to stitch together and were believed to heal less well. This is not the case. Tears can be avoided if a woman is encouraged to stop pushing while the head is being born, and is allowed to let her uterus ease the head gradually rather than quickly. When the head delivers too fast, an episiotomy may be performed because the perineum is thought to be under stress. If you wish to avoid an episiotomy, let your doctor know that don't want one unless absolutely necessary.

Help yourself through contractions
• Relax as much as possible, especially during contractions; concentrate on the out-breath as you exhale, and drop your shoulders.
• Keep moving around between contractions, then get into a position that feels right. These may include a supported squat, leaning against your partner, on all fours, or kneeling down and leaning forward on a pillow placed on a chair.
• Try counting backward from 100 through a contraction – the concentration needed takes your mind off the pain. Keep your eyes open to externalize the pain; focus on something in the room such as a picture.
• Take sips of flat mineral water from a sponge if your mouth is dry, and ask your partner to massage your back during a contraction.
• Don't be afraid to say – or shout – anything you want during labor; no one will hold it against you after the birth.

Water labor

Although still somewhat unusual, water labor is a growing trend. Many women are now using water to help them manage pain during the first stage of labor. Using a birthing pool during labor can help to relax you and reduce the pain of contractions. You are less likely to be subjected to intervention procedures because of imposed time limits. This in turn means that you will have the time needed for your tissues and muscles to open and stretch. Ideally, the water should be at

body temperature – any warmer and you may be at risk of dehydration. Some hospitals and birthing centers now have water labor facilities but they can be difficult to reserve in advance. You may have to hope one is free on the day. A water labor is not for everyone, but if it suits you, it is a good way your partner can share in the intimacy. There are companies that have portable pools for rent which can be used in some birthing centers.

"happiness
is about
coming to
terms with
reality"

life stages: 18 to 40 years

Living in the 21st century is about as stressful a form of life as you can think of. Human beings are not very well designed to live under such conditions, for every aspect of modern life has an element of stress. We live in a success oriented society in which it's impossible to escape from competitiveness and the desire to succeed. And during our 20s and 30s we may be particularly exposed to stress as we struggle to establish ourselves in careers and relationships.

Although many people still think of stress as wholly negative, it can, in fact, be either positive or negative. There is evidence to show that a moderate degree of stress can be good for us – it improves performance, efficiency, productivity, and many of us thrive on it. Indeed, there are some people who *need* stress and function at maximum efficiency when they are under pressure. But they are rare. For most of us, if stress goes beyond a certain point, everything disintegrates and this can lead to both mental and physical illness. It is, therefore, very important for all of us to come to terms with what causes us stress, to recognize the part that it plays in our health or, conversely, ill-health, and finally to try and find out how we can get rid of it or manage it.

Coping with stress

Actually taking action is one of the best ways of handling stress; doing something, doing almost anything. I have found one of the best ways to manage stress is to start analyzing the problem on paper. Define it, write down as many solutions as you can think of and select the most realistic two or three. Opt for one of these if you can and write down an action plan, taking into account each step you need to take to bring about a solution. Even just the act of writing everything down should help you see your problem in proportion and will scale down the stress-producing difficulty. Follow your plan through and you should feel less stressed. If you don't or it doesn't work, you can always try one of your other options.

Learn to love yourself

One of the greatest causes of stress and mental ill-health can be a disparity between expectation and achievement, between hope and actual result. Happiness and mental well-being are not about playing out a fictitious role conjured up by authors and journalists. Happiness is about coming to terms with reality. One of the most important parts of that is learning what you want to do, deciding to do it to the best of your ability, and not feeling inadequate because it doesn't happen to coincide with what you think you ought to do. Forget what you ought to do. Learn to live with yourself. Most important, learn to love yourself for who you are.

We don't stop developing at the age of 18. Most adults learn that the real growth period for us as people only begins after this age and that the achievement of true happiness may take another three decades of hard work. Going through a period of self-analysis, choice, and possibly change of lifestyle requires courage, so you must be brave. In the pages that follow I offer guidelines where appropriate, advice where I feel there may be a need, and strategies for dealing with potentially difficult situations.

Beating stress

● Make a list of your three best attributes. Do people describe you, for example, as generous, affectionate, and trustworthy? Carry the list with you and read it to yourself whenever you find yourself thinking unpleasant thoughts.

● Keep a list of affirmations to say to yourself when under pressure. It's amazing – chanting simple phrases such as "I really can handle this" can divert the stress response.

● Keep a daily diary of all the small, pleasant events that happen and talk about them with your partner or a friend each day. Write down what you did for enjoyment or fun. Look back at your diary every week to see what progress you have made and to make plans for what you intend to achieve next week.

" few couples
realize the
impact
a new baby
will have on
their lives "

"it's never too early to start taking care of your heart"

mental fitness is just as important as physical fitness

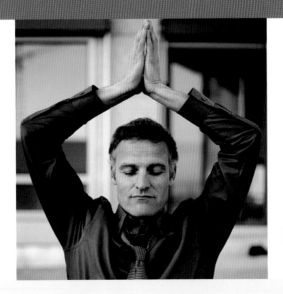

realize you can't totally control the world around you

healthy heart, healthy body

It's never too early to start taking care of your heart. Take action now to improve your general level of fitness and control your weight and you will have fewer health problems later in life.

Stop drastic dieting and start eating

The amount of energy you burn daily, besides any specific activities you undertake, is variable and you can make a positive impact on it. You can also do the opposite.

The popularity in the last few years of microdiets (diets where you consume only some 350 calories a day) has prompted concern that you end up losing too much lean muscle mass rather than mainly fat. But the most striking argument against them is their effect on your basal metabolism. If you put your body on a starvation diet, it thinks it really is starving and takes appropriate action. This is akin to hibernation, although not quite as drastic. The body simply slows down and burns about 15–20 percent less energy. You will still lose weight on these diets, but not in a healthy way. Nor do you learn anything about making the important lifestyle and behavioral changes needed to lose weight and keep it off in the long term.

A sensible eating pattern

Instead of starving yourself, eat a sensible amount each day of different kinds of foods – that is, very little fat, salt, sugar, red meat, and processed foods, but moderate amounts of poultry, eggs, and fish, and lots of fresh fruit and vegetables, beans, legumes, brown rice, and oats. By eating your food in six smaller installments, you will find that you burn off more calories than if you ate the same food as three larger meals. Eating little and often can also help regulate your glucose levels and appetite. And remember that if you don't exercise, you will lose weight more slowly, so get regular exercise.

Health checks

Women

● There are national screening programs for cervical cancer and breast cancer. Every woman from age 20 onward should do regular breast self examinations (see p. 243).
● To help prevent cervical cancer, any woman who becomes sexually active should be having regular pap tests.

Men

● Testicular cancer is the most common form of cancer in young men in the US and it is the most frequent cause of cancer-related deaths in males aged 15–35.
● The number of cases has tripled in the past 20 years.
● It's easily treated and if caught early, is nearly always curable. Every male from age 15 and up should do regular testicular self-examinations (see p. 264).
● More than 50 percent of testicular cancer sufferers consult their doctors too late, after the cancer has started to spread. This makes it more difficult to treat successfully and the side effects of the disease and the treatment become more unpleasant.

Keep your heart healthy

Heart disease is the biggest killer in the US. It's never too early to start taking care of your heart. Lack of physical activity is probably the most common risk factor for heart disease in the US. Seven out of 10 people in the US don't get enough regular exercise to achieve health benefits to protect their heart. You should aim for at least 30 minutes of activity that makes you slightly breathless three times a week.

Exercise has direct benefits for your heart.
● It helps improve your cholesterol levels.
● It helps prevent blood clotting.
● It helps lower blood pressure and prevent high blood pressure.
● It helps you reach and maintain a healthy weight.
● It helps your recovery after you have had a heart attack.

The risk raisers
● Physical inactivity.
● Smoking.
● High blood pressure.
● High cholesterol.
● Obesity.
● Drinking too much alcohol.

Cut out: smoking
Giving up smoking has immediate benefits for your heart.
● Within 20 minutes blood pressure and pulse rates fall.
● Within eight hours carbon monoxide

levels drop back to normal and the oxygen level goes back up to normal.
● Within 24 hours the risk of a heart attack decreases.
● Within 72 hours lung airways relax, making it easier to breathe and the volume of air the lungs can hold increases.
● Within one to three months circulation improves and lung function improves by up to a third.

Cut down: alcohol
Too much alcohol can damage your heart muscle, increase your blood pressure, and also lead to weight gain. Heavier drinking can contribute to heart ailments, including high blood pressure and stroke. Professional women are particularly prone to drinking too much – they're three times as likely to drink more than the recommended amount of alcohol than women in unskilled, manual jobs.

Cut down: salt
People who have a high salt intake seem more likely to have high blood pressure. Most people eat more salt than they need. On average we eat nine grams a day and the recommended maximum is six grams. The body only needs one gram.

Choose low-salt or reduced-salt foods, limit smoked foods, and try to eat as much unprocessed food as possible. Around three-quarters of the salt we eat comes from processed foods.

To cut down on salt, first try not to add it to your food at the table. Later, try cooking without adding any salt. Within a month your palate will have adjusted and you won't like salty foods.

Cut down: cholesterol
Lowering cholesterol levels by just 1 percent reduces the risk of coronary heart disease by 2 to 3 percent. To reduce your cholesterol level, cut right down on saturated fats such as fatty meats and dairy and replace them with small amounts of polyunsaturated fats and monounsaturated fats – for example, olive, grapeseed, and canola oil, nuts, avocados. Base meals on starchy foods (bread, pasta, rice, cereals, and potatoes) and remember to eat five or more fruits and vegetables each day.

● Foods such as oats, lentils, beans, and fruit contain soluble fiber and this is useful for mopping up cholesterol.
● A bowl of oatmeal made with skim milk every morning can help reduce your cholesterol levels.
● Garlic is useful too. Large doses of garlic (seven cloves a day) may help to prevent blood clots from forming. It may also lower total cholesterol levels.
● A portion of oily fish – mackerel, salmon, sardines – at least twice a week lowers triglycerides and reduces your risk of a heart attack.

Fit muscles help weight loss

When you are overweight, the problem is not as simple as you may at first think. Not only are you over your ideal weight, but you also probably have a disproportionate amount of fat instead of muscle. The point is this: when you diet, the more muscle you lose as a percentage of your body weight, the less energy you have and this leads to a further imbalance between fat and muscle.

However, if you combine a sensible diet with exercise, you will not only build up your muscle mass and tone up muscles that are out of condition,

you will also raise your metabolic rate and burn up more energy regardless of what you are doing. And by exercising, whether it's brisk walking, dancing, or marathon running, you will burn up energy over and above your basal metabolic requirements, which means that, once your weight is satisfactory, you can consume more calories and still stay at your ideal weight.

Exercise is therefore the key to weight loss. None of this is new information but it's surprising how easily it can be overlooked.

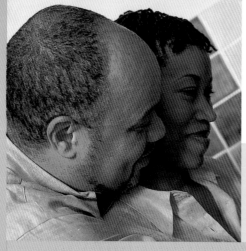

common worries

Both men and women in this age group may suffer anxieties about their appearance and their sexual performance, but there are ways you can help yourself.

Hair loss in men

Thinning hair can be a major cause of anxiety to men in this age group. Male baldness is an inherited condition and the most common form of alopecia (hair loss). The process starts when normal hair at the temples and crown is replaced by fine, downy hair. The hairline then gradually recedes. Only a trained dermatologist can determine if the hair follicle is so badly damaged that hair loss is permanent.

Over the years a number of different strategies have been used to help balding men with varying degrees of success. Here is a brief summary of those currently available.

Hairpieces

This is the safest and least painful way (in terms of health and money) to camouflage hair loss. Some hairpieces can be permanently attached to the head, either by being tied to existing hairs or by being sewn on to the scalp. The latter can cause infection and is not recommended

for that reason. The only possible side effect of hairpieces is that people may be sensitive to the adhesive that is sometimes used.

Hair weaving

This is a nonsurgical procedure that adds replacement hair to existing hair in order to cover bald patches. The new hair is braided strand by strand on to the edges of the hair. Hair weaving requires maintenance and careful cleansing.

Hair implant

This is a quasi-surgical procedure where strips of hair are attached to the scalp in the form of surgical threads implanted in the balding area. The implants are usually synthetic so a blow-dryer shouldn't be used.

Hair transplant

This is a surgical procedure that generally results in the permanent replacement of hair – though even when well established it is not as luxurious as the hair you've lost.

Plugs of hair are cut from remaining healthy hair on the sides and back of the head and implanted in bald spots. This hair normally falls out after transplant but is replaced by new hair. Quite a few hair follicles must be transplanted at the same session and the process needs to be repeated for bald areas to be covered.

Medication

During research on drugs to control high blood pressure, it was discovered that minoxidil promoted hair growth, and it is now available for this purpose. It has to be applied to the scalp twice daily for a minimum of four months for any effect to be noticeable. Treatment has to be continued or hair loss will recur.

A second drug, finasteride, used for treating benign enlargement of the prostate gland, has been found to help male baldness by reducing the effect of the enzyme alpha reductase which is thought to cause baldness.

Choosing celibacy

There is so much emphasis on sex and having successful sex, but it must be said that there is nothing wrong in not wanting sex at all. Sexual desire varies from none to

a lot, and all variations are normal. **There is absolutely nothing wrong with you if you don't want to have sex**. If you really don't want it, and are upset by having sex, be plain-

spoken about it and let it be known. Sex is supposed to be a pleasure, not a burden. If it is onerous and distasteful, don't have sex and don't feel guilty about it.

A woman's failure to orgasm

Probably the most common sexual problem seen in women is that of difficulty in reaching an orgasm (climax). There are two main groups: the first group consists of women who have never achieved orgasm, while the second group are women who have had orgasms but only in special circumstances.

Just because a woman is unable to reach a climax does not mean that she is frigid. She may well have a strong sex drive and be capable of falling in love. If a woman often fails to reach a climax, she is likely to become disappointed and eventually may lose interest in sex entirely.

A woman may find difficulty in reaching a climax if she is uncertain about her commitment toward her partner, or if she is frightened of losing control. If a woman has never reached a climax, this may just be due to the fact she has not had sufficient sexual stimulation for orgasm to take place. If she has had a lot of stimulation and she is still unable to reach a climax, either during sexual intercourse or by stimulation of the clitoris, then this is a problem which needs attention.

It has been found that it is easier for a woman to reach a climax on her own than when her partner is present. So to begin with, having ensured that she is alone and will not be disturbed, she should stimulate her clitoris by masturbation. She may well feel that it is wrong to reach an orgasm this way, but it is important that the woman should reach her first climax by whatever means possible. As soon as she is highly aroused she should contract her stomach muscles since this will help her reach a climax.

Achieving orgasm

She should continue with these masturbation sessions until she is able to achieve an orgasm fairly easily. At this stage, sexual intercourse may take place, but the woman should on no account make any attempt to achieve orgasm while the penis is in the vagina. Once the man has ejaculated, he should stimulate her clitoris so that, in her own time, she too can reach orgasm. She should concentrate only on her own sexual sensations.

There are many women who can reach orgasm by direct stimulation of the clitoris but, in spite of finding sexual intercourse an enjoyable experience, are yet unable to reach a climax with the penis in the vagina.

When there is a problem of this type, the couple should enjoy some foreplay until the woman is aroused, and at this point the man inserts his penis into the vagina and starts thrusting slowly. Then he withdraws the penis, and after a few minutes, he penetrates the vagina again.

If the woman is still unable to achieve orgasm by this method, then the man should stimulate his partner's clitoris with his finger between one insertion and the next. Again the man should wait until the woman is strongly aroused before penetrating again. As she comes closer to orgasm, she quickens her thrusting movements to help her reach climax.

Self-stimulation

If all these measures fail, then the woman should stimulate her own clitoris during sexual intercourse. She stops stimulating herself as she nears orgasm and finishes off by thrusting. Provided that care is taken in following these instructions, there is every likelihood that there will be a successful outcome. In a small number of cases where this is not sufficient, it is recommended that the couple consult an experienced therapist after discussion with their general practitioner.

It is a tremendously rewarding experience for a woman to reach a climax with the penis inside her vagina. This may well lead to a great improvement in the couple's relationship as a whole.

sexual problems

Premature ejaculation and anxiety about the size of his penis are common worries for a man and few manage to escape them entirely.

Penis size

A great many men worry about the size or shape of their penis, usually because they believe the size reflects their masculinity and manliness. The bigger the penis, the better the man. This is, of course, nonsense and is based on emotional responses rather than on hard fact. It compares with judging a woman by the size of her breasts and is just as senseless.

Besides its sexual function, the penis, like the breasts, has a physical job to do and, while it has to be big enough to get the job done, there is no advantage in hugeness. Penile size is not related to sexual potency – in fact, an overly large penis could cause a woman pain and this defeats the whole object.

What is the real problem?

It's hard to say if a lack of self-esteem causes anxiety about penis size or if penis size itself is the culprit. Either way, a loss of self-esteem is always present in those men who suffer from anxiety about the size of their penis.

Who really cares?

Penis size matters far more to men than it does to women. When it comes to being attracted to a member of the opposite sex, penis size is low priority. Women are more likely to seek kindness, warmth, generosity, and a sense of humor. Furthermore, most of a woman's sensations from intercourse come from the clitoris and from the nerve endings that are mainly in the first part of the vagina, so the length of the penis is really irrelevant. It is a man's skill and patience as a lover, not the size of his penis, that is responsible for giving his partner sexual satisfaction.

Is there any treatment?

There is no operation that will make a penis longer, but there is one that can increase the girth. Fat is taken from other parts of the body and used in a process called liposculpture. It is painful and is not a procedure usually covered by insurance. You would have to ask your doctor for a referral to an appropriate specialist.

It's more than possible that your doctor will be reluctant to make the referral for this operation. You can, if you want, visit another doctor for a second opinion. However, you should think closely and deeply about the risks associated with any surgical procedure and ask yourself if the end result is worth taking these risks.

What is the outlook?

Everybody cares about the way they look and most of us try to make the best of our appearance. But if concern about a particular aspect of bodily appearance prevents a person from enjoying their life fully, it is a symptom of a lack of self-confidence and self-esteem.

Sadly, some men allow their fear of failure to become an obsession and this can actually ruin their life. Penis size makes no difference at all to a man's personality and character and it is wrong to think that a bigger penis would, or even could, make a man better and more desirable than he already is. It simply wouldn't happen. If worrying about the size of your penis is a problem for you, it is your self-esteem that needs a boost.

Premature ejaculation

Premature ejaculation is the release of semen before or just after penetration. The most important aspect of premature ejaculation is that the man is unable to have any control over his ejaculation, so that once he is sexually aroused he reaches orgasm very quickly. The time between inserting the penis into the vagina and reaching orgasm is short – often less than 30 seconds. This does not allow the female partner sufficient time to become sexually aroused, especially if there has been no clitoral stimulation. This can lead to frustration in the woman and guilt in the man, and may well have a damaging effect on their relationship.

If premature ejaculation has always been present in a healthy man, then the cause is almost certainly psychological. But if a man develops premature ejaculation out of the blue, his doctor should exclude any physical disease. This latter type of premature ejaculation is rare.

What causes it?

Most men will experience premature ejaculation at some time in their lives, probably more than once, and for no apparent reason. Most will find that difficulties pass spontaneously as quickly as they appeared. Men who are young or inexperienced, who have abstained from sex for a long period of time or who are anxious and lack confidence are more likely to experience premature ejaculation.

What can I do about premature ejaculation?

When premature ejaculation is the result of a psychological problem, it is important that the man focuses all his attention on his own sexual sensations before orgasm is reached, using the "stop-start" method.

Try the following steps

1 First, the couple should engage in some foreplay so that the man gets an erection. He should then lie on his back and his partner should stimulate his penis with her hand. During this time, he should concentrate only on his own sexual sensations.
2 As soon as he feels that he is near to orgasm, he must tell his partner to stop stimulating him until the sensation disappears again. Before the erection is allowed to disappear completely, he asks his partner to stimulate him once more.
3 This cycle is then repeated, and ejaculation is only allowed on the fourth occasion. It is up to the man to signal to his partner when she should stop stimulating him and when to begin again.
4 Once the man is able to focus his attention on his own sexual feelings, and he is able to recognize the intense sensations immediately before orgasm, the couple can go on to the next stage.
5 This involves repeating the previous instructions but this time using a lubricating jelly, since orgasm occurs more rapidly in a moist situation. This is due to the similarity of the lubricant to the vaginal secretions.
6 The third stage is sexual intercourse. In the first instance the man lies on his back and his partner should sit astride him. He then lowers her onto his erect penis.
7 Again the "stop-start" method is used, and just before he reaches orgasm, all movement is stopped but the penis remains inside the vagina. When the sexual sensation subsides, but before the erection has gone, they begin to move again. As before, orgasm is only permitted on the fourth occasion.
8 As soon as the couple find that sexual intercourse is successful in this position, they then repeat the whole procedure in the side-to-side position, and finally with the man on top of the woman. You continue the stop-start exercises once every two weeks until he has fully recovered.

Outlook – good!

Provided that the couple follow these instructions carefully, practically all men with premature ejaculation are likely to make a complete recovery.

If the treatment is not successful, this may either be due to deep-seated emotional problems in the man, or because his partner finds difficulty in cooperating. It may help for the couple to seek expert advice from an experienced therapist, after first discussing this with their own doctor.

miscarriages and infertility

Both these problems are surprisingly common. One in five pregnancies ends in miscarriage. One in six couples have difficulty conceiving.

Miscarriage

Miscarriage is the spontaneous loss of a baby and can happen at any time from around the date of a missed period up to the 24th week of pregnancy. The anguish of the bereavement is more intense because all the hopes and expectations built on the arrival of a new baby are suddenly dashed.

What causes a miscarriage?

A miscarriage can result because of parental factors, fetal factors, or a combination of the two. These are the main things that can go wrong:
● A defective egg or sperm forms an abnormal fetus.
● An abnormally shaped uterus can't sustain a pregnancy.
● Fibroids in the uterus disturb the growing fetus.
● A weak cervix may open during pregnancy.
● A weak placenta may not develop properly.

● Diabetes or very severe high blood pressure may not be fully controlled by medication.
● Rhesus incompatibility.
● Maternal infections by bacteria or viruses damage the fetus.
● Pregnancy hormones aren't in balance and the fetus can't grow.

Should I see a doctor?

If you know you're pregnant, or think you might be, and experience any vaginal bleeding and/or cramping pain, call your doctor immediately.

While you're waiting, go to bed and keep your feet raised. Wear a sanitary pad if necessary.

What is the surgical treatment?

● If you have an incomplete miscarriage (when the fetus is expelled but parts of the placenta remain) a completion D&C (dilation and curettage) will be essential to

prevent serious infection. Infertility can result from such an infection if it is not treated.
● If the fetus dies in the uterus but remains there, the fetus will have to be taken away surgically.
● If you miscarry several times in a row, your doctor will perform tests to try to find the specific cause and prevent it from happening again.
● You may be given a test called a hysterosalpingogram (a procedure used to check out the condition of your uterus and fallopian tubes).
● Your doctor will examine the aborted fetus and placenta to make sure they're normal and treat you accordingly. In some cases, you may be referred to a fertility specialist for examination, testing, and advice.
● If you have a septic miscarriage (your internal organs have become infected) you'll be given antibiotics in large doses to deal with the infection.

Coping after a miscarriage

Whatever the reason for the miscarriage and whatever the treatment your doctor prescribes, the emotional effects can be devastating. As well as the natural feelings of grief, you'll probably feel angry that your body has let you down.

The one emotion you must try to quell is guilt. It's not your fault and, although you may be feeling like hiding yourself away and perhaps punishing yourself, this isn't the way to get back to normal. Try not to

isolate yourself and try to be positive about what you can do in the future.

Anxiety is one of the emotions that can prevent conception. Your doctor should give you an honest answer as soon as possible about whether you can carry a baby to full term without medical treatment. If he says it's possible, keep trying, but try not to become obsessive. If you have a problem that can be treated, don't waste time – seek treatment.

A miscarriage is a true bereavement and is difficult to cope with. Counseling might help and is available. If you think you'd benefit from it, ask your doctor to put you in touch with a therapist.

You can usually resume sexual intercourse within about 1-2 weeks, when the bleeding has stopped and the cervix has closed. But you'll probably be advised to wait about six months before trying to conceive again.

Difficulties in conceiving

Having problems conceiving doesn't always mean you are infertile. Most couples who think they are infertile are only subfertile and with help can conceive successfully.

What is infertility?
To most people infertility means the inability to have children but it's more complex than that. A couple may have no difficulty in conceiving their first child but find they cannot have a second; this means that they are suffering from secondary infertility. Another couple, who have both had children by their previous partners, may now find that they cannot conceive together. This is known as subfertility and happens because the fertility of a couple is the sum of their individual fertilities.

If both partners' fertilities are marginal, conception may not occur. But if one partner's fertility is strong, it still may be possible for the couple to conceive. Only 50 percent of couples conceive by the end of six months and 80 percent by the end of a year; if a couple hasn't conceived within six months and then approaches their doctor for advice, he

or she is most likely to send them away with encouraging words but advising them to come back if nothing has happened after a year.

Women produce lower quality eggs as they get older, so age is undoubtedly a factor. Statistics show that around 90 percent of women in their 20s will become pregnant within a year of trying, and the remainder still have a high statistical chance of becoming pregnant naturally within another year or so. But women in their 30s have a much lower statistical probability of becoming pregnant after a year of trying, so should seek help after that time has elapsed.

There are now many different ways in which a couple can be helped to conceive a child. These range from simple advice on sexual technique to drug treatment, surgery, and, ultimately, to the new assisted reproductive technologies (ART).

The importance of counseling
Given the tensions that surround the treatment of infertility, couples deserve and should get psychological support. When you decide to embark on investigation and treatment, ask your

doctor to refer you to a counselor trained in dealing with the stress of infertility at all stages of its management. You shouldn't have to wait until you find yourselves well on into secondary referral; you both need help and advice right from the start. Some procedures require a good deal of deep self-questioning and a couple will need a great deal of support because of the lengthy and invasive nature of the treatment, and especially the ethical issues surrounding assisted reproductive technologies, insemination, and any technique involving donors.

Psychological factors affecting fertility
The way you feel can in itself affect your fertility by causing a hormone disturbance or impotence. So, without proper support, fertility treatment may make matters worse. On the other hand, doctors have plenty of anecdotal evidence that couples suddenly conceive very soon after making the decision to have their infertility investigated, as if initiating an investigation releases the tensions that may have affected fertility all along.

Issues to consider about fertility

Even before you have counseling, it's worth asking yourselves some questions, so that some of the issues are out in the open.
- Would you tell friends and family, or would you attempt to keep your fertility treatment a complete secret?
- If you intend to keep it a secret, can you be sure that the truth won't come out, perhaps destructively, at a time of crisis?
- Could you cope with a multiple pregnancy?
- What if one, some, or all of the babies died?
- Having committed so much time and money to having a baby, how easy will you find it to let her go once she grows up?
- How long would you persist with infertility treatment?
- Would you consider donor eggs or sperm?
- Is adoption an option?

abortion

Opting for an abortion is never an easy decision. Some feel that it is morally, religiously, and biologically wrong to interfere with a pregnancy and are fervently opposed to abortion. Others are just as strongly in favor of the right to choose.

Deciding to have an abortion

Most of us would probably suffer a mixture of feelings were an unwanted pregnancy to be confirmed. We may be fearful that our families and friends will find out and that we may be punished. We may be fearful that we won't be able to decide what to do, and this indecision increases the circuit of anxiety. We are afraid that we will be alone in trying to decide what to do, and, of course, we are afraid of the prospects of motherhood.

We may also be afraid of abortion, even though we know it's legal and safe. "Will it cost more than I can pay?", "will my insurance cover it?", "will it be painful?", "will I be punished by suffering postoperative complications?", "will I be sterile afterward?", "I feel guilty now but will I carry around guilty feelings for the rest of my life?", "will I regret what I have done and wish that I had had the baby?", "will I fear sex and never be able to have a real relationship with a man again?".

Seek help and support

It is very normal for you to feel all of these fears and to be, in some instances, profoundly affected psychologically. But the reassuring news is that the majority of women feel relieved after an abortion although they may feel sad as well. You are going to have a fairly hard time and you need support, so establish it before you go into your abortion. Seek the help of a friend, make sure that your friend will stand by you and comfort you during and after the abortion. If this friend can be your doctor, that is even better; if it is one of your parents, you are very lucky; if it's your partner, you have the best of all worlds. Whoever you find, find someone because you are going to need them and you will pull through the post-abortion upset faster by having them close to you during this time.

Where can I go for advice?

First go along and see your family doctor (who should be well acquainted with your medical history), or go to an organization that specializes in giving help to people in your position. They offer a full, nonpressured counseling service. You will have the opportunity to ask all the questions you want to. You will be reminded about anything you have forgotten, all the various alternatives other than abortion will be discussed with you, and your personal domestic and financial commitments will be carefully considered.

Once you have decided on an abortion, your own doctor can make a second appointment with a gynecologist as soon as possible, or you can skip seeing your doctor and go directly to a gynecologist or contact Planned Parenthood. The abortion will then be arranged as soon as possible – most doctors and clinics prefer to perform an abortion sooner rather than later.

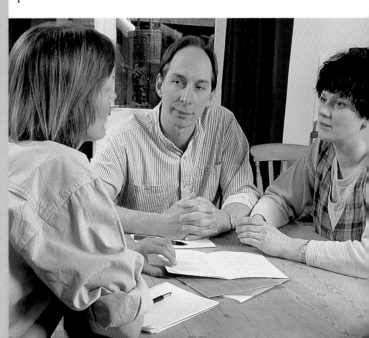

Legal requirements for abortion

In the US, a woman and her doctor may freely decide to opt for an abortion during her first trimester. State governments, however, can restrict access to an abortion after the first trimester with laws intended to protect the woman's health.

The laws governing teen abortion also vary from state to state and can be quite restrictive. In 30 states, laws mandate the involvement of one or both parents in the abortion decision. These parental consent or notification laws require teens, who

may be unable to tell both their parents about a pregnancy, or are unable to travel out of state, to get approval from a judge to obtain an abortion. This is known as a "judicial bypass" procedure and can be difficult to obtain for many teens.

The time to have an abortion

If you do decide on an abortion, you should arrange it as soon as you possibly can because the earlier it is done the safer it is. The later you let it go, the greater the chances are of complications.

There is no question that abortions are best performed before 12 weeks. After that time, and certainly after 20 weeks, it becomes not only more difficult, but also more dangerous to procure an abortion through the vagina. A D&E (dilation and evacuation) can be done up to 20 weeks under general anesthetic.

Late abortions
Only 1 in 100 abortions is undertaken after 20 weeks, and nearly all of those are done because a very severe abnormality of the fetus has been discovered or because of extreme distress or illness of the mother. In these instances, abortion is performed by hysterotomy – that is, an operation through the abdominal wall to open up the uterus similar to a cesarean section – or by a medical induction in which drugs are given to stimulate uterine contractions.

After an abortion

If you have your abortion performed within the first 12 weeks of pregnancy, you will be physically back to normal within a week.

Psychologically, though, it may take considerably longer for you to feel your usual self. It varies from individual to individual. Most women take three to four weeks to get over the psychological effects of an abortion. Some take several months. After an abortion it's common to feel withdrawn, tearful, and be unable to make decisions. But take heart; along with the sadness will come a sense of relief.

If your sadness persists, see your doctor. Most abortion clinics have a counselor you can confide in, and the right professional support can really help you to start feeling better about yourself.

How soon can I have sexual intercourse?
Provided you are using contraceptives, you can have sex again in about two to three weeks if you feel up to it. Do not have intercourse any earlier than this, because you are somewhat more prone to having an infection introduced into the genital tract immediately after an abortion.

do

 Take it easy
Look after yourself by taking things very easy and resting for at least a day.

 Checkup
Have a full medical checkup within a week of the abortion, even if you feel fine.

 Symptoms
Consult your doctor at once if you start to vomit or bleed heavily, if you have a prolonged or smelly vaginal discharge, or if you develop severe pain or fever.

don't

 No exercise
Don't do any strenuous exercise for at least three days.

 Tampons and pads
Don't use any tampons for two or three weeks to avoid the risk of infection; use sanitary pads instead.

 Next time...
Abortion is a tragedy, so make sure that there isn't going to be a "next time." Get advice about contraception now (see p. 118). And think of the results of all of your actions.

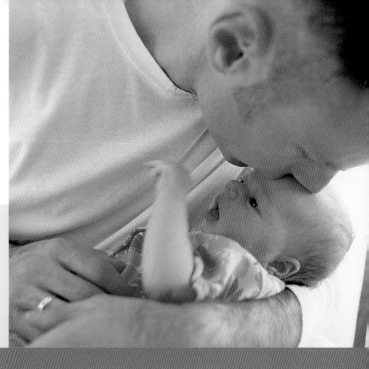

adjusting to parenthood

It's a huge leap from being a couple to becoming a family. Few couples realize how much impact their new baby will have on their lives, their work, their emotions, and their feelings for one another.

Tips for new dads

As a new father you may feel rather cut off from your partner. The best antidote is to get involved with the baby and to offer help at every opportunity. Even if at first your partner may seem a bit distant, your understanding and help will break down any barriers.

What you can do to help

● Take the initiative; don't wait to be asked to share your baby's care. Learn while your baby's still a newborn.

● Get to know your baby. Use these early days to establish a close relationship with your baby by changing her and learning to handle her. Hold your baby close to you so that she can focus on your face. Carry your baby around in a sling whenever possible, try to be there for the first bath and do regular feedings, changings, and bathtimes.

● Be ready for your partner's mood swings. At some point during the first week your partner will probably experience the so-called baby blues that come as a reaction to the sudden withdrawal of the pregnancy hormones and exhaustion after the labor. These baby blues are temporary; they subside in a week to 10 days.

● Never belittle or make light of your partner's feelings; she has a lot to cope with. Be sensitive to her needs and talk to her about them. If her depression lasts more than two weeks make sure she sees her doctor.

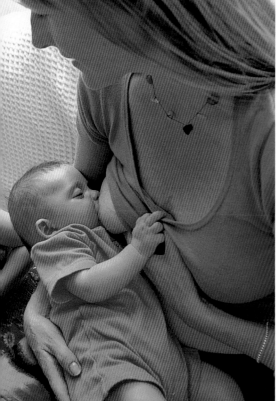

Tips for new moms

Even though you're longing to be home, try to take advantage of your time in the hospital to regain your strength and lean on your midwife, lactation consultant, and doctor for advice. Don't feel shy about asking – get as much help as you can. And friends and relations are also usually only too happy to help.

How you can adjust

● Share any aspect of your baby's care with your partner that you've been shown by a midwife or doctor. If you learn how to care for your baby together, you'll start out on an equal footing and he'll be more likely to take the initiative to help you once you are home.

● Prepare for time on your own. Build on the network of support that you have set up through prenatal classes before the baby was born. Within a week or two of the birth, your partner may have gone back to work, and friends and family will have withdrawn back to their own lives.

● Be ready for mood swings. At some point during the first few days you may experience tearful moments – and it often happens just as your milk comes in, three or four days after birth. The so-called baby blues are your normal reaction to the sudden withdrawal of pregnancy hormones and usually subside in a week to 10 days. Don't try to hide your feelings from your partner – be open about them.

● Make time for your partner. The baby may be time consuming but it's good for your relationship to reserve some time and attention for each other.

New parents

What a new mother wants from her partner

● Recognize her vulnerability. A father needs to recognize how vulnerable a new mother feels, both physically and emotionally, in the days after the birth.

● Appreciate the depth of her feelings. A father needs to accept the strength of his partner's overwhelming involvement in the baby and not to construe this as a rejection of him.

● Protect her privacy. One of the most important roles for a new father is to make sure that his partner isn't overwhelmed by visitors and to give her time and space to establish breast-feeding and recover from the physical stresses of labor and birth.

What a new father wants from his partner

● Recognize his difficulties. She should be ready to accept that this is also a confusing and emotional time for her partner.

● Allow him to make mistakes. After a hospital birth, a new mother necessarily has more time to get used to the baby, but she needs to allow her partner to handle and care for the baby, and not to criticize if he fumbles.

Sex and parenthood

There's no magic date when you can start to have sex again. One of the things that will help is to start your pelvic floor exercises immediately after delivery, even though your genital area may be a bit sore. Take it slowly and gently.

● The ideal time to start making love again is when you and your partner want to, so discuss it and try it out tentatively.

● If you both feel like it, there's no reason why you couldn't try sex that's non-penetrative but nonetheless entirely fulfilling and satisfying within a few days of delivery. Some women want to have orgasms a few days after birth. Having an orgasm can be beneficial because it seems to help the uterus shrink.

● You may find that you're a bit sore or tight, but waiting will not make you stretch. It helps, too, if the vagina is well relaxed before penetration, so concentrate on foreplay before entry.

● Try a different position than the woman lying on her back since the penis can press on the sensitive bruised rear wall of the vagina. Your partner can help by gentle manual dilatation if your vagina seems to be too tight. Don't be concerned about setbacks, they're normal; try again gently.

● Many couples resume sex at six weeks – the time of the postpartum checkup. If you've had an episiotomy you'll be sore and tender for longer and your partner should not attempt penetration until you feel comfortable. However, this doesn't bar gentle exploration. In fact, get your partner to feel your episiotomy scar. It's huge and he'll be sympathetic immediately.

● While you're breast-feeding, your breasts may feel sore and heavy and if you have cracked nipples fondling will be out of the question.

● The most important thing is to talk about your feelings and keep the channels of communication with your partner open.

● If, after several months, one of you is still feeling reluctant to resume your sexual relationship, ask for help. You'll be surprised how much easier it is once you've talked to someone.

Episiotomy aftereffects

An episiotomy scar is often painful and, particularly if large, can make sex so uncomfortable that women shrink even from an embrace that might lead to other sexual activities. Women may feel aroused and ready for sex but the scar hurts so much that penetration is impossible, often for up to six months after delivery.

new responsibilities

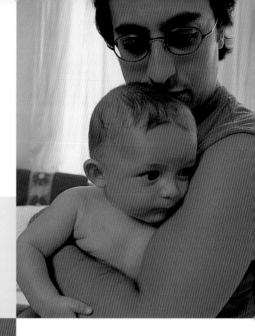

Parenthood is full of ups and downs, especially at first. Having a positive and equal relationship with your partner, or a good support network if you are a single parent, can make the transition that much easier.

Fatherhood

Be aware that barriers between you and your partner are likely to spring from the fact that, as one psychologist put it, "although men and women become parents at the same time, they don't become parents in the same way." There are many sociological, financial, and environmental reasons for this, but the result is often straightforward resentment or jealousy.

Jealous feelings

A man can quickly feel isolated within the family unit. He suddenly finds his partner's time monopolized by the new addition, and unless he is taking an active role in caring for the baby, he's no longer sure where he fits in. It is quite common to find a father becoming jealous of his own child. This situation may be exacerbated if there were differences of opinion about having the child in the first place (men often complain of being "pressured" into having a baby).

A father may find these feelings particularly difficult to deal with if he also feels rejected on a sexual level. Often men take a new mother's diminished sex drive as a personal rebuff. If it's not too late, discuss the effects this may have on your relationship before the baby arrives.

Many of us remember our fathers seeming more unapproachable and distant than our mothers, but there is no reason why a child cannot enjoy an equally close relationship with both parents. A baby's relationships do not operate on an either/or basis and parents should never worry that if a baby spends an equal amount of time with his father, he might love his mother less. All young children need as much love as they can get, and both parents should do their utmost to provide it.

For a father to take on an equal role as a parent, he will have to overcome cultural pressures, and perhaps change his own attitudes too. He will also have to recognize his role as a caregiver rather than just a provider. Some men confuse parenthood with taking care of the bills, because that is what they saw their own fathers doing.

Who's left holding the baby?

Today it may be economic factors that determine who is left holding the baby. If a woman earns more than her partner, or if he is unemployed, many couples can't afford to let misplaced male pride reduce their weekly income. While the rise of the house-husband has undoubtedly benefited lots of families, it is important to bear in mind that the man left at home with a small child may suffer from the same problems as a woman: isolation and boredom. Whatever your arrangement, when you're together try hard to talk about how you feel.

Single fathers

There are very few men who are the sole carergivers of a young baby, but for those who are, the pleasures and most of the problems will be the same as those of a single mother. Single men are at no more of a disadvantage in the practical care of their baby because they are male; the only thing they can't do that a woman can is breast-feed.

The benefits

Although it's not an ideal situation to be caring for a baby alone, a single father may benefit in ways that would not have happened had he been sharing the care with his partner. Research has shown that single fathers are more satisfied parents, feel closer to their children, and are more confident and effective than the average father.

The problems

The main problem that may occur for a single father is that of isolation. He may find that he has to battle for recognition in female-dominated environments and, sadly, there will be those who question his ability to bring up his baby properly. But over time, a full-time father will stop being the token male and become just another parent, who shares the same pleasures and problems of parenthood as his female friends.

Lifestyle changes

The arrival of a child means that choices become stark: beforehand, for instance, if neither partner wanted to clean the bathroom floor, it could be left until later. But a baby can never be left until later. His needs take priority and somebody has to take immediate responsibility for meeting them. Time that was previously spent on other things must now be given to the baby.

Ideally, these lifestyle changes are shared equally within a partnership, but in practice women very often end up taking on the main burden. Depending on individual expectations, this can lead to deep resentment within a relationship, causing a couple to move apart following the birth of their baby.

Increasing conflict
Research in America has shown that 1 in every 2 marriages goes into decline after the birth of the first child. All of the couples in the study, no matter how well-adjusted, experienced on average a 20 percent increase in conflict within their marriage during the first year of parenthood. Although conflict can sometimes be healthy, it is often not what new parents expect. To reduce the stress placed on a partnership, it is vital that each partner has at least some idea of what to expect and is able to compromise. Having a baby means rearranging your life.

Lone parenting

Being a single parent, you won't have the luxury of a partner to share the day-to-day care of your baby or the joys of watching him develop. Without a good support network, it can be physically and emotionally exhausting, but the knowledge that you've done it alone can also be hugely rewarding for you and beneficial to your baby.

Single parent by choice?

If you've chosen to be a single mother, you may be more prepared emotionally, practically, and financially for caring for a young baby and look forward to the prospect. If you've split up with your partner during the pregnancy or soon after the birth, you may have more difficulties. Coping with the emotional problems of separating from someone while caring for a young baby is bound to have an impact on your ability to cope. In this situation, it's more important for you to ask for and accept help.

Lone parenting can be positive

Being a single parent is by no means all doom and gloom. You and your baby can benefit in many ways from the special relationship you'll form.
● Single parents tend to develop a much closer bond with their babies; they do not have to share their love between a partner and a child.
● Extended family – grandparents, aunts, and uncles – often get more involved when there's only one parent. The baby can greatly benefit from this network of support and love.
● Caring for a baby alone is a great achievement. You'll strengthen as a person as you watch your baby develop.
● If you're single because your relationship has broken down, you have made the right decision; it may be better for the baby to live with one fairly contented person than two people who are at war.

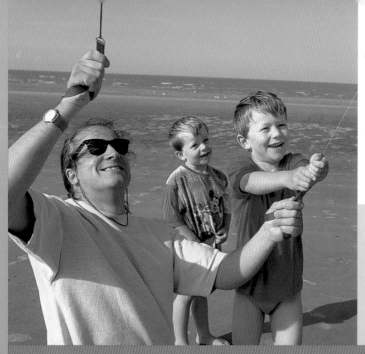

partnership problems

At some stage in every relationship, difficulties arise. In some cases couples live happily ever after, but many don't. Some problems can be overcome, but for others separation is the only answer.

Effects of divorce on your children

Research suggests that children are better off with two unhappy parents than with divorced parents. But the research gives no indication of the different divorce situations, which are critical in determining the effect on the child. An amicable divorce may be barely damaging and its effect entirely different from that of a bitter, acrimonious divorce. The main reason for this is that in an acrimonious situation, each parent usually does his or her best to turn the children against the other parent. This has a very negative and damaging effect on children, and should be avoided at all costs. Remember that a child has the right, indeed the need, to love and respect both parents, even though they're living apart. No child can split themselves in two.

Explaining to your children
A young child is like a sponge that soaks up emotional signals, whether or not they are directed at her. If you are happy, the chances are your child will be happy; if you are sad, she will be sad. Although it is always worth making an effort "for the sake of the children," don't fall into the trap of

thinking they won't know what is going on. They usually sense when something is wrong, whether or not you have a smile on your face.

Because of this it's always best to explain, at least partially, what is going on. If you don't, children will invent their own explanations, mistakenly blaming themselves for problems in the family. This is because children under 5 only conceive the world in relation to themselves. If you don't give a plausible explanation of why you and your partner are arguing or splitting up, they may come up with explanations that are inconceivable to an adult, but make perfect sense to a child, such as: "daddy has left because I don't clean my room properly," or "mommy is upset because I wet the bed."

Feelings of guilt are severely damaging, especially for a child already struggling to come to terms with the emotional turmoil and insecurity that marital breakups can trigger. Doubt is one of the worst fears in a child's mind, so never leave your child in any doubt that you love her and that you will look after her.

Access
Whatever your feelings are about your partner, it's best for your child if you're easygoing about access.
● Don't be stingy and don't be confrontational – it causes your child such anguish. Hand her over somewhere civilized like one of your homes, not somewhere like a park or shopping center, or your child will feel like a commodity.
● Plan well ahead, don't break promises at the last minute, and if your partner is late, be breezy about it, otherwise your child will worry about both of you. Don't make it an opportunity to denigrate her other parent; be offhand, and keep your child calm: "should we play a game of checkers until he gets here?"or "oh, I bet the traffic's bad."
● If your partner is consistently late or unreasonable, arrange a separate meeting to discuss this, out of earshot of your child. The only time to consider preventing your ex-partner having any access to your child is if you think she's at risk of being kidnapped or otherwise harmed. In such cases seek professional advice.

Separation and divorce

More and more couples are experiencing problems with their relationship. This doesn't necessarily reflect a lowering of moral values; it is more an indication of the complexities and pressures of modern life. Support systems are weaker and expectations higher.

Statistics show that today 2 in 3 divorces are initiated by women, many of whom feel they are asked to do too much without adequate support from their partners. The average marriage lasts eight years – a depressing fact of life for growing numbers of children brought up without two parents.

Periods of change

The problem for nearly all couples is that in the long term people change. Although this can be difficult, it can also be invigorating and constructive. If you learn to develop together, you will prevent boredom from building in your relationship.

At the end of periods of change, which are often fraught with emotional insecurity, you will either grow together or grow apart. Whatever happens, it is vital that your children always feel secure of their future. For young children, change within a family unit (or fear of that change) is very damaging. Children do not have the defense mechanisms to protect themselves from the severe emotional insecurity that a breakup can cause.

Domestic violence

Many women live with a partner who resorts to physical violence when he can't win an argument. He uses threats to control her freedom of speech and movement, and invades her privacy by spying and snooping. To the outside world he appears to be the ideal husband but behind closed doors it's a very different story. Research shows, about 1 woman in 4 is likely to be abused by a partner in her lifetime.

Making the break

Starting a new life alone is undeniably difficult. In ridding yourself of one set of problems, you'll inevitably find yourself with others you may not have expected. But you'll be in control of your own future and you may find that this more than compensates for the hardships you'll encounter. It may help to strengthen your resolve if you visualize the rest of your life as continuing on the same as it has been over recent years, then comparing this with how content you could be if left to your own devices.

There are no easy steps to changing one's life and little can be done to prevent the showdown you fear with your violent partner. The obstacles you have overcome to achieve your independence are very similar to obstacles an addict has to overcome. It's a matter of mustering the willpower and determination and once your mind is set, the rest will be surprisingly easy.

Your children

If you're a battered mother your first concern has to be the emotional well-being of your children, and how well they manage depends to a large extent on how you behave.

Brought up in a violent home, children rapidly come to think of masculine behavior as violent and women always appear weak and powerless. In a violent home, children desperately need a parent who's strong enough to continue, even when she's at her most vulnerable – a parent who still has the emotional capacity to love. Most women are strong and brave enough to do that, though they don't always see themselves that way at first.

Getting out of a violent relationship

● Acknowledge that it's happening to you and stop playing down the abuse you're experiencing. It's not unusual for some women to minimize or justify what's happening to them.
● Recognize that you're not to blame. No one deserves to be assaulted, humiliated, or abused, least of all by their partner in a supposedly caring relationship. Women often blame themselves because they have consistently been told it is their fault. Prolonged exposure to violence may convince you that you deserve to be hurt. But there is no justification for violence, ever.
● Begin seeking the help and support that's available. This step includes gaining emotional support and practical help. You can even start by talking to a friend you trust or calling an organization such as the National Domestic Violence Hotline or a local battered woman's shelter.
● You may want to think about moving somewhere safe, away from your abuser, or taking legal action that will protect you and stop the violence against you.

mental fitness

Many of us spend a great deal of time, energy, and even money trying to do something about our physical fitness. Unfortunately, the same does not always apply to mental fitness, although it is just as important.

Women and mental fitness

For women especially, mental fitness should be as important, if not more important, than physical fitness. Why? Because women, regardless of marital status, suffer from more depressive and anxiety disorders than men. Women take more drugs that affect mental activity than men and are more often diagnosed by doctors as suffering from mental health problems.

The reason for these phenomena is twofold. First, our physical condition makes us more vulnerable. Women are prone to psychological disturbances relating to hormonal behavior, not only monthly, but especially after pregnancy and childbirth, and we live longer to experience mourning, loneliness, and the depression of old age. Second, the status of women has meant that we haven't always been given sufficient freedom of choice in our lifestyles, which leads to frustration. No matter what lifestyle we choose, there are conflicts that can breed unhappiness such as balancing a family and a career – even marriage itself may be an ongoing mental trauma for us, much more than for men.

This remarkable bombardment of mental trauma means that we must strive to maintain a basic state of mental health – so that we can take knocks and not go under; so that we can rise to emergencies and cope well with them; so that we are resilient enough to survive long-term, stressful situations, so that we can deal with the possible loss of those closest to us.

Maintaining psychological equilibrium, however, requires a different sort of self-knowledge from physical fitness. It also requires supreme realism. It is essential that we realize our difficulties are not unique. We all go through periods of stress and, no matter how unpleasant, most of us survive. Adversity is normal, indeed it is a condition of living, and we must not overreact to it or feel that we've messed up our lives irretrievably and are failures because we're experiencing it.

When things go wrong, it is natural to think that we are to blame. **But we should keep in mind that difficulties in our environment, over which we have no control, might be a major factor.** Things such as overcrowding and violence in society are factors we can do little about. Poverty is a particularly powerful exacerbating factor and, as with physical illness, mental illness is much more common among poorer people.

Ways of coping

It is important that we achieve a certain measure of emotional growth. Coming to terms with the way we feel about things, being able to work with our own emotions, as well as other people's, in a nondestructive but helpful, even affectionate, frame of mind is a goal we should all try to achieve. Accepting ourselves for what we are and permitting ourselves a proper measure of self-esteem means that we can take responsibility for our own actions and seek and accept forgiveness from others, when necessary, without damage to our self-image. This process of independence is a long one and may even continue through life but is necessary to seek out the goodness within ourselves.

Another effort to make is not to set our standards too high; it's not necessary and it can be a great strain. It is acceptable for anyone to let go now and then, to have a good cry, to pour out troubles to a friend, or to rant and rave and let off steam. Better that than blowing a fuse and becoming ill.

But it is possible to prepare for catastrophes and the answer lies in yourself – you have to have the desire to cope and survive a bad patch. If you practice on manageable "disasters," you'll find the major ones cause you much less stress, keeping in mind that once your mental fitness is jeopardized it will take time to come back to normal. There are, however, two ways in which you can control your body and mind immediately: relax and breathe calmly and slowly (see p. 292 for relaxation techniques).

Combating stress

Dissociate

This means putting your worries out of your head. Try to ignore your problem for as long as possible. The longer you keep it at bay and remain calm, the more time there is for the body's fight and flight reaction to lessen, thereby reducing stress and anxiety.

Have fun

Enjoy yourself; go out to dinner with a friend, or simply take the afternoon off to go shopping, or snatch a weekend away in the country. While you are having fun, and even after it, notice how most problems diminish in size.

Physical activity

Work off stress through any kind of exercise that you enjoy and are physically able to do. Physical activity of almost any kind counteracts the effects of stress and nearly always leaves you feeling more relaxed and rational about your problem.

Get another opinion

Most problems which to us seem so overwhelming and individual are not uncommon. Getting advice from someone with experience in the situation, with no personal connection, can help to shed new light on the problem. A problem shared is a problem halved. Groups such as Weight Watchers, Alcoholics Anonymous, and other support groups are specially set up to deal with particular stressful situations.

Look at the way you manage your time

Stress is often caused by mismanagement of time such as getting behind in our work or jobs at home. Assign priorities to tasks and do the important ones first. Look at the way you spend your time. For a few days write down all your activities, the relevance they have to figuring out your problem and the result they achieved. At the end of this period it's astonishing to see how your time was spent – how much of it was wasted and how much of it was put to useful purpose.

Scale down your expectations

Recognize your own limitations and take on only what you can accomplish in the time you've allowed yourself. Realize that it isn't possible for you totally to control the world around you. Setting up and meeting realistic goals can lessen stress, while failing to live up to your expectations can bring it about.

Withdraw

A more radical alternative is to cut yourself off from the situation that is causing your stress. Withdrawal, however, may involve substantial effort. If, for example, you find you cannot get along with your boss, you may have to change your job. If you hate the house you live in, you may have to consider moving to a new one, possibly in another area.

FOCUS *on* cosmetic surgery

Few people regret having cosmetic surgery, though many regret not doing so. If you want, a good surgeon can change your appearance. But beware. Such an operation requires that you be well motivated or you could be unhappy with the results.

You'll have to endure quite a lot of discomfort and may be somewhat depressed until the effects become apparent. It's important that you have the operation for the right reasons and not because a critical partner pressures you into having surgery.

If you have serious psychological problems, cosmetic surgery isn't going to fix them. If a relationship is disintegrating or a marriage is falling apart, plastic surgery isn't going to remedy the situation. On the other hand, if you've suffered severe psychological stress because of your appearance, cosmetic surgery can have long-term benefits that will affect all aspects of your life. These days, a good reason for having surgery may simply be that your body looks older than you feel. You don't need to seek further justification.

After cosmetic surgery, people are often more at ease with themselves and feel more self-assured. That alone makes you look better.

CHOOSING A SURGEON

First step is to find a good cosmetic surgeon with whom you get along well. Don't be afraid to shop around. Here are some tips to help you find one:
• Get a sound recommendation from a doctor or a good friend.
• As a rule, don't select a surgeon from an advertisement in a newspaper, magazine, or on television.
• A surgeon who is trustworthy will advise you on which operation will give you the best results. Be suspicious of a surgeon who agrees to perform exactly the operation you request without giving you a professional opinion as to what you actually need.
• No good surgeon will give you a 100 percent guarantee of success. He should take time to explain in detail exactly what the operation involves, what can be achieved, and give a realistic estimate of the chances of success or failure. Be skeptical about a surgeon who's not realistic.

• Only entrust yourself to a surgeon if you get along with him or her from the beginning. If you don't like the surgeon at your first visit, you're unlikely to later.

REMOVING THE SIGNS OF AGE

Cosmetic surgeons say that typical face-lift patients are not vain, rich women with nothing better to do with their money, but energetic, active people who are less interested in hiding their age than in looking as youthful as they feel. These patients think that an obviously aging face erodes self-confidence and may even cause panic. A typical question such a patient should ask herself is "why should I go on looking like this when every other part of me feels young?"

Many women in their 40s and 50s are not ready to resign themselves to being thought of as aging. They feel that growing older would be easier to bear if they could avoid looking old in the process. Furthermore, they often feel it is unjust that they should start to show signs of deterioration when they are just beginning to reach intellectual and emotional maturity. Consequently, when fine lines, wrinkles, and sags appear on their faces, they fight back.

A woman having a face-lift does not want friends and relatives to gasp with surprise at their first sight of her afterward. She would prefer a natural look, an almost indefinable improvement in her appearance. For this reason, totally smooth skin is not the desired outcome. If the skin is overstretched, a false Asian look around the eyes may rob the face of much of its expressive quality. The best advertisement for a good cosmetic surgeon is a patient who looks naturally young for her age, not one whose smooth skin seems artificial.

IMPROVING THE FEATURES

In some instances, the decision to have cosmetic surgery has nothing to do with aging. Sometimes an obvious facial peculiarity, such as a long or bulbous nose, can have profound psychological effects that begin as early as adolescence. A teenager may find that no matter how she styles her hair or puts on make-up, the flaw is still apparent. This situation may make a good student feel inadequate and too restless to continue education, or lead the drop-out to a succession of jobs.

Facial operations

Face-lift – removes major wrinkles and lifts sagging skin.

Blepharoplasty – removes sagging skin that makes the eyes look puffy, raises drooping eyelids or reshapes eyebrows.

Cheek or chin augmentation – inserts molded implants to reshape chin or cheekbones.

Otoplasty – takes back protruding ears.

Double chin reduction – removes the sag of fat and loose skin under the chin.

Chin reduction – removes bone and cartilage to reshape the chin.

Lip augmentation – reshapes the lips, using fat cells to make them fuller.

Rhinoplasty – reshapes, smoothes out, or straightens the nose.

Before a face-lift

After a face-lift

At some point, matters reach a crisis: the patient may resort to psychotherapy, for example, because of her problems with self-confidence, indecisiveness, and inability to enjoy sex. She may find it impossible to relax with people because of her consciousness that she is not looking attractive. Often there is not so much an intense desire to have the offending feature improved as a continual feeling of depression caused by the knowledge that she is not looking good. It is not unreasonable to expect many of these feelings to diminish sharply, if not to disappear, once the deformity has been corrected by cosmetic surgery.

The same feelings, of course, may arise from a flaw so trivial that scarcely anyone else is aware of it. Even in these cases, cosmetic surgery can bring about a dramatic psychological improvement – although it is always possible that the patient's own feeling that her appearance has been altered for the better may vanish when no change in other people's reactions to her is apparent. The inner quality that makes some people attractive is something no surgeon can give, and it is not necessarily linked with having beautiful features.

LIPOSUCTION

Liposuction is one of the three most popular cosmetic surgery procedures, along with breast enlargement and removal of bags under the eyes. But liposuction is not to be taken lightly. You should investigate the implications before going ahead.

The number of obese people in the US increases all the time, and with magazines full of tall, thin models many women are tempted to strive for that kind of slender perfection. Not satisfied with dieting, you may be tempted to turn to a surgeon to give you a flat stomach and slim thighs. Liposuction may sound like a minor procedure but there are risks involved.

What is liposuction?

Liposuction is a way of removing fat from areas of the body such as hips, thighs, buttocks, chin, and male breasts. It was designed, not as a cure for obesity, but to remove pads of fat that don't respond to diet and exercise.

How liposuction is performed

● Liposuction is not a gentle procedure. Initially, a cold salt solution, which also contains adrenaline, a local anesthetic, and a chemical to break down fat cells, is injected into the fatty area of your body.
● Next, a large, hollow needle, usually about 3mm in diameter, attached to a powerful suction machine, is inserted through several small cuts in the skin. It is passed into pockets of fat, where it is moved around with considerable force. Fat is quite solid, and it needs some liquidizing to be sucked into the draining tube. The saline solution helps to loosen and liquidize the fat.
● It's dangerous to remove too much fat. All body fluids are in equilibrium and the body responds to loss of fat as it does to loss of

A wide range of cosmetic operations is now available to improve features such as brows, eyelids, chin, and lips, and to reduce fat on buttocks and stomach.

blood; if too much fat is removed, you'll go into surgical shock with very low blood pressure.

Recovery

There can be considerable discomfort and stiffness after the operation and the wider the needle used, the worse the pain and the longer it lasts. You can expect to resume normal activities within two to three days for minor liposuction, but it may take up to two or three weeks after major fat removal.

The operation can cause severe bruising so, to minimize this, special elasticated garments that compress the skin must be worn for two to three weeks after the operation to help skin contraction and support the operation site to prevent fluid from collecting.

Side effects

Liposuction results do vary. The procedure works best on women under 40, whose skin is elastic and springs back into shape relatively easily. Older women can be left with unsightly sags and folds. If too much fat is removed from one place, or if it's removed unevenly, ridges and dimples are the result. Common complaints are stretched skin not shrinking back to its former size, numbness in muscles surrounding the area operated on, and uneven fat removal, leaving lumps.

Breast surgery

There are several different ways in which cosmetic surgery can change the size, shape, and uplift of your breasts. These include breast lift (mastopexy), breast enlargement, and breast reduction. Make sure you understand exactly what your operation involves before you take the plunge.

BREAST LIFT

A breast-lift operation is usually for sagging breasts – it removes excess skin and raises the nipple. The smaller the breast the better the result. It can be combined with augmentation if your breasts are small, or reduction if your breasts are very large. Without reduction, mastopexy is not very effective on large breasts because gravity will pull them down again.

Be realistic. Mastopexy can't give you the pert breasts of a teenager, and it will leave scars. Discuss the operation with your surgeon in some detail before proceeding.

As with all breast operations, make sure you see before and after photographs so that you can check good, moderate, and poor results. Ask for a description of the kind of cuts that will be made, and even get the surgeon to draw on your breasts where the scars will be.

You should keep in mind that your breast-lift, just like a face-lift, is by no means permanent. Your breasts will continue to age and eventually sag all over again.

Ask your surgeon if the technique to be used gives you the option of breast-feeding if it's important to you. It's advisable to have a mammogram before you go ahead with any type of breast surgery.

The operation

A general anesthetic is usual. Your surgeon will remove excess skin and fat from under the breasts and move the nipple upward by pushing it through a hole in the skin higher up your chest.

Aftereffects and follow-up

Mastopexy is usually very successful and there are few side effects, although you may notice loss of sensation in your nipple and areola. There's a 50–50 chance you'll be able to breast-feed after the operation, as long as the milk ducts aren't cut. You can expect to have all the stitches removed after two weeks and, if you're an active person, you'll have full movement of your arms and shoulders and be able to take up sports after about three weeks.

Although it may be slightly uncomfortable, it's advisable to wear a good supporting bra after the operation to support the inflamed breast and skin and help healing. You should be prepared to wear your bra day and night for at least three months after surgery.

BREAST REDUCTION

There are two groups of women who look for breast reduction. The first group dislike their large breasts because of the inconvenience and social embarrassment. The second group want cosmetic breast reduction to achieve firm, well-positioned breasts, and are happy with C or D cups as long as the breasts look good.

The operation

While different surgeons have slightly different techniques for reducing the size of breasts, the basic operation is very much the same no matter who does it. It requires a general anaesthetic and it'll probably take as long as four hours. The nipples are important. Ask whether your surgeon's going to simply move your nipples up, or remove them and then graft them back in a different position.

You can request that your nipple is preserved on a stalk of tissue – called a pedicle – so the tissue is taken from the sides and the underside of this stalk. This is essential if you want to breast-feed in the future.

If you wish to know exactly what's going to be removed, ask your surgeon to draw the shape on your breast with a pen. The nipple can be lifted up and stitched into the breast at a higher level. The flaps of skin underneath are stitched together, resulting in reduction and some uplift.

You'll be left with scars around the areola, in a line from the nipple to the underside of the breast, and in the skin fold where the breast joins the skin of the chest.

Aftereffects and follow-up

The results of the operation are usually extremely good, but this is major surgery, so you can expect to have some discomfort for several weeks after. By the time you go home two or three days later, however, the pain should have subsided. Wear a bra day and night for support and to help healing. The stitches should be removed within about two weeks, after which you could restart work. After a month you'll virtually be back to normal.

BREAST ENLARGEMENT

Breast enlargement can only be accomplished with the aid of implants, which are inserted in front of or behind the muscles of the chest wall – the pecs – underneath the actual breast. Implants have received a lot of medical attention in recent years and their safety has been questioned. If you're considering breast augmentation, you owe it to yourself to become informed about these issues.

● Breast augmentation can have complications, so read as much as you can about it. Ask your surgeon if he can put you in touch with someone who's had the operation so that you can go into it with your eyes open.

● Have a detailed discussion about the size you'd like your breasts to be. Be realistic. If your frame is small and you already have tiny breasts, think twice before going for a D cup. Your surgeon will probably advise against it anyway. The best prostheses now are shaped and are of standard width. You will be measured for the appropriate size and shape of these biodimensional prostheses.

● Make sure that your doctor checks for cysts in the breast that might require treatment in future. It's difficult for a surgeon to interfere

with the breast once an implant is in place.
- Ask about the possibility of contracture (see below) and ask where the scars will be.
- Ask whether the incisions will interfere with breast-feeding or sensation in the nipple.
- Make sure that your surgeon tells you the size and the manufacturer of your implant in case it needs replacing at a future date.

The operation
The length of the operation is largely determined by where the implant is placed. If it goes underneath the muscles of the chest wall, the operation will take less time than if it is placed underneath the breast tissue but on top of the muscle layer, because there's less bleeding in the former operation. You might want to stay in hospital for 24 hours to recover from the anesthetic, but then you can go home. You'll be asked to return to the hospital in about 10 days to have any stitches removed.

The incision for an augmentation operation may be made in the armpit, around or across the areola, or under the breast. Scarring may occur in any of these areas depending on which incision your surgeon uses.

Aftereffects and follow-up
Make arrangements to take time off from work for at least 10 days to two weeks. Don't attempt to drive a car for a full two weeks and avoid overhead lifting for about four weeks. You should be back to normal in about three weeks, but it's best to avoid sports for about six weeks.

POTENTIAL WORRIES
Breast cancer
There's no proof of a link between silicone implants and cancer. The Food and Drug Administration (FDA) concluded in 1989 that a carcinogenic effect in humans could not be completely ruled out, but if such an effect did exist, the risk would be very low. Breast surgeons around the world have found this statement reassuring enough to continue using silicone implants.

Mammography
Implants can make it difficult to read mammograms precisely. This means that women who have a strong family history of

Types of implants

Silicone gel implants feel more natural than saline-filled ones and they're still the first choice of most surgeons in the US. The likelihood of contracture is about the same with both types, but obviously there's no risk of silicone leakage with saline-filled ones. If silicone implants leak, they'll deflate and will need to be replaced. All implants used to be smooth, but nowadays a textured surface is preferred as this seems to reduce the frequency of contracture. Alternative implant-fill materials are being researched. It's hoped that these new materials will be absorbed by the body if leakage occurs, won't react with breast tissue, and won't obscure mammography X-rays. One new implant available in the US contains triglyceride, which is similar to body fat, and has a built-in electronic chip with a unique code to identify it.

breast cancer should probably not use silicone implants. It's a good idea for all women to have a mammogram performed before any breast surgery. It's possible to get a good mammogram of a breast with implants, but more than one view will be needed.

Contracture
The capsule of scar tissue that forms naturally around any implant can be quite thin and pliable but it may contract and become as hard as wood. One research study puts the possibility of contracture as high as 7 out of 10 at two to four years after surgery. Massaging the breasts may reduce hardness, but if they're very hard, treatment can be quite complicated.

Your surgeon can ease the tension by cutting a wider space around the implant. Or, if the implant lies above the chest wall muscles, it can be removed and a new one inserted below the muscle, where contracture is less likely.

Other complications
Breast pain, loss of sensation in the breast, difficulty with breast-feeding, infection, and movement and leakage of an implant are all well-known complications. A more uncommon one is rupture of the implant, which can occur spontaneously or through physical force such as a blow. You'll need immediate surgery if this happens to remove all traces of silicone from the breast.

Some authorities say half of all breast augmentation patients will have some side effects by 10 years after the operation; others estimate a one-in-three chance. So it's not clear sailing, though none of the above side effects is life-threatening.

"life becomes fulfilling, satisfying, and, perhaps for the first time, contented"

life stages: 40 to 60 years

Adults have a series of milestones in their lives just like children. But whereas in your younger days you may have rushed past the markers with your eye constantly on the lookout for the next, as you grow older, you tend to look back, reflect on what you have done, and you may find that it is time to choose a new lifestyle.

The saying goes "life begins at 40" and so it does for some. However, many of us reach a crossroads around 35 when we take stock, and it may take two or three years before life restabilizes. The mid- and late 40s, therefore, can be looked forward to as a period of equilibrium. The major problems of life and your place in it, and the adjustments you have to make to feel at one with yourself, have been largely figured out and life becomes fulfilling, satisfying, and, perhaps for the first time, contented.

Whether you feel renewed or resigned will depend on the choices you made at your crossroads. If you refused to make any changes, then a sense of staleness may progress into resignation and a feeling of discontent. You will not be growing and you will be aware that you're standing still. What happens is that things in your life that have made you feel safe, and that have supported you, will be gradually withdrawn. Your children will grow up and leave you, your partner could develop faster than you and grow away from you, your career may seem less satisfying and merely become a job that has to be done.

What is more, each of these events will gradually become less and less tolerable and a crossroads will probably emerge again around the age of 50, and, be assured, it will hit you much harder than it did at 40.

A renewed sense of purpose

If, on the other hand, you faced your 35-year-old crossroads and made the necessary adjustments, you will find a renewed sense of purpose, and from within yourself a drive and energy to build a good lifestyle, and the knowledge that you are looking forward to the best years of your life. For most people who are prepared to take on this difficult passage, personal happiness soars. A self-confidence that you never suspected emerges, and you can take on problems and difficulties calmly and rationally. You become less possessive about your children, you become less possessive about your partner, you find yourself warming and mellowing toward life and other people. Priorities suddenly become clear and decisions easier to take.

Facing the 50s

The 50s are a time when, once again, people take stock of their lives. We may feel increasingly aware of the importance of remaining as physically and mentally fit as possible. For women, the menopause is undoubtedly the period's most significant biological and physiological event, but there is no reason why we shouldn't feel as healthy, if not even healthier, as ever. Our increased physical awareness can lead to increased emotional awareness and we become more reflective. We become more tolerant of our own abilities and those of others; our outlook becomes increasingly philosophical and by the end of our 50s, if we've managed to remain married, we're often closer to our partner than at any other time in our life.

Planning for the future

Making plans for the years ahead is like planning a trip. Remember your last big vacation. Half the fun was thinking about it a long time in advance. The further ahead you made your plans, the more you looked forward to going and the more you enjoyed the trip. There may have been some unexpected adventures along the way, but because you had prepared yourself thoroughly you were able to cope with any eventuality.

Life can be much the same. In the pages that follow I offer guidelines where appropriate, advice where I feel there may be a need and strategies for dealing with potentially difficult situations.

Body

Social

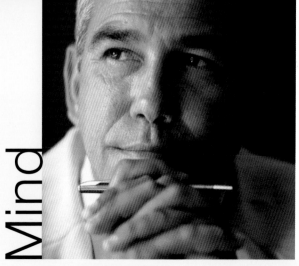

Mind

as we grow older we should be prepared to change our attitudes "exercise is particularly valuable as you get older"

"balancing work and family is a major issue for many people"

"if you don't think, your brain will slow and become feeble"

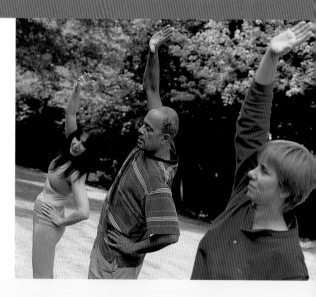

your changing body

Telltale signs such as wrinkling and changes in body shape may start to appear. But take good care of yourself and you can be as healthy as ever.

Increase in weight

Being very thin at any time of life means that a woman is unhealthy. Some fat is essential for true health and this is never more true than at the time of menopause. Being too thin can increase your risk of osteoporosis and gives you no "reserves" in case you become ill.

Slowing metabolic rate

Weight increase is gradual in both men and women as they age, but for women it may become especially noticeable during menopausal and postmenopausal years. There are at least two factors involved here. First, lack of estrogen leads to a change in body shape and fat distribution, so that the waist thickens and fat is deposited on the front of the abdomen (fat cells all over the body also increase in size). Second, the metabolic rate gradually slows down as we mature (by about 5 percent or 100 calories a day per decade) so that by the age of about 55, we need fewer calories.

Regular exercise

The main reason our metabolism declines with age is because we lose muscle strength through being less active. Unless we have a regular and frequent exercise regimen incorporated into our lives, continuing to eat at our usual rate will lead to weight gain. To combat this we need to eat sensibly and get regular exercise.

Although we need fewer calories, our body's nutritional needs remain the same. Calorie counting may be too time-consuming for anyone to maintain in the long term, so it's much better to eat a diet that is well-balanced and contains few "empty" high-calorie foods, such as sugar and fat.

Changing your eating patterns

It's within your power to change not only what you eat, but how you eat. As we get older, many of us find we can't manage three main meals a day. Try eating five or even six small meals at regular intervals so that the nutritional load is spread. This eating habit is very effective in terms of weight control because small frequent meals prevent troughs of low blood sugar, which are accompanied by cravings for food. By eating little and often you will gain confidence in your ability to control your appetite.

Many studies have been performed to show the differences between people who eat small, frequent meals and those who eat fewer and larger meals. The latter invariably have more body fat than the former. Some dieters find that a diet designed on a nibbling pattern helps to prevent hunger pangs, and there is evidence that this may actually speed up weight loss. Your digestive system will prefer a nibbling pattern, particularly if you suffer from indigestion.

Reducing the saturated fat content in your diet will also greatly help you to maintain your weight, and it will protect you from a range of diseases.

Avoid crash diets

Try not to attempt crash diets or long-term diets that are little more than starvation. The initial weight loss may be impressive – as high as 6–11lb (3–5kg) in the first week – but less than half of this will be fat; most of it will be water, and it could even include some of your precious body protein. A diet that restricts total calorie intake to below a thousand calories is only just adequate. Very strict diets, those around 500 calories, cannot provide all the required nutrients for an adult. You will even struggle with 1000 calories. There is much research to show that toward the end of a long period of this kind of dieting, the rate of weight loss not only decelerates, but the weight starts to go back on.

Eating binges

The fewer and fewer calories we give the body, the harder it is to maintain the diet. A return to a normal eating pattern will cause an inevitable increase in weight as body stores of glycogen are replaced. This is extremely depressing if you have made a great effort to shed excess weight. It is common for a person coming off a starvation diet to go on eating binges and find themselves on a treadmill of intermittent starving and bingeing that is extremely damaging to their health and self-image.

Changing body shape

One of the first changes in girls approaching adolescence is the appearance of fat on the hips, breasts, upper arms, and upper thighs. **Throughout fertile life, estrogen and progesterone are responsible for maintaining the female shape, with its narrow waist and rounded hips.** We now know that these proportions are more than simply an expression of the female gender. They have a much greater significance for both health and longevity.

The narrow waist and rounded hips pattern of fat distribution is closely and unequivocally related to coronary health. The usual ratio of the waist to hip measurement is less than one and this is associated with a low risk of a heart attack. If your waist to hip ratio creeps above 0.8, you are at much more risk.

After menopause, when levels of estrogen and progesterone are low or absent, one of the first things that a woman may notice is a thickening of the waist and the appearance of "middle-age spread." She may also notice abdominal swelling because of increased fat on the front of her abdomen. Her shape comes to resemble a more masculine outline, **and her risk of having a heart attack increases in relation to this increased fat distribution.**

The first place a man puts on weight is the abdomen, with an accompanying increase in girth. A similar rule about the ratio of waist to hips applies to women. If it goes up, then the risk of a heart attack goes up too.

Wrinkling

Wrinkling is traditionally thought to be the most obvious sign of aging skin. But wrinkling actually begins as early as our 20s and continues at a fairly steady pace for the rest of our lives. We use our facial expressions as a way of communicating with others and recording anger, rage, disappointment, happiness, surprise, consternation, and so on. These expressions are captured on our faces by lines which begin to form in the places that move most. Very few of us get to our 40s without any of these telltale signs.

Lessening the effect of wrinkling – both sexes

● Splash water on your face and keep it there with a moisturizer to prevent your skin from dehydrating.
● Never go out in the sun without wearing sunscreen – the higher the number, the greater the protection. Remember, a day on the ski slopes can do as much damage as a day at the beach.
● If you have tiny surface veins on your face, avoid eating hot, spicy food and drinking alcohol; these will aggravate face flushing.
● Stop smoking. Cigarette smoking may hasten crow's feet and causes deep lines. The skin is 10 years older in a smoker than a nonsmoker.
● Keep your body well rested by adequate sleep to improve your complexion.
● Facial exercises help to relax the facial muscles, which cause "tension" wrinkles and lines. They can also help keep facial and neck muscles mobile and relieve tension headaches. They cannot, however, stop wrinkles from forming. Try a smile all the time instead of a frown since it exercises more muscles.

For women

● If you don't wear makeup, be sure to wear a fairly liberal covering of rich moisturizer that prevents water loss.
● If you do put on some makeup, it will help reduce water loss from the skin. Avoid astringent toners; switch from cleansing soaps to creams.

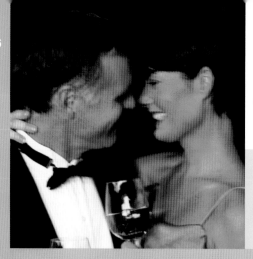

declining sexuality

High, medium, and low sex drives are all normal. All that matters is whether a couple can accommodate each other's needs, however limited or great these may be.

Vaginal dryness

A common myth about menopause is that it marks the beginning of a woman's sexual decline. Nothing could be further from the truth. **The majority of women can continue to experience sexual pleasure well into old age, indeed as long as their health remains good.** Some women even report that their sexual enjoyment starts to increase after menopause. This may be due to a higher testosterone to estrogen ratio than before.

Most menopausal women, however, notice some changes in the way their bodies respond during arousal and sex. This is often due to physical changes in the urogenital tract rather than a decreased psychological desire for sex. Research on sexual pleasure by Alfred Kinsey some decades ago has shown that women who have an enjoyable sex life before menopause are likely to continue to enjoy sex after it. On the other hand, for women who have not enjoyed sex throughout their lives, the menopause is more likely to be associated with a decrease in all kinds of sexual activity.

One of the most common sexual problems after menopause is lack of lubrication. In youth, blood flow out of the genitals is slow during arousal,

causing swelling and sensitivity to touch. After menopause, there is less engorgement of the clitoris, the vagina, and the vulva, leading to subdued arousal.

In a young woman, the vagina expands during sexual arousal to allow easy penetration. After menopause, the vagina does not expand so much, but it still remains large enough to accommodate an erect penis (as long as you allow time to achieve proper lubrication).

Healthy adrenal glands are also critical to sex drive. Long-term stress, such as bereavement and divorce, can adversely affect glandular activity. Sexual desire can also be diminished by drugs such as tranquilizers and antidepressants. Alcohol, smoking, coffee, overwork, tension, and depression have the same effect.

Self-help tips
● Before sex, put some sterile, water-soluble lubricant on your vaginal entrance. You may want to put a small amount inside your vagina and on your partner's penis or fingers. Water-based jellies are better than oil-based ones because they are less likely to promote bacterial growth and infections, and they will not cause the rubber of a condom to disintegrate.

● Avoid douches, talcum powder, perfumed toilet papers, and any fragranced bath oils and foams, which can irritate the vagina.
● Avoid washing the inside of your labia with soap since it will dry the skin.
● Avoid remedies for genital itchiness containing antihistamine or perfume.
● Spend longer on foreplay to give your body more time to produce its own lubrication. Gentle massage of the breasts, belly, thighs, and genitals can help and be extremely erotic.
● Research shows that regular sex or masturbation may help keep the vagina lubricated. This may be because sexual activity stimulates the adrenal glands that in turn help to keep the vagina lubricated.
● Women who have low histamine levels may find it difficult to reach orgasm, whereas women with high histamine levels achieve orgasm easily. Women who take antihistamines regularly need to be aware of the possibility of decreased sexual desire and delayed orgasm.
● Pelvic floor exercises (see p. 169) will make you more aware of your vagina and will increase your sexual enjoyment, as better-toned muscles will enable you to grip your partner's penis more tightly.

Loss of libido

Sex is a highly complex part of our lives and it is influenced by our current moods and emotions outside the bedroom. If we are depressed, tired, or ill, we will have little inclination for it. One of the most common and frustrating problems a couple can face is that one partner wants sex much more than the other. It is important to realize that no matter how well matched you are there will be times when your sex drives are out of sync with each other. Like any other appetite, desire for sex waxes and wanes. It is a popular myth that men are always ready and willing for sex, but they are not.

If you find there is a substantial difference in your appetites, you will need to work out some long-term strategy that prevents you from feeling continually dissatisfied, rejected, and unloved and for your partner not to feel he is continually under pressure to have sex more than he wants.

Remember sex doesn't necessarily involve intercourse. Even if your partner is not aroused himself he can still arouse you using manual or oral stimulation. To awaken desire for sex, the following suggestions may be helpful.
● Make love somewhere other than in bed (on a chair, sofa, etc).
● Take a bath or shower together.
● Create an intimate atmosphere with music and candlelight.
● Give each other a massage with scented body oils.
● Make love at an unusual time.
● Make love in the dark if you usually prefer some light and vice versa.
● Allow enough time for lovemaking.
Don't make an issue of masturbation because sometimes a man finds it easier to achieve and sustain an erection this way. It's possible that he's noticed some differences in his performance which are perfectly normal but worrying for him.

Aging does have an influence on sex. It takes a man longer to become sexually aroused and his erection may not be as strong. He may need much more direct manual or oral stimulation of his penis. His erection will not be quite as hard or its angle as acute as when he was younger. Orgasms themselves may be less intense than before. And because ejaculation generally becomes less powerful with age, semen seeps rather than spurts out.

Many men feel desire should be spontaneous, that they should not need direct stimulation in order to become aroused. This is not the case, even less so as as they grow older. So encourage your partner to let you arouse him.

Viagra

There are many treatments now available for the treatment of waning sexual potency: the best known is Viagra. It was hailed as the answer to a failing man's prayer but it can't be used by everyone to pep up their libido. It has side effects and for it to be effective a man's equipment must be in moderately good working order.

Health requirements

For starters, the blood vessels and nerves in the penis must be intact, otherwise no form of medication can bring about an erection. And the heart and blood pressure must be close to normal. With these provisos, men with the following conditions may experience an improvement in their sexual performance by taking Viagra: diabetes, multiple sclerosis, Parkinson's disease, poliomyelitis, prostate cancer, prostatectomy, radical pelvic surgery, renal failure treated by dialysis or transplant, severe pelvic injury, single gene neurological disease, spinal cord injury, and spina bifida.

Does it work?

Viagra isn't a miracle cure. In the original research, almost half of the subjects had better erections than previously, erections sufficient to allow penetrative sex, but not the rigidity of youth. Half did not.

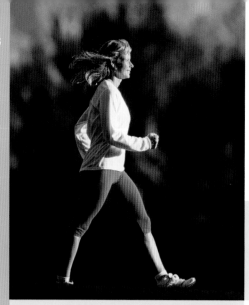

don't let your body fall apart

Don't fall into the trap of taking less and less care of yourself, otherwise your muscles will get slack, and your heart and lungs will be less able to deal with exertion.

Walking

Like other good habits, exercise should be undertaken regularly and be a lifelong habit. Doing a reasonable amount of walking – 20 or 30 minutes or so each day – is a good habit to develop, and you can build this up over a period of months. This kind of routine becomes important after retirement, when most people use up less energy but continue eating and drinking the same amounts they did before.

Tips for walking

● Do some gentle flexibility exercises before you go out.

● Begin by walking on level ground and progress to hill walking as you become more fit.

● Walk at a speed that makes you slightly short of breath but don't get too out of breath to talk.

● Never push yourself further than you feel you can comfortably go.

● Try to increase the distance or the time you spend walking, rather than the speed at which you walk.

● Don't walk into the wind since this requires more effort. If you suffer from heart disease, you should be able to walk quite comfortably in calm weather, but walking into the wind may cause angina pains.

Exercise as a mental tonic

Regular exercise may also have a significant effect on our mental agility by increasing the amount of oxygen supplied to the brain. In a comparison between sedentary older women and older women who got regular exercise, after four months the latter group processed information faster in tests. This effect of exercise is particularly marked in older people.

Besides increasing the oxygen supply to the brain, exercise may also slow down the loss of dopamine in the brain. Dopamine is a neurotransmitter that helps prevent the shaking and stiffness that can come with old age. A severe shortage of dopamine results in the exaggerated tremors of Parkinson's disease. Dopamine decreases in the brain by about one percent a year from our mid-20s, and if we lived to be 100, we would all appear to have Parkinson's disease. Since exercise can slow down dopamine loss, it is particularly beneficial as we grow older. Exercise can also prevent our reaction times from slowing down.

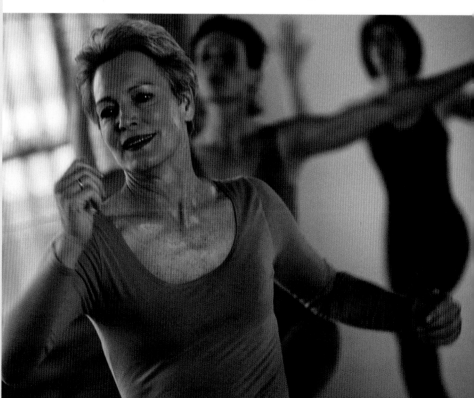

The benefits of regular exercise

Exercise is vital throughout your life, but as you get older these benefits are particularly valuable:
- a reduced risk of heart disease
- a lower chance of developing diabetes
- maintenance of muscle strength
- higher levels of the healthy type of cholesterol in the blood
- better bone health and less chance of developing osteoporosis (if you do weight-bearing exercise)
- a more efficient immune system
- reduced body fat
- better appetite control
- reduced risk of constipation
- increased mental agility
- fewer headaches
- improved sleep quality
- flexible joints.

The type of exercise you get will obviously depend largely on resources, how much time is available, and personal preference. To gain the best effects from exercise, try to find a form that you enjoy. There is a wide range of opportunities available in sports centers and exercise classes and, for those who need or prefer to exercise in their own home, there are a lot of books, videos, and tapes on the market.

You may prefer a sport such as tennis or raquetball, which offers the added attraction of meeting people. Likewise, joining a class may encourage you to exercise regularly. Less rigorous, more traditional forms of exercise such as brisk walking and swimming offer a viable alternative and keep the body fit and supple.

Recently, there has been a move away from aerobic training toward strength-training and weight-bearing exercise. Research suggests that any form of exercise involving weights can delay loss of bone and muscle tissue, which is a natural consequence of aging. Weight-bearing exercise also helps to normalize the flow of sugar from the blood into muscle tissue, where it can be properly metabolized. This may lower the risk of diabetes and heart disease.

Kegel exercises

Almost all women who've had children notice slight leakage when they cough or lift a heavy weight. But regular kegel exercises will do much to put things right. Here's how to do your kegel exercises.
- The first step is to find the group of muscles that form a figure of eight around the vagina, urethra, and anus. You can do this by stopping the flow several times while you're urinating.
- Tighten the muscles for five seconds, relax them for five seconds, then tense them again. Make sure you're not just tightening your buttocks and try not to tighten your stomach muscles at the

same time. You may not be able to hold the tension for the full five seconds at first, but you are likely to develop this ability once your pelvic floor muscles grow stronger.
- The next stage is to tighten and relax the muscles 10 times, as quickly as you can so that they seem to "flutter." You will probably need to practice for a while to control the muscles in this way.
- Next, contract the muscles long and steadily as though you were trying to draw an object into your vagina. Hold the contraction for five seconds.
- The final step is to bear down, as if emptying the bowels, but pushing more

through the vagina than the anus. Hold the tension for five seconds.

Gradually build up to 10 contractions, 10 times daily or more, spaced over several hours, and check your progress once or twice a week by stopping the flow when you urinate. After about six weeks of these exercises you should find stopping the flow is much easier than it was in the beginning. The beauty of kegel exercises is that, once you've mastered the technique, you can do them anywhere, any time – lying down, watching television, even when you're washing dishes or waiting for the bus!

looking good

Re-thinking hairstyles and makeup and modernizing skin-care routines can take 10 years off your looks. You need a look to suit the woman you are now rather than the woman you were.

Creams

No substance yet known to science can permanently restore the collagen, protein, fat, and moisture that we lose from the skin as we grow older. Nor is it possible to repair the fractures that develop in the collagen within the dermis as our faces start to wrinkle. Creams cannot hold lines and wrinkles at bay, no matter what exotic ingredients they contain, but rich cleansing creams and moisturizers may prevent the top layer of our skin from drying out.

Hair

After menopause, hair growth starts to slow down, the diameter of the hair shaft reduces and gray hairs become more prominent. It is a myth that gray hair is coarser. Gray hair only appears coarser because it starts to appear as the scalp becomes drier. This is due to the oil glands slowing down. Now is the time to switch your shampoo and conditioners to richer, more moisturizing formulas. They aren't sales gimmicks – they really can add moisture to your hair.

Tips on hair care

If you've had the same style for years, ask your hairdresser what style would update your look. Look through magazines and cut out pictures of styles you like. Contrary to popular belief, most hairdressers like to see pictures of the hairstyles you favor because if you simply describe them there is too much room for misinterpretation.

● To cover the first few gray hairs use a semi-permanent hair color one shade lighter than your natural color.
● The addition of highlights or lowlights can even out the effect of gray hairs.
● Never be tempted to stay the color you were when younger. Skin tones change along with hair color so lighter hair colors become more flattering.
● Soften salt-and-pepper hair coloring with a pale blond semi-permanent hair color. It gives the effect of expensive highlights.
● If you wish to gray gracefully but your hair has yellow tones, use pearl or silver shampoos and toners to enhance your hair.

Makeup colors

There are rainbows of shades to choose from, but fortunately nature tells us what colors suit us. Take a magnifying glass and look in a mirror for flecks of different colors in the iris of your eye. All of these, if used as an eyeshadow, will suit you. When selecting colors, take your skin tone into consideration. If you have a warm skin tone, choose warmer colors like golds and bronzes. Cooler skins should opt for cooler colors like silver and lilacs. If your skin is pale, avoid colors that are too dark. If you are olive-skinned, pale colors will be lost so more intense shades are better.

Brunettes

More intense shades suit you better. Try olive green, bronze, and terracotta eyeshadows teamed with warm peach or tawny-brown blush and rust, wine, or warm neutral corals on the lips.

Blondes with cool skin tones

Heather, soft grays, lilac, and ice blues are good eyeshadow shades to try, along with soft pinks or tea rose blushes. Try lipsticks in dusky rose or raspberry.

Gray hair

Slate blue or steel blue eyeshadows flatter gray hair, along with soft fuchsia blush. Lips can take raspberry or tea rose shades.

Black skin

Try jewel shades or coppers and bronze for eyeshadows, and rust and fuchsia blushes. Rich gold wine or bronze look good on lips.

Changing your makeup

When you were 17 you wore makeup to look older. If you are stuck in a makeup rut, you could still be making yourself look older. Go through your makeup bag and be ruthless. The colors that suited you a few years ago might not suit you now. As you get older your skin changes tone, so treat yourself to some new, more flattering colors. Look through magazines to see what's popular this year, what new products are around and how you can include them in your lifestyle. If you feel magazines cater only to the young, then book a consultation at a makeup counter and see what the trained beauticians recommend. Don't forget that they are there to sell their own products, so try a few different counters before deciding what you really need to buy.

One of the easiest ways to look younger is to re-think how you use foundation. A thick one won't hide the lines – just the opposite. Foundation collects in any tiny lines, emphasizing wrinkles. The older you get, the less you should use.

Makeup tips

● Try making up without using any foundation at all. Concealer can be used to hide under-eye shadows or broken veins and you can always use a little skin-toned pressed powder to take away any shine.
● If you feel you need foundation, choose light reflective formulas or switch to a tinted moisturizer.
● Don't be tempted to add color with foundation, leave that to the blush. Make sure foundation matches your skin tone exactly then you don't have to apply it all over your face, just where you need it, usually across the cheeks, chin, and nose area.
● Plucking the stray hairs from underneath your eyebrows can instantly open up eyes.
● If you have overplucked your brows in the past, try using brow powder makeup instead of filling in with pencil, which can look too hard. Apply the color with a small angled brush to create soft, more natural brows.
● Avoid frosted eyeshadows, which draw attention to any lines. Choose shadows with semi-sheen, since matt shadows can look dull.
● A hard line of eyeliner only looks good if you are 18. Use an eyeliner brush and a dark powder eyeshadow and brush a fine line as close to the lashes as possible. The effect is softer and much more flattering.
● Blush brushes can be too small and so narrow you end up with a stripe of color across your cheek. Use a powder brush instead since they tend to be fatter. Don't stop at the cheeks, brush on blush across the chin, temples, and forehead for a healthy glow.
● The perfect blush shade for your skin tone is the color your cheeks get when you're naturally flushed.
● Build up the color in gentle layers. Not only will it look more natural but it will last longer too.
● If your skin is naturally dry, switch from powder blush to cream. Dot along the cheekbone after moisturizing and blend while the skin is still dewy.
● Lips can loose their plumpness and the edges become less defined. Sharpen the outline with a lip pencil.
● Avoid lip liners darker than your lipstick; they look too hard. Choose a shade that matches your natural lip color. As well as sharpening the outline it also stops lipstick from bleeding.

Skin care

After menopause, skin becomes drier and thinner. Dead cells aren't shed as quickly, resulting in dull, dry patches. To keep skin as dewy as possible, switch to richer day moisturizers and night creams and exfoliate twice a week to remove sluggish dead cells.

Remember that the basic rule of cleanse, moisturize, and protect is more important than ever now.
● **Protect your skin from the sun.** About 80 percent of wrinkles are caused by earlier sun damage. Protect from further damage by using a SPF of at least 15.
● **Don't forget to protect both your neck and hands.** Both are just as much exposed to the sun as your face.
● **Increase your water intake** – water does aid the metabolic rate of the body. So does exercise, even if it is only walking or swimming.
● **Don't use rich moisturizers near your eyes.** You simply end up with puffy eyes in the morning. Use an eye cream for this area, dotting along the bone under your eye, and blend it by gently patting with your ring finger.

male menopause

Little is known about male menopause, or "male climacteric," other than it doesn't exist in the same form as a woman's: hormonally speaking it may not exist at all.

Is there a male menopause?

Do all men experience a menopause or "climacteric"? If there is such a thing, what are the symptoms? Drawing a parallel from menopausal symptoms in women, should men be the beneficiaries of hormone replacement therapy (HRT)? Once this question is advanced, others follow. What would happen to the male climacteric if HRT were widely used? What would the success rate be? What are the harmful effects? There are very few answers to any of these questions because so little research has been done in this area, though this is sure to change in the near future as more people take an interest in male symptoms.

Male menopause doesn't have the same drama as a woman's. It is more gradual, gentle, and in a way more insidious than a woman's; nor does it occur during exactly the same years. It is much better thought of as a male climacteric, which envelops all the changes going on in the body and mind as the male genital system begins to wane.

Fear of failure

There is no doubt that "fear of failure" plays a very important part in the aging man's withdrawal from sexual activities.

Once a man has noticed that his potency is declining, or he experiences one occasion when he is unable to achieve sexual satisfaction due to impotence, he may withdraw voluntarily from any kind of sexual activity. This is mainly because most men are unable to face the ego-shattering experience of repeated episodes of sexual inadequacy. Most men are unable to accept the fact that a lessening of sexual drive and a lowering of sexual performance are parts of the normal aging process, and they make all kinds of excuses and will blame many different kinds of external factors rather than face the truth that their bodies are maturing.

Researchers Masters and Johnson hypothesized in 1970 that a man who finds his potency declining may be showing signs of lowered levels of androgens that may amount to a deficiency. They went on to say that until studies had shown that there was a general requirement by the body for androgen (testosterone) replacement therapy during the male climacteric, cases had to be treated on an individual basis.

There are endocrinologists in many parts of the world who make a special study of the male climacteric, employing hormone replacement therapy for their male patients. The whole area, however, still awaits clear definition and guidelines. **Until then HRT for men will remain a highly specialized field not generally practiced.** In this respect women are better off than men. It may be because women are honest and courageous enough to declare that their bodies are deficient, whereas men, particularly in the sensitive area of sexual activities, have yet to come to terms with their bodily changes.

Work/family tensions

Most men between the ages of 40 and 60 are going through the most competitive stages of their careers. The tensions of work are not eased by the financial necessity to look after a growing family with many needs and activities. **On the one hand, men are striving for personal eminence, and on the other they are preoccupied with the security of the "family."** A man in this situation often finds that he spends more time following his professional career than with his family. This leaves a smaller amount of time for loving relationships with his partner, and the stress may lead to gradual lessening in sexual activity.

Both mental and physical fatigue have an ever-increasing influence on sexual activity. **An active sex life in the middle years means being in good condition**, for if a job requires a great deal of physical effort, a man may simply not be physically fit enough to have stamina left over at the end of a day to enjoy an active sex life. Sometimes, if a man is not fit, a weekend of recreation is more exhausting than the demands of his job, particularly in the age group of 50 and over. Again, this leaves very little energy for sexual activity. If a man is exposed to unaccustomed or excessive physical activity he may feel a loss of sexual responsiveness for a day or so, which will add to his feeling of despondency.

Sexuality in older men

Masters and Johnson, a pioneering research team in human sexuality, made a detailed study of the psychological and physiological factors that might contribute to a decline in a man's sexual prowess as he grows older. From their studies it became obvious that there are factors that affect a man's sexual responsiveness:
● monotony, described as being the result of repetitious sexual relationships
● preoccupation with career and economic pursuits
● mental or physical fatigue
● overindulgence in food and drink
● any physical or mental infirmities in either of the partners
● fear that his performance does not come up to scratch may be greater than at any other time in his life, especially during a time of stressful career decisions.

Monotony is quoted most often and most constantly as the factor that leads to a loss of interest in sex and sexual performance. The end result of this may be one of dutiful indulgence and the need for sexual release. This sometimes arises from a failure of the sexual part of a relationship to grow throughout the marriage. Overfamiliarity with a partner is often blamed; the female partner may no longer be stimulating to her man. She herself may be engrossed in caring for children, or busy with her career. Furthermore, women generally do age more during their 40s and 50s in terms of physical appearance than men. Without attention to her appearance, a woman may become older-looking than her partner.

Sexual problems

As men grow older they eat and drink more, which has a tendency to repress their sex drives. Also, if men feel satisfied from good food this lowers their capacity to achieve in other areas. Overindulgence in alcohol has a particularly negative effect on potency. Impotence developing in a hitherto potent man often makes him drink excessive alcohol and otherwise behave in a way that has not been in his nature.

Most men approaching middle age become concerned about performance. One of the ways of handling any concern is to withdraw from having to perform. This leads to total avoidance of sex within the marriage. If a man is also drinking heavily it only makes matters worse. A problem may arise within the marriage. A man may find that he is impotent with his wife but with another partner, who cannot measure present sexual performance against past, he is perfectly normal.

At any age, physical or mental infirmity can lower or even eliminate sexual drive. After the age of 40 physical or emotional difficulties have a much greater effect, and above the age of 60 a tremendously negative influence. Being physically disabled in the short or long term lowers sexual responsiveness in either sex, but if the illness is acute, such as pneumonia, loss of libido is usually transient and accepted by both partners. With more long-term disabilities, such as arthritis, interest in sex may decline slowly until it becomes nonexistent. Conditions such as long-term diabetes can lead to impotence in men for medical reasons, and such problems need to be discussed with a partner.

female menopause

For many women, menopause can be a psychological, emotional, and intellectual turning point as well as a physical one, but it does not have to mean a decline.

Overcoming stereotypes

Referring to menopause as "the change of life" is misleading and can be counterproductive. Menopause isn't the only change that will occur during your life and it is unlikely to be the most significant change. **Life is a series of gradual changes – we don't suddenly reach a turning point and start growing old when we reach midlife.** Aging is a continuous process that begins the moment we are born. I believe that a healthy attitude to menopause is to see it as a time in which to rediscover yourself, to assess your life and its purpose, and to establish new aims and goals.

Many of us have spent much of our lives trying to please other people. We put a great deal of effort into taking care of our children, husbands, parents, and friends. We try to be what they would like us to be, and very often we lose sight of who we

are and what we want. By trying to become everything to everyone, we can end up being nothing to ourselves. By the time we reach middle age most of us carry around the received "wisdom" of society, leftovers from old customs and traditions, fears that are often obsolete, and beliefs that may be borrowed. Without clearing up all these redundant feelings, we can lose touch with our inner selves.

It is important to resist negative stereotypes associated with menopause. These are often culturally created, and do not reflect the reality of our individual experiences. In countries where age is venerated and older women are respected for their experience and wisdom, fewer physical and psychological symptoms of menopause are reported. Many Asian, Arab, and African women

positively welcome the end of fertility and childbearing, and, perhaps as a result, they seem to encounter fewer difficulties than Western women. In countries that lack a tradition of myths and misconceptions about menopause, aging seems to be regarded as a more natural process; women aren't adversely affected by negative images and may feel less confused by what is happening.

If you believe that in order to be beautiful and successful you must be young, then you may not enjoy your middle age to the fullest. If you are convinced that the quality of life deteriorates from the age of 50 onward, this can become a self-fulfilling prophecy; because you believe it is going to happen, you may inadvertently make it happen by not taking care of yourself and adopting resigned, negative attitudes.

Menopause

The word "menopause" is usually used to describe the time in a woman's life between the ages of 45 and 55, when her fertility declines and her menstruation stops. The word literally means "cessation of menstruation."

Menopause has quite rightly been given a good deal of attention because it

is a dramatic event. There are many changes: hormonal, physical, mental, and emotional, which occur during the change, and there is the obvious and inescapable punctuation mark of no more menstrual periods. To feel confident, it is necessary that we know what is taking place in our bodies, so that we can understand that

the mechanism is normal (see p. 497).

Menopause is closely involved with gaining new insights, maturing, changing standards, choosing new lifestyles, and developing new opinions and priorities. It may be a confused state, or it may be clear sailing. We must draw on our reserves of serenity and maturity.

Developing a positive attitude

The first step in developing a positive attitude toward menopause is to look back and assess what we have already accomplished. This can reassure us and give us the impetus we need to make decisions about the future. If we forget to acknowledge what we've already done, we can make future goals seem much less attainable.

No matter how active we've been, or what contributions we have made to our work and our family, contemplation of the future can bring mixed emotions. We may find ourselves debating two alternatives: trying to continue living and working as we have always done; or starting to make changes, perhaps reducing our workload. You might justifiably say to yourself that you've been working all your life, so why should you feel guilty for not working now? **It's important as we get older to learn how to enjoy leisure time and to find new and varied diversions.**

Find out what excites and motivates you. Stop spending time on things that don't interest you, household chores for example. You have as much potential as when you were young, but now you are better equipped to harness it. **Make a list of things you "must" do in the rest of your life, things you may never have attempted before.**

Some women break out of their usual lifestyle after many years as wife, mother, and family caretaker to indulge an entrepreneurial spirit and branch out on their own, perhaps setting up a bed-and-breakfast, opening a store, or running a small business. You may remember your mother in her 50s claiming that she was growing old. If you're still alive at 85, as my mother is, 35 years is a long time to be old, and an intolerable length of time to be inactive.

We have a responsibility to ourselves to make the most of each month, year, and decade. Repeat this to yourself every day, and if you feel you lack energy, the best technique is to get angry, particularly if you feel you've stifled your anger and held back in the past. Put yourself in touch with your anger, and use it as fuel. It's absolutely crucial to respect and to trust who you are. You need self-respect before you can respect others and understand them as individuals. Older women are perceptive, experienced, and wise about relationships and life. We can benefit even more from joining a group of women of a similar age and sharing our experiences.

The strong interaction between your mind and your body means that you can make your menopause more difficult with negative thoughts. If you believe you're sick, you can start to behave like a sick person.

Repeat some of these statements like a mantra each day and you will gradually become convinced of their truth. Positive attitudes will maintain your self-esteem.

- My body is strong and healthy and can become healthier each day.
- My female organs are in good shape.
- My body chemistry is effective and balanced.
- I eat healthy, nourishing food.
- I'm learning to handle stress.
- I'm calm and relaxed.
- I work efficiently and competently.
- I have the freedom and confidence to enjoy life.
- I can be happy and optimistic at this time of my life.
- My life belongs to me and it brings me pleasure.
- I devote time to myself each day.
- My friends and family are more enjoyable than they have ever been.
- I'm going through menopause more easily and more comfortably with each passing day.

life changes

Some of today's 40-year-olds are deciding to start families, while others are dealing with the end of a long marriage. For many life in the 40s and 50s just gets better and better.

Older mothers

Though fertility does diminish with age, statistics show that the odds are greatly in favor of you having a successful pregnancy at almost any age provided you are healthy. Many studies have been done on normal pregnancies in women past the age of 40 and all of them concluded that the general health of the mother is much more important than age alone as a factor in predicting how the pregnancy will turn out. **If your health is good, the decision to have a baby should not be abandoned because of age alone.**

Age will always be a factor for you to consider when deciding to have a

baby but not the negative one that you might think. **Considerations of personal freedom and career moves are causing more and more women to wait until they are over 30 and even 40 to become pregnant,** but many still fear that they may be letting it go too long. This is because they may have heard that the longer they wait the greater is the chance of having a difficult pregnancy or even, possibly, a child with an abnormality. However, although the risk of having a Down syndrome baby increases with the age of the mother, carefully documented case studies show that it is not physically dangerous to the woman

herself if she defers pregnancy until she is well past 30.

The risks undoubtedly do increase with age but every decision to have a child is unique and the age of the parents is only one factor, and a very small one, in weighing the risks and benefits. The age of the father relates more to infertility than to a risk factor. Many other factors affect the risk factor ratio in each woman's case. Of course, what these statistics do is to lump all mothers over the age of say, 30, together, regardless of their health or financial background whereas an important factor in maternal risk is the mother's socioeconomic situation. **The complications during pregnancy and delivery for older mothers are not related to age but to other factors such as malnutrition;** a pregnant woman will need special care only if she is poorly nourished, regardless of age.

Although physically a woman may be better suited to childbirth when she is in her early 20s, emotionally she may not be ready to be a parent. When she is younger, a woman may be too involved with her career to have children or she may not have met the right person to be the father of her children.

Satisfaction with life

Gail Sheehy in her book *Pathfinders* describes a questionnaire relating to members of the American Bar Association. Those lawyers who were judged to be most happy and contented were almost all older than 47. Those who were older than 45 thought life was wonderful and were loving it, but the most contented age group of all consisted of lawyers over the age of 56.

Ages 37 to 45

"Not enough time for anything but work."
"Obsessed with money and material success."
"Feel this is my last chance to pull away from the pack."
"Worry about becoming trapped by others finding out I am not as good as they thought I was. About messing up my personal life."
"Uncertain about my objectives."
"Ambivalent about my values."
"Envy the spirituality of others."

Ages 46 to 55

"Finally feel I have it all together."
"Secure enough to stop running or struggling."
"Easy to relax, open myself to new feelings, take vacations."
"Not concerned about what others think of me."
"More willing to help others, not so competitive and compulsive."
"Feel that time is running out."
"Suddenly notice my friends are looking old and unhealthy."
"Was over-monitoring my own health."

Ages 56 to 65

"Delighted to see vigor of life is continuing."
"Pay more attention to my body and I am in better physical condition than I was five years ago."
"Sex is still important."
"Feel a new tolerance. Formed companionship with my partner."
"More focus on the spiritual dimension."
"Vacations are essential."
"Less concerned with money, more concerned with comfort."

Divorce

Divorce is often harder for people when they're older than it would have been if they had gone through it when they were young. In the aftermath of divorce many people feel that they are "over the hill" and unattractive. They may fear that no one will ever want them again. Many dislike going to dances and parties alone after so many years of living with a secure partner. Some people are bitter because they are left alone after 30 or more years.

The divorced woman
Women, especially after being deserted for someone younger, may feel ferociously protective about their alimony payments, particularly if they haven't been trained for a job and feel they are too old to begin a career. Salt is rubbed in the wound if a woman can remember it was she who put her student husband through his professional training so that he could earn a good salary for the two of them. Some women feel that after bringing up the family for a man and helping him achieve success in his career, they deserve every penny they can get.

This pessimistic approach may end up making women believe that divorce is the end of their lives. But having lived through the despair, pain, self-hatred, and even self-pity, many of us find that life is better after divorce. Some get their first full-time job to keep busy and sane. Some feel confident enough to have dates with other men. It is possible for women to discover sex for the first time after having been trapped in a claustrophobic marriage. Prior to divorce and meeting men,

some women wrongly believe that they have a low sex drive. They believe that sex can never really be enjoyable. Sometimes they feel reborn when they have a fulfilling relationship with a new and more sympathetic partner.

It's easy to feel cheated for having spent a long time with a rather stodgy partner, but the best view is that there are a number of good years ahead. It is the prime time of life, there is no worry about becoming pregnant, menopause has passed. The children are grown up, and therefore you don't have to worry about taking care of them. It is possible to have a small, efficient apartment that takes little time to maintain. You may find that the only worry you have is how best to go about having a good time – just like in your old single days.

The divorced man
Now that they have discovered that they can take care of themselves economically, women are leaving men more frequently than before. More and more men over 50 are being left behind by wives who always wanted to get out of the marriage.

It is not always the case that an older man who is divorced is the guilty party and has left his aging wife for a younger woman. On the contrary, his wife may have left him for a younger man. Men in this situation feel depressed and deserted and many seek a lasting relationship for the years ahead. Men seem to be very well suited to the marriage state. Health statistics show that they are happiest, in the best health, and least depressed when they are married. So they tend to re-marry.

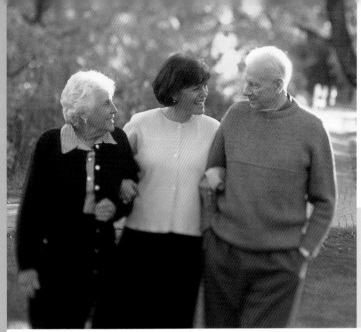

sandwich generation

People in this age group are often caught between caring for their growing children on the one hand and for their aging parents on the other.

Caring for a family and elderly parents

Although family relationships have changed radically in the last century, one thing that has remained fairly consistent is the way in which younger members of a family assume responsibility for older members. There is no doubt that this can place severe emotional, physical, and economic stress on the caretakers. The mobility of today's society means that the family is not always gathered in one place. Even a few minutes traveling time can make support difficult, especially if we have other commitments, such as work. Sometimes the combined responsibilities of taking care of a home, family, and aged parents, as well as dealing with postmenopausal symptoms, can seem overwhelming. Try to delegate as much as you can. Enlist the help of your partner, your children, and your siblings.

If you have very old or infirm parents, you may have to make the decision to house them in an assisted living center or nursing home. No family should feel guilty about this – it's a highly responsible option, ensuring that your parent is well cared for. No one has to sacrifice their own family to care for a parent.

Respite care

I get many letters from adult children stretched to the limit by having to look after sick, aging relatives. These old people may simply be frail, but remain pleasant and grateful. That's hard enough when the caretaking lasts seven days a week, but the strain is crushing if the elderly person is difficult, irascible, ungrateful, and worst, suffers dementia. Then caretaking can become an almost unbearable burden.

The people who write to me find themselves in the dilemma of being exhausted, unable to go on, but nonetheless wanting to go on taking care of their mother or father and wracked with guilt at the thought of turning them over to the care of others, even for a short time.

They write to me hoping I will give them permission to take a life-saving vacation, on their own, away from the demands of a bed-bound parent. I always do. No one should feel guilty about taking advantage of respite care. Indeed, I feel caretakers of old people should have at least a month of respite care each 12 months. Otherwise they will crack up. Someone must care for the caregivers.

The empty nest syndrome

I found it hard when it was time for my own sons to fly the nest. It's difficult to accept that from the day a baby is born a parent's mission is to prepare the child for that day. Some parents do feel excited and proud – or relieved – as the conflict and commotion of living with a young adult gives way to more peace and privacy. But many feel the loss of an all-consuming role in their lives, one that gave definition, activities and a sense of being needed. That's a pretty major event. After years raising, protecting, and nurturing a child it is tough letting go, but it has to be done. It's not fair to try to keep control or smother him with your love.

A sense of loss

The observation that women who react badly to menopause have a low opinion of themselves is not a new one. Particularly vulnerable are women who have defined their role in life in terms of pregnancy and motherhood. For such women menopause can take away part of their identity, and in some cases can make them feel purposeless. If motherhood was the focal point of your life, it is easy to understand how the climacteric can bring a sense of loss. The same is true for women who have never had children, but have wanted to.

Many women, to varying degrees, suppress their own desires, talents, and

personal growth, and invest all their energies in caring for their children, husbands, and families, so that they only express themselves through the activities and accomplishments of others. When their children leave home, they may undergo an emotional and intellectual trauma similar to bereavement.

Such women have to find a new focus to their lives, and the climacteric can be a time of major reassessment. Dependence signals the child in us.

If you remain overly involved it won't be for your child's good, it will be to indulge your own selfish needs. Feelings of depression, sadness, and/or grief and loss of purpose are normal reactions. If you can find someone to talk to, such as your partner or a friend, it may help.

Making new plans

The empty nest syndrome implies that once children have left home parents become redundant. Nothing could be further from the truth. It's simply time to create new roles for yourself. What interested you before you had children? Plan on bringing some of those interests into your life now. Remember, the more "hats" you wear, the happier your life. It helps to convert the children's bedrooms as soon as is feasible and affordable into practical and usable space. This will keep you from wandering into their rooms and getting melancholy over past times. For example, have you always wanted to take up a hobby like painting? Your son's room could become your studio. What about making plans to travel, moving to a smaller home – anything that keeps you busy.

Keep in mind that this can also be an invigorating time in your relationship with your child – a chance to go from being a parent to a young adult's vital, trusted friend.

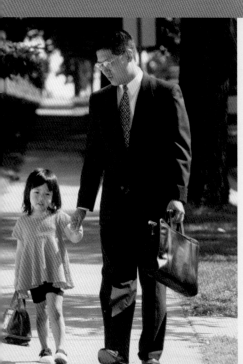

Work/life balance

One of the major issues of the first decade of the 21st century will be the need to find a balance between working and family life. Almost all people who work, men and women, are concerned about the encroachment of work on their leisure time and the problems of incorporating family and leisure activities into a professional working week.

Achieving a balance

Working parents are so exercised by trying to achieve this balance that some men refuse promotion if it means that the new job will curtail the time they have available for their families and the

pursuit of hobbies and sporting activities. Women, more and more, are choosing to work only for companies that are family friendly and offer good maternity benefits, flexible working hours, job sharing, and telecommuting as a matter of course.

The effect is seen in men as well as women employees because every man with a partner who has difficulty in finding a work-life balance has a problem of work-life balance himself. Responsible employers are sympathetic to the needs of parents of young families in their workforce and try to cater to them as much as possible.

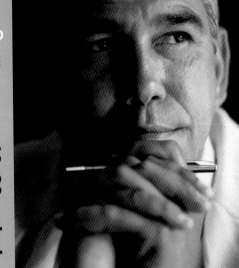

mental well-being

As we grow older, we should leave behind preconceptions and prejudices, and constantly be prepared to change our attitudes. We need to work with our emotions in a constructive and helpful way, and yet still be affectionate and tender with ourselves.

Maintaining memory

As we get older, our long-term memory gets clearer; it's our short-term memory that may suffer. You may forget where you put something, miss appointments, and things that used to be easy to remember can suddenly require enormous effort. If you are worried about becoming forgetful, there are several exercises and techniques that will help your short-term memory.

● When you read a book or a magazine article, summarize the plot or the points made in it to a friend. Refer to names, places, and dates.

● When you go shopping, try to collect as many items as you can without looking at your shopping list.

● If there are several things you want to remember, try to do it with a mnemonic. For example, tasks such as ironing, making a phone call, and typing a letter can be abbreviated into a single word. Take the first letters of each task, and make them into a word, for example "PIT" (Phone/Iron/Type), which will act as a memory aid.

● If you walk into a room and forget why you've gone into it, go back to the place that you came from and don't leave until you have remembered the reason for going there.

● If you have lost something, track it down by a process of elimination. Write down the last six things you did prior to losing it and where you were for each activity. If necessary, draw a grid on a piece of paper with what you were doing along one side and where you were along the bottom. The item you've lost lies in one of those squares; just check each one out and you should find it.

Staying mentally fit

Mental fitness can be as easy to maintain as physical fitness, and we must strive to maintain a basic state of mental health so that we can rise to challenges, cope with emergencies, and have the resilience to survive stressful situations in the long term. As we get older, we have to deal with emotional trauma, such as the loss of parents and possibly our partner.

Self-knowledge requires supreme realism: we have to learn that we are not unique in suffering, that difficult times come and go, that adversity is normal and that some failures are inevitable. We can learn a lot by observing the qualities of people whose mental and emotional resilience we admire. The following qualities result from emotional openness, flexibility and self-reliance:

● independence and recognition of others' independence, privacy, and peace

● lack of self-pity, so that when a problem arises it is looked at objectively

● the attitude that nothing is hopeless and problems are there to be solved

● a sense of inner security rather than security gained from controlling others

● being prepared to take on responsibility for your own mistakes

● a few close relationships rather than many superficial ones

● a sense of realism about the goals you can set yourself

● being in touch with your emotions, and feeling free to express them.

Just as a muscle becomes weak if it's not exercised, so your brain will slow and become feeble if you do not think. The best mental exercise is work. An experiment performed on Japanese octogenarians showed that those who kept going into their offices, even for one hour a day, had greater mental powers than those who had retired at 60 and given up disciplined thinking. It helps if your efforts are judged by your peers, but work of any kind provides mental stimuli. Interaction with other people forces you to assess what they are saying, and respond with questions and comments. Your brain has to assimilate information and your cognitive processes remain active.

Keep thinking

As we get older, we lose the ability to form new brain connections, so we have to make certain that old and well-established connections are continually used. The only way to do this is through thinking. Thinking is not a passive process – it means engaging in, questioning, and absorbing what is happening all around us. For example, arithmetic "exercises" are often encountered in daily life and you can engage in them more actively. Anticipate your supermarket bill by adding up the cost of your groceries, or estimate how much change you'll receive.

Try to add new words to your vocabulary. Keep a dictionary handy to check meanings, and use the word in subsequent conversations. Read a daily newspaper article or watch the television news and discuss the main events of the day with a friend.

If you have the opportunity, think about taking evening classes. The range of courses available to adults is huge – there are craft classes that take up a couple of hours a week, or you can take full-time courses in academic subjects such as history or literature.

How could I tell if my parent might have Alzheimer's?

As Alzheimer's disease is diagnosed more and more, many families find themselves wondering if a parent or relative is in the early stages of this condition. But they fear that seeking diagnosis may seem cruel. Trying this test, sensitively, might give you an idea of whether or not you need to see the doctor, but be very careful not to pressure or upset your relative.

Ask the following questions and score 1 point for each wrong answer, up to the maximum. The questions are weighted according to importance. Multiply the number of mistakes by the weight. Then add to get the final score.

How to read the score
The score can range from 0 (no mistakes) to 28 (all wrong). A score greater than 10 may be consistent with Alzheimer's.

Test 1: How good is his memory and concentration?

Questions	Maximum no. of errors	Multiply by	Points
1 What year is it now?	1	x 4	=
2 What month is it now?	1	x 3	=
Repeat this memory phrase after me: *Mary Smith, 20 Market Street, Springfield.*			
3 About what time is it? (within 1 hour).	1	x 3	=
4 Count backward from 20 to 10.	2	x 2	=
5 Say the months of the year in reverse order.	2	x 2	=
6 Repeat the memory phrase again.	5	x 2	=
		Score	

How independent is he?

This is how you can measure how dependent on others your relative has become. The higher the number, the more dependent.

From the following list, select the answer that best describes his current situation and allocate points accordingly. Add these points to get the score.

3 points: Dependent
2 points: Requires assistance
1 point: Does (or could do) by himself but with difficulty
0 points: Does (or could do) with no difficulty

How to read the score
The score can range from 0 (totally independent) to 30 (totally dependent). A score higher than 9 may indicate Alzheimer's.

Total score
Add the scores of tests one and two to make the total. A total of higher than 20 points may indicate Alzheimer's.

Test 2: Daily life

Questions	Points
1 Writing checks, paying bills, etc.	
2 Completing tax returns or papers, handling business affairs.	
3 Shopping alone for clothes, household necessities, or groceries.	
4 Playing game of skill, working on hobby.	
5 Heating water, making cup of coffee, turning off the stove.	
6 Preparing a balanced meal.	
7 Keeping track of current events.	
8 Paying attention to, understanding, discussing television, book, magazine.	
9 Remembering appointments, family occasions, holidays, medications.	
10 Traveling out of neighborhood, driving, arranging to take bus.	
	Score

"optimism is the most important personality trait to have if you want to live a long life"

life stages: 60+ years

The 60-plus age group is the largest and fastest growing in the Western world. Sixty is no longer old, and for the first time ever it's possible to say that aging isn't inevitable. The reason we age is not because we're programmed to die, but because our tissues accumulate a range of faults that eventually overwhelm us. Now that we know this, we can naturally enhance the body's own repair systems and extend life. There's more and more evidence to support this optimism that aging is controllable.

The two main supports of longevity are, and will always be, eating well and staying active. Of the two, being active is the more important because it keeps the brain alert, with the added bonus that fit muscles burn so many calories that weight gain is controlled. Furthermore, keeping muscles fit acts as a natural appetite suppressant in that active muscles "demand" healthy nutrients. The brain interprets that demand as a command to make healthy choices when you decide what to eat.

Remember – it's never too late to change; it's never too late to start. Alterations to your lifestyle take effect immediately.

Positive attitudes

There are other key factors in controlling aging. **Positive attitudes**, social networks and a strong spiritual life will increase your lifespan through a sense of well-being and life satisfaction. The stress-resistant personality lives longest. People who live to 100 are often strong-willed characters with youthful, can-do attitudes. These same people score high when it comes to self-confidence and resilience, which helps them cope with major stressful events such as war or death in the family.

Strong social networks are important for physical and spiritual well-being. Close ties with family and friends can actually strengthen the resilience of the immune system, which affects a person's resistance to disease, including cancer, and can protect against illness and premature death. Nonetheless, a fair amount of independence may be one of the reasons why the oldest folk can be active and self-supporting in the community until very old age.

Adaptability is another key to long life. Stress accelerates aging and it may do so by causing shrinkage of the hippocampus in the brain, the main area for memory. It's the negative responses to stress that do the harm in causing premature aging and there's convincing evidence that adapting to stressful life events through coping is one of the most important factors for successful aging. It would seem that the key to this talent for adapting is not to perceive events as stressful. So it's important how we react to modern life's stresses – excessive noise, air pollution, traffic jams, rude people, and time pressures. People who live to 100 are much better at managing stress than the average person.

Be optimistic

Optimism is the most important personality trait to have if you wish to live a long life. A recent study on men with AIDS showed that those who were optimistic about their future lived nine months longer than those who weren't. In other words, optimism about our health may influence our life expectancy. Optimism has a positive effect on the immune system too. Men undergoing coronary bypass surgery recover more quickly if their outlook is optimistic. The opposite is also true. The belief that we are powerless to influence situations – known as "learned helplessness" – describes a loss of willpower that promotes stress-induced illness. An emotionally stable, flexible personality helps us to stay healthy far into our senior years. Strength of will and assertiveness are an added bonus.

Today we expect to live much longer than our ancestors did. By taking care of ourselves well, we make sure we enjoy those years. In the pages that follow I offer guidelines where appropriate, advice where I feel there may be a need, and strategies for dealing with potentially difficult situations.

Body

Mind

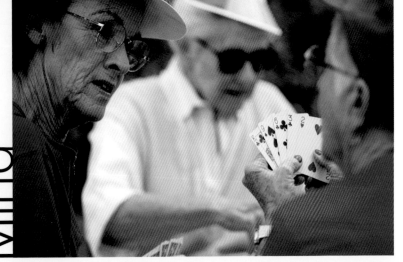

long life is determined more by a positive outlook than any other factor

Social

" about 80 percent of older people are sexually active "

" retirement is a time to acquire new skills and new interests "

planning for a long and enjoyable life

Eating the right things, exercising, and keeping active will help you get the most out of life when you're 60 plus.

Tips for living with chronic conditions

Few of us escape a touch of arthritis as we get older and for some it can be quite debilitating – but less so if you follow a few golden rules.

Osteoarthritis

● Use your whole hand, not just the first finger and thumb, to lift heavy objects, and be careful not to twist your hand when removing tight lids from jars or turning stiff door knobs.
● Exercise and walking are fine, but beware of standing and walking on hard surfaces for prolonged periods.
● Sitting in cramped seats becomes painful after half an hour or so. When this happens it is helpful if you stand up, walk around, or massage your knees.
● Sitting with your legs crossed is not good for your knees.
● Hips stiffen quickly if not exercised.

Sitting like Buddha, though bad for your knees, is good for your hips. An important exercise is for you to flex your knees to a right angle.
● Backs stiffen with age so it helps if you exercise your spine after a hot bath or shower. Swimming is also good.
● Necks stiffen if not exercised, so regular relaxation exercises keep your neck supple.
● Sensible footwear is essential. Avoid high heels and pointed shoes – they can push your big toe out of line.
● When lifting heavy objects, bend your knees and straighten your spine.
● Stay trim. Extra weight means less exercise and increased load and wear on your knees and hips.

Rheumatoid arthritis

● Energy is important so make sure you preserve it.

● Full range of movement exercises is necessary. Keep supple; exercise after a bath or shower. Not doing enough will lead to stiffness; doing too much will increase pain and swelling in the joints.
● Eat like other healthy people. Diet does not influence rheumatoid arthritis, except in people who have a gluten intolerance and benefit from a gluten-free diet.
● Maintain hobbies and interests. Lead as full a life as you are able. A good general rule to follow is if anything you do makes you ache badly for more than two hours or makes you feel bad next day, then you have done too much.
● Take medications as prescribed; if you have any side effects, tell your doctor.
● Don't expect any miracle cure. Great tolerance and patience are most needed.
● Ask your doctor for physical therapy to keep your joints from stiffening up.

Help your circulation

Our extremities are often the first to suffer as our blood circulation slows down, so it is important that we take care of our legs and feet. Do these exercises lying down.
Leg raising (20 times) Keeping your legs straight, point your feet and toes upward and raise one leg 45 degrees. Hold to a count of three and then slowly lower it to the floor. Repeat with your other leg.
Foot bending (10–15 times) Point your feet and toes upward as far as you can manage and then point them down. Repeat this action vigorously.
Foot circling (15 times) Working from your ankles, circle your feet in one direction. Repeat in the opposite direction.

Eating to stave off illness

The right diet is more important than ever once you're over 60 to reduce risks of cancer and heart disease. Make sure you have plenty of fruit and vegetables, fiber, oily fish, some nuts, legumes, and garlic. A Mediterranean-style diet is excellent.
● Reduce the amount of saturated fat in your diet. Replace most of the animal fat with unsaturated vegetable fat such as olive oil, corn oil, grapeseed oil, or soy bean oil. Do not have more than ¼oz (7g) of butter a day, and never use lard for cooking.
● Eat lean rather than fatty meat, for example chicken not beef. Always cut the fat off meat if possible. Never eat the skin;

fat is stored in a layer under the skin.
● Broil food when you can; never fry it.
● Try to eat less red and more white meat, such as poultry and fish.
● Eat oily fish at least twice a week – fish oils protect the heart. If you have heart disease, increase this to three or four times a week.
● Make sure you eat five portions of fruit and vegetables every day and some green or root vegetables to provide roughage.
● Eggs are okay – you can have three or four a week.
● Avoid cream whenever you can.
● Include three servings of whole grain breads and cereals a day.

Exercise to stave off stiffness

A decrease in physical activity is directly related to aging. Exercise helps the metabolism of food by the body, and relieves tension and promotes mental well-being as well. If for any reason our vigor decreases, our desire and ability to take part in physical activity is affected. Mental stress from depression and anxiety can further dampen down our desire to participate in any kind of physical activity. A chronic cycle of less activity and more stress, withdrawal, and depression may follow.

Inactivity-stress syndrome

The inactivity-stress syndrome becomes more common as we grow older. It adversely affects our energy and motivation no matter what we attempt to do. It pervades all aspects of our everyday living and it follows that we get less out of life. We are able to participate less, enjoy ourselves less, and we become less and less happy – no further argument is needed in favor of retaining our physical activity.

Benefits of exercise

But as we get older, we can no longer rely on having mobile joints, supple muscles, and strong bones. Our insurance policy is exercise. Exercise promotes an agile, healthy body which will respond quickly. We need to have strong muscles that can maintain effort and give us stamina. Just as important, we need to have healthy minds that are eager to encourage our bodies. None of this will happen if we neglect our bodies. They have to be put through their paces regularly to bring them up to a level of fitness that has to be maintained. Exercise keeps us young.

Anyone who has exercised will tell you about the sense of euphoria felt after completing an exercise program. This is not just due to the satisfaction of having done something well, it is a hormonal effect. If we exercise, we release many beneficial hormones and one of them affects our state of mind. It counteracts depression and makes us feel tranquil and generally content with life.

Calming effects

It is not a fallacy that if we let our bodies slow down, the brain slows down too. Regular exercise can speed up the rate at which your brain works and promotes recall so that the memory improves. Exercise is also one of the best medicines for anxiety. It has a calming effect throughout our bodies. It counteracts headaches and helps you sleep well.

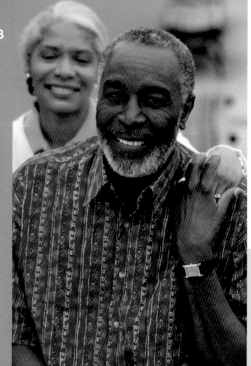

planning for a long and enjoyable sex life

There is nothing but good news about sexuality in our later years. In fact, recent research has confirmed that for many older people, sex drive and sexual pleasure are greater than when they were younger.

Adjusting your expectations

All-consuming, passionate lovemaking is a rare occurrence. If we set our sights on this romantic ideal and expect it to occur with any frequency, we are almost bound to be disappointed. **There are, though, many forms of enjoyable sex** and everyone can experience perfectly satisfying sex, which can be quite different on different occasions, with the same partner. This is one of the thrills of a long-term relationship – gradually discovering new ways of enjoying sex by being together over time. For many women an orgasm is not the be-all and end-all of enjoyable sex, and as a man gets older he may not experience an orgasm every time he has sexual intercourse. Many men

feel that they have to chase the elusive orgasm with every coital union, but **why, when there is so much satisfaction in warm, less passionate sex?**

Several pitfalls await us if we continue to believe that sex must be exciting and that only exciting sex is good. This makes us tend to avoid having it unless we are sure that excitement will be an ingredient and, in this way, we narrow the spectrum of attainable experiences and deprive ourselves of peaceful, relaxing, joyful sex. Another unfortunate result is that sex becomes hard work and, as such, is boring and dull.

Hostility, resentment, contempt, and distaste can all ruin a good relationship, even a sound marriage,

let alone sexual enjoyment. No good relationship requires an intense, permanent state of rapture or even a permanent emotional commitment. It does, however, require goodwill, caring, thoughtfulness, a desire to comfort, and shared intimacy. Problems are bound to arise when one partner has difficulty being warm and close with the other. There may be a steady pulling apart rather than a coming together if one person feels that the other is demanding more affection than he or she feels comfortable about giving. **No couple can be close and intimate if there is no basic mutual respect and affection between the partners.** In addition to this, any sex therapy cannot work.

Your diet and sex

Sex is improved if you are physically fit and eat a healthy diet. While there's no proof that certain nutrients improve desire or performance, several minerals are thought to be important.

When your zinc levels are low, your histamine levels are also low, which

may make it slightly more difficult for you to reach orgasm.
Zinc deficiency is not unknown in women because many don't eat enough zinc-rich foods such as red meats and whole grains – the process of refining grains and cereals removes 80 percent of their

zinc content. You can make up for this by eating seafood, such as clams, oysters, herrings, and sardines. **Seeds and nuts are also good sources of zinc.** Niacin, one of the B vitamins, is another nutrient that may be associated with histamine production.

Defying the myths

The years after 60 can be our prime time. The facts about sexual pleasure in older people challenge the widely believed myths that they are beyond having sex.

● Sex is commonly considered a crucial part of life during our older years and provides a sense of well-being and a positive feeling about ourselves.

● Sex makes older people feel beautiful, desirable, exhilarated, and mystical, and for some who attach importance to the youth cult, it makes them feel young. Also, sex is relaxing and relieves tension. It may be one of life's exquisite moments, driving every other problem and care out of our minds temporarily or even permanently.

● Only a minority of people (less than 30 percent) feel there is a decline in sexual response and feelings. This is especially true of men who have problems with erection and, therefore, withdraw from sexual activities.

● Nearly three-quarters of older people feel that sex is the same as it was when they were younger; more than one-third of older people say that sex is better than when they were younger.

● For those of us who find sex more gratifying when we are older, the key is having the right partner, loss of inhibitions and a greater understanding of sex.

● For couples who get married for the first time or remarry in later life, love, caring, and sharing and companionship are emphasized; so is sex. The majority of people consider that sex is very important later in life.

● Of those older people who are sexually active, half have sexual intercourse about once a week or more; 30 percent have sexual relations three times a week; 20 percent report sexual relations twice a week.

● Sex brings love, faith and trust, approval, and warmth; these are needs and desires that are the same for people of every age.

Maturing sexual responses

In both sexes, the sexual impulse does decline with age but the general pattern differs in men and women. A man's sex drive reaches a peak in his late teens and thereafter gradually diminishes. A woman's sexual feeling reaches a maximum much later in her adult life and is sustained on a plateau of responsiveness which, if it is going to decline, tends to do so only in her late 60s. **There is much research supporting the existence of a strong sexual urge in 70- and 80-year-old women, just as there is in some men.** There is not usually an abrupt loss of sexual feeling with menopause as many women fear.

About the time of menopause, a woman may become anxious about her loss of youthful attractiveness and the fact that any children she might have no longer need her maternal care. These insecurities may make her less ready to respond sexually.

Psychological benefits

At the same time of life, both men and women may have reached the most senior position they will attain in their careers. If early ambitions have not been fulfilled, older people may feel threatened by younger colleagues, and their feelings may find expression in a lack of sexual interest or a feeling of sexual inadequacy. Both men and women may seek escape from this sense of decline by engaging in sexual adventures in a forlorn attempt to recapture the experiences of youth. However, a satisfactory sexual relationship in an older couple is likely to be sustained if the couple enjoys a close understanding, companionship, and mutual respect throughout their middle age. This is entirely within the grasp of most couples and it is worth planning and working for.

sexual worries

Sex is a highly complex part of our lives, influenced by our current moods and emotions outside the bedroom. If we're anxious, tired, or ill we'll have little inclination for it, but there are strategies that can help.

Sexuality and heart disease

All in all, the news on heart disease and sex is extremely good. Doctors now realize that a normal sex life can actually benefit many men who suffer heart attacks, but it is important that they don't get overly tired. Here are the facts.

● There is absolutely no need to eliminate sexual activity altogether unless heart disease is very severe.

● Research has shown that fewer than one percent of all coronary deaths occur during, or after, intercourse. Most doctors believe that the therapeutic benefits outweigh the risks.

● Total abstinence can bring a great deal of psychological stress, which will worsen any heart condition.

● In many cases of heart disease sexual activity can be beneficial, since making love can be the equivalent of performing moderate exercises causing an increased heart rate, slightly increased blood pressure, and improved oxygen consumption.

● Try making love in the morning after a good night's sleep, when both partners are feeling rested. One of the great things about being retired is that you no longer have to jump out of bed at seven o'clock every morning.

● A change in position can also help people with heart conditions. Lying next to each other on your sides, face-to-face, is more restful than the missionary position. You can find positions that avoid muscle cramps and tension, with the woman on top so that she can do most of the moving, which will avoid the man's getting overly tired.

Keeping love alive

Sexual desire in everyone varies from day to day, and like the rest of our behavior, is dependent on what is going on around us. For example, there is no way that sexual desire can surmount a sudden shock, a severe illness, or a bereavement and it would be foolish to expect it to do so.

Sex may not be enjoyable all the time; just like any other sensory experience it can be good or bad. While it is realistic and healthy to accept that it can be less than good, having bad sex once does not mean that it will happen frequently or even again for some time. It is a natural variation and should be accepted as such.

It's a popular myth that men are always ready for sex, but they aren't. While a woman can participate even when she's not in the mood, it's not so easy for a man since he needs an erection.

Sensate focusing

When there are sexual problems, a sympathetic and patient partner is very important because the more a man worries about getting an erection, the more likely he is to fail. Sensate focusing helps a couple to focus on the sensations they feel when they gently explore and caress each other's bodies. There's no intercourse or genital contact at first. The heat is taken out of the situation so there's no reason to feel anxious about your ability to enjoy sex.

● **Stage one:** Explore your own body, massaging and stroking it to rediscover sensual feelings. You should concentrate on your feelings at this time and not worry about sexual intercourse.

● **Stage two:** Take turns massaging each other all over and talk about your feelings and what gives you pleasure. But at this stage you mustn't touch each other's genitals or highly sensitive parts of your bodies.

● **Stage three:** Touch one another's sexually sensitive zones and the genitals. Talk to each other all the time. During these sessions, your partner may be eager for intercourse but it's essential to wait until you're ready.

Sex and the older woman

Not only do some women write themselves off after they have gone through menopause, but so may society: both are quite wrong. **Up until the age of 60, whatever changes take place are extremely slow and gradual.** There are some physiological changes with age, such as vaginal lubrication, which from taking only 15 to 30 seconds in younger women may take one, two or even five minutes when older. There may be some thinning and loss of elasticity in the walls of the vagina, plus a shortening of vaginal length and width, changes that have little or no effect on sensation and orgasm. Some 80 percent of older women report no pain or discomfort on intercourse, even though it is a commonly accepted myth that intercourse in an older woman results in discomfort.

Studies show that women have a more stable sex drive than men. Women over 65 continue to seek out and respond to erotic encounters, have erotic dreams, and continue to be capable of orgasms, even multiple ones. Most aspects of arousal are the same for older women as for younger. Nipples still become erect and the clitoris is the main organ of sexual stimulation. The excitement generated by clitoral stimulation is exactly the same. **A woman of 80 has the same physical potential for orgasm as she did at 20.**

Sex and the older man

As a man ages it often takes longer to get an erection, or the erection may not be maintained for as long as the man would like. Moreover, the erection may not be as full or as hard as before. Many men see such limpness as the end.

It may be that a man needs stimulation to maintain an erection. Erection may refuse to occur for a multitude of reasons, and if it doesn't happen, a man tends to panic and think he is impotent.

Once a man starts to worry about his erection, he is in a vicious circle because anxiety leads to flaccidity. Insecurity is made worse by the fact that a man who fails to have erections is sometimes labeled impotent. **Once a man relaxes and stops worrying about his potency a return to normal sexual activity nearly always follows.**

It helps if he realizes that it is unnecessary for him to ejaculate every time; rest periods of several days between sexual encounters help both erection and orgasm. If older men respond to their natural rhythms instead of feeling forced by macho instincts to have frequent sex, then their own sex lives come more under their control. It is important for a man to be open and honest with himself and his partner to maintain a loving relationship.

planning for a healthy mind

The latest research suggests that a long life is determined more by a positive outlook and a determination to overcome obstacles than by any other single factor.

Tips for coping with loneliness

One of the best ways of handling loneliness is to face up to it. You will get great insight into just how lonely you are if you keep a diary. Write down the times when you feel you are at your lowest ebb, when you are the most lonely. For instance, you may realize that the worst times are evenings from about six o'clock, Sundays, and holidays. Once you have narrowed those times down, they may be much less frequent than you think.

Planning time

Start splitting up your evenings during the week by allocating them to different activities. You could go to night school on one and take up a new hobby, craft, or subject for study. You could make one evening a time for having some friends to your house, and another for visiting someone else. You could make another evening an occasion for going to the movies, theater, or a concert with a friend. Another could be devoted to keeping fit by going to a yoga class, playing a game of tennis, or going to the gym for a workout. One could be for a home hobby like painting, gardening, carpentry, or

odd jobs around the house. Saturday night could be something special. You could join a local club whose members are interested in the same things as you.

Sundays should be carefully planned. Unless you invite distractions or go out to meet others, it is a long day because it is less easy to shop or do errands. The best and most satisfying way of occupying your Sundays is to invite friends to your home for lunch or brunch. Make it a very relaxed occasion and arrange the food so that people can come and go as they like.

Finding new interests

You are never going to meet people staying at home alone. One of the best ways of getting yourself out of the house is to decide to take up one of your pet passions. Have you always been interested in politics? If so, go along to the next local political meeting. Have you always wanted to paint or sculpt? Enroll at evening classes at the local school. If you have oodles of self-confidence, go along to the local singles club. If you are interested in travel, you could go on a cruise or take up a travel-study program where you can learn while vacationing in a foreign country.

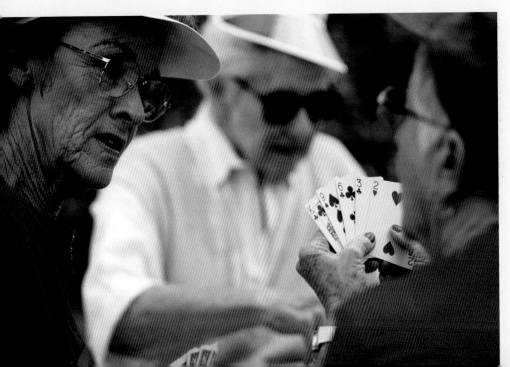

Successful and unsuccessful aging

Many of us are likely to have evolved ways of making personal adjustments that help us to avoid disturbing situations, but there are still factors that can make adjustment difficult. **Anxiety** increases steadily with age, especially among women. Anxiety arising from what psychologists call "cross pressures," which are typical of adolescence, probably diminishes with age because the older we get the more likely we are to have ironed out the difficulties and contradictions in our circumstances and relationships with others. We all differ as we get older, but many of us become more cautious and less confident.

Rigidity is the inability to modify habits. Naturally habitual ways of thinking and behaving increase with age, partly because the long familiarity with a stable environment has "shaped" behavior in this direction. Clinging to old ways will ultimately make aging a difficult transition.

Intelligence, too, is an important determinant of personal adjustment, so that changes in intelligence bring about changes in personality that make aging more or less difficult.

Personal adjustment is considered to be high if a person can overcome frustrations, resolve conflict, and achieve socially acceptable satisfactions and achievements. As you'd expect, good adjustment expresses itself in happiness, confidence, sociability, self-esteem, and productive activity.

Personal adjustment is felt to be low if the individual cannot overcome frustrations, resolve conflicts, or achieve satisfactory results by means of socially acceptable forms of behavior. Common signs of poor adjustment are hostility, unhappiness, fear of people, morbid anxiety, dependence, guilt, feelings of inferiority, apathy, withdrawal, or incompetence.

Our later years of life doesn't have to be static and unchanging. We can continue to learn and grow until the day we die. If we are prepared, personal adjustment should evolve smoothly and logically out of earlier patterns of behavior. If a sense of continuity and identity can be maintained in spite of physiological, social, and psychological changes, the process of re-engagement can proceed successfully. This is essential for adjustment and secures a more effective use of our reduced resources. Normal aging is gradual, by psychological standards at least, and with foresight, planning, and social support, much can be done to ease the problems of adjustment and improve the general level of achievement and happiness.

Adequate adjustment to old age requires certain abilities before we can be happy.

● Our mental state and external circumstances are in balance. There is a degree of continuity between past and present patterns of adjustment.

● We accept old age and death.

● We feel a degree of euphoria arising out of security and relief from responsibilities.

● We have security and adequate financial circumstances to maintain the lifestyle we are used to.

Keeping a tranquil mind

Tranquil young people will probably grow into tranquil old people; **as a general rule, our personalities don't change as we grow older.**

If we are placid and easygoing with a rather philosophical attitude to life, this attitude will almost certainly extend to our middle and later years. If we are excitable, enthusiastic, and precipitate, there is a good chance that we will remain this way. If we have been anxious, nervous, and inclined to worry, it will be similar later on. If we have had bouts of depression, moodiness, and withdrawal from society, the chances are we won't change as we get older.

As we grow older our mental well-being is threatened by all kinds of environmental stresses. We may suffer bouts of depression during and after disruptive life events such as retirement, breakdown of marriage, or bereavement.

As at any other time of life, we are much better equipped to cope with setbacks, even such serious ones as mentioned, if we are well prepared for them and know where to turn for help. **If you feel strong and supported, mental traumas will be less distressing** and enable you to face the future more calmly and confidently with a greater prospect of happiness.

overcoming depression

Depression isn't inevitable as we age, but the problems we may have to face as we get older, such as divorce, bereavement, and ill health, can predispose to it.

Depression and aging

At certain stages of our development we may become more vulnerable to external changes and we will show this internal strain by being depressed. Our own individual vulnerability will be based on hereditary factors, our own strengths and weaknesses, and our psychological makeup. It is possible to see how depression may express itself as we age and face a life of retirement.

It's lowering to find we can't do the things we used to, nor do we have the status of holding down a job. A woman entering menopause still cherishes her sexuality and her capacity to bear children. A man cherishes his power, largely represented by his earning capacity. **As we go through middle age we may start to feel that we are lagging behind.** As we reach retirement and get older, we begin to recognize that we are slower than we once were.

Depression is not inevitable at any critical stage of life, but it is usually those people who have suffered an early loss in infancy, or who have not had their needs met when they were young, who are more likely in later life to become depressed when either internal or external change exposes them to stress.

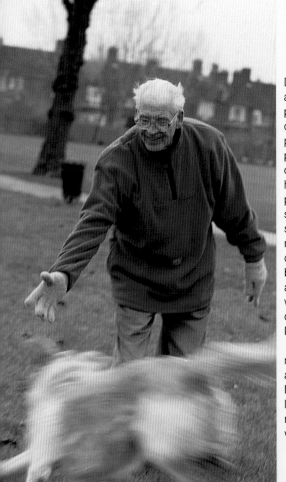

Causes of depression

Depression has physical, psychological, and social causes. In addition, some people have a genetic predisposition to depressive disorders. Some of the physical causes, including infections – particularly viral infections and most commonly influenza, encephalitis, and hepatitis – are frequently followed by a period of depression that lasts up to several months. Changes in the brain, such as epilepsy or a stroke, can lead to mood changes, alteration of behavior, and depression. Women undergo certain biochemical changes in their bodies such as those that occur during menopause, which can lead to depression. Some drugs while dealing with one illness can lead to depression as a side effect.

The social causes of depression are nearly always associated with separation and loss. Being poor does not necessarily lead to depression, but if poverty means a loss of status, it may. Bad weather doesn't necessarily lead to depression, but if bad weather means that you have to abandon

a treat, then it can. Belonging to a minority group doesn't cause depression, but if by being so you are cut off from others or persecuted then it wouldn't be surprising if you did get depressed.

Some people believe that there is one social factor – isolation – that seems to be linked very closely with a tendency to depression. Studies have shown that self-destructive acts are more common in people who are cut off from one another. The isolated spinster or bachelor, widow or widower is the one more likely to end up attempting suicide. Marriage, because it avoids social isolation, is less likely to cause suicide, despite the unhappiness it may bring.

As we get older, a wide range of social and psychological stresses may contribute to depression. Bereavement would be the most dramatic, but other causes of isolation, such as children getting married or their moving far away or our moving away from a familiar neighborhood, are examples that can cause disquiet.

Bereavement

The grief associated with bereavement is not always easy to describe. There may be a good deal of ambivalence at the time – for example, sorrow and disappointment may be mixed with anger, guilt, and anxiety. Bereavement is a stress that can precipitate psychiatric disorders, psychosomatic illness, or suicide. Many women, for example, experience guilt about their role in the events leading up to the death of their husbands, and widowhood reduces life expectancy.

The reorganization that is called for following the death of a spouse introduces an added source of stress with regard to emotional deprivation and living arrangements, and the increased risk of death of the bereaved person. There are good reasons for supposing that preparation and psychological support help to alleviate the distress that leads to personal conflict. In older people, the awareness of dying has developed slowly. There has been enough time to adapt to the prevailing circumstances and time to learn appropriate strategies of adjustment. Without such adaptation, bereavement and the awareness of dying may evoke feelings of dread associated with a sense of isolation or rejection.

The importance of grief

Bereavement is the loss of someone very precious; grief is the resulting emotional experience of being bereaved. Most people think of grief as a natural response to bereavement. Indeed, they are suspicious of those who deny their grief. Nearly all of us see grief as therapeutic, and we are often told "get it off your chest and have a good cry."

Grief is more complicated than that. It is dynamic and we live through it. We go through several steps, each of which is hard work. It is not a passive process of the letting out of pent-up feelings but an active process of adjustment. It is a positive "letting go" of something or someone that has been very precious to you for a long time.

Coping with bereavement

● It is important to realize that the feelings you are experiencing are normal. It is normal to feel rage and anger. You wouldn't be human if you didn't feel guilty, so don't spend a lot of emotional energy on self-recrimination.
● Try to find an understanding person to talk to. You can work through a lot of your anger, guilt, shame, and grief with someone who will just listen, correct you when you overreact, and sympathize with what you are going through. At this moment, when you are in the depths of despair, an objective viewpoint that doesn't see life as entirely white or entirely black is one of the best helps you can have.
● It is important to grieve. Grieve in your own time. Don't take any notice of people who encourage you to snap out of it or get back to normal. You will know when your grieving work is done, because you will feel it has worked its way out of your system and you will feel like starting afresh. So if you really want to have a good cry, if you want to have a conversation with your dead partner, go ahead and do so.
● Once the grieving is over, it is important that you start to think about regaining your identity, or even possibly building a new one. Resist the temptation to live in the past. Try to become your own person and to assert your own identity. Start shaping your life as it suits you by doing things that you are really interested in rather than continuing a past way of life.
● Don't make any big decisions quickly, rather let yourself grow into them gradually. Some decisions may be quite hard to take at first. If left for several months or a year, a problem that seemed insoluble will have a very ready solution.
● Whatever you do, try to stay mobile. Don't find yourself chained to the house, unable to get out. Not only see people, but also do essential shopping to give yourself vital changes of routine.
● Don't neglect your finances. This is not a time for them to get out of control and find yourself in debt. So keep an eye on them, budget your expenses and keep a good eye on all your sources of income.
● Though it seems unlikely while you are grieving, life does go on and you will live again. Meanwhile you should take good care of yourself. Reward yourself with a vacation. Spend some time in your favorite surroundings or take a class to study a hobby. Go and see members of your family and perhaps stay for a few days.

becoming a grandparent

One of the joys in store for many of us as we grow older is becoming a grandparent. There are few experiences as wonderful as those of being with, teaching, and learning from your grandchildren.

Grandparents – part of the family

To my mind, grandparents are an extremely important part of the family, be it nuclear or extended. I personally see a family as a fundamentally stable structure, encompassing strong and lasting relationships, linked to an extended group in which a child can grow up feeling secure and loved, to which she must contribute, and in which her voice is heard. I also think it's important for a child to be able to relate to people of all ages, and so to meet relatives and friends who are older.

Grandparents are vital in helping a child to do this. They also play a unique part in enabling children to develop their personalities and are a valuable asset to a family. By virtue of their age, they are generally more philosophical, long-

suffering, and sympathetic than parents. Long practice means that they have the knack of handling children with ease.

The best grandparents can interpret warning signs, anticipate problems, and head them off. They pacify by distraction not by insistence, and so obtain obedience more readily. Unlike those parents who rule by force, grandparents will more often than not persuade children with patience.

"Spoiling" children?

It is said that grandparents spoil their grandchildren. This must be a misuse of the world "spoil." If spoiling a child means giving explanations instead of dismissals, suggesting alternatives instead of negatives, and helping instead of ignoring,

then grandparents do spoil children. The presence of grandparents in the house can often be a boon to the family and, given that they don't cause friction with the parents, is often welcomed.

Grandparents can renew earlier joys with their grandchildren. A grandmother can teach her young grandchild the art of sewing or gardening. A grandfather can once again enjoy tranquility while he is teaching his grandchild to fish, and discover a new sense of purpose and usefulness if he can take the young baby for a walk and chat to his friends on the way. Grandparents should live with their grandchildren rather than through them. If they do the latter, they may suffer an emotional setback if misfortune strikes the younger generation.

Being a participant not an observer

Age is no reason to be sidelined. These days the majority of people expect to be just as much part of the swim as they get older as they were in their youth. The "swim" may be slightly different, but the participation is just as energetic and joyful.

Of course being a participant rather than an observer takes a bit of effort. First you have to be physically fit so that you can enjoy 16 hours a day rather than falling asleep in front of the television after 12. This means paying attention to what you eat and getting regular exercise. It also means you have to be something of a

self-starter, a get-up-and-go kind of person. If this sounds like too much, consider the benefits: vacations with the "children" because you can keep up; following a passionate hobby like salmon fishing that takes you abroad; enjoying the outdoors through energetic sports such as horseriding or skiing.

Yes, it requires determination and stamina, but who would want to stay at home and stiffen up? Added to which, you'll never be alone, you'll always have companionship because you're an interesting person.

Family upheavals

When things go wrong in our adult relationships, it is not uncommon to hide them from our parents for as long as possible, so as "not to worry or bother them." Usually there is another part of us that feels guilty. We often underestimate the capacity older people have for forgiving and forgetting. It is possible that our childhood anxieties linger on and stop us from communicating, even as middle-aged people, with our parents.

It is not only older people who experience their children's marriages breaking up – parents may be still middle-aged when family ties are broken. **In either case, the effects of family break up can be profound on the older members, who may feel helpless.**

Stresses and strains within the changing family will be, for the most part, private and handled between family members themselves. Very often there is no thought or place for social workers, but in matters of divorce and child custody, they do become involved.

Older family members may also be called upon to take an active part. Grandparents may have an important role to play in divorce. A social worker, thinking positively about what help could be offered to children of divorcing parents, might well recommend grandparental custody, with benefits to children, parents, and grandparents. **With increasingly close ties between children and grandparents**, this option of grandparental custody for children could become more and more common.

The role of grandparents

The best thing you can do is to show your children and grandchildren how to deal with change. You have lived longer than any of your family so you have had to cope with a rapidly changing society more than anyone who is close to you. Your young granddaughter may be very depressed because she can't get a job. Only you, with a historical perspective on unemployment and knowing how much it demoralizes people, can help her to develop a healthy critical distance between the refusals she gets at job interviews and her feelings about herself. You can share with her what you remember about unemployment in your time.

You can allow your grandchildren to see you as a real person for the first time, drawing a parallel between their development and yours. In a conversation on politics, for instance, you can stop being a wrinkled, white-haired old person and describe how you were a young soldier in the army during the Second World War. You can recount some of your experiences, possible moments of glory. There isn't a grandchild in the world who won't be riveted by that kind of story, and learn much from it.

You can show your family that you are not a doddering and useless grandparent. You can be independent and act it. You can be mobile and agile so that you can join younger members for a walk. You can also listen. Parents don't have a lot of time for that. But you can listen without giving advice; you can tell your family what experience you have had in your life and what it has led you to believe.

Grandparents and teenagers
You will also find that you have a lot more in common with teenage grandchildren than you ever had thought. At opposite ends of life you are both searching for changing identities, and both asking the same questions "who am I?" "what do I really want to do?" "how shall I do it?" Very often adolescents have more in common with grandparents than they do with their own parents. Parents often are too busy forging ahead in their careers to have time to be self-examining and introspective.

planning for retirement

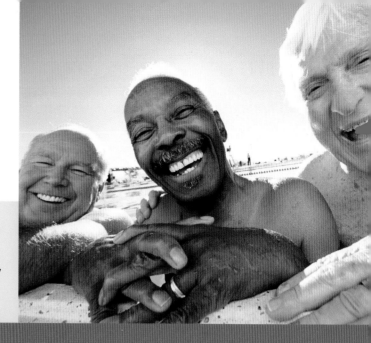

If you are healthy, with reasonable financial resources, and have planned for your retirement, then you will adapt both quickly and completely to your new life.

Preparing to give up work

As you near retirement, you may start to reduce your workload, seek financial advice, or decide to move to a smaller house. On a personal level, you may start to place more emphasis on your relationships with family and friends.

Whereas some people find retirement a natural transition, others, particularly those who have had very fulfilling careers, may find it harder. You need to prepare for this time because there may be little space for adjustment if you don't.

Retirement preparation is now a widely recognized need. Many firms, voluntary organizations, and adult education centers give advice or run classes about financial planning, buying and dispersing personal property and assets, attending to health needs, and organizing leisure time.

Financial planning

● Get the best advice you can to make your money work for you during your retirement years. Several years before you retire, think about investments, insurance, mortgages, and a will. An accountant or a bank manager will be happy to give you advice. Try to work out a comprehensive budget based on what your income will be after you leave work and what your expenses are likely to be.
● Start living on your projected retirement income about six months before you or your partner retire. If you ease into retirement this way, before you are under the strain of other changes that go with retirement, financial adjustments will be easier to cope with. You will also have saved up the money that you didn't use in the previous six months, which will give you a nest egg and a sense of security. You may get

a pleasant surprise and find out that it isn't nearly as difficult as you thought it would be.

Organizing your time

● If your partner retires and you continue working, or vice versa, you will find that your days are suddenly out of sync. Instead of both getting up early in the morning and going to bed at the same time, one of you will be tired while the other is still raring to go. If this becomes a problem, talk about it and find a solution that works for you both. Make a point of doing things together on weekends when your body clocks become synchronized again.
● If you find yourself at home with time on your hands and you feel at a loss for something to do, you are probably having problems making the emotional transition to retirement. Your partner may be able to help by adapting slightly. Discuss a rotation for the chores. Make a list of friends and relatives who are free at certain times during the week (perhaps people whom you haven't seen for several years), and share your interests with these people.
● If you've retired while your partner is still working, take up new projects and revive old hobbies. If you have lots of spare time, spend some of it pampering yourself. Sleep late, meet a friend for lunch, read in the afternoon, and put your feet up whenever you feel like it.

Commit yourself to action

It's never too late to make changes in your life. Once you've made up your mind about what you want to change and how to go about it, take the leap and commit yourself. This doesn't have to mean moving or filing for divorce, it just means taking a step in the right direction, whether it be looking around at other places you might live or spending more leisure time away from your partner.

Try to avoid thinking of yourself as selfish – others close to you, such as your partner, can also benefit from any changes that you decide to make. For instance, if you have spent most of your life at home bringing up a family, a new part-time job or a course could increase your sense of independence and make you feel more fulfilled, and this can have a positive effect on your relationship. Alternatively, if you've always worked full-time you may be looking forward to a restful retirement.

Remember, you have already made many decisions and experienced many changes in your life and you're well equipped to cope with new experiences. Think of retirement as a period of self-renewal and it shouldn't be the crushing change that people often perceive it to be.

When asked what they miss most about working life, many people mention money and the social environment of work. But there are many advantages to retiring: you can follow your own body clock – eating, sleeping, and studying when you feel like it; you no longer have to comply with authority; you have more time to spend on your family, friends, and hobbies; and being out of the rat race can dramatically reduce your stress levels.

Pre-retirement
- Other people can dictate your life.
- Your life is structured around work.
- Your leisure time is limited.
- Your tax burdens may be heavy.
- You worry about getting ahead.

Post-retirement
- You can live life as you please.
- You can set your own pace.
- You can choose your own friends.
- You have fewer expectations.
- You have time to be with your family.

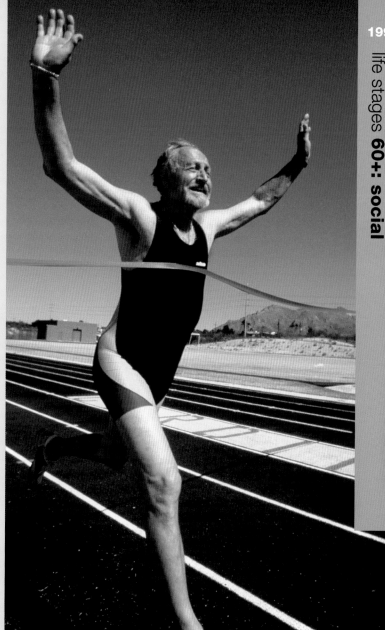

Changing for the better

As you grow older, you may go through a period of major reassessment. You may have a nagging feeling about something in your life you would like to change but, consciously or subconsciously, you have deferred making changes because the time was never right. You may be dissatisfied with where you live. You may feel that you don't spend enough time doing the things that you want to do. Your marriage may feel claustrophobic, and you may want to make some changes in your relationship, or even arrange some time away from your partner.

If any of the above apply to you, confront your feelings and try to be honest with yourself. Talk over your thoughts with your partner, friends, or perhaps even with a therapist. If you let people know what you are looking for, sharing your thoughts may open the door to new opportunities.

enjoying retirement

To make the most of your retirement you may want to acquire new skills, new attitudes, new interests, and, in some cases, new relationships. You stand the best chance of success if you approach life in a positive state of mind, with energy, resolve, and determination.

Marriages after retirement

Retirement can sometimes put a strain on marriages. **Couples who can live together quite happily in the evenings and on weekends find that it can be hard to talk to and tolerate each other all the time.** You might encounter problems that you never anticipated. Your partner might compensate for his loss of power and prestige at work by demanding excessive attention, and you might respond by nagging.

Alternatively, a man and a woman who are wrapped up in work and children may find that when they leave their jobs and the children leave home, they have fewer things in common than they imagined.

If a marriage has never been good and problems have never been resolved, the situation will be dramatically intensified when two people are thrown together for the greater part of every day. Emotional strain at this time can be great – but it is preventable if you tackle problems early on.

Tips for alleviating stressful situations.

● Plan separate, as well as joint, activities.
● Try to arrange your home so that you both have a place to escape to, for instance a television room and a study.
● Respect each other's friends, conversations, and routines.
● Develop a common interest, such as a shared hobby, a small business venture, or an evening class.
● Keep talking to each other. Your partner can be your closest friend.
● Maintain a wide circle of friends; you'll need to plan not only for today but for the future, when one of you may be alone.
● Plan your finances together.
● A full life includes physical love. If the frequency with which you and your partner make love declines, try to examine the reasons why and find solutions.

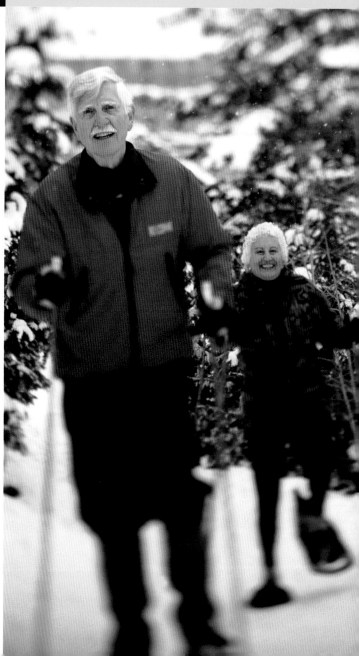

Making the most of retirement

Look at the years ahead in terms of possible problem areas, and to see what the most appropriate solutions to them are. Whatever the situation, it will help to look at it in terms of how it can be made to work for you, and how it can eventually enrich your life. It will help if you share the responsibility of planning with your partner; if you are single and feel that you need help, either join up with another single person or seek help from family, friends, or an organization.

Your partner's retirement
Whether or not you, yourself, have retired, it may be necessary to act as an emotional prop if your partner is unable to come to terms with retirement. Encourage your partner to talk about it, and to see the positive aspects; make plans for both of you.

Money
Once you have retired, use your money sensibly: never buy prepared meals; you have the time now to cook with low-cost cuts of meat and fresh vegetables. Keep your eyes open for bargains – whether food or clothing; book your vacations well in advance and take full advantage of reductions on all forms of transportation.

Moving
For some people, retirement is the ideal opportunity to make a break and move elsewhere, but it is a decision which should be carefully considered beforehand. If, for example, you do want to move, make sure that you know enough people in the new town for social contact. Check that there are facilities for your favorite hobbies or sports; make sure that the stores are easily accessible; and guarantee that you do, indeed, like the area, both day and night.

These suggestions may seem pedantic, but with your increased leisure time, it is doubly important that you enjoy your surroundings and are able to make the most of them.

Social relationships
If possible, continue some of your earlier working activities or social relationships with old colleagues. This will help you feel a sense of belonging and participation, and will avoid the traumatic, sudden withdrawal of all your professional relationships. At the same time, make use of any new contacts that you have.

Leisure time
Now, more than at any other time in your life, your time really is your own, but you must plan to make proper use of it. There is no truth in the adage "you can't teach an old dog new tricks," so, if you feel like going to day or evening classes to learn something unusual, do so. You can only benefit from the fact that your brain is being kept alert; indeed you will feel a sense of achievement, usefulness, and happiness. To enable you to make the most of all the new opportunities, make sure that you attend to your diet, physical fitness, and health.

Finding another job
Some people find that although they enjoy their new-found leisure time,

what they really want is another job. The idea of finding a job is an admirable one as it may restore any lost sense of self-esteem and will keep the mind alert. If you have both the business acumen, and financial backing, you may decide to start up a new business. Alternatively, you may not want this kind of responsibility and opt, instead, for a part-time job in a local business or store, or take up voluntary work. The only reservation would be if the job became too taxing or tiring, in which case it should be stopped or at least curtailed somewhat.

Travel
The period of retirement is an ideal one for travel as it is possible to journey at off-peak times and make full use of any fare concessions. If you feel like traveling – whether in your own country or abroad – it is an ideal way of not only "broadening the mind," but also of meeting new people in new situations.

What you must do, however, is make a plan well before you start, taking the advice of a travel agent if necessary. Make sure that you choose the travel arrangements that suit you best – do you want, for example, to have everything arranged for you, from flights and rooms to tours and restaurants, or would you rather buy an open-ended ticket and explore for yourself?

Avoid traveling alone if you can. Not only is it more fun going with someone else, but should there be any trouble, it can be a great help to have someone there to help. If you take regular medication, or if you have any allergies, keep a note of them in your wallet or on a medic-alert bracelet or necklace.

dying well

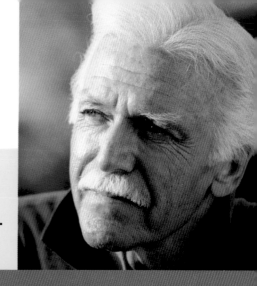

The living will – also known as an advance directive – lets you outline treatments you don't want if you are seriously ill in the future and can't indicate what you want to happen. A living will can help you die well.

Living will

Through a living will, you can make sure you're not given life-prolonging treatment if, for example you suffer from a massive stroke from which you won't get better. It's your chance to take control over your treatment and make sure that you're not kept alive in a situation that you would find intolerable. You can add to, or amend, the basic living will form to fit your personal feelings and beliefs.

Advantages of the living will

A living will makes sure you won't have any treatment you don't want, even if you cannot tell the doctors your decision at the time.
● A living will ensures that your family and friends are not left with difficult decisions because they are not what you would have wanted.
● Knowing what you want will help doctors to make the right decision in difficult situations.
● A living will gives you the chance to discuss your views calmly with doctors treating you and with your close family and friends long before a decision has to be made.
● When a medical team is faced with a difficult decision about what treatment or care to give you when you aren't able to make a decision, a living will helps the team understand what you would have wanted if you'd been conscious.
    However, the living will still has to be interpreted to make sure that the situation it describes applies to the patient. Besides allowing you to control the treatment you receive, the living will also gives you the opportunity to

discuss difficult issues with family and friends without any pressure.

Show your willpower

You never know what's around the corner or what lies in the future for you. By the time you find out, it may be too late to make any decisions for yourself because you're not physically or mentally able to do so. This leaves your friends and family caring for you with difficult decisions to make about your treatment, hampered by not knowing what you would have wanted. You may have a serious or terminal illness, brain damage due to stroke or injury, dementia, or Alzheimer's disease, or advanced nervous system disease, such as motor neuron disease.
    You could have severe or lasting brain damage due to an accident. You could be left on a life-support machine or in a deep coma being fed through a tube or intravenously, with all your bodily functions under the control of a machine to keep you alive. Treatments may offer you little or no chance of recovery and they may have side effects that you would consider worse than the illness itself, or leave you in a condition you would find unbearable.
    You may feel strongly that you don't want to go through this treatment. That is what a living will is for – to ask doctors not to subject you to any medical intervention designed to sustain your life beyond a certain point.
    A living will is a legal document. You can get a living will form from a hospital, from the U.S. Living Will Registry, or

from the Internet, or you can create your own with the help of a lawyer. In the US, on admission to the hospital, patients are asked to assign someone to act as their Health Care Proxy should the patient become unable to make informed decisions about medical care or life-prolonging treatment. Having a proxy in place can be extremely helpful, but sometimes the proxy does not know the patient's wishes regarding life-prolonging treatment. An advantage of a living will is that the patient's wishes are made explicit.

What does a living will do?

Many people fear that if they become ill they could face a situation where they may be given overzealous treatment when there's little or no chance of recovery, or given treatment which would leave them in a condition they couldn't deal with. A living will shows that, in the future, under clearly defined circumstances, you don't want treatment which will help you live longer – treatment such as antibiotics, tube feeding, and being kept alive indefinitely on a life-support machine.

Updating your living will

It's sensible to go through your living will every few years. Updating it isn't a legal requirement but it makes sense to review it, reassuring medical staff that it's current. Every three to five years, simply re-sign and re-date every copy of your living will. Make sure that your doctor has the most up-to-date version on file.

Is a living will legally binding?

Although there's no law that governs the use of living wills, in common law, refusing treatment before you need it will have a legal effect as long as it meets the following conditions.

● You were mentally able, not suffering any mental distress and over 18 when you made the request.

● You were fully informed about the nature and consequence of the living will at the time you made it.

● You're clear that the living will should apply to all situations or circumstances that arise later.

● You weren't pressured or influenced by anyone else when

you made the decisions outlined in your living will.

● The living will hasn't been changed, either verbally or in writing, since it was drawn up.

● You're now mentally incapable of making any decision because you are unconscious or otherwise unfit.

Adjusting to the idea of dying

It's possible to die badly and it's possible to die well. Having been close to two of each kind of death, it became clear to me that what distinguishes dying well from dying badly is the effect on those who are left behind after the death – partners, children, family, and friends.

When someone dies well, as my uncle did, we all felt whole, complete, happy for him, unashamed. None of us wished his death had been any different, none of us wished we had done more for him or felt there were things we wanted to say or do for him. This calm and serenity is impossible when someone dies badly. They leave us feeling uneasy, discomforted, guilty, ashamed, angry, cheated, unfulfilled.

Allowing "closure"

I have no easy recipe for how we should die well, but what I've noticed in those who do, and have the time, is that they put the comfort of their family and friends before selfish considerations. So they are open, accepting, generous. They talk intimately to those who surround them, allowing deep, spiritual conversations and contact before the moment of dying. They allow "closure" with all those who love them. They are physically open, too, hugging, kissing, and holding others. The flow of love and energy is tangible all around them and it makes for such peace for everyone. To create that peace is our responsibility as we face death.

Symptom Guides

SYMPTOM GUIDES

It can be difficult at times to decide whether you should see the doctor or whether you can treat an illness at home using self-help measures. The symptom guides in this section are designed to help you make that decision. They cover the main symptoms you and your family are likely to experience, and suggest the illnesses that the symptoms could denote. The symptom guides are NOT a substitute for medical advice, and you should always consult a doctor if you are concerned.

HOW TO USE THE SYMPTOM GUIDES
Symptoms are categorized by determining factors such as age, distinguishing features, and location. Where a category is not relevant in diagnosing the problem, it does not appear.

Starting with the age category, you can see at a glance which conditions might be relevant to your symptoms. By proceeding to the distinguishing features category, you can review features of your symptoms that are relevant to diagnosis. Finally, looking at the location map will help you to differentiate symptoms according to where they appear.

"Call" the doctor means just that: speak to him or her, by telephone, to get an opinion about what you should do. "See" the doctor means that you should seek an appointment with your doctor at the earliest opportunity.

RASHES
By location

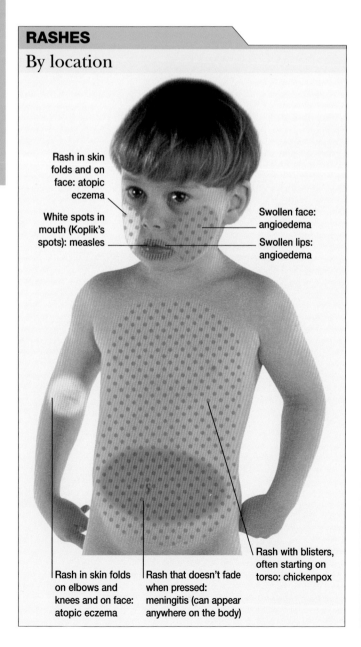

Rash in skin folds and on face: atopic eczema

White spots in mouth (Koplik's spots): measles

Swollen face: angioedema

Swollen lips: angioedema

Rash in skin folds on elbows and knees and on face: atopic eczema

Rash that doesn't fade when pressed: meningitis (can appear anywhere on the body)

Rash with blisters, often starting on torso: chickenpox

ITCHING
By age

In a baby or child
- If on fingers could be scabies (p. 452) **see doctor for whole family treatment**
- If rash all over body could be flea bites **see doctor; take cat or dog to veterinarian**
- If face, hands, skin creases affected probably baby eczema **self-help (see Eczema in babies and children, p. 313); see doctor and possibly dermatologist**
- If blotchy rash on cheeks, arms, and legs could be fifth disease **see doctor**
- If rash with fever **see doctor**

In an adult
Could be:
- Scabies (p. 452) **see doctor**
- Neurodermatitis (a form of atopic eczema, p. 312) due to chronic scratching **see doctor**
- Insect bites **self-help (see Bites and stings, p. 564)**

In an older person
The skin becomes more prone to itching with age.
- Neurodermatitis (a form of atopic eczema, p. 312) **see doctor**
- If persistent can be a sign of a hidden cancer **see doctor for investigation**

CHEST PAIN

By age

In a child

There are few causes of chest pain in children and young people, the main one being a strained muscle or bruise of some kind.

In a young adult

A healthy adult will rarely suffer from chest pain, with a few exceptions.

Could be:
- Pneumothorax (p. 395), most common in healthy young men **call doctor**
- Bronchitis (p. 390), pneumonia (p. 392) **call doctor**
- Bornholm disease or intercostal myalgia – a viral inflammation of the muscles between the ribs **see doctor**
- Pericarditis – an inflammation of the membrane that surrounds the heart **call doctor**

In an older person

Could be:
- Angina (p. 224), not relieved by rest (could be heart attack) **call ambulance**
- Heartburn (p. 350) (could be hiatus hernia, indigestion) **see doctor for endoscopy**
- Peptic ulcer (p. 353) **see doctor for endoscopy and biopsy**
- Gallstones (p. 357) **see doctor for cholecystography**
- Shingles (p. 335) **see doctor**
- Angina (p. 224), relieved by rest **call doctor for ECG immediately**
- Pleurisy (inflammation of the covering of the lungs, p. 393) causes pain that is worse when breathing and coughing **call doctor**
- Pulmonary embolism (p. 395) complicating deep vein thrombosis (p. 235) of leg or surgery **call doctor immediately**

By location

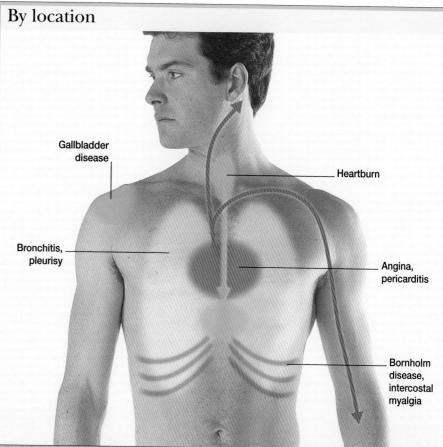

Gallbladder disease

Heartburn

Bronchitis, pleurisy

Angina, pericarditis

Bornholm disease, intercostal myalgia

Distinguishing features

Breathing is difficult

Could be:
- Pulmonary embolism (p. 395) **call doctor**
- Pneumothorax (p. 395) **call doctor**

Pain worse when breathing or coughing

Could be:
- Bornholm disease (viral inflammation of muscles between ribs) **see doctor**
- Bronchitis (p. 390) **call doctor**
- Pleurisy (p. 393) **call doctor**

Pain relieved by

- Alkaline food, could be peptic ulcer (p. 353) or heartburn (p. 350) **see doctor**
- Rest, could be angina (p. 224) **see doctor**
- Sitting forward, could be pericarditis (inflammation of the membrane that surrounds the heart) **call doctor**

Pain made worse by food

- Unrelieved by alkaline food Need to exclude stomach cancer (p. 354) **see doctor immediately**
- Especially by fatty food Could be gallstones (p. 357) **see doctor**

JOINT PAIN

By age

In an infant
Joint pain is always serious **call doctor**

In a young adult
Joint pain could be rheumatoid arthritis (p. 429) but is most commonly due to prolonged, unusual activity or body position or trauma e.g.:
- Home decorating
- Weeding the garden
- A sports injury **get X-ray**
- Transcontinental flight

In an older person
It's most probably a touch of osteoarthritis (p. 428) – the natural aging process of joints which we all have to some degree or other – but could also be:
- Sudden onset osteoarthritis in a joint which has been injured in the past and possibly overused **self-help (see Exercises for people with osteoarthritis, p. 429)**
- Unusual overuse such as hanging pictures, cleaning windows
- Osteoporosis (p. 423) if you're a woman and there's a family history of brittle bones or you're post-menopausal **get bone density scan**
- Osteoporotic fracture if you have osteoporosis and have had a fall or a bump **see doctor**

By location

Peripheral joints of the fingers, hands, and wrists, toes, feet, and ankle
- In a child could be a virus or rheumatic fever
- In a young adult can be caused by a virus or Lyme disease **see doctor**
- In an older adult could be rheumatoid arthritis (p. 429) or part of an autoimmune disorder like lupus (p. 324)
- Common in last trimester of pregnancy and disappears after the birth spontaneously

Weight-bearing joints, the knees, hips
- Nearly always osteoarthritis (p. 428) due to obesity or past injury **see doctor for diagnosis; try self-help (see Exercises for people with osteoarthritis, p.429)**
- Most commonly Lyme disease in young people in endemic areas

Joints of the trunk such as the neck, shoulders, spine, and lower back
- In a young adult could be part of an autoimmune disease like ankylosing spondylitis (p. 430) **see doctor**
- In an older adult probably osteoarthritis of spine (spondylosis; p.432) with or without inflammation (spondylitis; p. 430) **see doctor for diagnosis**
- Osteoarthritis (p. 428) of vertebrae with osteophyte (bony) formation of vertebrae causing nerve compression and referred pain (pain that originates elsewhere) to shoulder, arm and hand if in neck or sciatica if in lower back **get X-ray**
- Slipped disk (p. 437) occurs in the spine where most movement occurs, i.e. back and lower back, giving rise to nerve root pain, numbness, and tingling over the distribution of the nerve **get X-ray; try self-help (see Preventing back pain, p.436); try osteopath**
- Lower back pain could also indicate a bowel or bladder problem **seek immediate medical attention**

Distinguishing features

Joint is hot
Means that there is some kind of inflammation in the joint and the most common causes of inflammation are:
- Infection, usually a virus or Lyme disease
- Trauma
- An allergic reaction to an external allergen (a drug, say, or internal autoimmune reaction) **see doctor**
- Inflammatory arthritis

Joint is swollen
Means that there is fluid in the joint formed to protect the bony surfaces of the joint from injury – it's the body's response to injury to minimize further damage and always denotes pathology in the joint **see doctor**

Joint is red
Means that there is very active inflammation going on inside the joint Range of motion in a pain-free arc should be done. Lack of motion leads to stiffness **see doctor**

Joints are stiff/painful to move
- In the early morning nearly always signifies rheumatoid arthritis (p. 429) or a related condition
- Later on in the day is typical of an osteoarthritic joint after use **self-help (see Exercises for people with osteoarthritis, p. 429)**
- If there is a fracture the joint CAN'T be moved and SHOULDN'T be moved **call doctor**
- If there's a lot of fluid in the joint it's almost impossible to move for mechanical reasons **call doctor**
- Child is limping and won't walk or won't move joint; could signify a greenstick fracture near the joint or a bone condition and is always serious **call doctor**

Fever
Denotes that the joint pain is only a symptom of an illness which is affecting the rest of the body too and it's ALWAYS serious **call doctor**

Young adult:
ankylosing spondylitis
Older adult:
spondylosis, spondylitis

Older adult:
referred pain
from osteoarthritis

Osteoarthritis

Children:
rheumatic fever,
juvenile
rheumatoid
arthritis
Adults:
viral infection,
Lyme disease
Older adults:
rheumatoid
arthritis, lupus

Children:
rheumatic fever
Adults:
viral infection,
Lyme disease
Older adults:
rheumatoid
arthritis, lupus

Older adult:
referred pain
from osteoarthritis

Osteoarthritis,
trauma, Lyme
disease

Children:
rheumatic fever
Adults:
viral infection, Lyme
disease
Older adults:
rheumatoid arthritis, lupus

Slipped
disk

Sciatica due
to osteoarthritis
or disc herniation

Self-help

- Rest the joint.
- If suspected fracture, immobilize the joint
  (see Broken bones and soft tissue injuries, p. 560).
- If fever very high, lukewarm sponge **call your doctor**
  (see Fever in children, p. 540).
- For joints of ankles and feet, raise the joint when possible
  to prevent further swelling, ice.

- For joint stiffness get them working with heat
  (warm bath, infrared lamp, warm pad).
- For pain anti-inflammatory analgesic.
- For stiff spinal joints try gentle massage.

BACK PAIN

By location: back view

Spondylosis, spondylitis,
tension in neck muscles

Referred pain from
gallbladder disease

Fibromyalgia, fibromyositis,
referred pain fromspleen
injury

Shingles

Back strain, slipped
disk, osteoarthritis

Back strain, slipped
disk, osteoarthritis

Sciatica

Coccydinia

neck and
shoulders

shoulder blades
and rib cage

lower back
and coccyx

In neck and shoulder area
Could be:
- Osteoarthritis of cervical spine – cervical spondylosis (p. 432) or spondylitis (p. 430) **see doctor**
- Referred pain (pain that originates elsewhere) from gallbladder (p. 357) **see doctor immediately for sonogram of gallbladder**
- Tense neck muscles
  self-help (see Relaxation, p. 292)

In area of shoulder blade
Could be:
- Fibromyalgia or fibrositis **see doctor**

In area of rib cage
Could be:
- Shingles (p. 335) **see doctor**

In low back area
Could be:
- Kidney infection (pyelonephritis), if fever present **see doctor**
- Slipped disk, if pain came on suddenly **see doctor**
- Osteoarthritis of lumbar spine = lumbar spondylosis or spondylitis **see doctor, take analgesics**
- Back strain **self-help**

In area of coccyx
Could be:
- Coccydinia, if following a fall **see doctor**

If pain shoots down leg
Could be:
- Sciatica **see doctor**

By age

In a young person
- If pain worst when waking could be ankylosing spondylitis (p. 430) **see doctor**
- If pain stops you from moving could be slipped disk (p. 437) **call doctor**

In older woman
- If menopausal could be osteoporosis (p. 423) **see doctor immediately**

In very elderly man
- Osteoporosis **see doctor immediately**

ABDOMINAL PAIN

By age

In an infant
Could be:
- Intussusception (p. 546)
  emergency – take to the emergency room

In a child
Could be:
- Appendicitis (p. 547) (loss of appetite and fever) **emergency – take to the emergency room**
- Migrane with nausea (p. 408) (is there a family history?) **call doctor**
- Flatulence (goes in an hour) **self-help (see Flatulence and bloating, p. 390)**

In an adult
Could be:
- Kidney infection (p. 376) (accompanied by high temperature) **call doctor**
- Kidney or bladder stone (p. 377) (pain may start in your back) **call doctor**
- Shingles (p. 335) (pain on one side) **call doctor**
- Gallbladder disease (p. 357) **call doctor**
- Appendicitis (p. 547) **call doctor**
- Peptic ulcer (p. 353) **see doctor**
- Cystitis (p. 378) **see doctor**
- Flatulence (goes in an hour) **self-help (see Flatulence and bloating, p. 361)**
- May not originate in abdomen, may be in chest **(see By location, right)**

Distinguishing features

Hurts when breathing/coughing
Could be:
- Pleurisy (p. 393) **call doctor**

Goes up into neck, shoulder, down arm to elbow
Could be:
- Angina (p. 224) **call doctor**
- Heart attack (p. 230) **call doctor**

Accompanied by diarrhea, blood in stool, constipation
Could be:
- Irritable bowel syndrome (p. 362) **change diet; see doctor**
- Diverticulitis (p. 364) **change diet; see doctor**
- Ulcerative colitis (p. 367) **see doctor, specialist**
- Crohn's disease (p. 366) **see doctor, specialist**
- Colorectal cancer (p. 368) **see doctor, specialist**

By location

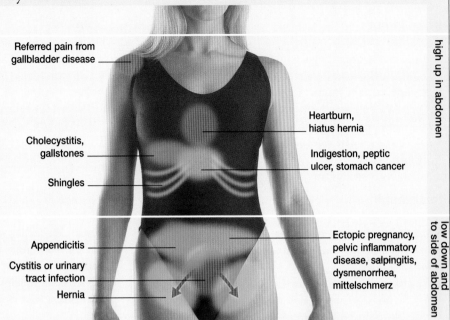

Referred pain from gallbladder disease
Cholecystitis, gallstones
Shingles
Appendicitis
Cystitis or urinary tract infection
Hernia
Heartburn, hiatus hernia
Indigestion, peptic ulcer, stomach cancer
Ectopic pregnancy, pelvic inflammatory disease, salpingitis, dysmenorrhea, mittelschmerz

high up in abdomen
low down and to side of abdomen

High up in abdomen
Could be:
- Under right ribs – cholecystitis (p.358), gallstones (p. 357) **change diet; see doctor**
- Behind sternum – heartburn, hiatus hernia (p. 350) **change diet; see doctor**
- In center between ribs – peptic ulcer (p. 353), stomach cancer (p. 354) **see doctor, specialist**
- Indigestion **self-help (see Indigestion, p. 352); if new, see doctor soon**
- Along ribs on one side – shingles (p. 335) **call doctor**

Low down in abdomen
Could be:
- Worst after passing urine – urinary tract infection (p. 378) **drink cranberry juice; see doctor**
- Missed a period – ectopic pregnancy, miscarriage **call doctor**
- Smelly vaginal discharge – pelvic inflammatory disease (PID; p. 251), salpingitis (inflammation of fallopian tubes) **call doctor**
- Accompanies a period – dysmenorrhea (p. 247) **take analgesics; call doctor**
- Swelling in groin – hernia or abscess (p. 371) **see doctor**

To side of abdomen
Could be:
- Loss of appetite, tender to touch – appendicitis (p. 547) **emergency – go to the emergency room**
- Middle of the month: ovulation (mittelschmerz pain) **take analgesics**

Involves your back
Could be:
- Comes from back – kidney infection (p. 376), kidney stone **call doctor**
- Goes through to your back – peptic ulcer, pancreatitis **see doctor**
- Goes up to your right shoulder – gallbladder disease **see doctor**

DIARRHEA

By age

In an infant
Could be:
- Travel to a foreign country and new bacteria, not necessarily harmful **call doctor, electrolyte solution for 24 hours to replace lost fluids**
- A viral infection (gastroenteritis) **call doctor**
- Food poisoning **see doctor**
- Celiac disease **see doctor**
- Lactose intolerance (sometimes following gastroenteritis and temporary) **see doctor**

In an adult
Could be:
- Anxiety (p. 287) **self-help (see Relaxation, p. 292)**
- Travel (see above) **call doctor, electrolyte solution for 24 hours**
- Food poisoning **call doctor**
- Irritable bowel syndrome **see doctor, self-help (see Irritable bowel syndrome, p. 362)**
- Ulcerative colitis (p. 367) or Crohn's disease (p. 366) especially with blood **see doctor and specialist**
- Side effect of medication **speak to doctor**

In an older person
Could be:
- Diverticulosis (p. 364) **change diet, see doctor**
- Diverticulitis (p. 364) **change diet, see doctor**
- Colorectal cancer (p. 368) **see doctor soon**

Accompanying symptoms

Vomiting
Could be:
- Food poisoning
- Gastroenteritis
- Food allergy (p. 320) **call doctor; 24 hours of electrolyte solution to replace lost fluids**

Fever
Could be:
- Dysentery
- Diarrhea and fever can lead to dehydration **get advice from your doctor soon; 24 hours of electrolyte solution to replace lost fluids**

Blood in the stool
In an infant:
Could be:
- Intussusception (p. 546) **emergency – go to the emergency room**

In an adult:
Could be:
- Hemorrhoids (p. 370) **see doctor soon**
- Crohn's disease (p. 366) **see doctor soon**
- Ulcerative colitis (p. 367) **see doctor soon**
- Colorectal cancer (p. 368) **see doctor soon**
- Anal fissure (p. 370) **see doctor soon**

Distinguishing features

After food
- Up to 6 hours after – Bacterium (probably staphylococcus)
- 6–12 hours after – Bacterium (probably clostridium)
- 12–48 hours after – Bacterium (probably salmonella)

Bowel habit
- A sudden change in bowel habit at any age requires immediate investigation **see doctor soon**

CONSTIPATION

Distinguishing features/frequency

Always had it
Could be:
- Too little fiber in diet **change diet**
- Overuse of laxatives leading to inactive bowel **stop laxatives; retrain bowel**
- Ignoring urge to defecate so it dries out in the rectum **heed urge to defecate**

Comes and goes
Could be:
- Irritable bowel syndrome (p. 362) **change diet, see doctor**
- Diverticulosis, diverticulitis (p. 364) **change diet, see doctor**

Recent origin
Could be:
- Hypothyroidism (p. 507) (you feel the cold) **see doctor for tests**
- Hemorrhoids (p. 370) **see doctor**
- Anal fissure (p. 370) (painful) **see doctor**
- Colorectal cancer (p. 368) **see doctor for tests**

LOSS OF APPETITE

By age

In a child
Always a serious sign especially if accompanied by any or all:
- Diarrhea **call doctor**
- Vomiting **call doctor**
- Abdominal pain **call doctor**
- Fever **call doctor**

In a young adult
Could be:
- Anorexia (see Eating disorders, p. 300) **see doctor**
- Anxiety disorder (p. 287) **see doctor**
- Depression (p. 298) **see doctor**
- Drug abuse **get advice from doctor**
- Kidney infection (p. 376; with back pain) **call doctor**
- Hangover
- Viral infection
- Food poisoning (with vomiting and diarrhea) **call doctor if no improvement in 48 hours**

In an older person
Could be:
- Gastric ulcer **see doctor**
- Alcohol abuse **see doctor**
- Liver disease **see doctor**
- Old age **home care**

WEIGHT LOSS

By age

In an infant
Failure to gain weight may be due to:
- Celiac disease (stools are clay-colored, bulky, small, and float) **see doctor with stool sample**
- Poor diet

In a teenager
The most common causes are:
- Dieting **see doctor and therapist**

- Anorexia (see Eating disorders, p. 300) **see doctor and therapist**
- Bulimia (see Eating disorders, p. 300) **see doctor and therapist**
- Juvenile diabetes (p. 504) (hungry, frequent urination) **see doctor soon**

In an adult
Could be:
- Dieting
- Malabsorption syndrome (p. 365)

(stools as for celiac disease) **see doctor with stool sample**
- Diabetes (p. 504) **see doctor soon**
- Cancer **see doctor soon**
- Hyperthyroidism (p. 506) (hot, palpitations, clammy palms) **see doctor**

In an older person
Could be:
- Not eating **get doctor's advice**
- Depression (p. 298) **get doctor's advice**

FEVER

By age

In an infant
- Always serious if it lasts longer than six hours **call doctor** (Remember, babies can become "feverish" for many reasons, not all of them serious, so if your child isn't listless, vomiting or having diarrhea try one dose of liquid acetaminophen)
- With vomiting and diarrhea (p. 364) **call doctor immediately**

In a child with loss of appetite
Can be the first signs of:
- Appendicitis (p. 547) confirmed by abdominal pain **call doctor**
- Any infection (including ear, nose, throat, urinary tract, stomach, bowel) **call doctor if not normal in 24 hours**
- Heatstroke, after sun **get advice from doctor,**

In an adult
The most common cause is a virus infection:
- Flu **self-help (see Influenza, p. 334)**
- A bacterial infection, e.g. food poisoning, bronchitis (p. 390) **call doctor if not better in 48 hours**

Up to 100°F. (38°C.)
- This is almost within the realm of normalcy **try liquid acetaminophen and monitor**

Up to 102°F. (39°C.)
- Definitely something wrong but not too serious, e.g. cold (p. 333), flu (p. 334) **try acetaminophen, call doctor if not better in 24 hours**

Up to 104°F. (40°C.)
- Could be a serious infection, e.g. kidney infection (p. 376) or salmonella **call doctor**

Over 104°F. (40°C. +)
- Could be very serious, such as malaria (p. 343) **call doctor or take to the emergency room**

Distinguishing features/frequency

Higher at night
- Everyone's temperature is higher at night than in the morning
- Night sweats are a symptom of menopause (p. 497) **see doctor**
- In a man, night sweats can be caused by lymphoma (p. 328) **see doctor**

Comes and goes
- Everyone's temperature is higher after exercise
- The fever of tuberculosis typically comes and goes **see doctor**

Long term
- A fever that stays around may signify a chronic infection like brucellosis (a rare bacterial infection) or AIDS **see doctor; keep temperature chart and show to doctor**

Middle of the month
- In women, temperature rises at ovulation and remains up for the rest of the month

Accompanying symptoms

Rash
- With fever in a child could be an infectious disease of childhood, e.g. measles (p. 544) or chickenpox (p. 335) **call doctor**

IMPORTANT A rash that doesn't fade with pressure (see Thrombocytopenia, p. 239) is a sign of meningitis (p. 404) **emergency – take to the emergency room**

Vomiting
- Always potentially serious if it continues for six hours or more because of risk of dehydration
- Vomiting can be a sign of brain irritation as in meningitis (p. 404), middle ear infection **call doctor**

Diarrhea
- Always potentially serious if it continues for six hours or more because of risk of dehydration **call doctor**

FATIGUE

By age

In a child
- Listlessness is always serious **see doctor**

In a teenager or young adult
Could be:
- Viral infection, e.g. flu (p.334)
- Post-viral fatigue, e.g. mononucleosis, which may take 6–9 months to clear up **wait a week or so before seeing a doctor**
- Depression

In an older person
Could be:
- As for teenager and young adult **wait a week or so before seeing a doctor**
- Anemia (p. 236) or other blood disorder **see doctor for blood test and cause**
- Malabsorption syndrome (p. 365) **take stool specimen to doctor**

- Depression (p. 298) **examine lifestyle for stress; see doctor for possible treatment with antidepressants; talking therapy; try self-help with yoga, relaxation exercises (see p. 292)**
- Hypothyroidism (p. 507) (feel cold, hair thinning, skin dry and coarse) **see doctor for thyroid tests and treatment**

Distinguishing features

Worse in early morning
Could be:
- the endogenous form of depression (i.e. not caused by external events) (p. 298), especially if it's accompanied by early waking **see doctor**

Worst just before periods
Could be:
- part of PMS (p. 302) (other symptoms – lack of concentration, tearfulness, insomnia) **see doctor; self-help (see Premenstrual syndrome, p. 302)**

Worst since periods stopped
Could be:
- menopause (p. 497) **see doctor for HRT (p.502); self-help without HRT, including diet, exercise, herbs (see Coping with menopause the non-hormonal way, p. 497)**

Worse at night
Could be:
- stress (p. 288), anxiety (p. 287), overwork **examine lifestyle for areas to change; self-help (see p. 288)**

FAINTNESS/DIZZINESS

By age

In an adult
Could be:
- Pregnancy **test**
- Low blood pressure (p. 234) **see doctor (no treatment)**
- Low blood sugar **eat regularly**
- Overbreathing as a reaction to anxiety, a shock **self-help (see Anxiety, p. 288)**
- Heatstroke (after sun) **get advice from doctor**

In an older person
Could be:
- High blood pressure (p. 226) **get advice from doctor**
- Ménière's disease (p. 477) **get advice from doctor**
- Labyrinthitis (p. 478) **get advice from doctor**
- Osteoarthritis (p. 428) of the neck **get advice from doctor, get X-ray**
- Transient ischemic attack (TIA; p. 402) **get advice from doctor**
- Brain tumor (p. 409) **call doctor**
- Dehydration
- Heart arrhythmias

BLURRED VISION

By distinguishing feature

- Followed by headache could be migraine (p. 408) **see doctor**
- Lasts only 20–30 minutes could be optical migraine (p. 470) **see doctor**
- Gradual onset, getting worse could be nearsightedness (p. 469) **see optometrist**
- Or farsightedness (p. 469) **see optometrist**
- Or astigmatism (p. 470) **see optometrist**
- Accompanied by dry eyes could be Sjögren's syndrome (p. 473) **see doctor**
- Loss of part of visual field with attacks of vertigo (p. 418), pins and needles or muscle stiffness could be multiple sclerosis (p. 412) **see doctor and neurologist**
- Very sudden onset in an older person, like a curtain falling, could be retinal detachment (p. 467) **see doctor and ophthalmologist**
- Diabetes

HEADACHE

By age

In a child
Could be:
- Migraine (p. 408) (is there a family history?) **get advice from doctor**
- Middle ear infection; sinusitis (p. 481) **call doctor**
- Meningitis (p. 404) (is there a rash?) **call doctor**
- Depression (p. 299) (is child a loner?) **get advice from doctor**
- School phobia **get advice from doctor**

In an adult
Could be:
- Side effect of drug you're taking **get advice from doctor**
- Sinusitis (p. 481) **see doctor**
- Migraine (p. 403) **get advice from doctor**
- TMJ (painful jaw) **call doctor**
- High blood pressure (p. 226) **check with doctor**
- Very rarely, if severe recurrent headaches start out of the blue, brain tumor (p. 409) is a possibility **see doctor**
- Tension due to stress (p. 288); anxiety (p. 287) **self-help (see Relaxation, p. 292)**

In an older person
Could be:
- Temporal arteritis (throbbing pain in temple(s) **see doctor soon**
- Postherpetic neuralgia (p. 408) (after shingles, p. 335) **see doctor**
- Trigeminal neuralgia (p. 408) **see doctor**

BREAST PAIN

By distinguishing feature

Cyclical prior to periods
Could be:
- Normal menstrual changes in breasts **keep pain calendar; see doctor; try high dose of evening primrose oil (see Breast pain, p. 243)**

Noncyclical or unrelated to periods
- If stabbing pain around nipple could be duct ectasia (p. 246) **see doctor**
- Tender spot in the breast could be a cyst (p. 246) **see doctor for ultrasound**
- Could be unrelated to breast such as intercostal myalgia (inflammation of muscles between ribs) **see doctor**
- Tietze's syndrome (arthritis in rib joints) **see doctor**
- Injury or strain to pectoral muscles **see doctor**
- Mastitis **see doctor**

EARACHE

By age

In a baby or a child
- If fever is present could be middle ear infection **call doctor immediately**
- With red spot on cheek and baby pulling her ear could be teething **get advice from doctor**
- If discharge from ear could be otitis externa (infection of outer ear) **see doctor**
- With cough, cold, sore throat could be tonsillitis (p. 536) **see doctor**
- If intermittent could be dental problem **see doctor, then dentist**

In an older person
Could be:
- Dental problem **see dentist**
- Temporomandibular joint disorder (p. 494) **see doctor**
- Shingles (p. 335) **see doctor**
- If persistent and constant (exclude cancer of pharynx) **see doctor**

LUMP IN SCROTUM

By anatomical criteria

Related to testis
Will probably be:
- Spermatocele (see Why it's important to check your testicles, p. 264) **see doctor soon**
- Cystocele (see Why it's important to check your testicles, p. 264) **see doctor soon**
- Hydrocele (see Why it's important to check your testicles, p. 264) **see doctor soon**

None of these is sinister.

- Exclude cancer **see doctor soon**

Unrelated to testis
Could be:
- Varicocele (see Why it's important to check your testicles, p. 264) (feels like a bag of worms) **see doctor**

Symptoms that may denote cancer if they arise suddenly

- **Headache**
- **Hoarseness**
- **Cough**
- **Blood in sputum**
- **Blood in stool**
- **Blood in urine**
- **Change in bowel habit**
- **Indigestion or heartburn**
- **Loss of weight**
- **Loss of appetite**
- **Breathlessness**

Directory 4

How to use this section

The Directory section covers a wide range of the medical conditions that you and your family may encounter. There are 16 chapters, including one on children's conditions, each devoted to a body system or an area of medical specialization. Each chapter has an introductory essay, which highlights the main conditions and serves as a personal overview of the body system. Conditions listed within each chapter are grouped into related topics, making it easier to find related conditions and to understand shared causes of a group of conditions. Sometimes a chapter will have sections of its own if this is helpful in explaining a group of conditions.

Each condition listed covers the reasons why it might arise (including any relevant risk factors, such as age or gender), how it is diagnosed, how your doctor might treat it, what you can do to help yourself, and what the outlook might be. Test and treatment boxes offer up-to-the-minute information on the latest diagnostic procedures and treatments, explaining each procedure in a patient-friendly way. Each chapter also features special "Focus On" topics, where issues of particular interest are discussed in greater depth. Cross-references to related topics appear at the end of entries, so that the flow of information is not interrupted.

How each chapter works

PERSONAL OVERVIEW   **ANATOMY**   **FOCUS ON**

▲ **Dr. Stoppard's** unique overview of each body system explains its basic concepts in a friendly way.

▲ **The anatomy** pages show the location of structures discussed in the articles in each section.

▲ **Focus on** articles give Dr. Stoppard's personal view on topics of special interest today.

Find your way around a typical spread

Common conditions are explained in full, with information on causes, symptoms, diagnosis, and treatment.

Self-help panels include essential information on what you can do to help yourself.

Warning boxes highlight important advice.

Cross-references Essential cross-references are clearly signposted in tinted boxes.

Tests and treatment boxes offer detailed, up-to-the-minute information on the latest diagnostic procedures and treatments, explaining in a patient-friendly way what each procedure involves.

Heart, Blood, and Circulation

Image shows a colored transmission electron micrograph of red and white blood cells

Miriam's overview

The headlines in this chapter are heart attacks and high blood pressure. The first can, by and large, be prevented. The second can't but can be successfully treated almost all the time.

Your heart health is in your hands once you've excluded a genetic cause for high cholesterol. All that's required is a heart-healthy lifestyle that encompasses healthy eating – including five fruits a day and if possible two more portions of vegetables.

It also means you won't allow yourself to succumb to a sedentary life. The body is like a muscle – it's better when exercised. Brisk walking is good enough, fast enough to pant a bit, done for half an hour three times a week.

The heart itself is entirely muscle and like any muscle it requires a workout, once a day if you can but three times a week will keep it in shape.

Without that kind of care, your coronary arteries could become clogged with fat, giving you coronary artery disease (CAD). It will invariably show up as angina and may then proceed to a heart attack that might, if the CAD is gross, lead to heart failure, or even death.

How will you know if you're a candidate for a heart attack? The best indicator is having a mother or father who had a heart attack. If so, you stand a chance of having inherited a gene that could increase your risk of developing heart disease.

A diet rich in folic acid from leafy green vegetables and whole grains is essential for a healthy heart because folic acid lowers homocysteine levels – a risk marker for heart attack.

Normal blood pressure is essential to lower your chance

"the body is *like a muscle* – it's *better* when *exercised*"

of ever having a stroke. High blood pressure is the major risk factor for stroke and if yours is high it's essential that you be assessed by your doctor for treatment.

The first line of treatment is very simple and cheap – a diuretic to get rid of any excess fluid. It alone can lower your chances of ever having a stroke.

With the emphasis these days on a balanced diet anemias of any kind are much less common than they used to be, but particularly those due to deficiencies, such as iron-deficiency anemia.

It has also meant that inherited anemias such as sickle-cell anemia have received the attention they deserve.

INSIDE your heart

The **heart** is a hollow muscular organ about the size of your fist whose function is to pump **blood** around the body. The heart itself is divided into four chambers: two upper chambers, called **atria**, and two lower chambers, called **ventricles**. When deoxygenated blood from the body enters the heart it collects in the right atrium, then flows into the right ventricle. From there it is pumped to the lungs. Oxygenated blood from the **lungs** enters the left atrium, then flows into the left ventricle. From there it is pumped around the body.

the structure of the heart

Aorta

Superior vena cava

Pulmonary artery

Pulmonary veins

Left atrium

Right atrium

Left ventricle

Right ventricle

Endocardium

Septum

Myocardium

Inferior vena cava

Descending aorta

KEY

Deoxygenated blood

Oxgenated blood

The heart is a powerful muscular organ that pumps the body's blood supply (about 6½ quarts/5 liters) around the entire body once every minute.

the major blood vessels

Jugular vein

Common carotid artery

Subclavian artery

Aorta

Subclavian vein

Inferior vena cava

Heart

Femoral artery

Femoral vein

Blood travels around the body via a complex network of blood vessels, which range in size from the large aorta in the center of the body to tiny capillaries in structures such as the lungs.

Blood typing

Your blood type is determined by the presence of certain proteins, called antigens, on the surface of your red blood cells. If you are given blood containing antigens that are incompatible with your own, your immune system will attack and destroy them. Blood typing ensures that your are given blood that is compatible with your own.

The major blood types are ABO and Rh (Rhesus). All blood, regardless of ABO type, is classified as either Rh positive or Rh negative. In pregnancy an Rh negative mother's blood may produce antibodies against her baby's blood if it is Rh positive. This problem can be successfully treated if it is identified before the birth.

The heart and atherosclerosis

BLOCKAGE OF THE WALLS OF THE ARTERIES WITH CHOLESTEROL AND OTHER FATTY SUBSTANCES
THAT CAUSE THEM TO NARROW IS A SERIOUS CONDITION CALLED ATHEROSCLEROSIS.

When the arteries of the heart and brain are affected by atherosclerosis, many common symptoms and diseases develop. **In the case of the heart**, common symptoms are **angina** and **palpitations**, and diseases include **coronary heart disease** and **heart attack**. **In the case of the brain**, symptoms are **dizziness**, **fainting spells**, and **memory loss**, and diseases include **stroke** and **dementia**. Seen like this, atherosclerosis is the common denominator of many important conditions and the explanation for many symptoms.

Because of its importance I start with atherosclerosis in this section on the heart and circulation. If you understand atherosclerosis you'll automatically understand a lot about heart (cardiovascular) disease and strokes (cerebrovascular disease).

You'll also become aware of how to lower your chances of getting it and much of the treatment and recommended changes in lifestyle will become obvious and logical.

I also feel a brief discussion of cholesterol is useful for understanding how your heart condition has come about and how you can manage it. Cholesterol has been demonized but not all of it is bad. Indeed, some cholesterol, namely high-density lipoproteins (HDL), is positively good for you and actually protects against heart disease.

Atherosclerosis is a disease that results in the arteries becoming narrowed. The condition can affect arteries in any area of the body and is a major cause of stroke, heart attack, and poor circulation in the legs. Platelets (tiny blood cells responsible for clotting) may collect in clumps on the surface of the fatty deposits and form blood clots. A large clot may then completely block the artery.

Atherosclerosis becomes more common with age. However, it rarely causes symptoms until around 45–50 years. The female sex hormone estrogen helps protect against the development of atherosclerosis. As a result, the incidence of atherosclerosis is much lower in women before they reach menopause than in men. By the age of 60, however, the risk of women developing atherosclerosis has increased until it is equal to the risk for men. The recent Women's Health Initiative study challenged the notion that hormone replacement therapy will protect you from heart disease.

WHAT ARE THE CAUSES?

The risk of developing atherosclerosis is determined largely by two things: the level of cholesterol in the bloodstream, which depends on dietary and genetic factors, and whether or not you have the tendency, partly genetic, for cholesterol to collect on the walls of the arteries.

Since cholesterol levels are closely linked with a diet high in fat, atherosclerosis is most common in Western countries where people eat a high-fat diet. In some conditions, such as diabetes mellitus, there is a high blood fat level regardless of diet. Some inherited disorders, such as inherited hyperlipidemia (see opposite), also cause a high blood fat level.

Factors that make atherosclerosis more likely are smoking, not exercising regularly, having high blood pressure, and being overweight, especially if fat accumulates around the waist.

WHAT ARE THE RISK FACTORS?

There are several proven risk factors for atherosclerosis and given that atherosclerosis precedes most heart disease, the risk factors for atherosclerosis apply to heart conditions such as angina, coronary heart disease, and heart attacks. These are:
- family history of angina or heart attack
- smoking
- diabetes mellitus
- high cholesterol
- not getting exercise or being overweight
- high blood pressure.

WHAT ARE THE SYMPTOMS?

There are usually no symptoms in the early stages of atherosclerosis. If the coronary arteries that supply the heart muscle become blocked, however, symptoms include the chest pain of angina. If atherosclerosis affects the arteries in the legs, the first symptom may be cramping pain when walking caused by poor blood flow to the leg muscles.

HOW IS IT DIAGNOSED?

Since atherosclerosis has no symptoms until blood flow has been restricted, it's important to screen for it, checking on cholesterol levels, blood pressure and diabetes mellitus. You should have your cholesterol levels measured at intervals of five years after the age of 20, if you are at risk (see above).

We have sophisticated imaging techniques using X-rays (angiography) and ultrasound (Doppler scanning) that show the blood flow in the blood vessels of the heart, brain, and lungs. An electrocardiogram (ECG) will monitor the electrical activity of the heart. Some of these tests may be performed while you exercise to check how your heart functions when it's put under stress.

WHAT IS THE TREATMENT?

■ **Preventive measures** include following a **healthy lifestyle** by eating a low-fat diet, not

Cholesterol

Cholesterol is a fatty substance made in the liver from the saturated fats in food. Too much cholesterol in the blood can increase your risk of getting coronary heart disease.

Cholesterol comes in two main forms:
- low-density lipoproteins (LDL), which carry cholesterol from the liver to the cells in the body, including the arteries
- high-density lipoproteins (HDL), which return excess cholesterol to the liver.

LDLs are the body's natural enemy. High LDLs are a serious risk factor for coronary heart disease, especially with a low HDL. HDLs on the other hand are the good guys and high levels are extremely healthy. The best position to be in therefore is to have a high HDL and a low LDL.

Now we come to the tricky role of diet. A diet high in saturated fat (i.e. animal fat, mainly from whole milk dairy products) raises your LDL and lowers your HDL – the opposite of

what you want. On the other hand, by changing your saturated fats to unsaturated fat (oils) you'll reverse this tendency. More than 25 percent of American adults have been told that they have high cholesterol. This is high compared to other countries. In China, for example, the average cholesterol level is lower than in the US. If your measurement is over 5.8mmol/l, your doctor will want you to try to reduce it with changes to your diet and lifestyle, and possibly by prescribing drugs.

Cholesterol is only one risk for getting heart disease. If you have any other risk factors, such as smoking, being overweight, or high blood pressure, then these risk factors multiply your chances of having a heart attack.

About 1 in 10 people has high cholesterol as the result of a familial condition called inherited hyperlipidemia. If this condition is left untreated it can lead to coronary artery disease and heart attack at an exceptionally young age.

TESTS

Blood chemistry and cholesterol

Blood chemistry tests

Blood chemistry tests measure the levels of certain chemicals and minerals in the blood and are a simple way of discovering whether particular cells and tissues are functioning normally. They are usually used to check the levels of chemicals produced by the kidneys, the liver or the muscles. The tests can also be used to check levels of bone minerals, such as calcium.

Cholesterol tests

Cholesterol tests measure levels of certain fatty substances, known as lipids, in the blood. High levels of lipids cholesterol and triglycerides cause fatty deposits to develop on the walls of the arteries, resulting in atherosclerosis. The fatty deposits interfere with blood flow and can cause coronary artery disease (CAD) and stroke.

As well as measuring the total level of cholesterol in the blood and the levels of other lipids such as triglycerides, the tests also measure the levels of two specific types

of cholesterol: high-density lipoprotein (HDL) and low-density lipoprotein (LDL). HDL seems to protect against atherosclerosis, while a high level of LDL is a risk factor for developing atherosclerosis. A result of 5.0 mmol/l (millimoles of cholesterol per 1 liter of blood) or lower is generally considered desirable. The ratio of HDL to LDL is also important; ideally the ratio should be less than 4. Depending on the results of blood cholesterol tests, your doctor may advise you to make diet and lifestyle changes or may prescribe lipid-lowering drugs, or both.

smoking, exercising regularly, and maintaining the recommended weight for your height.
■ If you are in a good state of health but have been found to have a high cholesterol level, your doctor will advise a **low-fat diet**.
■ You may also be offered **drugs** that decrease your cholesterol level.
For people who have had a heart attack, research has shown that there is a benefit in lowering cholesterol levels, even if the cholesterol level is within the average range for healthy people.
■ Your doctor may prescribe a drug such as **low-dose aspirin** to reduce the risk of blood

clots forming on the damaged artery lining.
■ If you are thought to be at a high risk of severe complications, your doctor may recommend other treatment, such as **coronary angioplasty**, in which a balloon is inflated inside the artery to widen it and improve blood flow.
■ If blood flow to the heart is seriously obstructed, you may have **coronary bypass surgery** to restore blood flow.

WHAT IS THE OUTLOOK?
A healthy diet and lifestyle can slow the development of atherosclerosis in most

people. If you do have a heart attack or a stroke, you can reduce the risk of having further complications by taking preventive measures.

See also:
• Angina p. 224 • Coronary angiography p. 224 • ECG p. 224

Inherited hyperlipidemia

THE CONDITION IN WHICH THE BLOOD CONTAINS ABNORMALLY HIGH LEVELS OF CHOLESTEROL AND/OR TRIGLYCERIDES (ANOTHER TYPE OF FAT) IS KNOWN AS INHERITED HYPERLIPIDEMIA.

Inherited hyperlipidemia is present from birth, but usually only becomes apparent in early childhood and is due to an abnormal gene inherited from one or both parents.
A high-fat diet and lack of exercise aggravate the condition. Elevated levels of triglycerides, or, especially, cholesterol increase the risk of **atherosclerosis** and **coronary artery disease**.

WHAT ARE THE RISKS?
■ The most common form affects about 1 in 500 people of European descent, who inherit one copy of an abnormal gene. Affected people have a cholesterol level **two or three times** higher than normal.
■ There is a **one in a million** risk that people will inherit the abnormal gene from both parents. If two copies of the gene are inherited, the cholesterol level is **six to eight times** higher than normal.

■ Affected people have a high probability of a **heart attack**, which may occur **even in childhood**.

WHAT ARE THE SYMPTOMS?
Besides the symptoms of atherosclerosis, very high cholesterol levels associated with inherited hyperlipidemia may cause some of the following symptoms, which develop gradually over a period of several years:
• yellow swellings under the skin (xanthomas) on the back of the hands
• swellings in the tendons around the ankle and wrist joints
• yellow swellings on the skin of the eyelids (xanthelasmas)
• pale yellow ring around the iris (the colored part of the eye).

Men with these disorders can develop symptoms of coronary artery disease, such as angina, as early as their 20s or 30s. In women,

estrogen usually gives protection from these problems until after menopause.

WHAT MIGHT BE DONE?
■ There is no cure for inherited hyperlipidemia so cholesterol lowering drugs must be given early.
■ Symptoms can be treated with a combination of exercise, a diet that is low in saturated fats, and medication.
■ The prognosis varies, but early treatment can reduce the risk of a heart attack.
■ Relatives of an affected person should be screened for the disorder.

See also:
• Angina p. 224
• The heart and atherosclerosis p. 222

Angina

THE TYPICAL CHEST PAIN OF ANGINA IS OFTEN DESCRIBED AS HEAVINESS OR TIGHTNESS IN THE CENTER OF THE CHEST SPREADING TO THE ARMS, ELBOWS, NECK, JAW, FACE, AND BACK, USUALLY BROUGHT ON BY EXERTION OR ANXIETY AND RELIEVED BY RESTING FOR ABOUT 10 MINUTES.

Coronary angiography

Coronary angiography is used to give a picture of the arteries that supply the heart muscle with blood. Angiography can show narrowed or blocked coronary arteries, which are not visible on a normal X-ray. A local anesthetic is injected to numb the skin, and a fine flexible catheter is passed into the femoral artery, through the aorta, and into a coronary artery. Contrast dye is injected through the catheter, and a series of X-rays is taken. The procedure is painless, but you may feel a flushing sensation as the dye is injected.

During the procedure

The catheter is positioned in the heart so that its tip rests in a coronary artery and contrast dye is then injected. The artery and the small vessels leading from it are visualized by a series of X-rays. The catheter may be repositioned and the procedure repeated to check all the coronary arteries.

Angina affects both sexes but rarely occurs in women before the age of 60 because estrogen protects against it. After menopause, however, the protective effect of estrogen gradually disappears and angina is as common in women as in men, as is heart disease.

Angina is the most common symptom caused by blockage of the coronary arteries (atherosclerosis). Since atherosclerosis precedes most heart conditions, angina is a warning sign for many different heart diseases.

WHAT BRINGS IT ON?

The pain originates in the heart muscle and is due to an inadequate supply of blood. It is a sign of coronary artery disease (CAD; see opposite) and coronary heart disease (CHD). It may come on when you're walking, particularly on a cold day or after a meal, but it can also come on when you're resting and may even wake you up at night. Some people notice that getting upset or anxious brings on angina.

WHAT DO I DO IF ANGINA COMES ON?

1. Stop what you're doing.
2. Rest. Don't move until the pain has completely gone.
3. Take your medication (e.g. a nitrate pill under your tongue) to relieve the pain.
4. If the pain lasts longer than 15 minutes or isn't relieved by a nitrate pill, call your doctor – it could be a heart attack. Also inform

your doctor if your angina comes on with less and less effort.

IS IT REALLY ANGINA?

There are many causes of central chest pain but they don't all have the significance of angina. Here are just a few:
- heartburn
- indigestion
- peptic ulcer
- gallstones
- anxiety
- muscle strain or inflammation.

Your doctor can usually distinguish these from a heart condition by the nature of the pain, but you may have electrocardiography (ECG), a radionuclide (thallium) scan, an angiogram, or coronary catheterization. An exercise ECG will show a heart that's under stress on exertion.

WHAT IS THE TREATMENT?
DRUG TREATMENT

■ Nitrate drugs increase the blood supply to your heart by widening the coronary arteries. You can get immediate relief by putting a glyceryl trinitrate (GTN) pill under your tongue. Always keep them with you and never run out. You can also use them as a preventive before exertion, such as before sex.

■ Beta blockers, calcium channel blockers, or potassium channel blockers reduce the amount of work your heart does by slowing down the heart rate and reducing the heart's

ECG

Electrocardiography (ECG) is used to record the electrical activity of the heart, to investigate the cause of chest pain, and to diagnose abnormal heart rhythms. Several electrodes are attached to the skin to transmit the electrical activity of the heart to an ECG machine. Each trace shows electrical activity in different areas of the heart. The test usually takes several minutes to complete and is safe and painless.

The trace (paper record) produced by the ECG machine shows the electrical activity of the heart as it contracts and relaxes.

need for oxygen. Side effects are uncommon but include impotence, so report anything unusual to your doctor and your pills could be changed.

SURGICAL TREATMENT
■ Coronary angioplasty will improve the flow of blood to your heart. This isn't major surgery and you'll be home in two days.
■ Coronary bypass is when the narrowed sections of your coronary arteries are bypassed by an artery or vein grafted from another part of your body, usually your leg. This is major surgery and you'll be in the hospital for a week.

LIFESTYLE CHANGES
An angina attack is an early warning sign. You must alter your lifestyle if you want to prevent another attack and stop your heart condition from getting worse.
■ Stop smoking.
■ Lose weight and eat a heart-healthy diet with more oily fish and fresh fruit and vegetables.
■ Start exercising gradually.
■ Control your blood pressure, under your doctor's supervision.
■ Keep an eye on your cholesterol (a level under 5mmol/l is best).

With these changes and treatment from your doctor you should be able to get back to normal life, work, and sex.

> **See also:**
> • **The heart and atherosclerosis p. 222**

Coronary artery disease

IN CORONARY ARTERY DISEASE, THE CORONARY ARTERIES (WHICH SUPPLY BLOOD TO THE HEART MUSCLE) HAVE BECOME SO CLOGGED WITH FATTY MATERIAL THAT THE BLOOD SUPPLY TO THE HEART MUSCLE IS COMPROMISED, LEADING TO HEART DAMAGE.

The underlying condition is atherosclerosis and the most prominent symptom is **angina** (chest pain). I've included a detailed discussion of risks, causes, investigations, treatment, and changes to lifestyle under those headings and I suggest you read them in conjunction with this one.

In coronary artery disease (CAD), which can progress to **coronary heart disease**, one or more of the coronary arteries is narrowed. Blood flow through the arteries is restricted, leading to damage to the heart muscle. Impending damage to the heart muscle is signaled by the chest pain angina. Serious heart disorders, including heart attacks, are usually caused by CAD. The condition is therefore a leading cause of death in many Western countries.

WHAT ARE THE CAUSES?
Coronary artery disease is usually due to **atherosclerosis**, in which fatty deposits accumulate on the inside of the artery walls. These deposits narrow the arteries restricting blood flow. If a blood clot forms or lodges in the narrowed area of an artery, it can become completely blocked. CAD caused by atherosclerosis is more likely if your cholesterol is high and you eat a diet high in animal fat. CAD is also linked to smoking, obesity, lack of exercise, diabetes mellitus, and high blood pressure.

In women, it is no longer thought that HRT reduces the risk of heart attacks, strokes, and blood clots.

WHAT ARE THE SYMPTOMS?
■ **Chest pain** (angina).
■ **Palpitations** (awareness of the heartbeat).
■ **Light-headedness** or **loss of consciousness.**
■ **Irregular heartbeats** in some people. These

are a result of an abnormality of the heart rhythm (arrhythmia). Some severe arrhythmias can cause the heart to stop pumping completely – cardiac arrest – which accounts for most of the sudden deaths from CAD.
■ In elderly people, CAD may lead to chronic heart failure, a condition in which the heart gradually becomes too weak to pump an adequate circulation of blood around the body. Chronic heart failure may then lead to the accumulation of **excess fluid in the lungs** and tissues, causing additional symptoms such as **shortness of breath** and **swollen ankles**.

WHAT IS THE TREATMENT?
■ Treatment for CAD falls into three categories: lifestyle changes, drug treatments, and surgical procedures.
■ If tests show that you have a high cholesterol level, you will be treated with lipid-lowering drugs to slow the progression of CAD and, as a consequence, reduce the risk of a heart attack.
■ Angina may be treated with drugs, such as nitrate drugs and beta blocker drugs, that improve the blood flow through the arteries and help the heart pump effectively. An abnormal heart rhythm is often treated using antiarrhythmic drugs.
■ Surgical treatment includes angioplasty and coronary bypass surgery.

> **See also:**
> • **Angina p. 224** • **Arrhythmias p. 231**
> • **The heart and atherosclerosis p. 222**
> • **Chronic heart failure p. 233**
> • **Heart attack p. 230**
> • **High blood pressure p. 226**

TEST

Exercise testing

Exercise testing is usually done when coronary artery disease is suspected. It is used to assess heart function when the heart is put under stress. The test involves raising your heart rate by exercising, generally using a treadmill with an adjustable slope or an exercise bicycle, and monitoring the heart's function. The exercise is tailored to ensure your heart is tested adequately without putting you at risk. Various methods of monitoring may be used, including radionuclide (thallium) scanning, which can image the heart's function, and electrocardiography (ECG), which monitors the heart's electrical activity.

Riding an exercise bicycle tests the heart safely.

FOCUS *on* high blood pressure

Persistently high blood pressure may damage the arteries and the heart. Untreated high blood pressure is the most common cause of a stroke. In the West, at least 1 in 5 people has high blood pressure, also known as hypertension.

High blood pressure is harmful because it strains the heart and arteries, resulting in damage to delicate tissues. If it's left untreated, high blood pressure may eventually affect the eyes and kidneys. The higher your blood pressure the greater the risk that complications, such as heart attack, coronary artery disease, and stroke, will shorten your life. Lowering your blood pressure even a little can cut your risk of having a heart attack by as much as 20 percent.

Your blood pressure varies naturally during the day with activity, rising when you exercise or feel stressed and falling when you rest and sleep. It also varies among people, gradually increasing with age and weight.

High blood pressure per se rarely makes you feel ill. A small number of people get headaches but only if their blood pressure is very high. If your blood pressure is that high, you may have dizziness, blurry vision, or nosebleeds. Hypertension is sometimes called the "silent killer" because people may have a fatal stroke or heart attack without warning.

However, if you know you have high blood pressure you're not alone and you're luckier than many because at least you're aware that you have it. Over one-third of people with high blood pressure aren't being treated and their health is at risk.

WHAT ARE THE CAUSES?
Even though high blood pressure is more common among men there is no single cause. All these factors can contribute:
- being overweight
- drinking large amounts of alcohol
- a stressful lifestyle
- excessive salt intake
- physical inactivity
- kidney disease.

In pregnant women, the development of high blood pressure can lead to the potentially life threatening conditions preeclampsia and eclampsia, in which the elevated blood pressure usually returns to normal after the birth.

WHAT MIGHT BE DONE?
- To detect high blood pressure it's important to have your blood pressure measured routinely at least every two years after the age of 30.
- If your blood pressure is more than 140/90mmHg, your doctor will ask you to return in a few weeks so that it can be checked again.
- A diagnosis of hypertension isn't usually made unless you have high blood pressure on three separate occasions.

Your doctor may arrange these other tests:
- heart tests including electrocardiography (ECG) or echocardiography
- eye tests to look for damaged blood vessels
- tests to identify the underlying cause. For example, urine and blood tests and ultrasound scanning may be ordered to look for kidney disease or a hormonal disorder.

ARE THERE COMPLICATIONS?
There is risk of damage to the arteries, heart, and kidneys with severe hypertension that's left untreated. Arteries that have been damaged are at greater risk of being affected by atherosclerosis, in which fatty deposits build up in blood vessel walls, causing them to narrow and restrict blood flow.

After many years, damage to the arteries in the kidneys may lead to chronic kidney failure. The arteries in the retina of the eye may also be damaged by hypertension.

WILL I NEED TREATMENT RIGHT AWAY?
The need for treatment is contingent on the level of blood pressure PLUS other risk factors

Measuring blood pressure

An inflatable cuff is wrapped around your upper arm and inflated using a bulb. The cuff is slowly deflated while the doctor listens to the blood flow through an artery in your arm using a stethoscope.

Blood pressure is expressed as two figures given in millimeters of mercury (mmHg). The blood pressure of a healthy young person who's been sitting down for five minutes shouldn't be more than 120/80mmHg. In general, a person is considered to have high blood pressure when their blood pressure is persistently higher than 140/90mmHg after three readings on separate occasions, even at rest.

140/90 – what it means
140 – Systolic pressure
The pressure when the contraction of the heart forces blood around the body
90 – Diastolic pressure
The lowest pressure occurring between heartbeats

• If self-help measures aren't effective your doctor may prescribe antihypertensive drugs. These drugs work in different ways, and you may be prescribed just one type of drug or a combination of several. There are many drugs for treating blood pressure and they'll lower your blood pressure gradually over several weeks or months.

DO ANY OF THESE DRUGS HAVE SIDE EFFECTS?

Most people will feel well but some will suffer side effects. Fortunately these are few but one of the most distressing is impotence. If you experience impotence ask your doctor if your pills could be responsible and whether you can change treatments.

WOMEN:

• with high blood pressure can take HRT
• who take the contraceptive pill should have blood pressure checkups every six months.

that may damage blood vessels, for example diabetes, continued smoking, or being overweight. So, treatment can vary from person to person and isn't always dependent on a certain level of blood pressure.
• Blood pressure that averages 160/100mmHg or higher over many readings is best treated with drugs (see table, below).
• Mild high blood pressure (between 140/90 and 159/99mmHg) may be checked regularly but not treated if the risk of damage to the arteries is low. This is often the case in young people, particularly in young women.
• On the other hand, mild blood pressure is best treated in older people and those who already have symptoms of blood pressure damage, such as those who suffer from angina.
• You'll probably be checked by your doctor for three or six months before starting treatment.
• For mild hypertension the first line of medical treatment is often water pills (diuretics).

WHAT IS THE TREATMENT?

• High blood pressure can't usually be cured but it can be controlled with treatment. If you have very mild hypertension, changing your lifestyle is often the most effective way of lowering your blood pressure.

WHAT IS THE OUTLOOK?

In most cases, lifestyle changes and drug treatment can control blood pressure and reduce the risk of complications. You'll probably have to stick to these measures for the rest of your life.

Drugs used to treat high blood pressure

Drug type	What they do	Used to treat	Not used to treat	Occasional side effects
DIURETICS	Get rid of salt and water	High blood pressure	Gout or diabetes	Gout Impotence
BETA BLOCKERS	Slow your heartbeat	High blood pressure or angina	Asthma	Cold fingers and toes Tired legs Vivid dreams, Impotence
ACE INHIBITORS	Relax walls of arteries	Diabetes or heart failure	Women who are or may be pregnant	Dry cough Throat discomfort, Diarrhea
CALCIUM CHANNEL BLOCKERS	Relax walls of arteries	Angina	Heart failure	Ankle swelling Skin flushing, Constipation
ALPHA BLOCKERS	Slow your heartbeat	Prostate problems	Asthma	Headaches, Dizziness Dry mouth
ANGIOTENSIN II ANTAGONISTS	Relax walls of arteries	High blood pressure heart failure	Women who are or may be pregnant	Ankle swelling Skin flushing

SELF-HELP: CHANGING YOUR LIFESTYLE

You can help yourself a great deal by changing your lifestyle. There's a strong link between being overweight and having high blood pressure.

If your weight's above normal for your height, you should try to lose the extra pounds and bring your blood pressure down. You don't need to aim for an ideal weight. Try to be within the healthy range for your height. Losing 22lbs (10kg) can reduce the bottom figure of your blood pressure by 20 points.

If you can't lose weight yourself, your doctor may refer you to a dietician for advice on ways to change how and what you eat. You don't have to give up eating all the food you enjoy. Some people find a diet or nutritional support group very helpful to give moral support.

DOS

Eat fish, white meat (for example, chicken without the skin), cottage cheese, low-fat yogurt, low-fat or skim milk. Try for seven items a day of fresh fruit and vegetables (eat seasonal vegetables and fruit when you can); when fresh vegetables are expensive eat frozen ones instead. When possible, broil food instead of frying it.

A diet containing plenty of fruit, vegetables and grains increases potassium intake, and this can help lower your blood pressure too.

DON'TS

Don't eat butter, cheese, and whole milk, fried foods and snacks, cakes, cookies, chocolate, and fatty meat.

KEEP YOUR ALCOHOL LEVELS DOWN

High alcohol intake increases your chance of developing high blood pressure.

- Limit your alcohol to no more than 21 units a week if you're a man, 14 units if you're a woman. One unit is equal to a glass of wine OR ten ounces of beer or lager OR a single shot of liquor.
- Try to spread your units evenly over the week and avoid a big drinking session.
- A large amount of alcohol the night before can raise your blood pressure significantly the following day.
- Talk to your doctor if you're drinking more alcohol than you should and finding it difficult to reduce the amount you drink.

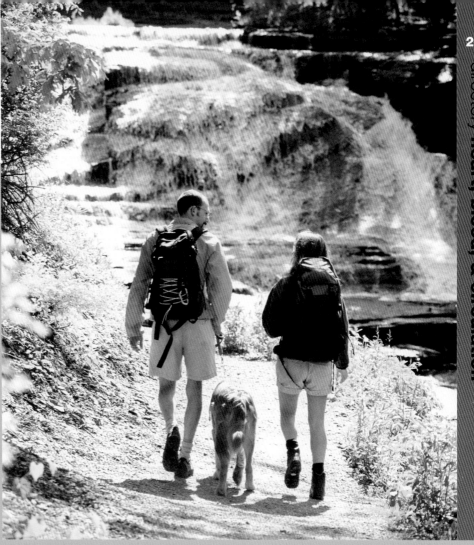

LIMIT YOUR SALT

A high salt intake raises your blood pressure
about 10 points. Salt can also increase the
amount of fluid that you retain in your body.

Fresh food contains very little salt. Most of
the salt we eat is in processed foods, or in salt
added to food while cooking or at the table.
So to reduce the amount of salt you eat:
- Look at food labels. If it says sodium
chloride (NaCl), sodium benzoate, or
monosodium glutamate then you may be
eating extra salt without realizing it.
- Cut down on processed foods. Salt is hidden
in many processed foods, e.g. canned or
packaged soups, breakfast cereals, bread,
canned or processed fish, potato chips, nuts,
hamburgers, and prepared meals.
- Look for low-salt bread.
- Cut down on corned beef, hard cheese, ham,
bacon, and sausages, which contain a lot of salt.
- Use salt very sparingly in cooking, if at all.
If you feel that you can't do without salt, you
might try a salt substitute (after checking with
your doctor). Rock salt and sea salt are not salt
substitutes.

It's preferable to avoid the taste of salt
altogether. You'll find fairly quickly that your
sense of taste adjusts so that you no longer
like the taste of salt, especially if you add herbs
such as basil, thyme, and rosemary to your
cooking, which release the natural salts in food.

EXERCISE

Exercise can help reduce your blood pressure
and keep your weight down. It is also a good
stress reliever. Stress isn't always a cause of
high blood pressure. It will, however, aggravate
high blood pressure.

If you haven't done any exercise recently,
check with your doctor first.

WHAT TYPE OF EXERCISE SHOULD I DO?

Any vigorous activity such as walking,
swimming, bicycling, jogging, dancing, or
gardening is good for you. The important
thing is to choose an activity that you enjoy –
if you don't like a particular form of exercise
you'll find it much harder to do regularly.

Exercise doesn't need to be too strenuous
either. You should start slowly and build up
the amount of exercise that you do. Start by
walking briskly. You don't have to jog unless
you want to. Walk the dog; use the stairs, not
the elevator, and keep active! Try to do 20–30
minutes of exercise at least three times a week.

For some people, it isn't advisable to lift very
heavy weights or to do certain very strenuous
activities such as playing raquetball. Check
with your doctor first if you're thinking of
taking up a new sport that is very strenuous.

STOP SMOKING

Giving up smoking won't lower your blood
pressure directly, but it lowers your risk factors
for high blood pressure by greatly reducing
the chance of blood vessel damage that can
lead to a heart attack or stroke.

It's so important that you stop smoking that
I suggest you make a plan and prepare yourself
to stop. Have an action plan, prepare well, and
you'll succeed.

Your pharmacist, doctor, or practical nurse
can advise you on stopping smoking and on
aids such as chewing gum and skin patches
that you might find helpful.

What about a home blood pressure monitor?

It's only worth monitoring your own blood
pressure if you stick to the correct
procedure, like resting for at least five
minutes before each reading and not taking
readings in isolation but averaging out three
consecutive readings.

There are two types of monitor:

- an inflatable cuff that can be pumped up
and the blood pressure is read from a dial.
- a digital electronic monitor that provides
a digitally displayed blood pressure reading.

Only buy a monitor that's approved
for use in the US.

Heart attack (myocardial infarction)

DEATH OF PART OF THE HEART MUSCLE, FOLLOWING A BLOCKAGE IN ITS BLOOD SUPPLY, IS COMMONLY CALLED A HEART ATTACK BUT IS ALSO KNOWN AS MYOCARDIAL INFARCTION.

A heart attack is the end result of **atherosclerosis** in the coronary arteries that supply heart muscle and it may have been preceded by **angina** (chest pain). Heart attack is one of the major causes of death in developed countries.

WHAT ARE THE CAUSES?

A heart attack is usually a result of coronary artery disease, which stems from atherosclerosis.

WHAT ARE THE SYMPTOMS?

The symptoms of a heart attack usually develop suddenly and include:
- severe, heavy, crushing pain just like angina but worse in the center of the chest spreading up to the neck and teeth and into the arms, especially in the left arm, sometimes centering on the elbow
- pale clammy skin
- shortness of breath

What can I do?

Making changes in your lifestyle after a heart attack can help your recovery and reduce the risk of another attack from occurring.

■ Stop smoking. This is the single most important factor in preventing another heart attack.
■ Eat a healthy diet and try to keep your weight within the ideal range for your height and build.
■ If you drink alcohol, take only moderate amounts. You should have not more than 1–2 small glasses of wine or beer a day.
■ Together with your doctor, agree on a program of increasing exercise until you are able to engage in moderate exercise, such as swimming regularly, for 30 minutes or more at a time.
■ Take the trouble to learn how to relax with relaxation exercises.

After a period of recovery, you can make a gradual return to your normal daily routine.
■ You will probably be able to return to work within six weeks, or sooner if you have a desk job. You might consider working part-time at first.
■ Try to avoid stressful situations.
■ You should be able to drive a car within four weeks.
■ You can resume having sexual intercourse about four weeks after a heart attack.

- nausea and, sometimes, vomiting
- anxiety, sometimes accompanied by a fear of dying
- restlessness.

ARE THERE COMPLICATIONS?

■ In the first few **minutes** the main danger is **acute heart failure** and **cardiac arrest**.
■ In the first few **hours** and **days** after a heart attack, the main risks are the development of an **irregular heartbeat** (arrythmia).
■ In the **weeks** or **months** after the attack, the pumping action of the heart muscle may be too weak, leading to a condition called **chronic heart failure**. Its symptoms include fatigue, shortness of breath, and swollen ankles. Less common complications include **damage to one of the heart valves** or inflammation of the membrane covering the heart's surface, the pericardium, leading to **pericarditis**, both of which may also lead to heart failure.

HOW IS IT DIAGNOSED?

An **electrocardiogram (ECG)** will show evidence of a heart attack. To confirm the diagnosis, **blood samples** may be taken to measure the levels of particular enzymes that leak into the blood from damaged heart muscle.

WHAT IS THE TREATMENT?

■ The immediate goals of treatment are to **relieve pain** and **restore the blood supply to the heart muscle** in order to minimize the amount of damage and prevent further complications. These goals are best achieved by immediate admission to an **intensive care unit** (ICU). You will be given an injection of a powerful painkiller, such as **morphine**, to relieve pain.
■ To help minimize damage to your heart within the first six hours of the attack, you may also be given a **drug** to dissolve the blood clot that is blocking the coronary artery.
■ Alternatively, you may have immediate **coronary angioplasty** to open the artery. If the blood flow to the damaged heart muscle can be restored within six hours, there is a greater likelihood of full recovery.
■ Once you have recovered from the attack, the condition of your coronary arteries and heart muscle is assessed. Tests such as **exercise ECG** and **echocardiography** are used to help decide on further treatment.
■ If the pumping action of the heart is impaired, you may be prescribed an **ACE inhibitor** and/or a **diuretic drug**.
■ If tests reveal that you have a persistent irregular heartbeat, you may need to have

a **pacemaker** implanted in your chest.
■ Certain drugs taken long-term can reduce the risk of another heart attack, and you may be prescribed a **beta blocker drug** and/or aspirin for this reason.
■ You may also be advised to eat a low-fat diet and to take **lipid lowering drugs** to lower your cholesterol level. These drugs are beneficial after a heart attack even if your cholesterol level is not elevated.
■ If a coronary artery is blocked, you may need **bypass surgery**.

WARNING:

■ An episode of angina that does not respond to your usual treatment or that lasts longer than 15 minutes may be a heart attack and requires immediate emergency hospital treatment.
■ About 1 in 5 people experiences no chest pain in a heart attack. However, there may be other symptoms, such as breathlessness, faintness, sweating, and pale skin. This pattern of symptoms is known as a "silent heart attack" or "silent infarction."

It is important to avoid becoming disabled by the fear of having another heart attack. Many hospitals offer ongoing cardiac rehabilitation programs after discharge from the hospital.

WHAT IS THE OUTLOOK?

If you have not had a previous heart attack, if you are treated quickly and if there are no complications, your outlook is good. After two weeks the risk of another heart attack is considerably reduced. The prognosis is better **if you stop smoking**, **reduce alcohol intake**, **exercise regularly,** and follow a **healthy diet**.

See also:
- Angina p. 224   • Arrythmias p. 231
- **The heart and atherosclerosis p. 222**
- **Coronary artery disease p. 225**
- **ECG p. 224**

Arrhythmias

AN ABNORMAL HEART RATE AND/OR RHYTHM OF THE HEARTBEAT IS CALLED AN ARRHYTHMIA, THE MOST DANGEROUS OF WHICH – VENTRICULAR FIBRILLATION – IS USUALLY THE END RESULT OF A HEART ATTACK.

A heart rate outside the usual range, however, is not always a cause for concern. For example, everyone's heart rate increases if they get excited or exercise.

Cause for greater concern is a rapid **irregular** heartbeat, although many people experience the odd irregularity and it has no significance. Arrhythmias of the heart's upper chambers, the **atria**, are nowhere near as serious as irregularities in the beat of the **ventricles**, the lower and more powerful chambers.

There are two types of arrhythmias: **tachycardias**, in which the heart rate is too high, and **bradycardias**, in which the rate is too low.

WHAT ARE THE CAUSES?

Most arrhythmias are caused by disease of the heart or its blood vessels. The most common underlying disorder is **coronary artery disease**. Less common causes include various **heart valve disorders** and **inflammation of the heart muscle**. Causes of arrhythmias that originate outside the heart include an **overactive thyroid** and a **lack of potassium**. Some **drugs**, such as **bronchodilators** and **digitalis** drugs, may cause arrhythmias, as may **caffeine** and **tobacco**.

WHAT ARE THE SYMPTOMS?

Symptoms do not always develop but if they do their onset is usually sudden and include:
- palpitations (awareness of an irregular heartbeat)
- light-headedness, sometimes leading to loss of consciousness
- shortness of breath
- pain in the chest or neck like angina.

Stroke and **heart failure** are possible complications.

WHAT MIGHT BE DONE?
- Electrocardiography (ECG).
- ECG over 24 hours to track the arrhythmia.
- Ambulatory ECG – a wearable device that's worn for 24 hours and detects intermittent arrhythmias.

WHAT IS THE TREATMENT?
- Antiarrhythmic drugs, such as **digoxin, beta blockers**, **calcium channel blockers**, **amiodarone**, **flecainide**, and **propafenone**.

- Cardioversion (defibrillation) – restoration of a regular heart rhythm by passing an electrical current through the heart under a general anesthetic.
- Cardiac **pacemaker**.

See also:
- **Coronary artery disease p. 225**
- **ECG p. 224** • **Heart attack p. 230**

TREATMENT

Cardiac pacemaker

Cardiac pacemakers stimulate the heart to maintain a regular heartbeat. Some pacemakers act continually, others send an impulse only when the heart rate falls too low.

A pacemaker is inserted just under the skin and stitched into position in the chest wall, usually under local anesthesia. Two wires from the pacemaker are passed into the large vein above the heart (superior vena cava). One wire is guided into the right atrium and the other into the right ventricle.

The latest pacemakers have batteries that last 8–10 years and are not affected by interference from radar and microwaves.

This X-ray photograph from the back shows a cardiac pacemaker in position in the chest wall, just below the right shoulder.

Palpitations

A FEELING THAT YOUR HEART IS THUMPING AT HIGH SPEED OR A SENSATION OF FLUTTERING IN YOUR CHEST OR A HAMMERING IN YOUR HEAD ARE ALL DESCRIPTIONS OF PALPITATIONS.

They don't necessarily denote anything serious – people who are anxious and tense frequently feel palpitations as a symptom of their anxiety – there's nothing wrong with their hearts. You can sometimes feel your heart beating after a heavy meal, after the effort of running hard, or when you lie down to go to sleep. These palpitations settle down very quickly. Those due to an overactive thyroid

gland rarely do and that's an important distinction. Cocaine and alcohol are both increasingly common causes of palpitations.

Palpitations in a person over 60 years old can be a symptom of a heart condition and should always be reported to a doctor for investigation and treatment.

Palpitations that arise from the atria, the upper chambers of the heart, and are regular

and can be uncomfortable but are hardly ever harmful, although you may feel dizzy and even faint.

Fast irregular beats are called **fibrillation** and, although not immediately dangerous if in the atria, they are unpleasant and must be investigated and treated promptly. Atrial fibrillation is the most common cause of irregular palpitations.

Atrial fibrillation

RAPID, UNCOORDINATED CONTRACTION OF THE UPPER CHAMBERS OF THE HEART,
THE ATRIA, IS A CONDITION CALLED ATRIAL FIBRILLATION.

Atrial fibrillation is the most common type of rapid, irregular heart rate, affecting up to 1 in 10 people over the age of 60 due to simple aging of the heart and coronary artery disease. During atrial fibrillation, the atria contract weakly at 300–500 beats per minute and so ventricular filling is inadequate. Since the atria and ventricles are no longer beating together, the heartbeat and pulse become irregular in timing and strength and less blood than normal is pumped out of the heart to the rest of the body, including the heart and brain.

The most dangerous complication of atrial fibrillation is a **stroke**. Since the atria do not empty properly during contractions, blood stagnates in them and may form a **clot**. If a part of the clot breaks off and enters the bloodstream, it may block an artery anywhere in the body. A stroke occurs when part of a clot blocks an artery supplying the brain.

WHAT ARE THE CAUSES?
Atrial fibrillation may occur for no apparent reason, especially in the elderly. **Smoking, lack of exercise,** a **high-fat diet,** and being **overweight** are risk factors for many of these disorders. Atrial fibrillation is also common in people with an **overactive thyroid gland** or **low potassium levels** in the blood. It may occur in people who drink to excess or use cocaine and crack.

WHAT ARE THE SYMPTOMS?
Symptoms do not always develop, but, if they do, their onset is usually sudden. The symptoms may be intermittent or persistent and typically include:
● palpitations (awareness of an irregular or abnormally rapid heartbeat)
● light-headedness
● shortness of breath
● shortness of breath at night that wakes you up
● chest pain (angina).

Stroke and **heart failure** are possible complications.

WHAT MIGHT BE DONE?
■ Electrocardiography (ECG).
■ Tests to look for an underlying cause such as hyperthyroidism.

WHAT IS THE TREATMENT?
■ You may be prescribed antiarrhythmic drugs, including digoxin, to slow a rapid heartbeat, and beta blocker drugs.
■ You may also be prescribed the **anticoagulant drug warfarin**, which reduces the risk of blood clot formation and thereby lowers the risk of a stroke.

See also:
● **Coronary artery disease p. 225**
● **Hyperthyroidism p. 506**

HEART FAILURE

The heart can fail suddenly and seriously, often as the result of a heart attack (myocardial infarction), and life is endangered. This is called acute heart failure.

The heart can also succumb to the long-term strain of an inadequate blood supply (coronary artery disease) or of pumping against resistance (high blood pressure). Such chronic heart failure comes on slowly and gradually.

Either way, whether heart failure is acute or chronic, it's almost always the left ventricle (the heart's main pumping chamber) that can't handle it, which means that the back pressure causes fluid to pool first in the lungs and later in the feet. This is why in acute heart failure the

person is said to "drown" in their own fluids since the lungs fill very rapidly and gaseous exchange is halted.

Doctors also describe RIGHT- and LEFT-sided heart failure. The right side of the heart serves the lungs via the pulmonary artery and a blockage there causes the **right ventricle** to fail. Lung disease, such as **chronic obstructive pulmonary disease**, also causes right-sided heart failure because the right ventricle eventually becomes too weak to overcome the resistance imposed by diseased lung tissue. Left-sided heart failure is due to persistently high blood pressure and coronary artery disease, particularly after a heart attack.

Acute heart failure

A SUDDEN DETERIORATION IN THE PUMPING ACTION OF THE HEART, USUALLY THE LEFT
VENTRICLE, IS CALLED ACUTE HEART FAILURE AND LEADS TO AN ACCUMULATION OF
FLUID IN THE LUNGS. IF NOT TREATED IMMEDIATELY, IT IS LIFE THREATENING.

WHAT ARE THE CAUSES?
The most common cause of acute heart failure is a heart attack that damages a large area of heart muscle. Right-sided acute heart failure is rare and is usually due to a blood clot blocking the pulmonary artery (pulmonary embolism).

WHAT ARE THE SYMPTOMS?
The symptoms of acute heart failure usually develop rapidly and include:
● severe shortness of breath
● wheezing
● cough with pink, frothy sputum

● pale skin and sweating.
If heart failure is caused by a **pulmonary embolism,** you may cough up blood and have sharp chest pain that is worse when breathing in.

WHAT MIGHT BE DONE?

■ **Acute heart failure** is a **medical emergency** and requires immediate hospital treatment.
■ You will be advised to sit in an **upright position** to make breathing easier, and **oxygen** may be given to you through a face mask.
■ You may need electrocardiography (ECG) and echocardiography to evaluate the function of the heart and to look for the cause of heart failure.
■ A chest X-ray usually confirms the presence of fluid in the lungs.
■ You may also have coronary angiography.

WHAT IS THE TREATMENT?

Diuretics given intravenously and appropriate medication to promote the efficiency of the heart, such as ACE inhibitors and beta blockers, usually bring relief.

Other common problems

Aortic aneurysm
Enlargement of a section of the aorta due to weakness in the artery wall. More common after age 65, more common in males, sometimes runs in families. Smoking, a high-fat diet, lack of exercise, and excess weight are risk factors.

Ectopic beats
Extra contractions of the heart that are out of the normal rhythmic pattern but are nonetheless normal. We all have them occasionally. Most people have at least one ectopic beat every day.

Superficial thrombophlebitis
Inflammation of a superficial vein (a vein just beneath the surface of the skin) that may cause a blood clot to form in it. More common after age 20, more common in women, and sometimes runs in families. Intravenous drug abuse is a risk factor. A blood clot of this kind rarely breaks off and travels because the inflammation holds it firmly within the vein.

Cardiac arrest
A sudden failure of the heart to pump blood, which is often fatal. The most common cause is a heart attack but excessive loss of blood, hypothermia, drug overdose, and shock can also result in cardiac arrest. A person with cardiac arrest collapses suddenly, with loss of consciousness, absence of pulse, and no breathing. Cardiac arrest is more common in males and more common with increasing age.

Chronic heart failure

PEOPLE WITH CHRONIC HEART FAILURE ARE SUFFERING FROM LONG-STANDING INEFFICIENT PUMPING ACTION OF THE HEART, WHICH LEADS TO POOR CIRCULATION OF THE BLOOD AND ACCUMULATION OF FLUID IN BODY TISSUES.

WHAT ARE THE SYMPTOMS?

The symptoms of chronic heart failure develop gradually, are often vague and may include:
● fatigue
● shortness of breath, which is worse during exertion or when lying flat
● loss of appetite
● nausea
● swelling of the feet and ankles
● in some cases, confusion.

People with chronic heart failure may also have sudden attacks of **acute heart failure**, with symptoms of severe shortness of breath, wheezing, and sweating. These attacks generally **occur during the night**. Occasionally, acute heart failure develops if the heart is put under additional strain due to a heart attack or a lung infection such as bronchitis. Acute heart failure is a medical emergency and needs immediate hospital treatment.

HOW MIGHT THE DOCTOR TREAT IT?

Your doctor will probably prescribe **diuretic** drugs, which turn excess water into urine, and **ACE inhibitors**, which cause blood vessels to widen and reduce the workload on the heart. In addition, drugs that increase the efficiency of the heart, such as **digoxin** or, in some cases, **beta blocker drugs**, may be prescribed. You may also be treated to prevent progression of any underlying cause. For example, if you have coronary artery disease, you may be advised to take a **daily dose of aspirin**, which reduces the risk of a heart attack. Your doctor will monitor your heart condition and adjust your drug treatments and the dosage as needed.

In some cases, drug treatment may not be effective, and a **heart transplant** may be considered if a person is otherwise in good health.

TREATMENT

A note on surgical operations

Most operations are performed using conventional surgery. An incision is made in the skin large enough to see the internal parts that require treatment and surrounding tissues. Although a large incision provides easy access, it may leave an obvious scar.

Most conventional surgery is performed under general anesthesia. Once you are anesthetized, the surgeon makes an incision through the skin, the layers of fat, and muscle below it. The skin and the muscles may be held back by clamps, and organs and tissues that are not being operated on are pulled out of the way by retractors. When the area to be worked on is clearly visible, the surgeon is then able to perform the procedure.

Blood vessels that have to be severed during surgery are sealed in order to prevent serious loss of blood. The surgeon checks that there is no internal bleeding before he or she sews up the wound. The wound may be covered with a sterile dressing.

All surgical procedures, whether major or minor, involve some risk. A general anesthetic can provoke changes in heart rhythm during or after surgery. An allergic reaction to the anesthetic may also occur. Rarely, if blood vessels are not fully sealed, excessive bleeding may occur during the operation, or there may be persistent bleeding afterward. In both cases, a blood transfusion may be required.

To avoid the risk of clots developing following surgery, you will be encouraged to move around as soon as you can afterward. You may be asked to wear pneumatic stockings, which rhythmically inflate and deflate to keep the blood flowing normally through your veins, or elastic support stockings. Drugs that prevent blood clotting may be necessary. Analgesics may also help prevent the formation of blood clots by relieving pain and allowing you to move around more easily. Antibiotics are often given before, during or after surgery to help prevent infection.

Low blood pressure (hypotension)

SOME PEOPLE HAVE BLOOD PRESSURE THAT IS PERSISTENTLY BELOW NORMAL LEVELS. IN MOST CIRCUMSTANCES, HOWEVER, SUCH LOW BLOOD PRESSURE OR HYPOTENSION IS HEALTHY AND THE LONGER YOUR BLOOD PRESSURE IS ON THE LOW SIDE THE HEALTHIER YOUR HEART WILL BE.

Except in very old people low blood pressure therefore shouldn't have to be treated.

A common type of low blood pressure is **postural hypotension**, in which suddenly standing or sitting up leads to light-headedness or fainting. This can be caused by several drugs, including those for high blood pressure. Shock is a serious form of low blood pressure due to rapid loss of fluids or blood or a heart attack, and requires emergency treatment.

WHAT ARE THE CAUSES?
Dehydration following loss of large amounts of fluid or salts from the body will lower the blood pressure. For example, heavy sweating, loss of blood, or profuse diarrhea may cause varying degrees of low blood pressure.

WHAT ARE THE SYMPTOMS?
You may not have any symptoms unless your blood pressure is very low. Symptoms that do occur may include:
- fatigue
- general weakness
- light-headedness and fainting
- blurry vision
- nausea.

SHOCK
However, if no pulse is present because the blood pressure is too low to provide an adequate blood supply to vital organs, it can be fatal. The low blood pressure that follows a heart attack, acute heart failure, and serious cardiac arrhythmias must be treated in an intensive care unit since life is threatened.

SELF-HELP FOR POSTURAL HYPOTENSION
1. Sit up slowly and rest for a few minutes.
2. Slowly lower your legs over the side of the bed and wait a few minutes.
3. Stand slowly holding firmly onto the bed or a chair to steady yourself.

These symptoms are usually temporary, and blood pressure rises when the cause is treated.

See also:
- **Shock p. 560**

CIRCULATION

Into this group of conditions fall disorders of the **peripheral blood vessels – the arteries and veins** of the **arms** and **legs**. Within the remit of this book I feel there's only room for the three most common conditions: one of the arteries, **Raynaud's disease and Raynaud's phenomenon**, and two of the veins, **varicose veins** and **deep vein thrombosis** (DVT).

It's worth just mentioning the word phlebitis, which is used to describe **inflammation** (not a clot) in a vein. It's important to distinguish between phlebitis and DVT. With the former, there's little risk of a clot breaking off and going to the lungs or heart; in the latter, there is. Treatment of the two conditions is therefore quite different.

Raynaud's phenomenon and Raynaud's disease

THESE TWO SIMILAR CONDITIONS CAUSE NUMBNESS, TINGLING, PAIN, AND CHANGE IN COLOR IN THE FINGERS OR TOES; THEY ARE MORE COMMON IN WOMEN AND SOMETIMES RUN IN FAMILIES.

The symptoms are due to sudden narrowing of the arteries in the hands or, rarely, the feet because of **hypersensitivity** to cold. **Smoking** and **exposure** to cold may trigger attacks.

In about half of all people with Raynaud's phenomenon, the condition is associated with another disorder such as rheumatoid arthritis. Certain drugs, such as beta blockers, are known to produce the symptoms of Raynaud's phenomenon as a side effect.

If there is no apparent cause for the condition, it's known as Raynaud's disease, which is most common in women between the ages of 15 and 45 and is usually mild. It can be triggered by smoking, because the nicotine in cigarettes constricts the arteries. Exposure to cold and handling frozen items can also trigger an attack.

Rarely the condition is due to abnormal proteins, **cold agglutinins**, in the blood, which show up when the extremities get cold or the body cools down.

WHAT ARE THE SYMPTOMS?
Both the hands and feet can be affected and an attack can last from a few minutes to a few hours. Symptoms include:
- numbness and tingling in the fingers or toes that may worsen and progress to a painful burning sensation
- progressive change of color in the fingers or toes, which initially turn white, then blue, and finally red again as blood returns to the tissues.

There may be a marked color difference between the affected area and the surrounding tissues. In severe untreated cases, skin ulcers or gangrene may form on the tips of the fingers or toes.

WHAT MIGHT BE DONE?
■ Your doctor will carry out tests to look for an underlying cause of your symptoms. For

example, blood tests may be performed to look for evidence of **rheumatoid arthritis** or **cold agglutinins**.

■ Your doctor may suggest that you take drugs to dilate the blood vessels during an attack.

■ If you smoke, you should stop immediately.
■ Keeping the body covered up with several layers of warm clothing is helpful.
■ Wearing a thermal hat, gloves, and socks in cold weather helps avoid the onset of symptoms.

■ Heating should keep the ambient temperature on the warm side.
■ If symptoms are very severe, surgery may be considered to cut the nerves that control arterial constriction.

Varicose veins

MANY PEOPLE HAVE VISIBLY SWOLLEN AND DISTORTED VEINS THAT LIE JUST
BENEATH THE SKIN, MAINLY IN THE LOWER LEGS.

These varicose veins may also be found at the **lower end of the esophagus** as the result of **liver disease** and in the **rectum** as **hemorrhoids** as the result of **constipation.** Varicose veins tend to run in families and pregnancy, excess weight and prolonged standing are risk factors. Sometimes they are a result of a deep vein thrombosis in the lower leg.

Varicose veins affect about 1 in 5 adults and are more common with increasing age. Although the condition may cause discomfort and appear unsightly, it's not usually harmful to your health. Varicose veins mainly affect the legs. Veins have one-way valves to stop blood from flowing backward down into the legs. If the valves in the deep veins do not close adequately, the blood flows back into the superficial veins near the skin. The pressure of returning blood causes these veins to become swollen and distorted, and they are then known as varicose veins. If left untreated, the condition often worsens. Sometimes **dermatitis** and even an **ulcer** may develop at the site of a varicose vein, often on the inner side of the ankle.

WHAT ARE THE CAUSES?
■ An inherited weakness of the valves in the veins can cause varicose veins to develop.
■ The female hormone **progesterone** – the pregnancy hormone – causes the veins to dilate and may encourage the formation of varicose veins. The condition is therefore more common during pregnancy. Increased pressure is placed on the veins in the pelvic

region during pregnancy as the uterus gradually grows larger.
■ Being overweight is a factor.
■ Occupations that involve standing still for long periods and little walking can be to blame.
■ A blood clot blocking a deep vein in the lower leg – deep vein thrombosis (DVT) – sometimes known as a "white leg." It may follow major surgery if the patient doesn't wear elastic stockings or remains immobile.

WHAT IS THE TREATMENT?
■ In the majority of cases, varicose veins do not require treatment. Self-help measures such as wearing elastic stockings may be enough.
■ If your varicose veins are small and below the knee, your doctor may recommend that the veins be injected with a solution to make their walls stick together and thus prevent blood from entering them.
■ For varicose veins above the knee, the usual treatment is to tie off the connection with the deep vein so that blood does not enter the varicose vein.
■ For entire varicose veins, surgical removal by "stripping" is an option. However, even after surgery, varicose veins may eventually recur, and treatment may need to be repeated.
■ **Varicose dermatitis** and/or **ulcer** requires special treatment with topical creams and supportive bandaging.
■ Varices at the **lower end of the esophagus**, usually as the result of alcohol-related liver cirrhosis, can bleed internally and must be treated as a medical emergency.

SELF-HELP

Coping with varicose veins

There are a number of measures you can take if you have troublesome symptoms caused by varicose veins.
■ Avoid prolonged standing.
■ Take regular walks to keep blood flowing in the legs.
■ Keep your legs elevated when sitting, if possible.
■ If your doctor has recommended that you wear elastic stockings, put them on before you get out of bed in the morning while your legs are still elevated.
■ Avoid clothing, such as girdles, that may restrict the flow of blood at the top of the legs.
■ If you are overweight, you should try to lose weight.

■ Varices in the rectum are **hemorrhoids** and they may cause rectal bleeding.

See also:
• **Cirrhosis p. 357**
• **Hemorrhoids p. 370**

Deep vein thrombosis

THE FORMATION OF A BLOOD CLOT IN A DEEP LYING VEIN, USUALLY IN THE LEG, IS CALLED DEEP
VEIN THROMBOSIS (DVT). DVT USED TO BE CALLED "WHITE LEG" BECAUSE IF A BLOOD
CLOT FORMS WITHIN A DEEP VEIN IN THE LEG IT SWELLS AND LOOKS WHITE.

DVT is more common over the age of 40 and slightly more common in females. It can run in families and risk factors include prolonged immobility after surgery or childbirth and excess weight. A combination of **age** (being

over 35 years), **cigarette smoking**, **obesity,** and the **oral contraceptive pill** increases the risk of DVT too.

The formation of a clot in a deep vein is usually not dangerous in itself. However,

there's a risk that a fragment of the clot may break off and travel to the heart via the circulation. If the fragment lodges in a vessel supplying the lungs, a potentially fatal blockage called a **pulmonary embolism** occurs.

WHAT ARE THE CAUSES?

Deep vein thrombosis is usually caused by a combination of:
- slow blood flow through a vein
- an increase in the natural tendency of the blood to clot, such as after surgery
- damage to the wall of the vein.

Long periods of immobility, such as those experienced during air or road **travel** or while **bedridden**, are a common cause of slow blood flow. Other causes include compression of a vein by the fetus during **pregnancy** or by a tumor. **Leg injury** may also cause a clot to form in the deep veins of the leg.

WHAT ARE THE SYMPTOMS?

A blood clot in a deep vein may produce:
- pain or tenderness in the calf of the leg
- swelling of the lower leg or thigh
- enlarged veins beneath the skin.

WHAT MIGHT BE DONE?

To confirm the diagnosis you may have **Doppler ultrasound scanning** to measure blood flow through the veins and sometimes a **venogram**, in which dye is injected into a vein and then X-rays are taken to reveal blood clots. A sample of your blood may be taken and analyzed to see how easily it clots.

WHAT IS THE TREATMENT?

- **Thrombolytic drugs** are used to **dissolve** the blood clot in the vein and reduce the risk of a pulmonary embolism.
- Injections of **anticoagulants** are administered to **prevent** more clots. Although treatment can take place in the hospital, you may be able to self-administer anticoagulant drugs at home.
- Rarely, the clot is removed surgically.

After you have had the initial treatment, your doctor will prescribe drugs to reduce the risk that the condition will recur.

CAN IT BE PREVENTED?

- If there is a high risk, low doses of short-acting anticoagulant drugs will probably be given before and after any surgery, to prevent the blood from clotting.
- Your doctor may also advise you to wear special elastic stockings for a few days after the operation to help maintain blood flow to the veins of the leg.
- Women who use a **combined oral contraceptive** should stop it two or three months before surgery and will need to switch to an alternative form of contraception.
- If you are **confined to bed**, you should regularly stretch your legs and flex your ankles. Your doctor may also recommend that you **wear elastic stockings**.
- **During a flight**, walk around at least once an hour, and, during a long drive, stop regularly to stretch your legs. If you're going to undertake a **long journey** and you'll be sitting most of the time, discuss with your doctor the possibility of **taking a small dose of aspirin** just before, during, and after the trip.

ARE THERE COMPLICATIONS?

- A fragment of the clot may break off and find its way to the lungs. Such a **pulmonary embolism occurs in about 1 in 5 cases of deep vein thrombosis**. The seriousness depends on the size of the fragment. The symptoms associated with pulmonary embolism usually include shortness of breath and chest pain. Rarely, if the clot is large enough to compromise the blood supply to the lungs severely, the condition is life threatening.
- In some cases, thrombosis causes permanent damage to the vein and **varicose veins may appear later**.

WHAT IS THE OUTLOOK?

Usually, if deep vein thrombosis is diagnosed in its early stages, treatment with **thrombolytic drugs** and **anticoagulants** is successful. However, if the affected vein is permanently damaged, persistent swelling of the leg or varicose veins may develop and there's a risk that the condition may recur.

See also:
- Pulmonary embolism p. 395

BLOOD

There are textbooks devoted to this subject but here I only have space for the most common, the **anemias**, and those that are lodged in the public consciousness, the **leukemias. Hemophilia** is mentioned because it's inherited and **thrombocytopenia** because it causes the classical rash of **meningitis** and all parents should be on the look out for it if their child becomes ill with a high temperature. They should know how to recognize the rash of thrombocytopenia, which is called **purpura**, with tiny hemorrhages in the skin called **petechiae** that remain visible if a glass is pressed onto the skin.

Anemias

THERE ARE FOUR MAIN TYPES OF ANEMIA, WHICH IS A DISORDER OF THE BLOOD IN WHICH HEMOGLOBIN (THE OXYGEN CARRYING PIGMENT IN RED BLOOD CELLS) IS DEFICIENT OR ABNORMAL.

As the oxygen carrying power of the blood is reduced, the tissues of the body may not receive sufficient oxygen giving rise to the classical symptoms of anemia – **paleness, fatigue,** and **shortness of breath**.

WHAT ARE THE TYPES?

There are four forms of anemia.
- By far the most common type is **deficiency anemia**, one of which results from low levels of **iron** in the body – **iron-deficiency anemia.** Low levels of other substances, such as vitamin B_{12} and folic acid, can lead to another deficiency anemia – **megaloblastic anemia.**
- Inherited abnormalities of hemoglobin production, such as **sickle-cell anemia** and **thalassemia.** The hemoglobin is abnormal from shortly after birth, but symptoms of anemia may not develop until later in childhood.
- Excessively rapid destruction of red blood cells (hemolysis) is called **hemolytic anemia.**
- Failure of the bone marrow to produce enough normal red blood cells and often all the other types of blood cells as well. One form, **aplastic anemia,** can be congenital or,

rarely, can be brought on by exposure to poisons, such as benzene, and certain drugs.

WHAT ARE THE SYMPTOMS?

All anemias have the same symptoms:
- fatigue and a feeling of faintness
- pale skin
- shortness of breath on mild exertion
- palpitations.

If the anemia is severe and long term, stress on the heart may result in **chronic heart failure**, with swollen ankles and increasing shortness of breath.

WHAT MIGHT BE DONE?

Tests are aimed at discovering two things.
1. Finding out what kind of anemia you have.
2. Finding out why you have that particular anemia, i.e. the cause.

Investigation starts with simple **blood tests** but sometimes more complicated tests, such as taking a specimen of **bone marrow from the hip bone**, may be needed.

WHAT IS THE TREATMENT?

Most anemias respond well to treatment, although some severe cases may require blood transfusion to ensure immediate improvement. If there is an underlying condition, such as a chronic peptic ulcer, your doctor will treat it too.

IRON-DEFICIENCY ANEMIA

Iron-deficiency anemia is the most common form of anemia. Iron is an essential component of hemoglobin. If insufficient iron is available, the production of hemoglobin and its incorporation into red blood cells in the bone marrow are reduced. As a result, there is less hemoglobin to bind with oxygen in the lungs and carry it to the body tissues. Consequently, the tissues receive insufficient oxygen.

WHAT ARE THE CAUSES?

■ Iron-deficiency anemia is most commonly caused by the loss of significant amounts of iron through persistent bleeding. Iron-deficiency anemia occurs mainly in women who experience regular blood loss over a period of time from heavy menstrual bleeding. Persistent loss of blood may also be due to peptic ulcers. The prolonged use of aspirin or long-term use of nonsteroidal anti-inflammatory drugs (NSAIDS) are possible causes of bleeding from the stomach lining. In people over the age of 60, a common cause of blood loss is cancer of the bowel. Bleeding in the stomach or upper intestine may go unnoticed, while blood lost from the lower part of the intestine or rectum may be visible in the feces.
■ The second cause of iron-deficiency anemia is insufficient iron in the diet. People whose diet contains little or no iron, such as vegans, may be at particular risk of developing this condition.

■ Iron-deficiency anemia is also more likely to develop when the body needs higher levels of iron than normal and these extra demands are not met by the existing diet. For example, women who are pregnant and children who are growing rapidly, especially adolescents, have an increased risk of developing iron-deficiency anemia if their diet does not contain plenty of iron.
■ Some other causes of iron-deficiency anemia include disorders that prevent absorption of iron from the diet. Iron is absorbed from food while it passes through the small intestine and conditions that damage it, such as celiac disease, may result in iron deficiency.

WHAT ARE THE SYMPTOMS?

You may experience the symptoms of an underlying disorder, along with the general symptoms of anemia, such as:
- fatigue and a feeling of faintness
- pale skin
- shortness of breath on mild exertion
- palpitations.

You may also have symptoms that are specifically due to a marked deficiency of iron. These include:
- brittle, concave-shaped nails
- painful cracks in the skin at the side of the mouth
- a smooth, reddened tongue.

If your anemia is severe you may be at risk of chronic heart failure because your heart has to work harder to supply blood to the rest of the body.

WHAT MIGHT BE DONE?

Your doctor will order for blood tests to measure the levels of haemoglobin and iron in your blood. If the cause of the iron deficiency is not obvious, other laboratory tests may also be necessary. For example, a sample of feces may be tested for signs of intestinal bleeding.

Your doctor will treat any underlying disorder such as a stomach ulcer. Iron pills (syrup for children) or, less commonly, iron injections for several months will replace iron reserves. Severe cases of anemia may require blood transfusion.

MEGALOBLASTIC ANEMIA

Megaloblastic anemia is a type of anemia caused by lack of vitamin B_{12} or folic acid. These two important vitamins play an essential role in the production of healthy red blood cells. Deficiency of either vitamin may lead to megaloblastic anemia, in which large, abnormal red blood cells (megaloblasts) form in the bone marrow and the production of normal red blood cells is reduced.

WHAT ARE THE CAUSES?

In the West, lack of vitamin B_{12} is rarely due to a dietary deficiency. The problem is usually

due to an autoimmune disorder, in which antibodies damage the stomach lining and prevent it from forming intrinsic factor, which is vital for absorption of vitamin B_{12} from food in the intestines. The resulting anemia, called pernicious anemia, tends to run in families and is more common in women and in people with other autoimmune disorders. Intestinal disorders such as celiac disease, infection, or surgery on the stomach can also interfere with vitamin B_{12} absorption.

Folic acid deficiency is often due to a poor diet. People who abuse alcohol are at particular risk because alcohol interferes with the absorption of folic acid. Pregnant women may also be at risk because folic acid requirements are higher in pregnancy. Disorders causing a rapid turnover of cells, including severe psoriasis, may also cause folic acid deficiency. In rare cases, the deficiency is a side effect of certain drugs, such as anticonvulsants and cancer fighting drugs.

WHAT ARE THE SYMPTOMS?

The initial symptoms of megaloblastic anemia, which are common to all anemias, develop slowly and may include:

- fatigue and a feeling of faintness
- pale skin
- shortness of breath on mild exertion
- palpitations.

These symptoms of megaloblastic anemia may worsen over time. Although lack of folic acid does not produce additional symptoms, lack of vitamin B_{12} may eventually damage the nervous system, possibly leading to:
- tingling of the hands and feet
- weakness and loss of balance
- loss of memory and confusion
- numbness of feet.

WHAT MIGHT BE DONE?

The diagnosis requires blood tests to look for megaloblasts and to measure the levels of vitamin B_{12} and folic acid. You may also have a bone marrow aspiration and biopsy to obtain tissue samples for further examination.

Megaloblastic anemia caused by an inability to absorb vitamin B_{12} may be improved by treating the underlying disorder, but some people, such as those with pernicious anemia and malabsorption caused by surgery, need life-long monthly injections of vitamin B_{12}. Symptoms should begin to subside within days, but nervous system damage may be irreversible.

If megaloblastic anemia is caused by an inadequate diet, the condition usually disappears with an improved diet and a short course of folic acid pills.

SICKLE-CELL ANEMIA

Sickle-cell anemia is an inherited condition caused by an abnormal form of hemoglobin in the blood. The inheritance is recessive; that is, both parents carry an abnormal gene but are themselves healthy. The anemia that results from the blood condition is not present at birth but develops in the first six months. Sickle-cell anemia is more common in people of African descent.

WHAT ARE THE CAUSES?

Hemoglobin is the protein contained in red cells in the blood. It picks up oxygen from the blood and carries it to various parts of the body. Sickle-cell anemia occurs when the abnormal hemoglobin causes the red blood cells to become sickle-shaped as a result of low oxygen levels. This may lead to a sickle-cell crisis, involving severe joint and abdominal pain or even a stroke. Immediate medical attention is needed.

WHAT ARE THE SYMPTOMS?

People with sickle-cell anemia may have the following symptoms:
- anemia
- fatigue
- mild jaundice – the whites of the eyes may be slightly yellowed
- pain in the limbs and abdomen
- susceptibility to infection leading to frequent colds and illnesses
- acute chest pain.

WHAT MIGHT BE DONE?

It is essential for people with sickle-cell anemia to be fully immunized against all infectious diseases and to take any prescribed vitamin supplements. Some people may need to take penicillin regularly to prevent certain bacterial infections. A sickle-cell crisis may be precipitated by strenuous exercise, particularly in the cold and damp, and this should be avoided. If a sickle-cell crisis occurs, it will be treated with painkilling drugs.

Since sickle-cell anemia is inherited, it is important for potential carriers to seek genetic counseling before deciding to have a baby. A blood test will show if the prospective parents are carriers of the disease.

THALASSEMIA

Thalassemia is a form of genetically inherited anemia. It occurs mostly in people from the Mediterranean area but it can also affect people from India and Southeast Asia. Thalassemia can be passed on to a child if both parents carry the faulty gene.

In thalassemia, the body cannot make normal hemoglobin, the substance in the blood that makes the cells red and carries oxygen through the body. The problem reveals itself when a baby is about three months old with symptoms of severe anemia.

WHAT ARE THE SYMPTOMS?

Thalassemia causes the following symptoms:
- fatigue
- breathlessness
- pallor of the lips, tongue, hands, and feet
- loss of appetite accompanied by a swollen abdomen.

WHAT MIGHT BE DONE?

Treatment for thalassemia requires regular blood transfusions, usually every 6–8 weeks, to prevent severe anemia from developing. The spleen is also sometimes removed, reducing the need for frequent transfusions. If a person with thalassemia has too many transfusions, iron can build up in the body and damage the liver, pancreas, and heart. There is now a drug available that helps the body get rid of excess iron; the treatment is sometimes carried out overnight by means of a continuous injection into the skin.

If you are from a group particularly susceptible to the disease, you and your partner may wish to seek genetic counseling before trying to conceive to find out if one or both of you might be a carrier of the gene responsible for thalassemia.

See also:
- **Malabsorption p. 365**

Hemophilia

NORMALLY A CUT STOPS BLEEDING WITHIN 10 MINUTES UNLESS IT IS VERY SERIOUS. IN HEMOPHILIA, AN INHERITED DEFICIENCY OF BLOOD CLOTTING FACTORS DUE TO ABNORMAL GENES, EVEN A SMALL CUT MAY BLEED FOR HOURS OR DAYS, AND THERE MAY BE EPISODES OF SPONTANEOUS BLEEDING.

The much rarer **Christmas disease** has similar features and is named after the person in whom the disease was first diagnosed. Both conditions affect only **males.**

WHAT ARE THE CAUSES?

Hemophilia and Christmas disease are both due to a deficiency of a protein involved in blood clotting. In hemophilia, the deficient protein is **Factor VIII**; in Christmas disease, the protein is **Factor IX**. In both these

conditions, the deficiency is the result of a faulty gene. The particular gene involved is different in the two disorders.

In both disorders, the abnormal gene is located on an X chromosome (X- or sex-linked inheritance). Women do not develop the disease because they have two X chromosomes and the normal gene on the other X chromosome compensates for the abnormal gene. Men with the abnormal gene do develop the disease because they have only

one X chromosome (the other is a Y chromosome) and so do not have a normal copy of the gene to compensate for the abnormal one. Women, however, may pass on the faulty gene to their children. Each child, male or female, has a 1 in 2 chance of inheriting the faulty gene.

In one-third of all cases, the conditions are due to a spontaneity gene abnormality and there is no family history of hemophilia or Christmas disease.

WHAT ARE THE SYMPTOMS?
The symptoms are highly variable, and their severity depends on how much Factor VIII or IX is actually produced. The symptoms usually develop in infancy and include:
● easy bruising, even after minor injury
● sudden, painful swelling of muscles and joints due to internal bleeding
● prolonged bleeding after an injury or a minor surgical operation
● blood in the urine.

Without treatment, prolonged episodes of bleeding into the joints may result in long-term damage and, eventually, may lead to **deformity** of the joints.

WHAT MIGHT BE DONE?
The doctor will arrange for tests to see how long your blood takes to clot and to measure the level of Factor VIII or IX.

The goal of treatment is to maintain the clotting factors at a high enough level to prevent bleeding. If you have a severe form of either condition, you will probably need regular **intravenous injections of Factor VIII or IX** to boost the levels of these factors in the blood. If you have a mild form of either condition, you may need injections only after an injury or before surgery. You may also be prescribed **desmopressin**, which contains **pituitary hormone**, to boost levels of Factor VIII. Some people develop antibodies to Factor VIII supplements, which makes

treatment difficult. These people may need to take an immunosuppressant drug to destroy the antibodies.

WHAT IS THE OUTLOOK?
If you have hemophilia or Christmas disease, you can lead an active life but need to avoid sustaining any injuries. Activities such as swimming, running, and walking are beneficial, but contact sports, such as wrestling and football, should be avoided. Regular dental care is necessary to avoid the risk of bleeding from inflamed gums.

If you have a family history of either disorder, you should obtain medical advice when planning a pregnancy.

Leukemia

IN EVERY TYPE OF LEUKEMIA (BONE MARROW CANCER), ABNORMAL OR VERY IMMATURE WHITE BLOOD CELLS MULTIPLY RAPIDLY AND ACCUMULATE WITHIN THE BONE MARROW, WHERE ALL TYPES OF BLOOD CELLS ARE NORMALLY PRODUCED.

The usual production of normal white blood cells, normal red blood cells, and platelets within the bone marrow is reduced by the invading cancerous white cells leading to symptoms of **anemia** and **purpura** (bleeding under the skin that may appear as unprovoked bruising). Leukemia may therefore show up as anemia. Other symptoms may include weight loss, fever, night sweats, excessive bleeding, and recurrent infections.

In most of the leukemias, the cancerous white blood cells spread, causing enlargement of the lymph nodes (glands), liver, and spleen.

WHAT ARE THE TYPES?
The two main types of leukemia are **acute leukemia**, in which the symptoms develop rapidly, and **chronic leukemia**, in which symptoms may take years to develop.

1. Adults may develop either type but children usually have the acute form. Acute leukemia can be divided into acute lymphoblastic and acute myeloid leukemia, depending on which type of white blood cell is involved.
2. Chronic leukemia is also divided into two types: chronic lymphocytic leukemia and chronic myeloid leuaemia.

HOW IS IT DIAGNOSED?
Leukemia may be diagnosed from blood tests and examination of the bone marrow.

WHAT IS THE TREATMENT?
■ Treatment is tailored to each kind of leukemia and often to each individual case.
■ Chemotherapy is usually given, often as combinations or "cocktails" of several drugs.
■ In some cases, radiation therapy is given.

■ Blood transfusions are sometimes necessary.
■ In some cases, a bone marrow transplant will be done, provided a suitable donor is found.

WHAT IS THE OUTLOOK?
The prognosis varies depending on the type of leukemia and its severity. For instance, chronic lymphocytic leukemia may run a long, benign course and need little radical treatment.

Treatment of leukemia in children is a success story. Decades of intensive research into chemotherapeutic regimens, mean the majority of children will be successfully treated.

TREATMENT

Bone marrow transplants

To perform a bone marrow transplant, cells in the center of certain bones are collected from a living donor and are then transfused directly into one of the recipient's veins after his or her existing bone marrow has been destroyed. Alternatively, cells may be collected from the recipient's own bone marrow during a period when his or her underlying disease is in remission and frozen for later use. The stored bone marrow may then be thawed and used to replace abnormal bone marrow in the recipient's body if disease recurs.

Thrombocytopenia

Thrombocytopenia is a reduced level of cells called platelets in the blood. Platelets are necessary for blood to clot normally, therefore platelet deficiency causes bleeding into the skin and internal organs. Bleeding into the skin causes bruising and a rash called purpura where there are tiny hemorrhages (petechiae) into the skin. There are many causes of thrombocytopenia but I want to mention only one here, meningitis.

Meningitis
■ Thrombocytopenia may be an early

complication of meningitis and shows up in the skin as a purpuric rash.
■ The rash is simple to distinguish from all others: because it's caused by small hemorrhages in the skin, it therefore DOESN'T DISAPPEAR WHEN APPLYING PRESSURE as almost all other rashes do.
■ If your child is ill with a high temperature and a rash appears, use a glass to press down on the skin. If the rash remains, take your child immediately to the hospital.
■ The thrombocytopenia of meningitis will correct itself when the infection is treated. It needs no specific treatment.

Sexuality and Fertility

Image shows computer artwork of human sperm

Miriam's overview

This topic is so huge, taking in, as it does, all of gynecology, I hardly know where to begin. The span is the whole of reproductive life and beyond, starting at perhaps the age of 10 with the appearance of menstruation and stretching to the end of our lives in the case of our sexuality.

Oh yes, sex may diminish in importance and frequency as we age and performance may slump, but it remains the greatest source of comfort and companionship there is until we die.

Indeed all the news on sex is good. In one study 80-year-old women confessed to still being very enthusiastic about sex. All they lacked was a suitable partner.

As we entered the second millennium a very interesting finding emerged from demographic research. It revealed that 1 in 6 girls is menstruating by the age of 8, and 1 in 14 boys of a similar age is producing sperm.

I can remember thinking when the average age of menarche fell to 11.5 years, it couldn't get any younger, but it has, with implications for society in general, and for teachers and parents in particular.

If your daughter is fertile at the age of 8 when do you start sex education? If your child might be sexually active at 9 or 10 when do you give them advice on contraception? Fertile 8-year-olds raises the specter of parents aged 10 or even less. This possibility forces us to change our approach to burgeoning sexuality in our children.

"all the *news* on sex *is good*"

Two new vaginal infections have received, rightly in my view, much attention of late. One is usually self-induced, albeit unwittingly – bacterial vaginosis – due to over-zealous personal hygiene with vaginal deodorants, cleansers, and disinfectants in bath water. They all change the protective bacterial population of the vagina, leading to unhealthy overgrowth of certain bacteria with a characteristic unpleasant odor. Only antibiotics will bring it under control.

The second is chlamydia, often a hidden infection because it's symptomless and used to be difficult to diagnose. Chlamydia can cause pelvic inflammatory disease and subsequent infertility. When this was realized, research focused on devising a reliable diagnostic test so that treatment can be started before any damage is done.

We tend to take for granted that our wishes will be considered when facing mutilating surgery such as mastectomy and hysterectomy but as little as five years ago it wasn't so, and in pockets around the country it still isn't.

In the last 10 years we've seen a revolution in patient power that's been paralleled by a more humane approach by surgeons. In a matter of a few years mastectomy became largely a thing of the past when research showed that the less disfiguring lumpectomy had the same cure rate.

And when it was realized a woman could retain her uterus, women drove surgeons to question hysterectomy as a routine (and often unnecessary) operation in middle age. Suddenly women were directing their surgeons to leave behind their ovaries and cervix – which may be helpful if you wish to remain orgasmic – when hysterectomy was discussed.

For the first time ever, the cure rate for breast cancer is improving and, in the US, 97 percent of women survive five years if diagnosed early. Tamoxifen, a cancer fighting drug, is single-handedly responsible for this turnaround. Given routinely to all women whose cancers are sensitive to estrogen it will control the cancer and prevent spread and regrowth. There's probably never been as powerful an cancer fighting drug.

Most women are aware of breast self-examination but few men are aware of testicular self-examination or the importance of it to detect testicular cancer early, when the cure rate is over 90 percent.

Nor are many men aware that there is a screening test, PSA, for cancer of the prostate and that it's available to men who have prostatic symptoms.

INSIDE
your reproductive system

Male reproductive system

The external parts of the male reproductive system include the **penis**, **scrotum,** and the two **testicles**, which hang in the scrotum. Behind each testicle is a coiled tube known as the **epididymis**, which leads to another tube called the **vas deferens**. The top of each vas deferens is joined by a duct that drains from the seminal vesicle. These join the **urethra**, where they are surrounded by the **prostate gland**, and the urethra passes through the penis to the outside.

After puberty, the two testicles manufacture sperm continuously at the rate of about 125 million sperm a day. Sperm mature in the **epididymis**, and travel from there through the vas deferens before ejaculation. On this journey sperm are mixed with secretions from other glands to form semen. Semen contains about 50 million sperm per milliliter.

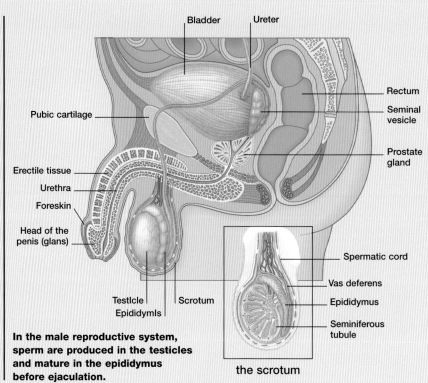

In the male reproductive system, sperm are produced in the testicles and mature in the epididymus before ejaculation.

the scrotum

Female reproductive system

The external organs of the female reproductive system consist of the **clitoris** and the **labia**, which surround it – together they are known as the **vulva**. Inside the labia are the entrances to the **vagina** and the **urethra**. In the lower part of the abdomen are the two **ovaries**. These organs store eggs and, following puberty, release them into the **fallopian tubes**, which in turn lead to the **uterus**. The neck of the uterus, called the **cervix**, projects down into the vagina.

Fertilization of an egg by a sperm usually takes place in one of the fallopian tubes, after which the fertilized egg travels down the tube into the uterus. It implants in the uterine lining and continues development there.

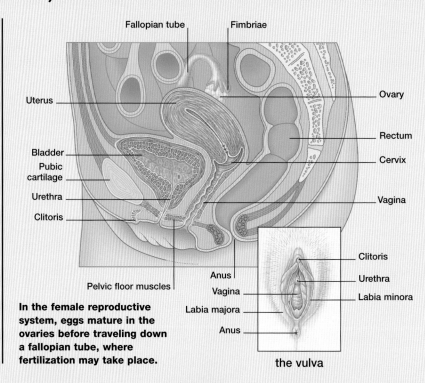

In the female reproductive system, eggs mature in the ovaries before traveling down a fallopian tube, where fertilization may take place.

the vulva

THE BREASTS

I recommend breast awareness (see box, below) for all women, at all stages of their lives. More checkups are advisable for older women, who have a higher risk of breast cancer, and for women in other high-risk groups – those with breast cancer in the family, for example. There's now clear evidence that early detection by screening cuts down the number of women dying from breast cancer. Studies in Sweden and the US show that screening can reduce deaths from breast cancer by up to one-third in women between the ages of 50 and 65. Early detection automatically means earlier treatment and increases the chances of a full recovery if a lump turns out to be breast cancer. Early detection also means you have greater choice over how your cancer will be treated. It's understandable to feel anxious about having regular mammograms. However, the chances are you'll be one of the 99 women out of every 100 routinely screened who are found not to have cancer.

Breast pain

BREAST PAIN, OR MASTALGIA, IS PAIN OR DISCOMFORT IN ONE OR BOTH BREASTS. SIXTY PERCENT OF WOMEN SUFFER SOME KIND OF BREAST DISCOMFORT. BREAST PAIN CAN BE DIVIDED INTO TWO TYPES: CYCLICAL, WHICH IS ASSOCIATED WITH MENSTRUAL PERIODS, AND NONCYCLICAL.

Noncyclical pain may originate in the breast or in the nearby muscles and joints, in which case it is not true breast pain.

CYCLICAL BREAST PAIN

The most common kind of breast pain is associated with the menstrual cycle, and is nearly always related to fluctuations in hormone levels, which every woman experiences as part of the cycle. Pain is probably related to the sensitivity of breast tissue to hormones and this can differ within a breast and between your two breasts. Hormones aren't the whole story, however, because in the majority of women the pain is more severe in one breast than in the other. Most women experience some degree of breast pain when their breasts become sensitive just prior to menstruation. Some women, however, may experience soreness and tenderness starting with ovulation, in the middle of the cycle, and continuing for about two weeks until menstruation takes place. Others find that this premenstrual soreness becomes even worse after the birth of their first child.

WHAT IS THE TREATMENT?

■ **Evening primrose oil**: this natural remedy has to be taken in a large dose (starting at 1g daily, working up to 3g) to be effective. It also has to be taken over a long period of time since its effects build up slowly; in most cases, it takes as long as four months to see if there are benefits. Notwithstanding the large dose and prolonged usage, evening primrose oil has very few side effects, which is why it should be the first line of treatment.

■ **Danazol**: this drug, has a success rate of nearly 80 percent, making it the ideal second choice of treatment. Despite its success, it is not suitable for everyone: some women may experience side effects such as weight gain and irregular periods. Danazol is given in a dose of 200mg daily for two months; if this is effective, the dose will be gradually reduced.

■ **Tamoxifen**: this drug is only rarely prescribed for women with severe breast pain. The usual dose in this case is 10mg, which may cause hot flashes but does not cause more severe side effects that are seen with higher doses. Tamoxifen may be used continuously or may be restricted to the second half of the menstrual cycle.

NONCYCLICAL BREAST PAIN

There are two types of noncyclical breast pain: true breast pain, which comes from the

Breast awareness

Women used to be advised to examine their breasts every month at the same point in their menstrual cycle. However, this made some women anxious and others felt guilty if they didn't do it or responsible if there was a problem. Now doctors are advising women that it is more important for them to be familiar with the shape and texture of their breasts than to examine them on a regular basis. This "breast awareness" means that you will be able to spot any unexpected changes in your breasts and can consult your doctor right away.

In order to be breast aware, you need to know what your breasts look like. Try to get into the habit of looking at your breasts in the mirror from time to time – you can easily do this after a bath or shower or before you get dressed.

Raise your arms over your head and notice how your breasts move, so that you know what is normal for you. Possible changes to watch out for include a difference in the shape of the breast, such as puckering or pulling of the skin, areas of swelling in the breast, or changes in the nipple, such as puckering.

You also need to be aware of how your breasts feel. So that you can identify changes, feel your breasts every day for several days until you are aware of their usual texture and how it changes throughout your menstrual cycle. Most women's breasts are a bit lumpy, especially in the days before a period. After your period lumpiness may lessen and disappear entirely.

If you note any unusual changes in your breasts, see your doctor as soon as possible.
It's normal to feel anxious, but remember that 9 out of 10 breast lumps turn out not to be cancerous.

breast but is unrelated to the menstrual cycle, and pain that is felt in the region of the breast but is actually coming from somewhere else. This latter kind nearly always involves the muscles, bones, or joints and for this reason it is called **musculoskeletal pain**. Two-thirds of noncyclical mastalgia is pain of musculoskeletal origin. Rarely what appears to be breast pain is due to underlying **lung** or **gallbladder disease**.

TRUE NONCYCLICAL BREAST PAIN

Some benign breast conditions may be associated with true breast pain. Burning or stabbing pains centered around or under the nipple may be due to dilatation of the ducts (duct ectasia) and tend to run an intermittent, though harmless, course. They may also be due to periductal mastitis, a condition that affects young women, the majority of whom are smokers.

A tender spot with occasional stabbing pain or an ache is common. Its cause is unknown, but it is no reason for anxiety. The pain can be relieved by an injection of local anesthetic mixed with prednisone to help to reduce any inflammation. A cyst occasionally underlies a tender spot; removal of fluid from the cyst can ease the pain.

PAIN OF NONBREAST ORIGIN

Pain originating in the chest wall or spine may be felt in the breast area. The most usual cause is a form of **arthritis**, called **costochondritis**, which affects the ends of the ribs where they join the breastbone; this condition is called **Tietze's syndrome**. If your pain is worse when you take a deep breath or press on your breastbone and ribs, it's likely to be costochondritis. Taking a painkiller, such as acetaminophen, or a nonsteroidal anti-inflammatory drug (NSAID), such as ibuprofen, is often effective.

Breast lumps

BREAST LUMPS ARE ANY MASSES OR SWELLINGS IN THE BREAST TISSUE. WHEN YOU FIND A LUMP IN YOUR BREAST, DOCTORS USE MANY INVESTIGATIVE TECHNIQUES TO ARRIVE AT AS SPECIFIC A DIAGNOSIS AS POSSIBLE.

The initial test sequence varies, depending on whether you have found the lump yourself or it has been detected during routine mammogram screening, in which case it may be too small to feel. In all cases, however, a sample of cells or tissue will have to be examined under a microscope to determine whether the lump is malignant. If it is, further tests will be done to assess the precise origin of the tumor and to see if it has spread.

CONSIDERATIONS

When you find any lump in your breast, look for the best possible treatment. You should expect the following things.
■ A prompt referral by your family doctor to a team specializing in the diagnosis and treatment of breast cancer, including a breast specialist.
■ A firm diagnosis soon after being examined.

■ The opportunity to have a confirmed diagnosis before consenting to any form of treatment, including surgery.
■ Full information about types of surgery (including breast reconstruction where appropriate) and the role of additional treatments such as radiation therapy, chemotherapy, hormone therapy, and so on.
■ A clear and detailed explanation of the goals and benefits of the proposed treatments and any possible side effects, including long-term ones.

HOW IS IT DIAGNOSED?

Your doctor will start the examination by looking at your breasts while you sit with your hands by your sides and then with your arms raised above your head, so that asymmetry between the breasts, nipple retraction (the nipple will appear drawn in), difference in level between nipples, or dimpling of the skin can easily be seen. You'll then be asked to lie back with your arms above your head while the doctor examines your breasts carefully, feeling each quadrant of both breasts with the flat of the hand.

The aim is to decide whether there's an obvious lump and if the breasts are just generally lumpy – and many are!

FINE-NEEDLE ASPIRATION CYTOLOGY (FNAC)

One of the three procedures in assessing a breast lump is **FNAC**. It's used to sample cells from the lump.

Under mammography or ultrasound guidance, a fine needle is inserted painlessly into your lump. If fluid is withdrawn, the lump is a cyst; the fluid can be drained and the cyst will disappear. If your lump is solid, a sample of cells is removed and spread on a glass slide for microscopic examination.

CORE NEEDLE BIOPSY

FNAC yields only a tiny sample of cells from breast tissue, so it's impossible to be specific about where they've come from. A core needle biopsy provides a sample of cells from the lump that can be analyzed to make this distinction.
1. Under a local anesthetic, a special needle with a sheath is painlessly inserted into your lump in order to withdraw a fine core of tissue from it.
2. The sheath is drawn back and some tissue from your lump falls into the notch.
3. The sheath is closed, trapping a tiny core of tissue from your lump inside the notch and the needle is withdrawn.
4. The skin is left virtually intact; although there may be a little bruising afterward, there's hardly any discomfort.

Fibroadenomas

Common in teenagers and women in their 20s, fibroadenomas are simply overdeveloped lobules and are completely benign. You don't always need to have one removed, as long as you agree to another ultrasound scan and examination in six months. The majority of women, when offered excision or observation, opt for the latter.

Fibroadenomas can be very large – they vary from pea size to larger than a lemon. While they can grow anywhere in the breast, quite often they're found near the nipple. They feel smooth and firm and quite distinct, and move freely in your breast. Most doctors can recognize one simply by feeling it, but

the diagnosis should be confirmed with mammography or ultrasound and fine-needle aspiration cytology (**FNAC**) or core needle biopsy.

Although they are most common in young women, fibroadenomas can occur at any age up to menopause (or later if you are on **HRT**). Most women who get a fibroadenoma will never get another one, but a few women will have several over a lifetime. It is possible to have more than one at a time or a single large fibroadenoma involving more than one lobule. In very rare cases there may be a tendency for them to run in families.

Mammograms

A mammogram is a low-dose X-ray of the breast. It's such a refined method of imaging the breast that it can pick up small cancers and other abnormalities that neither you nor your doctor can feel.

Why after 50?
Mammograms are not done with the same frequency in all age groups. In the US, mammograms are routinely given after the age of 40, either annually or every two years. Women who fall into high-risk groups may be offered yearly mammograms at an earlier age.

What about younger women?
Mammography is less effective in women under 50, since their breast tissue is more dense and abnormalities don't show up so well, but it's still more sensitive than self-examination.

This is why it can be used as a diagnostic tool, to investigate a lump found in physical examination, for example, or to look for more lumps when one has already been found. **Ultrasound scans** may be used to investigate breast lumps found in women aged 35 and below.

How often?
Currently, mammography is offered to women over 50 annually, although there's a continuing debate about this.

Getting the results
After your screening, the films are developed and examined by a radiologist who specializes in interpreting mammograms.

The results usually take only a few days to come through and most women will be told that they're fine and just need regular screening. A small number will be asked to come back for more tests. This can be worrying, but the chances of getting an all-clear are still high.

Although mammograms are good for detecting small lumps, they cannot determine a lump's precise character, so extra tests may be needed to pin that down. **Microcalcifications** are tiny deposits of calcium that show up as very fine specks on a mammogram. They may be quite normal

and many women have them but, because they have been occasionally linked with cancer, the radiologist will always mention their presence and you'll wonder why. They're only worrying if they suddenly appear in a cluster in one breast.

If it's your first mammogram, your doctor may wait six months before doing another one to see if there's any change. If the pattern of microcalcifications is very abnormal, a biopsy will be performed immediately.

If a lump is found
If your mammogram shows any kind of lump, further tests will be necessary.
■ If the lump is large enough to feel easily with your fingers, a fine needle can be inserted to draw off some of the cells. This is called **fine-needle aspiration cytology**, or **FNAC**.
■ If the lump is fluid filled it's a cyst, which is nearly always perfectly harmless. Your specialist will draw off the fluid with a needle and will usually discard it. A sample will be sent for laboratory tests only rarely.
■ If the lump is solid, some of the cells that have been drawn off will be smeared on a

slide, stained, and examined in the laboratory.
■ If the lump isn't easy to feel, you'll probably have an ultrasound scan to determine whether it's a solid lump or a cyst. Either way it will be investigated with FNAC or cutting-needle biopsy.

When a lump can't be felt, FNAC and core needle biopsy are done with guidance of ultrasound so that the tumor can be precisely located.

Putting you in the picture
To have a mammogram done:
1. You'll be asked to strip to the waist and remove any deodorant or talc from your breasts. The reason for this is that they may show up as microcalcifications.
2. You will then be asked to stand in front of the machine and the radiologist will compress your breast between two plates. The procedure is not without a degree of discomfort, particularly if the plates are cold. The sensation lasts no more than 10 or 15 seconds, however, so it's easily bearable.
3. Two views of each breast will usually be taken. The radiologist compresses each breast in turn between two plates so that a good image is obtained.

Having a mammogram takes only a few minutes and is not painful, although some women may find the procedure uncomfortable.

OPEN BIOPSY
This kind of biopsy is an alternative to a core needle biopsy. As the name implies, the skin is cut open to reveal the lump, which is then removed with a margin of healthy breast tissue. In practical terms, open biopsy nearly always

means removing the whole lump – **lumpectomy**. It is performed in an outpatient clinic with I.V. sedation.

Not every woman over age 30 with an obvious breast lump should have it removed. The goal is to diagnose the lump – those

that are benign are usually left alone and not excised.

Analyzing the biopsy
The biopsy or lump is sent to the pathology laboratory where it's very finely sliced,

stained to show up the cells, and examined under a microscope, a test known as **histology**.

If the tissue is found to be cancerous, a very precise diagnosis of the type of cancer can be made. The tumor is also **graded**, giving information on how malignant it is.

Diagnosis of secondary spread – staging the tumor

Spread of the cancer to lymph nodes in the armpit and further afield in the body is checked by a series of simple tests, generally performed during the initial assessment, so that the tumor can be staged (1, 2, 3, or 4).

WHAT IS THE TREATMENT?

If your symptoms are lumpiness of the breasts and pain or both, but no obvious lump is found when the doctor examines you, further treatment

depends on your age. If you're under 40, cancer is unlikely, and you may be asked to return in six weeks. If you still have pain from a lumpy breast, medication may be prescribed. If you're over 35, a mammogram and possibly an ultrasound scan may be advised to ensure that no hidden cancer is present.

CONSIDERATIONS

Whatever your doctors advise, you should take the right to time, space, and get counseling when considering treatment. You also can involve your partner, who can visit the doctor's office with you for moral support. Your care should include:
● access to a specialist breast-care nurse trained to give you information and emotional and psychological support
● as much time as you need to consider

your treatment options and gather information
● a sensitive and complete breast prosthesis service, where appropriate
● the opportunity to meet a former breast cancer patient trained to offer practical, psychological, and emotional support
● information on all support services (including local and national groups) available to breast cancer patients and their families through organizations such as Y-Me and the American Cancer Society.

> **See also:**
> ● Breast cancer p. 261 ● Ultrasound scanning p. 277 ● X-rays p. 422

Breast cysts

A BREAST CYST IS A FIRM, FLUID-FILLED SWELLING WITHIN THE BREAST TISSUE. CYSTS ARE NEARLY ALWAYS A VARIATION OF NORMAL ANATOMY, NOT SERIOUS DISEASE.

Breast cysts are most commonly found in women in their 30s, 40s and 50s, with the peak just prior to menopause. It's possible, although rare, for cysts to occur in young women or in postmenopausal women.

Your doctor will probably suggest fine-needle aspiration cytology (FNAC) or an ultrasound scan as the next step to confirm the diagnosis.

WHAT IS THE TREATMENT?

With cysts, FNAC serves as both diagnosis and treatment in one. Aspiration can be done quickly, simply, and painlessly as a routine procedure in a doctor's office. The whole procedure may be performed under **ultrasonic guidance,** allowing you to watch as your doctor inserts the needle, aspirates the cyst and it disappears. Large cysts that are easily felt

can be aspirated without the help of ultrasound. Cysts are rarely malignant, or not harmfully so. If any evidence of cell growth is found in the cyst, your surgeon will operate and remove it.

> **See also:**
> ● Ultrasound scanning p. 277

Nipple conditions

THE PRIMARY FUNCTION OF THE NIPPLES IS TO DELIVER MILK TO A BABY, BUT THEY ALSO PLAY A ROLE IN SEXUAL AROUSAL. IN THE COURSE OF A WOMAN'S LIFE THE NIPPLES ARE PRONE TO CERTAIN CHANGES AND CONDITIONS, SOME OF WHICH ARE DISCUSSED BELOW.

ECTASIA – DILATATION OF THE MILK DUCTS

The underlying change in the normal anatomy of the milk ducts as a woman grows older is called ectasia, or dilatation. Ectasia occurs in the last part of the breast's development cycle, and if the dilatation is excessive the nipple may retract, making it slitlike in appearance. The condition is normal and may affect both breasts. By the age of 70, 40 percent of women have substantial ectasia.

Sometimes ectasia is accompanied by nipple discharge or lumpiness. Although the cause of this discharge or lumpiness is very rarely cancer, you should always consult your doctor if you discover either of these things. You may be offered surgery to correct ectasia if nipple

discharge or the nipple's inverted appearance bother you.

NIPPLE DISCHARGE

Nipple discharge is far less common than pain and lumps, and is of no consequence when it only appears if the breast and nipple are squeezed. It's also normal for premenopausal women who have had children and for women who smoke to produce nipple secretions. The cause of nipple discharge is very rarely cancer, especially if both breasts are involved. To establish the cause it is important to find out if the discharge is coming from one duct or several. Always consult your doctor if you notice a discharge from your nipple.

CRACKED NIPPLES

During breast-feeding, the skin around the nipples is exposed to milk and vigorous sucking, both of which can damage the skin. Prevention is the best approach: the nipples should be gently dabbed clean after each feeding and a baby who is properly latched on will not need to suck hard to feed well. Applying a drop of baby lotion to your breast pad can also help. If the nipples become cracked, it's important to get advice on positioning the baby correctly on the breast and taking her off. This is best done by pushing down gently on the baby's chin to break the airtight seal between her mouth and the nipple. Treatment for cracked nipples with antibiotics must be prompt, since they are vulnerable to infections.

MENSTRUATION

Menstruation is the beginning (not the end) of the menstrual cycle. Day 1 of the cycle is the day bleeding begins. Though the cycle on average is said to be 28 days, few women cycle regularly for this time. A normal cycle can last anything between 21 and 35 days depending on our hormones. Not every cycle is smooth sailing.

For the first few years periods can be painful, sufficiently painful to make you ill and keep you out of work or school. But proper medication taken the day before your period can prevent discomfort. Periods quite often become very heavy as you approach menopause – often the first sign that your menopause has started.

Dysmenorrhea

THIS IS THE MEDICAL NAME FOR PAINFUL MENSTRUAL PERIODS. APPROXIMATELY 75 PERCENT OF WOMEN EXPERIENCE DYSMENORRHEA AT SOME POINT IN THEIR REPRODUCTIVE LIVES.

WHAT ARE THE TYPES?
Dysmenorrhea is categorized by doctors into two types.
■ **Primary dysmenorrhea** tends to start two or three years after menstruation begins, once ovulation is established. There is usually no underlying disease to account for it and the problem often diminishes after the age of about 25 and is rare following childbirth. However, it **can** continue after childbirth and into the mid-30s.
■ **Secondary dysmenorrhea** is more common later in life and causes stomach cramps 1 or 2 weeks before the period starts. It is usually a symptom of some underlying condition such as **endometriosis** or **adhesions**.

Either type of dysmenorrhea may or may not be accompanied by **premenstrual syndrome**, a bloated feeling, irritability, depression, and other changes that commonly occur in the days preceding menstruation.

WHAT ARE THE SYMPTOMS?
■ Violent abdominal cramps starting at the onset of menstruation and lasting up to three days.
■ Diarrhea.
■ Frequent urination.
■ Sweating.
■ Pelvic soreness with pain radiating down into the upper thighs and into the back.
■ Abdominal distension.
■ Backache.
■ Nausea and vomiting.

WHAT CAUSES IT?
Research has shown that women suffering from primary dysmenorrhea produce excessive quantities of the hormone **prostaglandin** at the time of menstruation or they're extremely sensitive to it. Prostaglandin is one of the hormones released during labor and is in part responsible for uterine contractions. Dysmenorrhea can therefore be seen as a **mini-labor**, with the prostaglandin causing uterine muscle to go into **spasm** producing cramplike

pain similar to labor pains. Pain may also be due to a small amount of menstrual blood flowing back through the fallopian tubes, which causes irritation.

WHAT IS THE TREATMENT?
Some doctors may imply that the pain of menstrual cramps is psychosomatic, but that isn't so. Don't be put off from consulting your doctor by the hope that the pain will pass as you get older or if you have children. Every woman deserves relief from dysmenorrhea.
■ Insist on a trial of **antiprostaglandin drugs**, such as naproxen, which should be taken just prior to and for the first two to three days of menstruation.
■ The **contraceptive pill** is often prescribed to relieve dysmenorrhea because it inhibits ovulation, alters hormonal balance, and reduces the thickness of the womb lining, so it's a highly effective treatment. The **progesterone IUD** also helps dysmenorrhea.

If you develop painful periods after several years of pain-free menstruation, your doctor will examine you and recommend treatment according to the underlying condition.

WHAT CAN I DO?
■ Most of us have our own methods of relieving this sort of pain and a heating pad is the favorite option for many women. Hot baths and bed rest also help.
■ I would encourage you to experiment with herbal teas that reduce spasmodic pain such as **mint** or **camomile** infusions. **Ginger** infusion is another common remedy. Add a cup of hot water to 1 teaspoon of fresh grated ginger, infuse for 10 minutes and drink when needed.
■ You can also try over-the-counter pain relievers, such as ibuprofen.

RELAXATION AND YOGA
Relaxation or special yoga-type exercises can also relieve the pain. For example, the bow and cobra positions may help (see below).

MASSAGE
Massage of the lower abdomen, the lower back, and the legs relieves period pain. You can massage your lower abdomen yourself:
1. Lie on the floor or on a bed with your knees bent.

The bow (left) and the cobra (right) positions can help relieve period pain by gently stretching the abdomen. Breathe while holding each pose for a few seconds. Do not perform these positions if you have a history of back problems.

THE BOW

THE COBRA

2. Place your right palm on the lower right side of your abdomen and place your left hand on top of it.

3. Press in with the fingers of both hands and make small circular movements.

4. Gradually move your hands up the right of the abdomen to the waist, across under the ribs, and back down and across the lower abdomen above the pubic hair.

AROMATHERAPY

Soaking in a warm bath to which 3 drops each of **essential oils** of **camomile** and **sweet marjoram** combined with ¼ fl oz (10ml) of carrier oil or lotion (available from health food shops and pharmacies) have been added, can reduce discomfort.

EXERCISE

I know that exercise may be the last thing on your mind, but if you can bear it, exercise can relieve pelvic congestion and ease menstrual cramps. Walking is really good, followed by as hot a bath as you can comfortably tolerate.

> **See also:**
> • **Premenstrual syndrome p. 302**

Heavy periods (menorrhagia)

HEAVY PERIODS ARE HEAVIER THAN NORMAL MENSTRUAL PERIODS. THE NAME WE GIVE TO UNUSUALLY HEAVY MENSTRUATION IS MENORRHAGIA.

Menorrhagia could be a single bout of flooding, a period that goes on for a long time (more than seven days) or very frequent periods so that the blood loss in any given month is excessive.

The main problem in diagnosing heavy menstruation is differentiating between bleeding that's heavier than you're used to, and heavy bleeding that's abnormal.

In a normal menstrual bleed 1–2 fl oz (30–50ml) of blood is lost, whereas in an abnormal bleed 2–3 fl oz (80ml) or more is lost.

WHO IS AT RISK?

Menorrhagia is common and may affect the following groups:
• women approaching menopause – the lining of the womb becomes extremely thick and there's a heavier blood loss as the lining is shed
• women who have been fitted with an IUD, which increases blood loss
• women with fibroids, because they increase the surface of the womb and its lining.

WHAT CAUSES IT?

Heavy periods are due to the absence of progesterone, the hormone that's responsible for controlling menstrual blood loss. It usually means that **ovulation is failing**. As a result the uterine lining builds up until finally it breaks down naturally, resulting in a heavy, uncontrolled bleed.

Bleeding of this type that occurs around the time of menopause can often be successfully treated using certain types of hormone replacement therapy (HRT).

WHAT MIGHT BE DONE?

Normally a doctor will want to exclude any womb problems and check on normal blood clotting. The following will be carried out:
• blood tests
• a general gynecological examination
• an ultrasound scan
• if the ultrasound reveals any abnormality, the uterine lining should be checked to exclude cancer by the removal of small samples of the lining.
• if the bleeding has an unusual pattern as well as being heavy, a doctor may decide to look directly inside the uterus in a procedure called **hysteroscopy** under a general anesthetic.

WHAT IS THE TREATMENT?
FIRST OPTION

Drugs are the first option in the treatment of menorrhagia – NOT a hysterectomy.

Hormones, such as **progestogen** and the **combined contraceptive pill**, may control bleeding. Less effective, but sometimes helpful, are the antiprostaglandin group of drugs, for example **Ponstel**.

A new form of hormone treatment has just become available that will be a boon to women with heavy bleeding. It's a **progestogen IUD**, known as the **Mirena**. The Mirena alters hormone levels less drastically than the combined pill, so there are few side effects. It seems ideal for women who have had their children because:
• it treats the heavy bleeding
• it's a virtually 100 percent effective contraceptive
• it remains during menopause and is part of your HRT treatment.
• Hysterectomy should be seen as a last resort and if our doctor advises it, get a second opinion.

OTHER OPTIONS
Endometrial Ablation

The cavity of the womb is viewed using a small telescope that is inserted via the vagina and cervix. At the same time, the lining of the womb can be removed using an electrical loop. This way periods are minimized or even stopped completely and no abdominal surgery is involved. There are many advantages to an ednometrial ablation.
■ It's an alternative to long-term drug therapy.
■ The major surgery of a hysterectomy is avoided.
■ Hospital stay and recovery time are much shorter than for hysterectomy.
■ There's no surgical incision and therefore no scar.

Hysterectomy: a warning

If you're considering a hysterectomy (see p.256) I should mention some serious but poorly publicized side effects.

■ Loss of sexual desire is rare if your ovaries are left intact but more common if they are removed. If taking HRT doesn't help, testosterone implants may be effective. Some women who have had a total hysterectomy have found there was a significant loss in their capacity for orgasm. The emotional consequences of hysterectomy, if a woman feels defeminized, may affect sexuality. Sensitive nerve endings in the cervix may play a crucial role in ability to have an orgasm; ask if you can keep your cervix.

■ A significant number of women suffer depression after hysterectomy. They're mainly those who weren't convinced of the necessity for the operation, who didn't have the alternatives explained, who didn't try drug therapy first, and who didn't seek a second opinion when there was doubt in their mind. Personally, I would never agree to a hysterectomy without a second opinion. Make sure you understand all of the options. The choice remains yours.

Uterine balloon therapy

The latest treatment for menorrhagia is performed under local anesthesia. It's designed to destroy the lining of the uterus with heat and so make periods lighter.

A soft flexible balloon attached to a thin catheter is inserted into the vagina through the cervix and placed in the uterus. The balloon is inflated with a sterile fluid and heated to 188°F (87°C) for about 8 minutes.

After treatment you have a period over the next 7–10 days.

SELF-HELP

Claims are made of certain foods and supplements but there is no proof of their usefulness. **Bioflavonoids**, which are found in citrus fruits, are said to alleviate heavy bleeding. Regular **strenuous exercise** and keeping **weight** down may also be helpful. **Avoiding alcohol** may help relieve menorrhagia, since heavy drinking can inhibit the formation of blood platelets, which means blood does not clot as well as it should and may flow more profusely during menstruation. The same is true of aspirin. **Hot showers or baths** during menstruation can also increase bleeding because

heat dilates the uterine blood vessels and increases flow.
Your blood should be checked regularly for signs of **anemia** and if your hemoglobin is low you should eat more **iron-rich foods** such as

nuts, liver, red meats, egg yolk, leafy green vegetables, and dried fruits.

TEST

Hysteroscopy

Hysteroscopy involves examining the inside of the uterus with a small telescopic camera that is passed through the cervix. It can be performed under a general anesthetic, when it is often combined with a dilatation and curettage (D&C), or in an outpatient clinic. Various hysteroscopic procedures have been developed to treat specific problems.

How is it done?

■ The procedure involves passing the hysteroscope through the cervix (neck of the womb) into the cavity of the uterus. If the procedure is being performed in an outpatient clinic you may be given painkillers about 1–2 hours beforehand, and occasionally a local anesthetic will be injected in and around the cervix to help relieve any discomfort.
■ In order to obtain a good view of the cavity, it has to be distended using either a harmless gas such as carbon dioxide, or liquid.
■ Most women go home the day of the operation. For a few days afterward you may notice some spotting. Some women may be required to stay in the hospital for a few days if the hysteroscopy has been combined with another operative procedure.

Make sure that you understand why the procedure is being performed and what is going to be achieved. Hysteroscopy is usually not performed if you are pregnant and is best avoided if you are suffering from pelvic inflammatory disease.

Amenorrhea

AMENORRHEA IS THE MEDICAL TERM FOR THE ABSENCE OF MENSTRUAL PERIODS. IT IS DESCRIBED AS PRIMARY IF PERIODS HAVE NEVER STARTED, AND SECONDARY WHEN NORMAL MENSTRUATION IS INTERRUPTED FOR FOUR MONTHS OR MORE.

Amenorrhea does not necessarily mean you are ill but it does usually mean that you are not producing eggs and so cannot conceive.

WHAT CAUSES IT?

Primary amenorrhea is usually due to **late onset of puberty**, although it can also be caused by a disorder of the reproductive or hormonal system. The most common reason for secondary amenorrhea is **pregnancy**. If the hormonal balance is interrupted for any other reason, however, periods may stop. So, for example, many women who **breast-feed** find that their periods do not start again until they wean their babies.

More seriously, amenorrhea can be a side effect of being **grossly underweight**, such as with anorexia nervosa. This will be suspected if your weight is as much as 26lb (12kg) below average for your height and frame. **Stress, chronic ailments** such as thyroid disease, and **long-term medication** with drugs such as antidepressants can also cause amenorrhea, as can **excessive physical training** if it reduces body mass index (weight in kilograms divided by height in meters) to less than 20.

Amenorrhea is, of course, a permanent condition after **menopause**, or if you undergo a **hysterectomy**.

WHAT ARE THE SYMPTOMS?

■ **Primary amenorrhea** – a failure to start menstruation and pubertal development; no development of sexual characteristics such as body hair, breasts, and pelvic broadening.
■ **Secondary amenorrhea** – periods stop suddenly or gradually cease with each successive month until the flow dries up.

SHOULD I SEE THE DOCTOR?

The tendency to start menstruation late may be inherited, so if your mother started her periods late, don't worry if you aren't developing at the same rate as your friends. However, if you are 16 and have not yet menstruated, contact your doctor to check that there is no abnormality. If your periods suddenly stop and you are sexually active pregnancy could be the cause, so do a pregnancy test first before contacting the doctor. See your doctor if your periods have been absent for six months and you are not pregnant or menopausal.

WHAT WILL THE DOCTOR DO?

■ If you have never had a period, your doctor will probably give you a physical examination and take a blood sample to measure the level of **pituitary hormones.** (The pituitary hormones include those responsible for menstruation.)
■ With secondary amenorrhea, once pregnancy is excluded, you should receive a full medical examination by a gynecologist, and if you are taking any long-term medications, these should be checked and stopped if necessary.
■ Your doctor may arrange for you to have an X-ray or an MRI to make sure that your pituitary gland is of normal appearance.
■ If you are not ovulating and wish to conceive, he may suggest that you take a course of **fertility drugs** or **pituitary hormones.**

WHAT CAN I DO?

■ The lack of periods is not dangerous and in most cases there is no cause for alarm; be patient and they will start up naturally.
■ You may need to change your lifestyle to correct any dietary or physical problem, if either is thought to be the cause.

VAGINAL INFECTIONS

Vaginal infections are important because some of them have the habit of "ascending," meaning they travel upward through the uterus and into the fallopian tubes and then even into the pelvis. Here they can give rise to **pelvic inflammatory disease** (PID), which can result in **chronic pelvic pain** and more alarmingly, infertility.

A vaginal infection due to chlamydia or gonorrhea therefore must be eradicated by vigorous treatment not just for you but for your partner too. Many women with chronic infections are being reinfected by their largely symptomless partners. Men must accept this and be assessed and treated at the same time.

Chronic pelvic pain

CHRONIC PELVIC PAIN IS LONG-TERM PAIN IN THE LOWER ABDOMEN OR PELVIS. THE PAIN MUST HAVE LASTED FOR AT LEAST SIX MONTHS AND ISN'T LINKED TO MENSTRUATION OR SEXUAL INTERCOURSE. ABOUT 1 IN 6 WOMEN HAS CHRONIC PELVIC PAIN.

Recent studies suggest that chronic pelvic pain may even be more common than low back pain.

Chronic pelvic pain may account for as much as ten percent of all outpatient gynecologic visits and women with this condition may need several days off work every month.

There's much that can be done to relieve their misery, yet women often feel they have to fight to get anything done.

Most doctors do refer women with undiagnosed chronic pelvic pain to a gynecologist but, even so, women often feel dismissed and find that their symptoms are not taken seriously.

Armed with some information, it's important for every woman to insist on investigation and treatment because the alternative may be the inability to have children some time in the future.

WHAT ARE THE CAUSES?

Several conditions may give rise to the condition, including **endometriosis**, **irritable bowel syndrome**, **pelvic inflammatory disease** (see opposite) and **musculoskeletal damage**.

Women are often aware that stress increases their pain, and some researchers have shown that deep-rooted psychological trauma, such as sexual abuse, may reveal itself as pelvic pain.

Sometimes several of these factors may

be present at the same time, making investigation and diagnosis of chronic pelvic pain quite difficult.

HOW IS IT DIAGNOSED?

You may need a specialist to figure out the cause, so I advise going to a gynecologist early. Don't wait and suffer.

LAPAROSCOPY

Your gynecologist will probably suggest an investigation called diagnostic laparoscopy (see box, left). It can be done as an outpatient under a general anesthetic, using a thin viewing instrument inserted through a small incision just below your navel. This allows the gynecologist to see your pelvic organs directly.

To see the pelvic organs clearly, carbon dioxide gas is pumped into the abdominal cavity so that the abdominal wall is lifted out of the way.

Don't be surprised if it takes you a week or two to recover fully. Relatively minor complications, such as nausea and pain, occur after about 3 in 100 laparoscopies. More serious complications are rare but bowel perforation or blood vessel damage, requiring further surgery and a longer hospital stay, occur after about 1 in 500 laparoscopies.

ULTRASOUND

Adhesions (scar tissue) and endometriosis don't show up clearly on an ultrasound scan, so ultrasound isn't much use in investigating pelvic pain unless an ovarian cyst is suspected.

MRI

Magnetic resonance imaging (MRI) can help identify endometriosis.

WHAT MIGHT BE DIAGNOSED?
ENDOMETRIOSIS AND ADHESIONS
The purpose of the laparoscopy is to look for endometriosis and adhesions resulting from

TEST

Laparoscopy

Certain conditions can be diagnosed accurately only if the organs are directly seen. Laparoscopy is a procedure that enables a doctor to see the inside of the abdominal cavity and organs such as the gallbladder, liver, and uterus through an instrument called a laparoscope. The most common use of laparoscopy is in gynecology, where it is commonly used for the following:
• tubal surgery, including sterilization
• infertility investigations
• ovarian cysts
• fibroids
• ectopic pregnancy
• laparoscopic hysterectomy
• bladder operations for stress incontinence.

How is it done?
■ The procedure is usually done under a general anesthetic. A tiny cut is made in the abdomen, usually just below the navel so that no scar is visible afterward. A needle is inserted into the abdomen and carbon dioxide gas is pumped into the abdominal cavity so that organs can be visualized.
■ The laparoscope is passed in and the doctor can angle it to get a clear view. If other instruments are being used, these are inserted through a second incision above the pubic line.
■ The procedure takes about 30–40 minutes and you will have one or two stitches in the skin. After about two hours, depending on the reason for the laparoscopy, you should be allowed to go home.

You may have a little discomfort from any gas that remains in your pelvic cavity, and the incision site may be sore. However, laparoscopy is very safe and you should have few problems.

pelvic infection, but in over 50 percent of cases no cause for the pain is found. Even when adhesions or endometriosis are detected, gynecologists disagree about whether either of these conditions is really the cause of the pain.

IRRITABLE BOWEL SYNDROME (IBS)

IBS can be detected reliably using a checklist of symptoms called the Rome Criteria.

This is a set of symptoms that includes pain relieved by defecation, bloating, and a change in bowel habit associated with pain.

MUSCULOSKELETAL CAUSES OF PAIN

If the pain is worse when moving and bending, musculoskeletal causes of pain, such as a trapped nerve, may be the cause. A skilled physical therapist, chiropractor, or osteopath can offer the best help if this is the case. Your doctor may offer you an appointment with a psychologist, too.

If your gynecologist fails to pinpoint the cause of your pain, it is possible that it may not be of gynecological origin. Unfortunately, gynecologists aren't always well trained to detect nongynecological causes of pelvic pain. In one study of women attending a gynecology clinic with pain, half had symptoms of IBS, but they were less likely than the other women to

receive a diagnosis and more likely to have pain persisting 12 months later.

But you need to get to the bottom of it, so if your gynecologist can't find the cause of the pain, seek referral to a gastroenterologist.

WHAT IS THE TREATMENT?

It depends on the diagnosis.

■ Endometriosis can be removed surgically, or treated by suppressing the ovaries using drugs such as the **combined oral contraceptive** or a group of drugs called **GnRH analogues**.

■ However, endometriosis is a recurrent disease and some women eventually choose **hysterectomy** with removal of their ovaries. This relieves the symptoms but does not cure the endometriosis.

■ Surgical division of adhesions works for some but not all women. Quite often the adhesions simply grow back again in time.

■ IBS often responds well to dietary changes or **antispasmodic drugs** and **bulking agents**.

■ Musculoskeletal pain is probably best treated with painkilling drugs, particularly nonsteroidal anti-inflammatory drugs (NSAIDs), manipulation, and a graded exercise program from a physical therapist.

■ If psychological factors play a part, they need to be recognized and sympathetically addressed along with any other treatment.

DRUGS TO COMBAT PAIN

For some women, no clear diagnosis is reached. Nonetheless, much can be done to relieve symptoms.

■ The most effective painkillers are NSAIDs such as ibuprofen. They may be used in combination with other types of painkillers such as acetaminophen or dihydrocodeine.

■ Drugs such as **amitriptyline** (an antidepressant) or **carbamazepine** (an anticonvulsant) can be used for chronic pelvic pain; they are also effective in conditions such as acute low back pain. This is because they have an effect on pain in addition to their other effects.

■ Some women find pain management, with careful pacing of activities and physical fitness training, can help them to live with chronic pelvic pain. And many derive great comfort and support from support groups. In many women the pain resolves on its own.

See also:
• **Endometriosis** p. 254
• **Irritable bowel syndrome** p. 362
• **MRI** p. 409
• **Ultrasound scanning** p. 277

Pelvic inflammatory disease

PELVIC INFLAMMATORY DISEASE (PID) IS AN INFECTION OR INFLAMMATION
OF ANY OF THE PELVIC ORGANS – THE UTERUS, FALLOPIAN TUBES, AND OVARIES.
PELVIC INFLAMMATORY DISEASE IS A POWERFUL THREAT TO FERTILITY.

Irrevocable scarring of the fallopian tubes and ovaries is the most serious complication because it causes sterility. Other complications include **painful intercourse** (dyspareunia). At one time, the most common cause of PID was tuberculosis. Now it is **chlamydia**. There is a little evidence that the use of **intrauterine contraceptive devices** (IUDs) may be a contributing factor.

WHAT ARE THE SYMPTOMS?
■ Abdominal pain.
■ Back pain.
■ Persistent menstrual-like cramps.
■ Vaginal spotting of blood.
■ Fatigue.
■ Pain during and after intercourse.
■ Foul-smelling vaginal discharge.
■ Flulike symptoms of fever and chills.
■ Sub-fertility or infertility.

PID must be treated early to prevent long-term problems. The symptoms can be those of an **acute infection** with fever, nausea, discomfort, and pain, which should alert you

to the fact that there is something wrong. A chronic infection may only cause recurrent mild pain and sometimes backache. But both kinds must be investigated. Don't wait for it to go away, see your doctor as soon as possible. If you have an IUD, go to your doctor immediately.

WHAT WILL THE DOCTOR DO?
■ You will be examined and tested to identify the organism causing the infection. Your doctor will probably prescribe antibiotics and bed rest. Eat well and don't have sexual intercourse during the course of treatment. If antibiotics are not appropriate for you, you may have to have other treatment.

■ If PID develops into a chronic infection, it can be difficult to eradicate. You may need investigative laparoscopy (see box, opposite) to confirm the diagnosis. In severe cases, for a long-term infection, **hysterectomy** with removal of the fallopian tubes can be the only course of action, although you should look into the alternatives fully before agreeing to this operation.

WHAT CAN I DO?
■ Don't let any vaginal discharge continue for any length of time without full investigation and treatment. Because PID can recur, have a full checkup to confirm that your infection has been completely eradicated.

■ If you suspect that you or your partner may have a sexually transmitted disease, go to a doctor or an STD clinic right away.

See also:
• **Chlamydia** p. 278
• **Hysterectomy** p. 256

UTERUS AND OVARIES

One of the most modern advances in this area has been the definition of polycystic ovarian syndrome (PCOS). It's a great step forward largely because once diagnosed there are several treatments to be tried, each with a degree of success.

PCOS is an important diagnosis to make. The usual clues are a tendency to excess weight, excessive hair and light, irregular periods, sometimes absent entirely. Ovulation may be missing but can usually be induced with clomiphene.

Ovarian cysts

OVARIAN CYSTS ARE FLUID-FILLED SACS THAT GROW ON OR IN ONE OR BOTH OVARIES. OVARIAN CYSTS ARE NEARLY ALWAYS BENIGN AND A SIGNIFICANT PROPORTION OF WOMEN SUFFER FROM THEM.

Benign cysts may be subdivided into two major categories. **Functional cysts** are merely small cysts (more correctly, follicles) that occur normally in a woman's monthly cycles. They do not usually cause any problems, but there may be several and they may be present in both ovaries. They rarely grow larger than about 1–2in (3–4cm) in diameter and commonly shrink back to normal size spontaneously. They are usually detected with routine ultrasound screening.

The second type are true benign ovarian cysts, of which the **dermoid cyst** is the most common. These are most often found in women in their 30s. Dermoid cysts may occasionally be present in both ovaries. They do not usually cause any problems unless they cause the ovary to twist or if the cyst leaks.

Dermoid cysts contain immature cells that are capable of growing into various types of tissue, and it is therefore not uncommon for dermoid cysts to contain bone, teeth, and hair. There are also other less common benign cysts.

WHAT ARE THE SYMPTOMS?
- Pain during intercourse.
- Painful, heavy periods.
- If a cyst twists or ruptures, it results in severe abdominal pain, nausea, and fever.

- Urinary problems due to pressure on the bladder.

While ovarian cysts are small, they produce few symptoms. Functional cysts disappear without treatment and you may never even know you had them. As true cysts get larger, however, they may cause pain and discomfort and may also affect your menstrual cycle.

The severe pain of a twisted ovary requires an emergency operation, so see your doctor as soon as possible if you suffer any of the symptoms listed.

WHAT IS THE TREATMENT?
- Your doctor will examine you both externally and internally in order to assess the size of the ovarian cyst. More tests will be arranged depending on what your doctor finds, and on your age.
- These tests will probably include an ultrasound examination of your ovaries, plus blood tests and an MRI.
- Laparoscopic surgery may be attempted to help diagnose the type of cyst present and, in younger women, to remove the cyst if it is benign.
- In older women, in women in whom the cyst is too large to be removed by laparoscopic surgery, or if there is a suspicion of malignancy, an abdominal operation will be performed. Both ovaries are always examined and checked during surgery. If malignancy is confirmed, it is usual to remove both ovaries and the uterus (hysterectomy).

Polycystic ovarian syndrome

Polycystic ovaries are ovaries in which multiple benign "cysts" form; these are not true cysts but small follicles. They are found in 15–20 percent of women. Women with the condition may have other symptoms, which include a tendency to obesity, excessive body hair, and acne. The ovary seems to produce an excessive amount of male hormones. The condition may cause fertility problems and sufferers may have irregular periods.

What causes it?
The exact cause is not known, but there is growing evidence that it is due to a resistance to insulin, leading to high levels of insulin in the blood. This stimulates the ovaries, disrupting normal ovulation.

What will the doctor do?
Polycystic ovaries are often discovered because of one of the complaints listed above. The doctor will examine you internally and may order an ultrasound examination of your ovaries and blood tests to confirm the diagnosis. You may be given the pill to stimulate a normal monthly period and combat the excessive male hormones. An oral contraceptive can help many of the symptoms, especially acne. If you want to conceive but are having difficulty, fertility treatment could be necessary.

What can I do?
Discuss the symptoms fully with your doctor so you understand the nature of all the treatments that are offered to you.

What is the outlook?
The outlook depends on the severity of the problems encountered. Currently available treatments provide good control of the majority of symptoms.

See also:
- Hysterectomy p. 256
- Laparoscopy p. 250
- Ultrasound scanning p. 277
- X-rays p. 426

Fibroids

FIBROIDS ARE BENIGN TUMORS OF THE UTERINE MUSCLE. THEY VARY IN SIZE AND NUMBER; THEY CAN BE ANYTHING FROM THE SIZE OF A PEA TO LARGER THAN A TENNIS BALL.

About 1 woman in 5 develops fibroids by the time she is 45 years old.

There is often no reason for concern because fibroids may never grow large enough to distort the uterus or cause symptoms. Large fibroids cause the surface of the uterus to feel lumpy and bumpy to the doctor when he examines your abdomen during routine pelvic examinations.

WHAT ARE THE SYMPTOMS?

About a quarter of women have no symptoms at all. Otherwise, symptoms include:
● heavy or abnormal menstrual bleeding
● swelling and a feeling of fullness in the abdomen
● discomfort or pain during intercourse
● pressure on the bladder and bowel, leading to urinary problems and backache.

If you have increasing pain or bleeding with your periods or if you have any other change in your normal menstrual cycle, see your doctor at once.

WHAT MIGHT BE DONE?

Your doctor will first perform a routine pelvic examination and question you about any symptoms you may have experienced.

If he feels that your condition warrants it, he may then order more specific tests, which will probably include an **ultrasound scan** of your uterus, a **hysteroscopy,** or **laparoscopy**.

Fibroids are treated according to the seriousness of the symptoms. Once you are past your childbearing years, the fibroids usually shrink and may disappear, unless you take HRT.
● **Antiestrogen** hormone treatments may be given to shrink your fibroids. This treatment can only be given for a period of about six months because of the risk of osteoporosis.
● If you want to start a family and your fibroids are numerous, your doctor may suggest an operation to remove them (**myomectomy**), leaving the uterus normal and intact.
● If your symptoms are really troublesome and you have already completed your family, a **hysterectomy** might be advised. It should be

considered as a last resort and only after you've had a second opinion and involved your partner in discussions with your doctors.

WHAT CAN I DO?

■ Fibroids are the most common reason for hysterectomy operations in the US, so be on your guard against having an unnecessary operation of such a radical nature. If you are suffering from profound anemia or have unbearable symptoms, obviously you should consider it; otherwise, look for alternatives.
■ A very few women with fibroids develop uterine cancer, so any unusual bleeding or other irregularity of your periods should be reported immediately to your doctor.

See also:
● **Hysterectomy p. 256**
● **Laparoscopy p. 250**
● **Ultrasound scanning p. 277**

The female snip – tubal ligation

TUBAL LIGATION IS A METHOD OF FEMALE STERILIZATION. IT REMAINS A POPULAR FORM OF BIRTH CONTROL IN THE US AND IS NOW PERFORMED MORE OFTEN THAN VASECTOMIES.

For the most part, sterilization is a permanent means of birth control making it impossible for an egg to be fertilized and conception to take place.

Tubal ligation closes off the fallopian tubes. This creates an obstruction that stops the ovum moving through the tubes to the uterus, or sperm from reaching the ovum via the tubes, and conception is prevented. Since it's a permanent operation that is very difficult to reverse, doctors usually advise childless women or women under 30 against this operation.

For some women, the decision is a difficult one. While they may be freed from the fear of having an unwanted pregnancy, they need to come to terms with their feelings about taking this irrevocable step. They may also have to deal with their partner's refusal to have a vasectomy, which is a far less invasive procedure and should always be considered first.

HOW IS IT DONE?

■ There are several different methods of female sterilization, using either the abdominal or vaginal approach. Most are performed under general anesthetic or, occasionally, under an epidural or local anesthetic.

■ Carbon dioxide gas may be introduced into the abdomen to inflate it so internal organs can be seen more clearly. While all procedures involve tying or closing the tubes, a small portion of the tube itself is almost invariably removed.
■ The tubes are closed using electrocautery which can be done with endoscopic ("keyhole") surgery.

WHAT ARE THE RISKS?

Sterilization has few serious risks or complications except those normally expected of any surgery or anesthetic. The vaginal route of sterilization has a slightly increased risk of infection, but is rarely used in the US.

IS IT EFFECTIVE?

■ Sterilization has a high efficiency rate and it's permanent.
■ Female sterilization has a very low failure rate – one pregnancy per 200–300 women per year.
■ It won't affect your sex drive or sex life.

IS STERILIZATION REVERSIBLE?

In some cases, microsurgical techniques may succeed in restoring fertility in a woman who

has been sterilized, but this does involve major surgery. About 70–75 percent of women later achieve pregnancy.

AFTER EFFECTS

■ After sterilization, you won't notice any change in your menstrual pattern, and you'll have a normal menopause when it occurs because your ovaries haven't been touched.
■ Some women have a routine dilatation and curettage (D&C) when they're sterilized to check the uterus for any abnormalities. Usually there's bleeding from the vagina for 1–2 days.
■ If you had a vaginal sterilization, you won't be able to have intercourse for a couple of weeks because of danger of infection, but you'll have no external scar.
■ You must use contraception during the cycle in which you are sterilized, because there is a risk of a tubal pregnancy if a fertilized egg cannot enter the uterus after the operation.

See also:
● **Microsurgery p. 467**
● **The male snip – vasectomy p. 269**

Endometriosis

ENDOMETRIOSIS IS A VERY COMMON CONDITION, DEFINED
AS THE PRESENCE OF CELLS FROM THE LINING OF
THE UTERUS AT OTHER SITES IN THE PELVIS.

The principal route of spread for these "seedlings" is via the fallopian tubes. Deposits find their way to the ovaries, bowel, bladder, and the pelvis, forming very small cysts and localized scarring. The seedlings respond to the cyclical changes of ovarian hormones, so bleeding occurs into the cysts when you are menstruating, but the blood cannot escape. The cysts become swollen and tender, and in the ovary may enlarge to 2–3in (5–6cm) in diameter, causing menstrual pain, painful sexual intercourse, and generalized pelvic tenderness. Adhesions may form around the cysts, interfering with ovulation and, possibly, conception.

WHAT ARE THE SYMPTOMS?

■ Heavy or abnormal bleeding.
■ Severe abdominal and pelvic pain, often leading to painful intercourse.
■ Severe cramping pain, starting before the period is due and continuing during menstruation, after which it gradually eases.
■ Urinary or bowel pain, including diarrhea.
■ Fertility problems.

If you are in your late 20s and have been unable to conceive, or if you suffer very painful periods or pain deep in your pelvis during intercourse, you should see your doctor as soon as possible. If you have never suffered from **dysmenorrhea** (painful periods) before, it is very unlikely to develop in your late 20s without there being a major reason.

WHAT MIGHT THE DOCTOR DO?

The drugs used to treat endometriosis suppress ovulation and menstruation, thus permitting the disease to regress. The drugs include the continuous use of high-dose estrogens and/or progestogens or drugs, called **GnRH analogues**, to suppress ovarian-stimulating hormones. All these treatments prevent pregnancy though backup contraception should be used.

Medical treatment of endometriosis is usually only offered to women who are not trying to conceive; it has not been shown to improve fertility rates.

For women wishing to conceive, surgical treatment, usually laparoscopic, includes **diathermy** or **laser vaporization** of the endometriosis deposits (see box, right) and **adhesiolysis** (removal of adhesions).

Radical surgery with removal of the uterus and ovaries (**hysterectomy**) may be necessary in older patients with advanced disease who don't want to have more children.

NB In vitro fertilization (IVF) should be offered immediately to women trying to conceive who have dense, widespread adhesions that are not amenable to, or recur after, surgery.

SELF-HELP

Join a support group where you can share your experience with other women and discuss the latest treatments and side effects of treatment.

See also:
• **Dysmenorrhea p. 247**
• **Hysterectomy p. 256**
• **Infertility p. 274**
• **Laparoscopy p. 250**

TREATMENT

Laser treatment

Light from a laser beam can cut or destroy tissue or repair damaged tissue by fusing together torn edges. This allows lasers to be used in a number of surgical procedures in place of scalpels, scissors, and stitches. Since laser beams can be focused precisely, small sections of tissue can be treated without causing damage to the surrounding tissues.

Laser treatment is commonly used in gynecological procedures. A laser beam can be directed into the body through an endoscope to remove scar tissue inside the fallopian tubes, which may be a cause of infertility. Lasers are also used to remove cysts that form in the pelvic area due to endometriosis and to destroy abnormal cells on the cervix which, if untreated, may develop into cancer. Similarly, small tumors or precancerous cells in other internal body areas, such as the larynx or inside the digestive tract, can be destroyed by laser beams directed through an endoscope. The technique can also be used to open arteries that have been narrowed by fatty deposits. In ophthalmic surgery, laser beams can be used to seal small tears in the retina, the light-sensitive layer at the back of the eye.

Laser treatment is often used on the skin, especially on the face, for reducing scar tissue and birthmarks, noncancerous moles, tattoos, or wrinkles. The results depend on the extent of the problem but in most cases scarring is minimal, and the appearance of the skin is much improved. External laser treatment can also be used to treat conditions such as spider veins and to remove warts on the skin and genital warts.

Most forms of laser treatment are done under either local or general anesthesia, depending on the type of surgery and the area to be treated. However, for minor skin conditions, laser treatment causes little discomfort and may be performed without anesthesia. There may be some swelling, redness, and blistering, which usually disappear within a week. Large areas of skin may have to be treated over several sessions.

A support group can help women with endometriosis cope with the psychological impact of the condition.

Prolapse of the uterus

PROLAPSE IS WHEN ONE OR SEVERAL PELVIC ORGANS DROP DOWN INTO THE VAGINA.
IF THE PELVIC FLOOR MUSCLES ARE WEAKENED, THE VAGINAL WALLS
BECOME DISPLACED, RESULTING IN A PROLAPSE.

Any of the pelvic organs, including the **uterus**, **bladder**, **rectum**, **bowel**, and **urethra**, can prolapse into the vagina, but prolapse of the uterus is the most common.

Depending on the severity, the cervix may drop and actually protrude from the vagina. Prolapse tends to occur in older women, and hardly ever occurs in those who haven't had children.

Pelvic floor muscles can weaken with age, but prolapse is nearly always caused by earlier injury to the pelvic floor muscles **during labor**.

This happens especially if you had a rapid delivery, you were allowed to go on too long in labor, or if your babies were on the large side.

To understand what your doctor is talking about these names can be helpful.

■ If the **rectum** bulges into the back of the vaginal wall, it is called a **rectocele**.

■ When the **urethra** bulges into the front of the vaginal wall, it is called a **urethrocele**.

■ If the **bladder** drops into the front of the vaginal wall, it is called a **cystocele**.

WHAT ARE THE SYMPTOMS?

■ Backache.

■ A feeling of something bulging from the vagina; difficulty inserting and removing a tampon.

■ Stress incontinence – leaking urine when you lift a heavy weight, cough, or sneeze.

■ With uterine prolapse, a dragging down feeling in the pelvis.

■ With a urethrocele or a cystocele, frequent urination and an urgent need to pass urine.

■ With a rectocele, discomfort on moving the bowels and difficulty in passing a stool.

Don't wait for symptoms to become really troublesome; consult your doctor as soon as possible.

WHAT MIGHT THE DOCTOR DO?

■ Your doctor will give you an internal pelvic examination to confirm a prolapse and to determine which type you have.

■ You'll be asked about the births you've had, whether they were difficult, if your babies were larger than normal, if the second stage of labor lasted a long time and if forceps were used to aid delivery of any of your babies.

■ Being overweight makes a prolapse worse, so you'll be advised to lose weight.

■ If you have a severe prolapse, your doctor will recommend surgery (see box, right). It will improve your quality of life by controlling incontinence and improving your sexual enjoyment. Surgery, in the form of a

hysterectomy, has been the treatment of choice in the US. In some cases, treatment options include a support device called a pessary which relieves symptoms by pushing the uterus back up to its regular position.

■ Most prolapse repairs are performed through the vagina and involve a general anesthetic. Occasionally, the operation may be performed with an epidural anesthetic, especially if the patient is old and infirm.

■ You will probably stay in hospital for 1–2 days. An outpatient appointment is usually made six weeks later, after which sexual intercourse can be resumed if there are no problems.

SELF-HELP

■ If you suffer from backache, try to avoid standing for long periods at a time. Wear a tight girdle to counteract any dragging feeling you may have in your pelvis.

■ If you are having difficulty with sexual intercourse, you and your partner may need to explore alternative nonpenetrative ways of achieving sexual pleasure.

■ Wear panty liners if you are troubled by leakage (stress incontinence). If the leakage becomes worse, see your doctor.

■ The most important preventative treatment is being conscientious about doing Kegel exercises regularly during pregnancy and

especially after the birth of your baby, whether or not you have stitches.

■ You should continue Kegel exercises until the day you die, each day going through them on five or six separate occasions.

■ If you stop your Kegel exercises for a few weeks, start again.

■ Mild incontinence can be controlled with Kegel exercises alone done five times a day for a couple of weeks.

Retroverted uterus

A mobile retroverted uterus is a harmless variation of normal in which the uterus is tilted backward. It is often blamed for failure to conceive but is in no way responsible.

See also:
● **Kegel exercises p.375**

TREATMENT

Surgery and Pessary

A hysterectomy is the most common form of treatment for a woman experiencing significant symptoms as the result of a prolapsed uterus. To correct a prolapse, a hysterectomy, in which the uterus is removed, is performed under general anesthesia. The surgery may be done through an incision made in the vagina (vaginal hysterectomy) or through the abdomen (abdominal hysterectomy). An abdominal hysterectomy generally requires a four to six day stay in the hospital followed by four to six weeks' recuperation time at home. A vaginal hysterectomy typically means a shorter hospital stay.

The decision to correct a prolapse with a hysterectomy depends on the woman's age, general health, desire for future pregnancies,

and the degree of the prolapse.

While not a permanent cure, a vaginal pessary is another treatment option for some women with a prolapsed uterus.

A pessary is rubber disk that is placed in the upper vagina and acts as a support device. Pessaries come in a variety of shapes and sizes and so, must be fitted for each woman individually. The decision to treat with a vaginal pessary depends on the extent of the prolapse and vaginal wall relaxation.

Vaginal pessaries do have drawbacks which include, irritation, discharge, and the need for frequent removal and cleaning, usually performed by your gynecologist. Some types of pessaries may interfere with normal sexual intercourse.

Hysterectomy

HYSTERECTOMY IS THE SURGICAL REMOVAL OF THE UTERUS. IN THE US, A SHOCKING 25 PERCENT OF ALL WOMEN OVER THE AGE OF 50 HAVE HAD A HYSTERECTOMY. THE OPERATION IS OFTEN PERFORMED FOR NO GOOD REASON, SUCH AS THE REMOVAL OF SMALL FIBROIDS.

America has a comparatively high rate of hysterectomies. In Great Britain, for example, there has been a reluctance by doctors to remove the uterus unless symptoms warrant it. The decision to have a hysterectomy should never be taken lightly and in young women the instant menopause that follows a hysterectomy in which the ovaries are removed must be treated with hormone replacement therapy (HRT); conception is never an option.

WHAT ARE THE TYPES?

■ **Subtotal abdominal hysterectomy**, in which the uterus and sometimes the ovaries and fallopian tubes are removed, but the cervix is left intact.
■ **Total abdominal hysterectomy**, in which the ovaries, fallopian tubes, uterus, and cervix are removed.
■ **Radical hysterectomy**, in which the uterus, cervix and pelvic lymph nodes are removed through an abdominal incision.
■ **Vaginal hysterectomy**, in which a hysterectomy is performed through the vagina instead of through an abdominal incision.

If the ovaries are removed, a woman no longer produces the female sex hormones and HRT must be considered.

WHY IS IT DONE?

Hysterectomy can be done for any of the following reasons:
● to remove **cancer** in the pelvic organs

● to treat any severe and uncontrollable **pelvic infection**
● to stop life threatening **uterine hemorrhage**
● in certain life threatening **conditions affecting the intestines and bladder**, when it's impossible to deal with the primary problem without removal of the uterus
● to remove multiple **fibroids** that are causing **excessive bleeding** and **pain**
● to treat **prolapse**
● to treat severe **endometriosis**
● in repairing **uterine and vaginal prolapse**.
● Hysterectomy should never be the first line of treatment for heavy, long periods.

HOW IS IT DONE?

■ Under general anesthesia, an incision is made in the lower abdomen, and the uterus, and if required the ovaries and fallopian tubes, are removed.
■ After the operation you'll have an IV drip for fluids and perhaps a catheter to drain urine. There'll be some discharge from the vagina for a day or two.
■ If your ovaries were removed, HRT will soon be started. If not, ask about it.
■ Alternatively, you may have a vaginal hysterectomy, in which the abdominal cavity isn't opened but the uterus is removed through the vagina. Recovery is quicker this way and complications are minimized or avoided entirely. This is the ideal operation to correct uncomplicated uterine prolapse.

Vaginal hysterectomy is only performed if the uterus is not too bulky and if the supporting structures aren't too tight.

WHAT ABOUT AFTERWARD?

■ When you go home after the operation, maintain a moderate level of activity, but stop the minute you feel any discomfort.
■ Gradually build up your strength. Gentle activities can be started by the fourth week after the operation; moderate activity such as light shopping or housework can be undertaken by about the fifth week. By the sixth week, you should start to feel nearly back to normal, although you may still feel tired.
■ By the sixth week, you can resume sexual intercourse since the top of the vagina will have healed. If you've kept your cervix there is no reason why sex should be any different for you.

ARE THERE PSYCHOLOGICAL CHANGES?

■ Most women who are appropriately counseled and have hysterectomies are happy with the operation. The vagina will be the same size as it was before unless it was a radical hysterectomy, when it will be slightly shorter.
■ Dissatisfaction is related to whether the operation was done for a very good reason and after full consideration by the woman and her partner of the options available.
■ Women who wanted more children find it difficult, as do some whose ovaries are removed premenopausally.
■ The women who suffer from depression after hysterectomy are usually those who weren't convinced that the operation was necessary, especially if it was done for a condition that was not life threatening. It's easier to adjust if you know the operation saved your life.

What should I do if hysterectomy is suggested?

■ Question your gynecologist very carefully about the reasons for your hysterectomy and be satisfied in your mind that it's absolutely necessary.
■ Don't make a decision quickly – complications after a hysterectomy are most common in women who remain unconvinced the operation was necessary.
■ If you are in doubt about the advice or wish to avoid hysterectomy, seek a second opinion from another gynecologist. Many conditions respond

to much less radical approaches than hysterectomy.
■ Check to see whether your ovaries need to be removed in addition to your uterus, and find out about hormone replacement treatments available for premature menopause, which will occur if your ovaries are removed. It's no longer medically accepted that the ovaries should be removed in case cancer should develop, so don't be persuaded by this argument.

FEMALE CANCERS

Cancer of the cervix and breast cancer are two of the most common cancers seen in women. Fortunately, cancer of the cervix can largely be prevented provided women attend appointments for regular Pap smears.

Breast awareness and screening can also help detect breast cancer while it is still at a curable stage. Cancer of the ovary and cancer of the uterus are two rarer forms of cancer that also affect women.

Cervical precancer and cancer

CANCER OF THE CERVIX IS THE SECOND MOST COMMON FEMALE CANCER (BREAST CANCER IS THE FIRST) AND IT'S BECOMING MORE COMMON, PARTICULARLY AMONG YOUNG WOMEN. UNTREATED, IT MAY SPREAD TO MOST OF THE ORGANS IN THE PELVIS.

The chances of a cure for cervical cancer depend very much on what stage the cancer has reached when first detected.

Cervical cancer has a **precancerous stage**, often called **cervical intraepithelial neoplasia**

(CIN), during which time abnormal cells grow but are not cancerous. As this precancerous stage may last for several years, any woman who has regular Pap smears will be identified early enough for the abnormal cells to be

totally removed by simply taking out the tissue from the cervix long before there's any threat of cancer.

Despite the fact that precancerous changes

continued on page 259

TREATMENT

Chemotherapy

Chemotherapy uses powerful chemicals in the form of pills, injections or an IV drip to kill cancer cells. Chemotherapy drugs interrupt cell growth, so they end up killing large numbers of cells, both cancerous ones and healthy ones. Many "normal" body cells (such as the bone marrow and

the lining of the intestine and mouth) divide rapidly and are therefore vulnerable to cancer drugs, giving rise to many of the side effects of chemotherapy.

Most chemotherapy is given as outpatient treatment, either as a short injection into a vein

or as an IV drip over an hour or so. It rarely involves staying in the hospital overnight.

Depending on the type of cancer being treated, chemotherapy is usually given once every three or four weeks, but some treatments may be given weekly. You'll probably receive 6–8 courses of treatment, and treatment usually lasts 5–6 months.

Hormonal drugs

For certain types of cancer, special hormonal drugs may be used. One of the best known of these drugs is tamoxifen, which is used to block the effect of estrogen, implicated in the growth of certain tumors (and especially in breast cancer). In women with a family history of breast cancer, tamoxifen may be given as a preventive measure, but the risks have not yet been fully investigated.

In chemotherapy, cancer cells are killed off faster than normal cells, until no cancer cells are detectable.

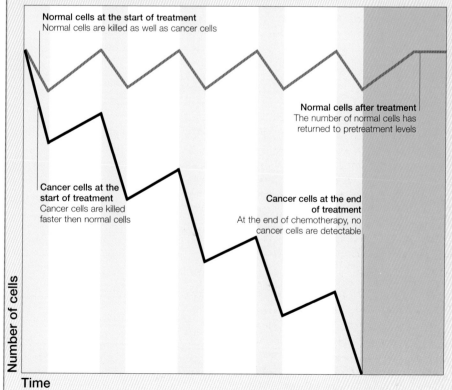

Normal cells at the start of treatment
Normal cells are killed as well as cancer cells

Normal cells after treatment
The number of normal cells has returned to pretreatment levels

Cancer cells at the start of treatment
Cancer cells are killed faster then normal cells

Cancer cells at the end of treatment
At the end of chemotherapy, no cancer cells are detectable

Number of cells

Time

Key
- .... Normal cells
- —— Cancer cells
- ▢ Treatment period
- ▢ No treatment
- ▢ Remission

FOCUS *on* Pap smears

Nearly all of us harbor some trepidation about having a Pap smear. It's natural to feel vulnerable about exposing ourselves to a stranger, and there's also the added fear the test may show a worrying result. But it's up to us all to take responsibility for our own health.

A Pap smear done regularly can detect the earliest precancerous changes, which can be treated promptly so the cancer never develops.

Since cervical cancer is one of the few cancers over which we can exert some positive control, it's crazy to allow a few minutes of embarrassment to prevent us from having regular checkups. It's a very quick procedure and before you know it, it will be over.

DID YOU KNOW?
● The human papilloma virus (HPV) raises the risk of cervical cancer.

Colposcopy

Colposcopy is a simple, noninvasive procedure and can be used as a treatment as well as a diagnostic tool following an abnormal Pap smear. It requires no anesthetic and can be done in your gynecologist's office or outpatient clinic. The colposcope, a kind of microscope, is placed at the entrance to the vagina. The doctor examines the tissue to identify the precise area of abnormal cells. (A Pap smear doesn't pinpoint this exactly.) He'll then remove the speculum slowly so that he can inspect the vaginal walls.

Abnormal cells inside the cervical canal can't be detected with a colposcope. If these are suspected, a cone biopsy (in which a cone of cervical tissue is removed) will be recommended.

Areas confirmed as abnormal by biopsy are treated by electrocoagulation or laser (both use heat to destroy tissue), by cryosurgery (which uses cold to destroy tissue) or may be removed by diathermy loop excision (DLE). Treatment may be carried out at the same time as colposcopy if the abnormal area is small and well-defined. If a woman is pregnant, treatment is usually delayed.

● 95 percent of women with cervical cancer carry HPV.
● HPV is symptomless in many women.
● Having many sexual partners puts you at risk as it increases your likelihood of being exposed to HPV.
● Cervical cancer won't have time to develop if you have regular Pap smears.

A Pap smear, also known as a **cervical smear**, is named after the doctor (Papanicolau) who invented it, and is done during a pelvic examination. It's primarily used to detect precancerous and cancerous cells on the cervix – the neck of the uterus.

It detects very early abnormal changes in the cells of the cervix, which can be destroyed thus preventing cervical cancer from developing.

Cancerous change is even more likely if you have several partners. Promiscuous sex also increases the risk of being infected with HPV, the virus that promotes cervical cancer.

The test offers a 95 percent chance of detecting **CIN** (abnormal cell changes which, if not discovered and treated, could become cancerous).

WHAT IS THE CERVIX?
The cervix is small, cylindrical, several centimeters in length and forms the lower part and neck of the uterus. The cervix dips down into the vagina. Running through the center of the cervix is a canal through which sperm pass from the vagina into the uterus on their way to fertilize an egg and through which blood passes during menstruation.

WHO SHOULD HAVE PAP SMEARS?
Pap smears should be performed on all women once they begin having intercourse and then every three years throughout life, even after age 65. The test is also important for women who have or have had infection with the human papilloma virus (HPV). A Pap smear may incidentally detect sexually transmitted diseases.

WHEN AND WHERE IS IT DONE?
A woman should have a Pap smear within a year of her 20th birthday. Pap smears may be performed by your gynecologist or at a family planning clinic. You shouldn't be menstruating or have had intercourse within 24 hours of having your test since blood and semen make the result unreliable. Ideally you should be at mid-cycle to obtain the best quality Pap smear.

HOW IS IT DONE?
You lie on your back with your knees bent. A warmed speculum is passed into the vagina to separate the walls so the doctor can see your cervix.

A wooden swab is wiped across the cervix to collect cells, and the smear is transferred to a glass slide and sent to a laboratory. The whole thing takes less than a minute and, although uncomfortable, isn't painful. The results should be available within 6 weeks.

THE RESULTS
Results of a Pap smear are classified into three categories:
● **Negative** gives you the all-clear.
● **Mild dysplasia** or CIN I means that you have some infection and should be screened more frequently.
● A **positive** Pap smear test, although not always indicating cancer, means there is a detectable change in the cells necessitating further investigation.

The table below gives you a comprehensive run down of the sort of results you're likely to get and what you'll need to do in response.

Result	Action
Negative	No follow-up needed: next smear in three years
Mild dysplasia or CIN I	Another smear in no more than 6 months
Moderate dysplasia or CIN II	Colposcopy
Severe dysplasia	Colposcopy

See also:
● **Cervical precancer and cancer p. 257**

continued from page 257
can be detected by **regular Pap smears** and treated, each year about 25 percent of women with cervical cancer die, usually because they have not had a Pap smear. Since the condition has no early warning symptoms it can only be detected by routine Pap smear screening.

STAGES OF CERVICAL PRECANCER AND CANCER
PRECANCER
- The mildest stage is known as CIN I.
- More severe changes, NOT CANCER, is called CIN II.
- The most severe stage is called CIN III.

CANCER
- Stage 1: cancer confined to the cervix.
- Stage 2: cancer extends beyond the cervix to involve the top of the vagina and/or tissue immediately surrounding the cervix.
- Stage 3: cancer extends to the lower part of the vagina and/or the side wall of the pelvis.
- Stage 4: cancer extends beyond the pelvis and/or involves the bladder or rectum.

TEST

Tissue tests

Some disorders change the number of different types of cell within an organ or make individual cells abnormal. Tissue tests can show these changes. In a tissue test, a small sample of a particular tissue is removed and examined under a microscope. One of the most frequently performed tissue tests is the Pap or cervical smear, in which a sample of tissue is taken from the cervix to look for pre-cancerous changes in the cells.

Biopsy

The procedure in which a sample of tissue is taken specifically for testing is known as a biopsy. Biopsy may be done to confirm a diagnosis or to investigate a suspicious lump or a tumor. For example, if cirrhosis is suspected, a biopsy of liver tissue may be done and if characteristic changes are found, the diagnosis is confirmed. If it is not known whether a tumor is malignant (cancerous) or benign (noncancerous), a biopsy can provide tissue that can be tested for cancerous changes. More tests are sometimes needed if tissue tests do not provide a definitive diagnosis.

WHAT ARE THE SYMPTOMS?
- In its early precancerous stages (CIN I and II), there are no symptoms.
- By Stage 1 or 2, **intermenstrual bleeding** and **spotting after intercourse** can show up as a warning sign that must always be investigated.
- An **offensive vaginal discharge** may be a symptom of cervical cancer and needs medical assessment.

WHAT ARE THE CAUSES?
While the exact cause of cervical cancer is not known, certain risk factors have been identified. These include infection with certain types of the human papilloma virus (HPV), which is linked with 95 percent of all cases of cervical cancer. Other risk factors include having multiple sexual partners, smoking, long-term use of the contraceptive pill, early pregnancy, and many pregnancies. Women who have not recently had a Pap smear are most at risk of developing cervical cancer simply because these women will not receive treatment for any precancerous changes to the cervix. Thus the biggest risk factor for cervical cancer is non-attendance for cervical screening.

WHAT'S THE TREATMENT?
MEDICAL
- All stages of CIN should be treated, although some doctors adopt a "wait and see" approach, involving repeat Pap smears for early CIN.
- Treatment of CIN involves performing a **colposcopy** usually in the outpatient department, when the cervix is viewed with a special microscope. Areas with abnormal cells may be identified and, if necessary, a biopsy may be taken to examine the tissue in the laboratory.
- Following a colposcopy a woman will either be reassured, or have a follow-up Pap smear or have further treatment.

SURGICAL
- The simplest surgical treatment of CIN involves removing the precancerous tissue under a local anesthetic with a **laser**, or **freezing** or **cutting** away the tissue with an electric loop (known as large loop excision of the transformation zones, or LLETZ, or diathermy loop excision, or DLE).
- A **cone biopsy** involves removing a larger piece of tissue and this may require a general anesthetic. This may be done with a scalpel or a laser beam. A cone of cervical tissue is taken out to remove all abnormal tissue plus a wedge of surrounding normal tissue. After the tissue is examined microscopically, doctors decide if you require any further treatment.

Treatment of full-blown cancer of the cervix depends on the stage that the disease has reached. Treatment may involve either **surgery**

or **radiation therapy**, or both. As a general rule radiation therapy is more often used for older women and surgery for younger, healthier patients, regardless of the stage of the disease.
- Surgery involves removing all affected tissue and organs. A **radical hysterectomy** is most often performed. This involves removing the uterus, the cervix, the upper vagina, and the surrounding tissues, including some lymph nodes.
- If the cancer involves the bladder or bowel, major surgery involving removal of the bladder or bowel, in addition to a hysterectomy, may be necessary.

Nearly half of all cases of cervical cancer are treated with radiation therapy. The goal is to give a fatal dose of radiation to the center of the cancer. Radiation also kills those parts of the growth that were invading other areas. However, surgery alone with conservation of the ovaries is preferred for younger women because of the adverse effect of radiation therapy on bowel and sexual function.

WHAT IS THE OUTLOOK?
- You'll be required to have regular checkups over the next five years or so to make sure the cancer spread has been stopped.
- You'll almost certainly not be able to have any or any more children and, if your ovaries are removed, you'll go through a **premature menopause**. You must be aware of this because you'll need HRT from day one after the operation, so ask your doctor about it.

Remember

If you maintain regular appointments for **Pap smears**, most cancers will be caught at a time when chances of a cure are high. Even if cancerous cells are found, try to take an interest in the disease and cooperate with your medical team as much as possible to fight it. Cancer cures do depend to a certain extent on your determination to beat the disease.

See also:
- HRT p. 502
- Hysterectomy p. 256
- Pap smears p. 258

Cancer of the ovary

CANCER OF THE OVARY IS A MALIGNANT TUMOR THAT CAN DEVELOP IN ONE OR BOTH OVARIES,
USUALLY IN WOMEN AFTER MENOPAUSE BUT OCCASIONALLY IN YOUNGER WOMEN.

Unfortunately ovarian cancer does not usually cause any symptoms until it is advanced, by which time it may be very difficult to treat effectively. Ovarian cancer is usually aggressive and can spread quite early in the course of the disease.

WHAT ARE THE CAUSES?
There are many theories about what causes ovarian cancer to develop. It is more common in older women and in women who have not had any children, and less common in women who have used the oral contraceptive pill or HRT for a number of years and in those women who had a late start to their periods and an early menopause.

"Resting" the ovary by suppressing ovulation, for example during pregnancy or while on the pill, may protect a woman against developing ovarian cancer. Genetic factors are important in ovarian cancer: sometimes it runs in families. A triad of cancers – ovary, breast, and colon – run through some cancer families where a gene is at work.

WHAT ARE THE SYMPTOMS?
■ Abdominal pain.
■ Swelling of the abdomen.
■ A hard lump in the abdomen.
■ If the tumor is large, pressure on the bladder can cause frequent urination.
■ Occasional breathlessness if the tumor presses upward on the diaphragm.

WHAT MIGHT BE DONE?
Some families carry a **gene** called BRCA1 and BRCA2 that increases the likelihood of both ovarian and breast cancer. Genetic tests for this gene are now available to help identify those women at risk of developing ovarian and breast cancer.

If you have a strong history of ovarian or breast cancer in your family, it is important to tell your doctor.

Treatment of ovarian cancer usually involves several things.
■ Your surgeon will attempt to remove the whole tumor and any local spread. The extent of surgery depends on the type of tumor found.

■ Minimal surgery involves the removal of both ovaries and the fallopian tubes as well as the uterus.
■ If the disease has already spread beyond the reproductive organs, much more extensive surgery may be necessary. This may involve surgery to other organs, such as removing part of the bowel and bladder.
■ Drugs containing platinum are commonly used to treat ovarian cancer, but radiation therapy has been found to have limited effect.
■ More surgery may be performed to remove any recurrences.

WHAT IS THE OUTLOOK?
The outlook in the longer term depends on the stage of the disease and the type of malignant cell present in the ovary, but the figures are not reassuring. If the cancer is restricted to the ovary, 60–70 percent of women can expect to live for five years; if the growth has spread, the five-year survival rate is only 10–20 percent.

Cancer of the uterus

CANCER OF THE UTERUS IS A TUMOR THAT GROWS IN THE LINING OF THE
UTERUS, THE ENDOMETRIUM, AND IS SOMETIMES KNOWN AS ENDOMETRIAL CANCER.
IT HAS A RELATIVELY LOW MALIGNANCY.

WHAT CAUSES IT?
Cancer of the uterus is more common in obese women and those taking the drug tamoxifen, which is used to prevent or treat breast cancer. Hormone replacement therapy (HRT) using estrogen alone also increases the risk but addition of a progestogen for 14 days at least every three months prevents this, and the continuous "nonbleeding" form of HRT actually reduces the risk of developing this cancer.

There has been a lot of controversy in recent years about the possible association of uterine cancer with taking HRT for menopausal symptoms. If a menstrual period is induced at least every three months by a 14-day course of progestogen, endometrial overgrowth is avoided. Inserting a progesterone IUD that can be left in place for five years accomplishes the same goal.

WHAT ARE THE SYMPTOMS?
■ Postmenopausal bleeding or brown discharge.
■ Discomfort in the lower abdomen.
■ Bleeding after intercourse.
■ Heavy menstrual periods.

WHAT WILL THE DOCTOR DO?
If you have any postmenopausal vaginal bleeding or any change in your normal menstrual pattern, consult your doctor immediately.
■ If your doctor suspects that you have a growth in your uterus, the only effective way to check whether there is any malignancy is to undergo an investigation. You are likely to have an ultrasound scan; if this shows a thickened endometrium, an endometrial biopsy may done via the cervix, or the inside of the uterus may be examined using hysteroscopy with a biopsy at the same time.

■ If the uterine lining contains cancerous cells, your doctor will recommend a total hysterectomy with removal of the ovaries and fallopian tubes as well as the cervix. Radiation therapy may be advised if the tumor has spread through the wall of the uterus.
■ If the growth is advanced, a radical hysterectomy will be performed to remove some vagina and the lymph nodes of the pelvis too.

WHAT IS THE OUTLOOK?
The news is good. The overall cure rate is as high as 90 percent when the cancer is localized to the lining of the uterus itself. If the spread is beyond the lining and the muscles of the uterus, the figure after five years is reduced to 40 percent.

FOCUS *on* breast cancer

I wish I could wave a magic wand and make women less afraid of breast cancer. I feel you, and every woman, would be less fearful if you knew the good news, and could take the reassuring facts on board. Fear can stop you from doing this.

I want to try to reassure women by starting with this very positive statistic, and then following with a lot more. **Of every 15 women referred, 14 do not have cancer.**

Understanding breast cancer can greatly improve your chances of avoiding it and defeating it. You can reduce the risk of ever getting breast cancer by knowing how to prevent it. This includes making life choices such as having your first baby before 30. Lifestyle changes, such as keeping your weight down and your consumption of alcohol low, may help. You should also eat at least five fresh fruits and vegetables every day.

Early detection and diagnosis play an important role in the successful treatment of breast cancer, and in the long-term outlook.

It's important to know that, even when a diagnosis of breast cancer is made, there are different types. Not all cancers have the same degree of invasiveness or potential to spread, so not all, by any means, have a poor outlook.

A positive attitude is a real asset, possibly as vital as some medical treatments.

PUTTING BREAST CANCER INTO PERSPECTIVE

- For every breast lump found to be cancerous, approximately eight others will prove to be benign and therefore harmless.
- If the lump is diagnosed and treated early, you'll have a better chance of a successful outcome.
- Even with cancerous lumps, 6 or 7 out of 10 will be treated without removing the breast.
- In postmenopausal women, deaths from breast cancer pale into insignificance when compared with the number of deaths caused by heart disease – **four** times as many!
- Five times more women suffer from the disease than die from it. In a given year, of 100,000 women with breast cancer, 80,000 **do not die.**
- More than 70 percent of women who have operable disease will be alive and well five years after diagnosis.
- By the age of 50, your chances of dying from breast cancer, compared to other causes of death such as heart disease, will have dropped dramatically from 1 in 12 to 1 in 70, and the odds get better with every year you live after that without developing it.
- By the time you are in your sixties, your chances of dying from breast cancer are probably less than half what they were when you were 50.

HORMONE REPLACEMENT THERAPY (HRT) AND BREAST CANCER

The risk of breast cancer increases slightly if you take HRT. The increase rises a little depending on the time you are on HRT. Here are the real figures:

Women aged 50 (per 1,000 women)	Breast cancer risk over next 10 years
No HRT (baseline risk we all have)	None
5 years HRT	0.2%
10 years HRT	0.6%
15 years HRT	1.2%

A woman who stops HRT treatment returns to the normal risk rate after five years. However, the risk of breast cancer should be weighed against the benefits of HRT.

Four times as many women die from coronary artery disease and the consequences of osteoporosis, both of which HRT may help guard against.

FAMILY HISTORY

About 5 percent of breast cancers may be due to genes inherited from your family. Women are at increased risk if their mother or sister developed breast cancer before the age of 40, if two of these relatives developed it before the age of 60, or if three relatives developed breast cancer at any age.

Any woman who's worried should ask her gynecologist for advice.

WHAT IS A TUMOR?

The word tumor simply means a lump. Most breast tumors aren't cancerous. They're usually benign, i.e. the growth of cells is confined to the area where the tumor starts. Tumors whose cells don't spread to other parts of the body aren't fatal.

In contrast, the cells that make up cancerous tumors are invasive. They spread beyond their original location, not just into adjacent tissues but to other distant parts of the body and as they invade they destroy.

The original tumor is known as the **primary**. Tumors that arise from cancerous cells that have spread elsewhere are called **secondaries** or **metastases**.

continued on page 262

What happens to your sex life if you lose a breast?

It's quite natural for the loss of one of your breasts to radically change your self-image and lower your self-esteem.

You may feel unattractive or embarrassed by it and not surprisingly you may become inhibited and lose your sex drive.

About 1 in 5 women has a loss of sexual interest a few months after mastectomy and at two years the figure rises to 1 in 3. Interest in sex declines in over a quarter of sexually active women, regardless of the kind of surgical treatment they have.

The psychological impact of knowing you have cancer and coping with its treatment may preoccupy you with thoughts of survival, so that sexual desire is at the bottom of your priority list.

Some couples will, however, find the trauma of breast cancer brings them closer together, especially if you involve your partner in every step from day one.

To determine how aggressive cancer cells are, and how far they have spread, if at all, grading and staging tests are done, which are also a basis for deciding on treatment.

SPREAD

Invasive cancers tend to spread first into the **regional glands** – the axillary lymph nodes in the armpits in the case of the breasts – causing swellings. They may also spread to lymph nodes under the breastbone and above the collarbone.

Spread via the bloodstream, through "seeds," is probably more important in determining the long-term outlook. This is why modern treatments, such as hormonal therapy and chemotherapy, are designed to eradicate cancer cells from the body as a whole rather than just dealing with the tumor locally.

1 IN 11

You may have heard that 1 in 11 women develops breast cancer. This figure, although true, may be misleading because it doesn't tell the whole story, only the alarming part of it.

1 in 11 represents the lifetime risk. This means 1 in 11 women will develop breast cancer during the course of their whole lives – that means over 70 or 80 years.

Not today, not this week, not this month. Since risk increases with age, the risk at any point in time is much lower than 1 in 11; in point of fact, it's closer to 1 in 1,000.

HOPE FOR THE FUTURE

● Women who have treatment for early breast cancer can expect to live a normal life span.
● For women who get local recurrences, radiation therapy can sometimes cure without the need for other treatment.
● While breast cancer is predominantly a disease of older women, many women live to die from causes other than their breast cancer.

SURGERY

Mastectomy, the removal of a breast, is less common these days – or should be. Radical surgery is no longer the norm for breast cancer and there are currently several possible variations of mastectomy.

More than 80 percent of breast cancers are localized and caught early enough to be suitable for lumpectomy – removal of the lump alone leaving the breast virtually intact.

The type of surgery selected to treat cancer depends on the size of the tumor and other factors.

The majority of women qualify for additional treatments after surgery. It's called **adjuvant therapy**.

CHEMOTHERAPY

Several drugs are designed to target rapidly dividing cancer cells anywhere in the body, and the use of these drugs can increase the cure rate by 10 percent.

Side effects, including hair loss and nausea, are unpleasant but usually only temporary.

Other noncancerous cells that are rapidly dividing, such as those in bone marrow, are susceptible to damage from chemotherapy.

HORMONAL DRUGS

Tamoxifen, a very promising hormonal drug, can block tumor growth in certain patients and is used widely. Tamoxifen may even be given as a preventive measure in women who are at high risk of getting breast cancer. The latest British figures show that tamoxifen has cut the death rate from breast cancer by nearly 40 percent.

Because it has an antiestrogenic effect, tamoxifen has side effects when taken for long periods, including menopausal symptoms. It slightly increases the risk of uterine cancer.

RADIATION THERAPY

Radiation destroys or slows the development of cancerous cells.

It's usually given after surgery, to kill any remaining cancerous cells, but may be used in place of surgery to reduce the size of breast tumors and thus to relieve symptoms.

Lumpectomy

Lumpectomy (also called breast-conserving surgery) is the removal of a breast lump along with some surrounding normal tissue. If the procedure is done to remove a cancerous lump, some of the lymph nodes in the armpit are usually also removed. The procedure is done in hospital under either a local or, more usually, a general anesthetic. Lumpectomy to remove a cancerous lump is usually followed by 3–5 weeks of radiation therapy to ensure that the cancer is eradicated.

Sites of incisions

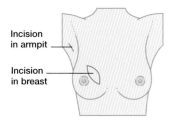

Incision in armpit

Incision in breast

The breast lump, some surrounding normal tissue, and some lymph nodes are usually removed during a lumpectomy.

Areas treated in a lumpectomy

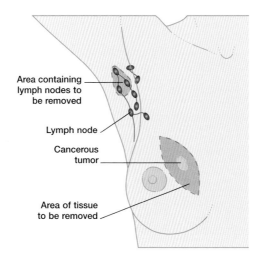

Area containing lymph nodes to be removed

Lymph node

Cancerous tumor

Area of tissue to be removed

A certain percentage of women may be left with discomfort and stiffness in the shoulders and arms following radiation therapy and you may lose some sensation in the treated breast; it may also be slightly swollen and feel different. If your breasts were an important source of sexual stimulation prior to surgery, counseling could help you to find other means of enhancing your enjoyment of lovemaking.

BREAST RECONSTRUCTION

Woman who have had a mastectomy should consider a new, reconstructed breast. It can be done at the same time as mastectomy or at a later date.

Most breast reconstructions involve a flap of skin, fat, and muscle swung around from the back that's folded into a breast shape. An implant may be inserted too.

New nipples can be created by tissue grafting and tattooing. The new breast is often better than the breast that's left!

FALSE BREASTS OR PROSTHESES

Breast prostheses are very sophisticated now and feel like a natural breast. They can be fitted into a bra or swimsuit. Bras containing breast prostheses can also be obtained. Prostheses are designed to simulate the appearance and feel of a natural breast.

WHAT IS THE OUTLOOK?

Remember, modern techniques mean that doctors can tailor treatment to the particular needs of each woman, so you will be given every chance of a cure. Rigorous follow-up will be necessary to pick up any problems and to check for recurrence of cancer. After months of intensive medical attention you may feel alone and fearful, and this is a time when a network such as a local breast cancer support group can be invaluable.

In conclusion, keep in mind that 1 in 3 women who have treatment for early breast cancer can expect to live a normal life span.

Being aware of the normal appearance and texture of your breasts enables you to bring any changes to your doctor's attention promptly.

MEN'S CONDITIONS

With some famous men going public and owning up to testicular and prostatic disease, men's conditions are much more high profile than they were, and it's about time too.

Men need a lot of encouragement to be open about their health problems, particularly intimate ones such as testicular and prostatic cancer.

Men don't easily talk about themselves. They are sometimes loath to consult a doctor because they see expressing concern about their health as somehow un-macho.

That's not only a great shame but also dangerous, especially since testicular cancer, caught early, is one of the most curable cancers there is.

Why it's important to check your testicles

WOMEN ARE GETTING THE MESSAGE THAT IT MAKES GOOD HEALTH SENSE TO CHECK THEIR BREASTS REGULARLY FOR LUMPS. BY COMPARISON, ONLY 1 IN 30 MEN EXAMINES HIS TESTICLES.

It's a pity more men don't do testicular self-examination because testicular cancer is **highly curable** when detected at an early stage. And self-examination couldn't be simpler, it only takes a few minutes every month. It's best done after a bath or shower when the scrotum is warm and relaxed since this will increase the chances of detecting any abnormality. Self-examination is really worth doing – the latest treatments mean 9 out of 10 men will make a complete recovery.

Men need to check their bodies for cancer, just as women do. Here's the simple self-examination you can use to test for first signs of testicular cancer.
1. Stand in front of a mirror and look for **any swelling** on the skin of the scrotum. One testicle may appear larger than the other and one may hang lower, which is usually normal.
2. Hold each testicle gently between the thumb and fingertips of both hands and slowly bring the thumb and fingertips of one hand together while relaxing the fingertips of the other.
3. Alternate this several times so the testicle glides smoothly between both sets of fingers. This lets you assess its shape and texture.
4. You shouldn't press too hard and you must be careful not to twist the testicle.
5. Each testicle should feel soft and smooth, like a hard-boiled egg without its shell.

WHAT YOU'RE LOOKING FOR
Any lump, swelling, irregularity, abnormal hardness, tenderness, or any change within the body of the testicle itself. Testicular cancer almost always occurs in only one testicle.

WHAT YOU MIGHT FIND
There are causes of testicular swellings other than sinister ones; these include a **hydrocele, epididymal cyst**, **spermatocele** or **varicocele**.
■ A **hydrocele** is a soft painless cyst surrounding the testicle. During development, the lining of the abdomen pouches down into the scrotum as the testicle descends. This closes off to leave an empty remnant in the scrotum.

In middle age, this remnant often fills with fluid and can grow quite large. In most cases there is no underlying cause, but occasionally a hydrocele forms as a result of inflammation, infection, injury or, rarely, an underlying tumor of the testicle on that side.

A doctor tests for a hydrocele by holding a **pen light** next to the scrotal skin. The swelling will light up if it is due to a fluid-filled hydrocele and you can do this for yourself. Small hydroceles are often left alone and larger ones may be drained under a local anesthetic, though they may recur, so surgery is the most effective treatment.
■ An **epididymal cyst** is a harmless swelling arising from the epididymis, the coiled collecting tube attached to the back of each testis. Small, pea-sized epididymal cysts are common in men over the age of 40. These cysts are often multiple and may affect both sides. They are filled with a clear, colorless fluid and are usually left in place rather than removed.
■ A **spermatocele** is similar to an epididymal cyst, but instead of containing clear fluid it is filled with milky semen and sperm. If you shine a light through it, it doesn't light up like a hydrocele. The two can only be differentiated if fluid is drained for examination.

Spermatoceles are harmless and are usually left in place unless they become troublesome.
■ A **varicocele** is a collection of **varicose veins** surrounding a testicle and is one of the most common reasons for an enlarged testicle.

It feels like a warm tangle of worms in the scrotum and it's a condition that affects about 10–15 percent of men; it is usually harmless although there may be aching discomfort in the scrotum or an abnormally low sperm count. Diagnosis is confirmed by examination of the scrotum while the patient is standing. Any aching may be relieved by wearing an athletic support or tight underpants.

WHAT CAUSES TESTICULAR CANCER?
Testicular cancer is still quite rare, accounting for only one percent of all tumors in males. However, it is one of the most curable cancers, with 90 percent making a complete recovery. We don't know what causes it yet, but we do know that men who were born with an **undescended, or partly descended, testicle are between 3 and 14 times** more likely to develop testicular cancer. Other research has suggested that there may be a **hereditary** factor involved. Treatment shouldn't affect your sex life or fertility in the long term.

> **See also:**
> • **Testicular cancer p. 270**

Younger men are at risk

■ Testicular cancer is the most common form of cancer in young men in the US and it occurs mostly in those aged between 19 and 44.
■ It's easily treated and, if caught at an early stage, testicular cancer is nearly always curable.
■ The risk of developing it has risen by 70 percent in the past 20 years.
■ Only 3 percent of young men check their testicles; most are unaware of this simple method of early detection of cancer.
■ More than 50 percent of sufferers consult their doctors after the cancer has started to spread. This makes it more difficult to treat successfully and the side effects of treatment become more unpleasant.

Gynecomastia

GYNECOMASTIA IS COMMON, NORMAL ENLARGEMENT OF ONE OR BOTH BREASTS IN MALES AND
HAS NO SINISTER SIGNIFICANCE. IT'S MOST OFTEN SEEN IN NEWBORN BABIES AND OLDER MEN.

All men produce small amounts of the female sex hormone estrogen. If estrogen levels are higher than normal, breast enlargement – gynecomastia – occurs. Either one or both breasts may become enlarged. Gynecomastia is common in newborn boys because of their mother's estrogen crossing the placenta. It affects a fair number of male adolescents too,

because their own estrogen levels are swinging around. In babies and adolescent boys it is almost always temporary. Gynecomastia can also affect older men when they have stopped producing the male hormone testosterone but their adrenal glands and fat are still producing estrogen. The condition may also be a side effect of certain drugs, for example digoxin.

WHAT MIGHT BE DONE?
In baby boys the swelling settles down after a week or so and in adolescent boys it disappears when their hormones level out. In these cases no treatment is usually needed. In older men, the doctor will ask about lifestyle factors and do an examination to exclude breast lumps. If a drug is the cause, it may be changed.

Peyronie's disease

PEYRONIE'S DISEASE IS A CONDITION IN WHICH THE SHAPE OF THE PENIS IS DISTORTED,
CAUSING IT TO BEND TO ONE SIDE OR UP AND DOWN WHEN ERECT. IT'S VERY
RARE UNDER THE AGE OF 40 AND SOMETIMES RUNS IN FAMILIES.

Some penises **always** bend when erect and this is just a variation of normal. In Peyronie's disease, the fibrous tissue of the penis becomes thickened, causing it to bend during erection. The penis may bend so much that sexual intercourse is difficult and painful. Peyronie's disease occurs in about 1 in 100 men.

Often no cause can be identified, but previous damage to the penis may be a risk factor. Peyronie's disease is also associated with **Dupuytren's contracture**, a condition in which the fibrous tissue in the palm of the hand becomes thick and shortened, causing the fingers to bend inward. Peyronie's disease can run in families, which implies that a genetic factor is involved.

WHAT ARE THE SYMPTOMS?
The symptoms of Peyronie's disease develop gradually and include:
● curvature of the penis to one side during an erection
● pain in the penis on erection
● a thickened area in the penis, usually be felt as a firm nodule when the penis is flaccid.
  Eventually, the thickened region of the penis may extend to include parts of the erectile tissue. In this case, Peyronie's disease may lead to impotence if it is not treated.

WHAT IS THE TREATMENT?
In some cases, Peyronie's disease improves without treatment. In other cases, vitamin E or

drug therapy may be of some benefit. Some surgeons **excise** the fibrosed tissue, others **remove a wedge** on the opposite side to encourage a straight erection. A vein patch may be inserted. Poor results are usually due to disease progression or scarring. If the condition is advanced, the best solution may be to implant a **penile prosthesis**.

Prostate cancer

THE PROSTATE GLAND IS ONE OF THE ORGANS THAT CAN DEVELOP CANCEROUS
TUMORS, AND THIS FORM OF CANCER CAN HIT ANY MAN.

HOW DOES PROSTATE CANCER GROW?
At first, the tumor stays inside the prostate's outer capsule but, as it enlarges, it may spread through the capsule and grow into the surrounding tissue around the prostate gland.
  Cancer cells can also break off from the primary tumor. They are trapped by the lymph glands near the prostate and here they can grow into secondary tumors or **metastases**.
  The tumor can also spread via blood vessels, giving rise to **metastases** in the **bones of the back, spine and pelvis**.

HOW IS PROSTATE CANCER DIAGNOSED?
A doctor will suspect a tumor if, when he does a **rectal examination**, he finds a hard, irregular lump in the prostate or if the whole prostate feels hard and uneven. As with breast cancer, very small tumors may be impossible to feel.

HOW COMMON IS PROSTATE CANCER?
It's much more common than we used to think. We now know that almost **three-quarters** of men over the age of 80 have it, but in many of these men the cancer is quiescent and most will die of something else.

Prostate cancer is the second most common cancer in American men. The risk of developing prostate cancer is about 1 in 10.
  As with breast cancer in women, it's important to catch the disease **early**, especially in men who are at high risk. A **family history** of prostate cancer, or even breast cancer, would put a man in the high-risk group.
  Prostate cancer may be preventable. A study published last year from Finland suggests that taking **vitamin E supplements** may reduce the chance of developing the disease by about a third and of dying from it by nearly a half. There's also some evidence that **selenium**

continued on page 268

FOCUS *on* prostate problems

Most men will suffer from an enlarged prostate to some degree. It's part of normal male aging and Western men suffer from it more than Asian men. What is the prostate anyway? Most people have heard of it, but have little idea what it's for, and many people don't even know where it is.

Indeed doctors and scientists don't fully understand its functions, and there's still a lot to be learned about the prostate and about the diseases affecting it.

The prostate gland lies underneath the bladder. Its main job is to produce a thin, clear fluid that nourishes sperm while they're being stored in the seminal vesicles awaiting release through ejaculation. The prostate needs hormones from the testicles (mainly **testosterone** but also **prostaglandin**) so that it can work properly, and if they're low the prostate shrinks.

Close to the prostate are two important bladder muscles called sphincters, one above and one below the prostate. They control the outlet from the bladder, stopping it from leaking urine. They also help to expel semen at ejaculation.

WHY DOES THE PROSTATE CAUSE TROUBLE?

A man's prostate usually becomes larger after the age of 50. The fact that the prostate grows isn't important in itself, and indeed the trouble it causes doesn't depend on its actual size.

However, the prostate surrounds the tube from the bladder called the **urethra** and as it enlarges it squeezes the urethra and narrows the opening out of the bladder. This is called **obstruction** and it impedes the flow of urine. 25 percent of men aged 50 and over will experience urinary symptoms due to prostate enlargement.

SYMPTOMS OF OBSTRUCTION

As obstruction occurs gradually, many men don't realize it's happening. They may notice that their urine stream doesn't travel as far as it did when they were young and they may be aware that it's less forceful.

Then there may be a delay in getting started (called **hesitancy**), and the urine stream tails off at the end, sometimes causing troublesome dribbling.

There may be a feeling that the bladder isn't quite empty, known as incomplete emptying.

WHY DOES THE PROSTATE GET BIGGER?

The main cause is simply **age**. The benign noncancerous enlargement is called benign prostatic hyperplasia (BPH).

The exact reason for enlargement is uncertain, but male hormones are required so it doesn't occur in men castrated at an early age.

Most men over the age of 80 have the condition, and about half will have some symptoms from it.

WHAT HAPPENS TO THE PROSTATE?

BPH starts in the inner part of the gland and, as it enlarges, it squashes the rest of the gland into a fairly thin shell, called the capsule. BPH never spreads outside the gland. However big the prostate, it remains covered by the capsule somewhat like a chestnut in its shell.

A doctor examines a prostate by doing a rectal examination (the prostate lies right up against the back passage). A prostate with BPH has a smooth surface with an even shape and feels rubbery, rather than hard.

PROSTATITIS

Inflammation of the prostate (prostatitis) from infection or other causes is not uncommon and can occur at most ages, affecting approximately 1 man in 10. Sometimes it causes symptoms like **cystitis** – such as **burning pain while passing urine**. In older men it might cause a sudden increase in prostate symptoms. The prostate is very **tender** when the doctor does an internal rectal examination.

DO I HAVE AN ENLARGED PROSTATE?

If you've read this far and you're a man of the right age for prostate problems, you'll probably be wondering whether you need to have your prostate checked, so ask yourself some questions.
● Do you have difficulty starting to pass urine?
● Does it take longer to pass urine than it did?
● Do you stop and start?
● Do you need to pass urine twice or more during the night?
● Are you sometimes caught short?
If your answer to two or more questions is yes, see your doctor.

TREATMENT OF AN ENLARGED PROSTATE

If you have a prostate problem, your doctor will ask you about your symptoms then do a rectal examination to assess the size of your prostate. Tests will be arranged for confirmation and to help plan your treatment.

You'll be asked to give a sample of your urine and a blood sample is usually taken to check how your kidneys are working and to measure a substance called **prostate-specific antigen (PSA)** (see opposite).

WHAT ARE MY TREATMENT OPTIONS?

Until very recently, virtually the only treatment for benign enlargement of the prostate was an operation. Operations on the prostate are usually very successful if a man has severe symptoms, but are sometimes disappointing if symptoms are only mild.

SURGERY

Transurethral versus open surgery
The earliest operations on the prostate were done as conventional surgery – removing the enlarged part of the gland through a surgical incision in the front of the abdomen.

Just before World War II, urologists in

America started doing an operation called **transurethral resection** (TUR).

It was one of the earliest types of endoscopic or **"keyhole" surgery** and now nearly all prostate operations are done this way.

An instrument called a **resectoscope** is passed into the prostate via the urethra.

The urologist can see the prostate directly and sends a special type of localized electric current through a metal loop to cut the prostate out in pieces, leaving a cavity in the middle of the gland through which urine will pass easily.

A general anesthetic may be used, but since the operation only takes about half an hour, it's often done with the patient awake but numb from the waist down under an epidural anesthetic, given through a needle in the back.

It's quite possible for a man to watch his operation being performed on a video screen in front of him if he wants to.

DRUG TREATMENT

Drug treatment of BPH is usually for mild symptoms where the obstruction isn't too bad. Drugs may be tried in more severe cases if there are medical reasons to avoid surgery, or for temporary relief while waitng for surgery.

HORMONE TREATMENT

• The drugs that shrink the prostate interfere with the action of the male hormone testosterone, which is part of the cause of BPH.

Only one, called **finasteride**, is used currently, given as a single pill once a day. It may take three months or more before the prostate shrinks enough to improve the symptoms, so don't stop taking it after a week or two because it doesn't seem to be working. A small number of men do experience failure of erections and other sexual difficulties. If sex is very important, you might feel that this treatment isn't right for you – although sexual

problems are more common with a TUR and then they aren't reversible.

As soon as the drug is stopped, the prostate grows again very rapidly, so if it is working, keep on taking it.

ALPHA BLOCKER DRUGS

The other type of drug used for treating BPH is called an alpha blocker. Alpha blockers relax the muscle, reduce the obstruction, and improve symptoms almost immediately, although they can cause side effects such as faintness, weakness, and fatigue.

OTHER TREATMENTS

• **Laser treatment** is more like a TUR and is an alternative way of removing the enlarged part of the prostate or of simply widening the urethra: it can be done as an outpatient or in a short stay and is associated with less bleeding.
• Microwave or thermotherapy, where heat treatment is used to destroy prostate tissue, may help some patients with less severe symptoms. This is performed in the doctor's office.

PROSTATE-SPECIFIC ANTIGEN TESTING

Any man with an enlarged prostate will have a fairly new test that measures the level of prostate-specific antigen (PSA) in the blood. The test has been given a lot of publicity as a method of early diagnosis of prostate cancer. Just because your doctor does a PSA test doesn't mean he suspects cancer. He's just being thorough.

Think of the PSA in the blood as if it's "leaking" out of the prostate. More PSA will come from a large prostate than from a small one, so as you get older the PSA can increase quite normally as the prostate enlarges. PSA is **prostate** specific but not **cancer** specific. So if your PSA is higher than normal, it doesn't mean you have cancer.

Since older men have larger prostates and also more have noncancerous diseases of the prostate, the average PSA is higher in men of 75 than in men of 55.

After the operation

• Will it be painful?

Postoperative pain is uncommon but the **catheter** can be uncomfortable, and may make the bladder feel full.

Sometimes painful spasms occur.

If they're severe you'll get drugs to control them. You'll be asked to drink a lot of water each day to help flush out your bladder.

• Getting back to normal

It's usual to have some **frequency** for a day or two, and often it's difficult to control the urine at first. A physical therapist (or a nurse) will teach you some **exercises** to help control the urine flow.

Sometimes it's difficult to start passing urine but persevering for a few hours usually does the trick. If not, the catheter may be reinserted. Don't despair – usually everything's fine when it's taken out again. Inside, the prostate is raw and needs time to heal. Continue to drink plenty of fluid (but no alcohol). Avoid driving, heavy lifting, and sex for two to three weeks.

You'll see some bits of tissue and blood in

the urine from time to time – this is like a scab coming off the skin and, as when a scab comes off, there's sometimes a little bleeding.

Frequency (an abnormally short time between passing urine) may take longer to improve and may not return completely to normal. Needing to pass urine **at night** may persist after the operation but it's a symptom of getting old as much as it is prostate trouble.

Leakage at the end of passing urine may persist, but can usually be controlled by being a little careful.

• Interference with sex

At the end of sex, a man may have a normal climax but no semen is ejaculated. This is called **retrograde ejaculation. "Having a dry run"** describes exactly what happens and it's because semen is leaking back into the bladder rather than coming out normally. A few men do experience difficulty in getting an **erection** after the operation, so ask your surgeon before having the operation for his opinion.

See also:
• **Endoscopic surgery p. 358**

continued from page 265

and **lycopene** (a substance found in **tomatoes**), **high soy intake** and a **low-fat diet** may help too.

HOW FAR MIGHT THE CANCER HAVE SPREAD?

Doctors can do tests that show how advanced the prostate cancer is, the most important being **PSA** and **Gleason scores**.

PSA measures the amount of a protein called prostate-specific antigen in the blood. Because this protein is produced by prostate cancer cells, its level is an indication of the severity of the disease.

As a general rule, **PSAs above 10** are considered indicative of advanced cancers that have spread. **Gleason scores**, based on a biopsy, measure the **aggressive** nature of cancer cells, and may be even more helpful in deciding the best individual treatment. A number below 7 usually means it's safe to opt for not such aggressive treatment. The higher the score, the greater the risk to the patient.

SCREENING FOR CANCER OF THE PROSTATE

Pap smears are used to screen for cancer of the cervix in women. So, you may be asking, can PSA be used as a test to screen for cancer of the prostate in men?

This is a difficult question to answer because there's no clear difference between the amount of PSA found in the blood of men with cancer and of men with simple benign prostatic hyperplasia (BPH) and other benign conditions.

It's not straightforward – noncancerous prostate cells can produce PSA too. So don't get alarmed if your PSA is high – it could be nothing more than a benign growth or an inflammation of the prostate.

WHAT ARE THE TREATMENT OPTIONS?

Once a patient has an idea of the type and state of his cancer, he has several treatment options to choose from.

SURGERY

Taking out the prostate is still considered by many to be the mainstay of treatment for cancers confined to the prostate. It's highly effective, but will probably not suffice on its own if the cancer has spread. This has to be weighed against the fact that the aftereffects of this operation can be severe. Additional surgical options include removal of one or both testicles to stop production of testosterone, which feeds the cancer.

RADIATION THERAPY

This is usually used to treat prostate cancer that's still contained within the gland. Side effects can be quite severe and include impotence, diarrhea, vomiting, and pain when passing urine.

A new version of this treatment restricts radiation to the exact shape of the tumor. It's expected to cut down on unpleasant side effects.

RADIOACTIVE SEED THERAPY

A relatively new treatment involves placing time-release radioactive seeds in specific areas of the prostate.

The procedure is performed on an outpatient basis and takes about an hour. It's popular too: up to **90 percent of radioactive seed recipients remain sexually active after treatment**.

For less aggressive prostate cancers, there's evidence that seeds may be as effective as more radical surgery. Men with advanced cancers, however, would not be helped by this treatment, although experimental treatments are currently being tried.

HORMONAL TREATMENT

Prostate cancer needs the male hormone testosterone, so it's logical to use hormonal treatments to lower its level in the body, especially for advanced prostate cancers.

Hormone treatments are often used in combination with other treatments, such as radiation therapy or surgery. Sexual function suffers substantially during treatment but will probably disappear once therapy is complete. Removal of the testicles would fall into the category of hormonal treatments, but are not as popular today.

TREATMENTS STILL IN RESEARCH

Medical advances are being made all the time in the field of prostate cancer and if a man is willing, he may wish to enroll in clinical trials for treatments not yet approved for general use.

These would include **vaccines** designed to induce the body's own immune system to attack the cancer, and techniques to shrink tumors by choking their blood supply.

If someone feels inclined to go this route he should talk to his doctor about it.

See also:
- **Chemotherapy p. 257**
- **Radiation therapy p. 395**

Balanitis

BALANITIS IS INFLAMMATION OF THE HEAD OF THE PENIS AND FORESKIN. IT'S MORE COMMON IN BOYS AND NOT BEING CIRCUMCIZED IS A RISK FACTOR.

In balanitis, the head of the penis (the glans) and the foreskin become itchy, sore, and inflamed. There may be a discharge and a rash. The disorder can be caused by a **bacterial infection**, a **fungal infection** such as yeast (candidiasis), or an **allergic reaction**.

WHAT ARE THE RISKS?

■ Men with **diabetes mellitus** are more susceptible to the condition because their urine contains high levels of glucose, which can encourage the growth of microorganisms. This leads to infection and inflammation at the opening of the urethra.
■ Excessive **antibiotics** can increase the risk of a fungal infection by temporarily lowering the body's defenses against this type of infection.

■ **Boys** are especially vulnerable to balanitis.
■ The condition may also occur as a result of **sensitivity** of the penis to certain chemicals, such as those found in some **condoms**, **contraceptive creams**, **detergents**, and **laundry soaps**.

WHAT MIGHT BE DONE?

If the head of your penis or your foreskin is inflamed, you should consult your doctor. The area will be examined and a swab taken to look for evidence of infection. The doctor may also test your urine to check for the presence of glucose.

WHAT IS THE TREATMENT?

The treatment of balanitis depends on the cause.

■ For example, if you have a **bacterial infection**, antibiotics may be prescribed.
■ If the infection is due to a **tight foreskin**, circumcision may be recommended to prevent balanitis from recurring.
■ If the condition is the result of a **sexually transmitted disease** (STD), your partner should be checked for evidence of infection and treated if necessary to prevent recurrence.
■ If the cause seems to be **sensitivity to a chemical**, the irritant should be identified, if possible, so that you can avoid it.

The inflamed area should be kept clean, dry, and free of irritants. Most cases of balanitis clear up rapidly once the cause has been found and appropriate treatment has been started.

TREATMENT

Circumcision

Circumcision is the surgical removal of the foreskin, which is the skin covering the head of the penis (the glans). The operation may be done if the foreskin is too tight to be pulled back over the glans (a condition known as **phimosis**). Circumcision may also be carried out for religious reasons or, less often now, for hygienic purposes. In boys and men, circumcision is usually performed under general anesthesia. However, in newborn boys it is more often done under local anesthesia. In the operation, the inner and outer layers of the foreskin are cut away and their edges are then stitched together. No dressing is needed while the wound heals.

Before the operation

location

Foreskin

Mucosa

Area of tissue to be removed (shaded)

Head of the penis

The foreskin covers the head of the penis (the glans) and is normally retractable.

After the operation

Remnant of foreskin stitched to skin of the penis

After circumcision, in which the foreskin is surgically removed, the head of the penis is exposed.

The male snip – vasectomy

STERILIZATION IS NOW A MORE COMMON CONTRACEPTIVE THAN CONDOMS – WITH APROXIMATELY 500,000 VASECTOMIES PERFORMED IN THE US EACH YEAR.

The decision to be sterilized should be considered carefully by any couple because it should always be thought of as irreversible. No surgeon will guarantee the snip can be reversed.

Couples who've completed their families may choose to be sterilized to avoid the inconvenience or side effects of other methods of contraception. Male sterilization provides a method of contraception that's safe and close to 100 percent effective; plus, the risk of complications is lower than for female sterilization.

The simplest sterilization is that done on men. The two tubes (**vas deferens**) that connect the testicles to the penis are tied or, more usually, cut (snipped). The operation is performed under a local anesthetic in about 20 minutes. It doesn't affect virility or sexual performance, nor does it increase susceptibility to illness. After the operation, ejaculation is the same during orgasm, but it contains no sperm and therefore isn't capable of fertilizing an egg.

WHAT ARE THE RISKS?
Sterilization has few serious risks or complications except those normally expected of any surgery or anesthetic.

IS IT EFFECTIVE?
■ Sterilization has a higher efficiency rate than any other form of contraception and it's permanent.

■ There'll be no effect on your sex life. Men often feel their potency has been interfered with after vasectomy, but this is only in the mind.
■ In 1 in approximately 2,000 men, sperm reappear and, if this happens, a man can safely have another vasectomy operation.

IS STERILIZATION REVERSIBLE?
About 50 percent of vasectomy reversal operations are successful.

AFTEREFFECTS
After a vasectomy, a man remains fertile until the sperm already present in each vas deferens are ejaculated or die. **Only after two consecutive specimens of semen are analyzed** (about three months after the operation) **and found to be sperm-free, is a man considered sterile**. Until that time, either he or his partner needs to use some other form of contraception.

TREATMENT

The procedure

Vasectomy is performed under a local anesthetic as an outpatient procedure. Small incisions are made on either side of the pelvis near the penis and a length of each vas deferens (spermatic duct) is usually removed. The cut ends are turned back and secured with stitches; this prevents the ends from rejoining. The skin incisions are then closed with stitches. After the operation, there may be slight bruising and mild pain, and patients should rest for 24 hours. Most men are able to return to work within a few days and can resume sexual intercourse within 7–10 days.

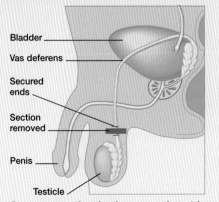

Bladder

Vas deferens

Secured ends

Section removed

Penis

Testicle

In a vasectomy, the tubes that connect the testicles to the ejaculatory duct of the penis are cut or tied off, preventing sperm from being ejaculated.

FOCUS *on* testicular cancer

Testicular cancer is a tumor that develops within the testicle. Men are vastly underinformed about male cancers. Despite the fact that testicular cancer is the most common cancer to affect young men, more than two-thirds of men know little or nothing about it.

And that's worrying, because if testicular cancer is caught early enough there is more than a 90 percent chance of a cure. Just as women should examine their breasts regularly, men should do a monthly self-examination for testicular cancer. But 50 percent never check their testicles for lumps and bumps.

Interestingly, more than one-third of men know how to check their testicles but don't. There seems to be a reluctance on the part of men to examine themselves intimately.

There's also a reluctance among young men to talk about their personal health – less than 1 in 10 does – whereas 6 out of 10 women do. This reluctance could be due to widely held misconceptions about testicular cancer, its treatment and future outlook:
- Many men think infertility and impotence are possible complications of testicular cancer when, in fact, neither has a high risk of occurrence.
- Many men thought the cure rate was much lower (6 out of 10) than it really is – a very encouraging 9 out of 10, if it's caught early.

WHAT ARE THE RISKS?
- In Europe, testicular cancer is most common in Denmark, Ireland, and Norway, and rarest in Finland and Spain. Worldwide, Japan, India, and South America also have low frequencies. The reasons for its different rates of occurrence in different countries aren't known.
- The most significant risk factor is undescended testis with 10 percent of patients having a history of this condition.
- Testicular cancer can have a strong inherited component. First-degree relatives (brothers, fathers, or sons) of testicular cancer patients have up to a tenfold increase in the risk of developing the condition.

WHAT ARE THE CAUSES?
- The first cancer gene, probably one of many, implicated in testicular cancer was located in the 1990s by an international collaboration of scientists, including the Institute of Cancer Research, the Cancer Research Campaign and Imperial Cancer Research Fund.

- Scientists don't know what percentage of cases are caused by an inherited genetic susceptibility, but some estimates place the figure as high as 30 percent of all cases.
- We know very little about the detailed gene mechanism for developing testicular cancer. More work is required to isolate the key genes involved in testicular cancer.

WHAT CAN I DO?
Testicular cancer normally shows up as a lump in the testicle. Regular examination of the testicles can, in most instances, detect testicular

Facts

- Testicular cancer affects young men, mostly between the ages of 19 and 44, although it can develop in boys as young as 15.
- The prevalence of testicular cancer has risen by 70 percent over the last 20 years.
- Between the ages of 15 and 50, about 1 man in every 500 will develop this problem.
- It's still quite rare, and accounts for only one percent of all cancers in males. But this figure could rise if current trends continue.
- The causes of the increase are unknown. Exposure to female hormones in the environment, in water, or in baby milk, have been suggested. In Spain, and most Asian countries, there has been no significant increase. Men with one or both testes undescended have a greatly increased risk.
- Many types of testicular cancer can be cured in more than 90 percent of cases if caught at an early stage. Even when the tumor spreads, it can be cured in 80 percent of cases.
- The most common type of testicular cancer is treated by removal of the testis followed by radiation therapy and, when needed, various drug treatments.

cancer at an early stage, but neglecting self-examination means it can grow and spread.

YOUR PLAN OF ACTION
Since testicular cancer can affect both younger and older men, it's important that everyone should be aware of it and how to detect it.

Since it can affect adolescent boys, there's an important role for parents to play. Wives, girlfriends, and partners can also help to try to encourage awareness in their men.

Men should perform a regular self-examination, similar to the way in which women, aware of breast cancer, do breast self-examination.

The best place to do a self-examination is in the shower. The heat relaxes the scrotum and makes it easier to check for any lumps of abnormalities. Men can also ask their partner to give them a helping hand.

The scrotum should be supported in the palm of the hand and the size and weight of each testicle noted. Each testicle should be examined by rolling it between the fingers and thumb. Press gently and feel for any lumps, swellings, or changes in firmness. Don't confuse the testicles with the epididymis, the sausage-shaped structure that lies along the top and back of each testicle. Lumps found here are likely to be cysts and blockages, which become more common as a man gets older.

While most lumps in the testicles are benign, any change in size, shape, and weight may mean something's wrong, and it's important to discuss it with your doctor as soon as possible.

WHAT MIGHT BE DONE?
Diagnosis and treatment of testicular cancer is helped by substances in the blood (markers) that are found in a large proportion of patients with testicular cancer. There's a new drug, carboplatin, which is highly successful in treating testicular cancer and has led to today's high cure rate.

Treatment for testicular cancer may be very intensive, but most patients cured of testicular cancer have no long-term side effects. A small number of patients will become infertile after chemotherapy treatment.

Other side effects are uncommon but may include damage to the nerve endings and hearing, spasms in the blood vessels, and possibly heart disease. There may be a small risk of developing other cancers, but all risks are lower if testicular cancer is treated early.

SEX LIFE

Sex is one of the greatest human pleasures but also one of the most problematic. I receive thousands of letters from men and women whose lives are severely upset because of sexual dissatisfaction in one form or another.

There is rarely a perfect balance between partners. One invariably wants more sex than the other. To the other, that's seen as their partner wanting less sex than they do. Each thinks the other is abnormal or being difficult. It's nearly impossible to see each other's point of view and find common ground.

Sex, more than any other area of human communication, demands understanding, compromise, and compassion.

If both partners can manage that, the rewards of sex are possibly greater than any other form of human interaction. So compromise is worth working for.

Painful intercourse in women (dyspareunia)

PAINFUL INTERCOURSE IN WOMEN, ALSO KNOWN AS DYSPAREUNIA, IS PAIN EXPERIENCED IN THE GENITAL OR PELVIC REGION DURING INTERCOURSE. MANY WOMEN EXPERIENCE PAINFUL SEXUAL INTERCOURSE AT SOME POINT IN THEIR LIVES.

The pain may be **superficial**, in the vulva or vagina, or deep in the pelvis. It may have either a **psychological** or a **physical** cause.

WHAT ARE THE CAUSES?
For many women, superficial pain during sexual intercourse may be caused by **psychological factors**, such as **anxiety disorders**, **guilt**, or **fear of sexual penetration**. These factors can also result in **vaginismus** (see below).

A fairly common cause is **vaginal dryness**, especially in women of **premenopausal**, **menopausal**, and **postmenopausal** age. Superficial pain during intercourse may also be caused by **infections** of the urinary tract or the genitals.

Pain that is felt deep within the pelvis during intercourse may be due to a disorder of the pelvic cavity or of the pelvic organs, such as **pelvic inflammatory disease**.

SELF-HELP
If you think your pain is due to vaginal dryness caused by lack of arousal, talk to your partner about spending more time on foreplay. You could also try a lubricating jelly. In menopausal women estrogen creams or suppositories inserted into the vagina help tremendously.

WHAT MIGHT THE DOCTOR DO?
If you consult your doctor, he or she may take swabs from your vagina and cervix to test for infection and may order an ultrasound scan and computerized tomography (CT) scan of the pelvis to look for abnormalities. If none are found you must consider that the cause could be psychological.

See also:
- CT scanning p. 401
- Pelvic inflammatory disease p. 251
- Ultrasound scanning p. 277

Vaginismus

VAGINISMUS IS AN INVOLUNTARY SPASM OF THE MUSCLES SURROUNDING THE VAGINAL ENTRANCE. IT MAY OCCUR WHEN SEXUAL INTERCOURSE IS ATTEMPTED, BUT MAY ALSO HAPPEN WHEN THE WOMAN TRIES TO INSERT A TAMPON OR GOES FOR A VAGINAL EXAMINATION.

Whenever the man tries to penetrate his partner, the opening of the vagina closes up so tightly that sexual intercourse is just impossible, and even a vaginal examination by a gynecologist may have to be carried out under general anesthesia.

WHAT CAUSES IT?
Most women with vaginismus think they're "too small" for sex, but this is hardly ever the case. The basic cause is fear: fear of sex, fear of penetration, fear of pain, fear of reliving a painful sexual experience, such as rape or sexual abuse.

HOW IT AFFECTS WOMEN
Vaginismus is a common cause of **unconsummated marriages**, and the couple often continue for several years before they do anything about it. Women who suffer from vaginismus are **terrified of sexual intercourse**, so that any attempts at penetration are frustrating and painful experiences.

Vaginismus may be associated with a **general lack of interest in sex**, but this is not necessarily the case. Many such women are **sexually responsive** and may be able to reach orgasm when the clitoris is stimulated. They may also enjoy sexual foreplay, always providing that this does not lead to sexual intercourse.

To be certain that a woman is suffering from vaginismus, she should go to her doctor, to exclude physical conditions causing an obstruction to the vagina that need to be treated.

THE RESULTS OF VAGINISMUS
Because involuntary spasm of the vaginal muscles makes sexual intercourse impossible, this may cause considerable distress to both partners. Attempts at sexual intercourse, while causing the woman a great deal of pain, may also frighten, humiliate, and frustrate her.

Recurring failure at sexual intercourse makes any woman feel inadequate and may lead to fears that she might be abandoned by her partner. It is not surprising therefore that such women may try to avoid sexual contact entirely.

The man frequently becomes frustrated by his inability to penetrate his partner, and often feels she is rejecting him.

WHAT CAN I DO?

The first stage in correcting vaginismus is to reduce the anxiety connected with sexual intercourse. This should be done by using a **relaxation technique**.

1. The woman should lie on the bed, close her eyes, and then relax all the muscles in her body, starting from the toes and working upward, until all the other muscles in the body are relaxed as well.

2. When she is fully relaxed, **she should first imagine** being in bed with her partner, and then gradually increase the degree of intimacy until she can imagine him penetrating her without this making her anxious. She may then go on to the next stage.

3. This involves gently inserting either **one of her own fingers** or letting her partner insert one of his fingers into her vagina, whichever

produces less anxiety. The finger should remain there quite still until all her feelings of discomfort have subsided. Then the finger should be moved forward and backward in the vagina until she can tolerate this without any discomfort.

4. The next stage is the insertion of two fingers, and if this is successful, the woman or the couple can then try moving the fingers around and around in her vagina. It is helpful if she can be encouraged to deal with her feelings of discomfort rather than avoiding them.

5. Sexual intercourse must on no account take place until the woman can tolerate her own or her partner's fingers in the vagina without any discomfort whatsoever. It is helpful if she learns to tense and relax her vaginal muscles because this gives her the feeling that she has got some control over her own vagina. **Kegel exercises** show a woman where her vagina is and let her feel it tightening up then loosening.

6. Also, it is helpful **if she "bears down"** when her partner inserts the penis for the first time.

7. It is extremely important that the first attempt at sexual intercourse should be

carried out very gently, with the assistance of a lubricating jelly.

8. The woman should **guide the man's penis into her vagina**, and once inserted, it should be held there without any movement taking place at all. Then he should start slow thrusting movements at her signal, and should withdraw his penis immediately if she wants him to do so.

9. All these stages may need **to be repeated several times** before she is sufficiently confident to allow normal sexual intercourse to take place.

10. **Thrusting to orgasm** should not take place on the first occasion and it is far better for the couple to wait until they are less anxious about sexual intercourse before either of them reach orgasm.

If the couple still find that they are having problems with sexual intercourse, then it is recommended that they seek expert advice from an experienced therapist, after discussion with their doctor.

See also:
• **Kegel exercises p. 375**

Impotence

IMPOTENCE IS INABILITY TO ACHIEVE OR MAINTAIN AN ERECTION. DON'T PANIC, IT'S VERY COMMON… DESPITE THE FACT THAT 1 IN 10 MEN OVER THE AGE OF 21 SUFFERS FROM IMPOTENCE, VERY FEW UNDERSTAND HOW IT HAPPENS.

Impotence can be a side effect of **accidents**, **disease,** and most important, of **prescription drugs**. This latter cause would fall into the category of medically-induced, or **iatrogenic**, impotence. A quarter of all cases of impotence occur as a side effect of drugs given to treat other conditions. The list of drugs that can interfere with erection (see opposite) is really very long. If you're on any one of them it could be the cause.

Impotence can be a feature of many conditions, including **heart diseases** such as **high blood pressure** and **angina**, **liver disease**, **thyroid disease**, **diabetes**, **chronic bronchitis**, and **emphysema**.

HOW ERECTION WORKS

In youth, no man worries about how his erection might work. He takes erections as a matter of course and never expects his penis to fail him. But erection is quite a complicated physiological event and a lot can go wrong.
■ The stiffness of an erection depends on blood being pumped into specially designed spaces (the corpus cavernosum) in the penis, in much the same way as we blow up a balloon with air.

■ To keep the spaces full of blood, and an erection stiff, blood must be prevented from escaping from the spaces by valves snapping shut.
■ Both of these events are controlled by nerves running down the sides of the penis that are in direct connection with the brain. Therefore a man can see a sexual image and a split second later feel his erection begin – the **brain–penis connection**.
■ Any interference with that connection, or damage to the penile nerves themselves, can result in too little blood getting into the penis to bring about erection (or only a limp erection). Alternatively, once in the penis, the blood necessary to maintain turgidity can simply seep away through leaky valves.
■ It also has to be said that, if the arteries bringing blood into the penis get clogged up, there's insufficient blood to stretch the corpus cavernosum and expand the penis, so erection will be a pretty half-hearted affair. This could happen to any man who has hardening of the arteries.
■ Given the importance of the brain in the complicated circuit of an erection it's not surprising that emotional or psychological disturbance can interfere with a man's potency.

Given this interaction of the brain, the nerves and a healthy blood supply, it isn't difficult to see how the complicated mechanism of erection could go wrong. And go wrong it will, if anything damages either the health of the nerves and arteries of the penis.

WHAT ARE THE CAUSES?
ACCIDENTS
Any accident that involves a **fractured penis** could, theoretically, cause impotence, either by damaging nerves, arteries, and veins, or by causing scars to form when injuries heal that distort the normal anatomy.

SURGERY
It's estimated that roughly **half of all men having a radical prostatectomy for cancer** will end up with a degree of impotence, in some due to nerve damage, in some due to scarring, and in some due to leakage of blood away from the penis in veins that form as the result of surgery. In other prostate surgeries, the incidence of impotence is 1 to 10 percent.

So, if you're contemplating having surgery for prostate troubles, ask your surgeon about his record of postoperative impotence.

Drugs that can cause impotence

Sleeping pills and tranquilizers
- Phenothiazines: sedatives, antinausea medications
- Benzodiazepines: tranquilizers and sleeping pills
- Lithium – antimanic drug

Antidepressants
- Tricyclic antidepressants, e.g. amitriptyline
- Monoamine oxidase inhibitors (MAOIs)

Almost all antihypertensives for high blood pressure and some heart drugs
- Digoxin ■ Diuretics (water pills)
- Beta blockers ■ ACE inhibitors

Endocrine drugs
- Antiandrogens ■ Estrogens

Cholesterol-lowering drugs
- Statins ■ Fibrates

Any drugs used to treat an enlarged prostate gland

Others
- Cimetidine – antiulcer drug
- Phenytoin – antiepileptic drug
- Carbamazepine – antithyroid drug

Recreational drugs
- Alcohol ■ Nicotine ■ Marijuana
- Amphetamines ■ Barbiturates

RADIATION THERAPY
Radical radiation therapy treatment for cancer of the prostate, bladder, or rectum can lead to impotence. The radiation therapy probably causes damage to the penile nerves.

INFECTIONS
Any virus has the potential to cause nerve damage, anywhere. But some viruses seem to go for the nerves supplying the penis. The most common ones are the **mumps virus** and the virus of **mononucleosis**. Recovery may take 1–2 years but impotence may be permanent.

DYSFUNCTION OF THE PENILE NERVES
- **Diabetes** causes nerve damage and doesn't spare the penis. Impotence is common in diabetes.
- **Multiple sclerosis** causes patchy inflammation of the nerves – sometimes in the penis, which can lead to impotence.
- **Motor neuron disease** and a stroke can also damage penile nerves.

HARDENING OF THE ARTERIES (ATHEROSCLEROSIS)
If you have **hardening of the arteries** then the arteries supplying your penis are hardened too and you could experience impotence. Warning signs are: **angina**, **high blood pressure**, **kidney disease**.

LIFESTYLE
The mildest impotence is made worse by heavy smoking and heavy drinking.

WHAT IS THE TREATMENT?
Doctors divide impotence into two main categories. First, men who have never been able to produce a satisfactory erection, and second, men who have had a good and active sex life, but who then find that they can no longer produce an adequate erection.

Men in the first category will need to seek professional help since impotence may be the expression of a **deep-seated emotional problem** that is unlikely to respond to simple measures. However, most men who complain of impotence will fall into the second category and are likely to benefit from a straightforward approach. Sometimes a couple have only to make a few lifestyle changes to see a surprising improvement.

LIFESTYLE
Time of day
Choose your moment carefully. The first important step when tackling impotence is to make sure that the man is not overly tired. Fatigue is death to an erection.

Many men find that they are able to produce an erection in the morning, but that it is quite impossible for them to do so at night. Also, it is well to remember that alcohol may well increase sexual desire, but at the same time, it reduces the capacity to produce an erection.

Reduce anxiety
It is extremely important to reduce the amount of anxiety and in the early stages, the couple should not even attempt sexual intercourse and just enjoy each other's bodies again without trying to reach orgasm. In this way, the erection will be strengthened.

Fear of failure
Often the man fears that he will not perform properly and he is overly concerned about what his partner may think of him. It is extremely helpful if the man is allowed just to concentrate all his energies on his own sexual desires instead of being overly concerned with what his partner is feeling. He should just abandon himself to his own sexual feelings, and temporarily think of nothing else at all.

A relaxing bath
It may be helpful for the couple to have a bath before attempting sexual activity, or for him to ask her to put on his favorite perfume, since smell is an extremely important aspect of sexual arousal. Some men will find that the

---

SELF-HELP

What you can do

Sexual positions
I'd like to suggest you take a fresh look at the positions you're using for intercourse. Traditionally, the missionary position has been the most popular with couples. This is where the man lies on top of his partner, supporting his weight on his arms. **For the older man,** this can be quite tiring and for the woman uncomfortable if her partner is much heavier than she is. **Lying side by side** with the man behind is probably a more suitable position since it is less tiring and also provides the opportunity for maximum manual stimulation.

Kind of lovemaking
All women know that wonderful orgasms can be achieved without penetration. If a man transfers his concern from his penis to his partner's enjoyment, he'll go a long way toward forgetting about his male obsession with erection. Concentrating on non-penetrative sex is one of the best cures for impotence.

What about complementary methods?
There are many herbal remedies that claim to help impotence. I stress the word "claim" because none of them has been really tested; most of the evidence is anecdotal. They claim to "tone up the genital tissues" or "promote healthy testosterone production" or "stimulate the circulation to the penis." This is all pseudoscience aimed at seducing you to buy the products. And they're not cheap. Most of them cost $30 or more. My advice is to save your money.

playing of soft music is helpful, others may prefer to make love in the dark. You should use any measures that are likely to increase sexual desire and remove anything likely to reduce it.

Give it time
No two men will respond to these measures in the same way, and your partner will have to be patient. It may be several weeks before you can get an adequate erection. Take your time.

ERECTION AIDS
There's a wide range of implants available, from relatively simple, rigid supports to sophisticated pumps that can inflate a tube in the penis to make it erect. These implants do not increase a man's desire for sex but they do make sex play and intercourse possible. Again, your doctor can help you here.

No matter how tempting, I wouldn't respond to newspaper advertisements. They promise the world and deliver very little.

DRUGS
In 1982 it was discovered that some drugs when injected into the penis could provoke an erection and this revolutionized the diagnosis and treatment of impotence. The latest drug,

alprostadil, relaxes the muscles in the erectile tissue of the penis, allowing increased blood flow, which is the basis of a normal erection.

Injectables
The idea of injecting the penis with anything makes me wince, but men do. Injectable alprostadil is available and it comes in a box containing a syringe with the dry, sterile powder form of the drug. The solution must be carefully prepared and the correct dose injected into the side of the penis through a very fine needle. Some discomfort is common but it's seldom troublesome. Overdosage may lead to a prolonged erection. If the erection lasts more than six hours, seek medical advice.

Pellets
Developed in the US, MUSE (medicated urethral system for erection) is a fairly new addition to the treatment of impotence. It's alprostadil in the form of a small pellet. The pellet is pushed directly into the urethra by a urethral stick – so there are no needles.

When this kind of treatment is effective, an erection generally lasts 30 to 60 minutes. Not more than two doses are recommended in 24 hours. It's available by prescription. Possible side effects include burning and bleeding.

Viagra warning
There's been a lot of hype about Viagra but the reality is quite sobering. For Viagra to work, the penis should have adequately healthy nerves and arteries. So while it may be worth a try if you have diabetes, in trials, only half the diabetic men tested had an improvement in their erections. If your pelvic nerves or pelvic arteries have been damaged by an accident or by surgery, Viagra might not perform miracles for you either; the success rate is only 40–50 percent.

In addition to normal nerves and arteries, you need to have normal sexual desire for Viagra to work. If you don't want sex, Viagra won't give you an erection.

Infertility

AS MANY AS 1 IN 6 COUPLES CONSULT THEIR DOCTOR BECAUSE OF AN INABILITY TO CONCEIVE. MOST DOCTORS WOULD FEEL THAT INVESTIGATION IS CALLED FOR IF NO PREGNANCY OCCURS AFTER A YEAR OF REGULAR, UNPROTECTED SEXUAL INTERCOURSE.

That, of itself, isn't a cause for gloom – most couples who are infertile after trying for a year do eventually conceive a child.

In addition, fertility isn't always a straightforward case of being able, or unable, to conceive.

WHAT ARE THE CAUSES?
Of all the cases of infertility, about 40 percent are due to the man, about 30 percent are due to the woman and about 20 percent are the result of combined factors. Ten percent remain unexplained.

Female infertility has been studied for years by gynecologists, whereas the study of male fertility, known as andrology, is relatively new.

Given the ready availability of sperm, however, **a semen analysis should always be the first investigation of infertility**. This includes a sperm count and tests the motility and quality of sperm.

Remember, infertility should **always be investigated as a couple – the fertility of a couple is the sum of their individual fertilities**.

MALE INFERTILITY
■ **Hormonal problems.** The brain sex hormones (gonadotrophins) of a man, luteinizing hormone (LH) and follicle-stimulating hormone (FSH), need to be in balance for sperm to be produced.
■ **Anatomical problems** with the penis or testicles, or the man's ability to ejaculate, can affect fertility.
■ **Immunological problems**, when a man's immune system produces antibodies that attack and destroy his sperm, reducing their ability to fertilize an egg.
■ **Decreasing sperm counts.** Studies suggest that sperm counts decreased over the course of the 20th century, due to environmental factors such as exposure to estrogens in foodstuffs and indestructible chemicals such as polychlorinated biphenyls (PCBs), used in the plastics industry, that enter the food chain. But, despite lower numbers of sperm, **actual fertility remains unaffected**, presumably because sperm are produced in such excessive numbers. **Smoking**, **alcohol,** and **stress** lower the quantity and quality of sperm. **Coffee** and

social drugs may produce abnormal sperm.

FEMALE INFERTILITY
Female infertility has many different causes such as the **inability to ovulate**, **endometriosis**, **blocked fallopian tubes**, **ovarian cysts,** or an **abnormal uterus**. A woman's **cervical mucus** may also be hostile to her partner's sperm.

When a woman's fertility is marginal, as when ovulation is irregular, it's known as subfertility. Usually this only becomes a problem if her partner's fertility is also marginal – if a man has a low to average sperm count, for instance – because subfertility in one partner can be balanced by strong fertility in the other.

HORMONAL PROBLEMS
About one-third of female infertility is due to a **failure to ovulate**. Ovulation is controlled by the same finely orchestrated release of hormones that controls the menstrual cycle. If the precise reason for a failure to ovulate can be pinpointed, it can be treated using synthetic hormones (fertility drugs).

A hormonal imbalance can result in two problems:

1. The ovary fails to produce properly mature follicles in which the ova can develop fully.

2. A slightly different hormonal imbalance can mean that, although the ovum matures, the ovary isn't triggered to release it.

Deep in the brains of both men and women, the **hypothalamus** is responsible for sending signals to the pituitary gland, which then sends hormonal messages to the ovaries and testicles triggering them to produce ova and sperm. A malfunctioning **hypothalamus**, therefore, may result in infertility of both men and women.

A malfunctioning **pituitary gland** – underactive, overactive, or injured in some way – may not produce the precise amount of follicle-stimulating hormone (FSH) and luteinizing hormone (LH) necessary for normal ovulation and sperm production.

REPRODUCTIVE ORGAN PROBLEMS
Ovaries
In addition to hormonal problems, the ovaries may be affected by **cysts**, **past surgery**, **radiation,** or **chemotherapy**, and **lifestyle** factors such as smoking (passive smoking too).

Fallopian tubes
About 50 percent of infertile women have blocked fallopian tubes. Healthy fallopian tubes are essential for conception because they're the pathways that allow the ovum and sperm to meet and fuse, and then enable the resulting fertilized ovum to reach the uterus. The fallopian tubes usually become blocked because of **pelvic inflammation** from an STD infection such as **chlamydia**. They're extremely delicate structures and it's difficult for them to be made fully functional once damaged.

Uterus
Uterine problems account for 10 percent of all cases of female infertility and may be due to fibroids or an abnormally shaped uterus. Other, more rare, uterine problems

Reasons for female infertility

Primary reason	Frequency	Causes	Results
FAILURE TO OVULATE	30 percent	• Underactive pituitary gland • Polycystic ovary syndrome	• No ova • Ova not maturing • Mature ova not able to be released
PROBLEMS WITH TRANSPORT OF OVA	50 percent	• Abnormalities of fallopian tubes, pelvic disease, or surgery • Endometriosis	• Ova cannot reach uterus
UTERINE PROBLEMS	10 percent	• Fibroids • Abnormally shaped uterus • Adhesions in uterus	• Fertilized ovum unable to develop properly

include polyps and internal adhesions that make the walls of the uterus stick together. The majority of these problems can be treated successfully.

Fibroids
Fibroids, benign muscle tumors of the uterine wall, don't necessarily affect fertility. 1 in 5 women over the age of 30 has them, and 1 in 3 women over 35, but many conceive nonetheless.

Cervix
Cervical mucus that is hostile to sperm may play a part in infertility.

INVESTIGATING THE PROBLEM
The investigation of infertility may try your patience and resolve. It may even humiliate you. Whichever partner is found to have low fertility will feel threatened and guilty. Be prepared to be long-suffering and very generous. And please see a counselor affiliated with your fertility doctor's office if offered.

Tracking down the cause of infertility proceeds logically.

PART ONE: YOUR DOCTOR
One couple in six consults their doctor about infertility. Your doctor first assesses how healthy you both are and will ask about your sex life.

The woman will be asked for dates of her last six periods to establish she's menstruating regularly.

If further investigation is needed, the couple will be referred to a fertility specialist and further tests will be done there.

PART TWO: A SPECIAL FERTILITY CLINIC
Women may be asked to keep an ovulation temperature chart and will have a blood test to check that ovulation has occurred. Men will have tests too. You can expect the following steps to be taken.

■ **Checking on ovulation:** If your doctor suspects there's a problem with ovulation, you'll be tested for the level of **progesterone in your blood on day 21 of a 28-day cycle**, or seven days before an expected period if your cycles are usually shorter or longer than 28 days. This is because progesterone levels rise after ovulation and a high level will indicate that if you're ovulating. You may be asked to keep a record of your basal body temperature (BBT) each morning for several cycles. Ovulation prediction kits can also be useful.

■ **The man is asked to provide a semen sample.**

■ **If a man's sperm are normal**, the woman

Ovulation chart

cycle in which ovulation occurs

anovulatory cycle

Basal body temperature (BBT) drops sharply before ovulation occurs and rises sharply afterward. Keeping a chart helps track ovulation.

Secondary infertility

The term secondary infertility applies if a woman already has a child but is unable to conceive another. The problem may be caused by an infection of the fallopian tubes, which are particularly vulnerable to STDs such as chlamydia, but may also be due to failure to ovulate or may be unexplained.

will then be offered an **ultrasound scan** and possibly **laparoscopy** if she's ovulating.

Once the cause of infertility is pinpointed an appropriate treatment will be suggested.

CHECKING MALE INFERTILITY
SPERM ASSESSMENT

Your doctor will arrange for preliminary tests on your semen before making more detailed investigations of your fertility. The semen samples are examined by a trained technician, using a microscope and a computer assisted semen motility analyzer.

Sperm tests

Sperm tests are performed to assess whether your sperm appear normal and are capable of swimming to and penetrating your partner's egg.

■ In the **sperm invasion test** the interaction between your sperm and your partner's cervical mucus is examined under a microscope. If sperm are unable to cross into the mucus or cannot move through it properly, the finding doesn't itself indicate whether the problem lies with the sperm or the mucus.

■ The **crossover sperm invasion test** is performed to answer that question. This uses exactly the same procedure as the sperm invasion test – but first, your sperm and normal mucus from a donor female will be used, and second, the normal sperm from a donor male will be combined with your partner's mucus.

These may reveal the problem but, if not, further tests such as the egg penetration test may be necessary.

■ The **egg penetration test** examines the potential of sperm to fertilize an egg. The test involves introducing the sperm to hamster eggs (yes, I know it sounds strange, but read on) and measuring how well the sperm penetrate and fuse with them.

The use of hamster eggs means that your partner doesn't have to go through stressful IVF treatment in order to provide eggs for testing. There's no danger of an embryo resulting from the fusion of sperm and hamster eggs.

CHECKING FEMALE INFERTILITY
LAPAROSCOPY

A slender telescope that's equipped with fiber optics, a laparoscope is about the width of a pen.

It can be inserted through a tiny incision in the navel to view the abdominal cavity directly.

In addition to offering the surgeon a superb view of the organs, high-quality videos can be taken through the laparoscope for later reference.

Laparoscopy allows the condition of the reproductive organs to be assessed under direct vision. The procedure is often timed for

the second half of the cycle to confirm that ovulation has occurred.

HYSTEROSALPINGOGRAPHY

Hysterosalpingography (HSG) is usually reserved for women found to have damaged fallopian tubes, or if doctors suspect there's something wrong with the uterus – say, a cyst.

HSG is an X-ray picture of the uterus and tubes and can show problems within the cavity of the womb and within the tubes.

Dye is useful for checking the fallopian tubes since it will only enter and travel through open tubes, thus showing any damage, distortion, or complete blockage. The injected dye is monitored on an X-ray screen. Ultrasound may be used to do a similar test since it does not expose the ovaries to X-rays.

ENDOMETRIAL BIOPSY

In this procedure a tiny amount of the endometrium (uterine lining) is removed and then examined for any changes.

An endometrial biopsy is performed in order to assess whether a woman's hormones are bringing about normal alterations to her endometrium during the second half of her cycle in preparation for conception.

When the hormones are balanced correctly, there's an increase in the production of progesterone, which thickens the endometrium.

If progesterone is being underproduced, the uterine lining won't develop sufficiently for an embryo to implant. If there's little or no alteration, then fertility drugs are an option.

ULTRASOUND SCANNING

Ultrasound scanning is used to check the development of ovarian follicles, so that doctors can track the growth of follicles and the release of the ovum or ova at ovulation.

WHAT IS THE TREATMENT?

Though you're desperate for a baby, if you're a candidate for fertility treatment of any kind, try to be rational and balanced. Get the success rate for any treatment from your doctors so that your expectations are reasonable.

Some treatments involve complicated regimens that will test your emotional and physical stamina. As a couple, you're going to have to be strong, so take advantage of any counseling service attached to your fertility clinic.

FERTILITY DRUGS
Step one

A woman's ovaries can nearly always be encouraged to produce good-quality eggs using fertility drugs, so when failure to ovulate is the reason for female infertility, fertility drugs are the usual treatment.

■ The most common fertility drug is clomiphene, which is taken for five days

at the beginning of each menstrual cycle.

■ Clomiphene stimulates the release of follicle-stimulating hormone (FSH) by the pituitary gland. This acts on the ovaries and often initiates the ripening of a follicle and then ovulation.

■ Clomiphene's advantages are that it's free from major side effects and has a low multiple pregnancy rate – only 5–10 percent – usually twins and occasionally triplets; quadruplets and quintuplets are now very rare because we know so much more about the correct dosage.

■ Clomiphene is an **antiestrogen** (the drug was first developed as a contraceptive), so it may impede conception if prescribed inappropriately.

Step two

If clomiphene fails, it's usual to try daily injections of human menopausal gonadotrophin (hMG), which is similar in action and effect to FSH, followed by an injection of **human chorionic gonadotrophin** (hCG).

This complicated treatment requires close monitoring of the ovaries with blood tests and daily ultrasounds in order to avoid the risk of multiple pregnancy. Some women require even more complex medical management in order to achieve ovulation.

OTHER METHODS
Artificial insemination

In this procedure, a partner's sperm (artificial insemination by husband, or AIH) or a donor's sperm (artificial insemination donor, or AID) is introduced into the cervix from a syringe. Insemination is done just before or during ovulation.

DI may be considered when a man has a very low sperm count, is sterile, or is known to be a carrier of a hereditary abnormality (see Sperm donation, below).

Single women who want a baby also consider DI. There are no legal barriers preventing single women in the US from becoming mothers through donor insemination. Women in other countries, though, may face obstacles.

Sperm donation

The best sperm donor is your partner, but, if not, sperm donors should be healthy, fertile men who have children of their own.

All sperm is screened for infectious diseases, such as AIDS, and all donors are asked about their genetic family background.

Clinics also try to match the donor's physical characteristics to those of the couple but, because a different donor's sperm is usually used at every attempt, the closest match may not be the one that actually results in pregnancy.

Egg donation

More complicated than sperm donation, this involves the female donor using fertility drugs so that her ovaries will be stimulated to produce several ova at once.

A couple of trips to the fertility clinic will be necessary and perhaps an overnight stay when the ova are collected. For this reason, many ovum donors are women who are undergoing in vitro fertilization (IVF).

The degree of medical data that is archived on each donor varies from state to state, as does its availability to the resulting child.

In vitro fertilization (IVF)

For IVF to work, two things are necessary.

1. Eggs from the female partner, if necessary harvested after clomiphene or hMG/hCG treatment.

2. Sperm from the male partner, if necessary isolated microscopically from a specimen of semen or the testicles themselves.

Both, of course, can be obtained from donors (see opposite).

Children conceived by IVF used to be known as test-tube babies. IVF was pioneered by British doctors Patrick Steptoe and Robert Edwards in 1978, when the very first IVF baby, Louise Brown, was born.

Since 1981, more than 45,000 IVF babies have been born in the US. Although this figure sounds high, IVF only has about a 20 percent success rate per cycle of treatment, although it can be as high as 30 percent under the best circumstances. Everyone contemplating IVF should know that it's physically and emotionally very demanding and stressful. You should always have **counseling** before and during IVF if it's available at your IVF clinic.

1. Once her partner's sperm have been tested for viability, the woman is given fertility drugs to stimulate her ovaries into producing ova.

She's then carefully monitored using ultrasound until the follicles are ripe, when the ova will be collected by her gynecologist using laparoscopy.

2. A long hollow needle will be inserted through the upper vagina or the abdominal wall to reach the ovaries, under constant monitoring with ultrasound.

The ova are gently suctioned out of the follicles into the probe, transferred to a culture medium in a petri dish, and then stored in an incubator, where they continue to grow.

3. Once they have reached full maturity (within 2–24 hours), the sperm are introduced. Fertilization usually occurs within 18 hours.

The fertilized ova are then kept inside the incubator for an additional 48 hours, by which time each will have divided into about four cells.

A maximum of three embryos can then be transferred into the woman's uterus. Additional embryos can be stored.

GIFT and ZIFT

Gamete intrafallopian transfer (GIFT) and zygote intrafallopian transfer (ZIFT) are two variations on IVF. In GIFT, the egg and sperm (both medically known as gametes) are transferred to one of the woman's fallopian tubes, where conception may then take place naturally. In ZIFT, the fertilized egg (medically known as a zygote) is transferred to one of the fallopian tubes before it has begun to grow into an embryo. There seems to be a slightly higher chance that an embryo will implant in the uterine wall if it travels down the fallopian tube at the correct time in a woman's cycle as it would if conception had occurred naturally. For both of these procedures, a woman must have at least one open and undamaged fallopian tube. Pregnancy success rates for GIFT and ZIFT are thought to be about 25–30 percent per cycle.

ICSI

Intracytoplasmic sperm injection (ICSI) is a new technique, not available everywhere, allowing a man with a very low sperm count to father a baby.

Sperm are sucked up into a syringe and, under a microscope, are injected into a harvested ovum to fertilize it. After 48 hours of incubation, the resulting embryo is replaced in the woman's body using the procedure for IVF.

TEST

Ultrasound scanning

Ultrasound scanning is a way of producing a photographic picture by using sound waves. The picture is formed by the echoes of sound waves bouncing off different parts of the body. The echoes differ in their waves according to the density of the organ. Ultrasound scanning can give pictures of soft tissue in great detail. If it is done during pregnancy, it will show fetal heartbeat and movement and can be used as a noninvasive means of examining the fetus. An accurate picture of the fetus in utero may be printed out.

Ultrasound is used in many areas of medicine as a diagnostic tool, particularly to detect breast lumps and the cause of abdominal pains, such as gallstones or hiatus hernia. It can also sometimes be used to treat abnormalities. For example, high levels of ultrasound waves can destroy stones in the bladder. Ultrasound scanning is also used widely in fertility treatment and to tell whether a pregnancy is viable or not.

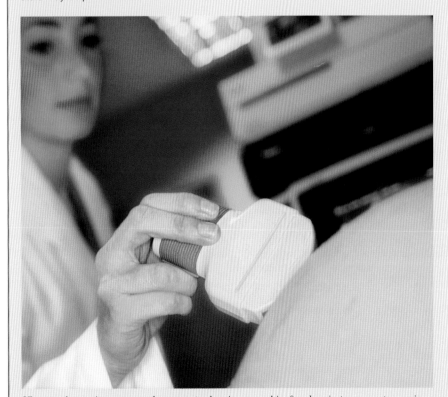

Ultrasound scanning uses sound waves to produce images and is often done in pregnancy to examine the fetus. The procedure is quick and painless and does not involve exposure to radiation.

SEXUAL HEALTH

The group of diseases classed as sexually transmitted are those that are passed on primarily by sexual contact between people. Many people delay seeking treatment for these diseases because of embarrassment, but if you suspect that either you or your partner are suffering from a sexually transmitted disease (STD), it's essential to seek help from your doctor, state department of health, or family planning clinic as soon as you can.

I begin with chlamydia, an STD that's on the rise and is especially dangerous because it can rob a woman of her fertility if not treated promptly. Next I cover yeast, which affects many people and is not necessarily sexually transmitted. Then come genital herpes and genital warts, followed by bacterial vaginosis and trichomoniasis. Syphilis and gonorrhea are also covered. I also discuss the importance of safe sex in preventing STDs.

Chlamydia

CHLAMYDIA IS THE MOST COMMON BACTERIAL SEXUALLY TRANSMITTED INFECTION AND IT'S ON THE RISE. THE ESTIMATED NUMBER OF NEW CASES OF CHLAMYDIA IN THE US IS OVER THREE MILLION EACH YEAR.

Rates have been consistently higher in women than men, and particularly in those aged 16–24. Part of this increase is due to new diagnostic methods and publicity, which mean that more people are being screened and seeking care. Up to 70 percent of women and at least 25 percent of men infected with chlamydia have no symptoms, so a substantial number of infections remain undiagnosed and untreated. Where there are symptoms, **women** may have discharge, pain when passing urine, heavy periods, or bleeding between periods, low abdominal pain, or abdominal pain during vaginal sex. **Men** may notice discharge from the penis and/or burning when passing urine.

New methods of testing for chlamydia are now available that will allow easier and more widespread detection and treatment. Chlamydia is the most frequenty reported infectious disease in the US. An estimated three million cases occur annually with teenage girls having the highest rate of infection.

HOW IS CHLAMYDIA PASSED ON?
Chlamydia is almost always transmitted through vaginal or anal sex, and very occasionally through oral-genital contact. Occasionally a pregnant woman can pass the infection to her baby. In this case infection is usually limited to the eyes, but can rarely cause pneumonia.

HOW DOES CHLAMYDIA HARM YOU?
After infection with chlamydia, the fine hairs that waft the fertilized egg down the fallopian tube to the uterus, can be destroyed. This sets the scene for tubal or ectopic pregnancy.

The rate of ectopic pregnancy in the US increased fivefold since 1970, but deaths from ectopic pregnancy are decreasing. The damage can also set up tubal inflammation, swelling,

Who should be tested for chlamydia?

- All sexually active women under 25 and women over 25 with a new sexual partner.
- Those with more than two sexual partners a year.
- All men and women attending STD clinics: nearly 1 in 5 has chlamydia.
- Women seeking termination of pregnancy: nearly 1 in 10 has chlamydia.

and complete blockage of the tubes, though why this develops in some women and not others isn't known. **Teenagers** are more vulnerable to this bacterial attack, threatening the fertility of future generations of mothers.

LONG-TERM EFFECTS
Chlamydia infection in women has serious fall-out. Untreated infections can persist for a long time and up to one-third of inadequately treated women may go on to develop **pelvic inflammatory disease**.

Up to half of all cases of pelvic inflammatory disease can be attributed to chlamydia.

Among women with pelvic inflammatory disease, **one-fifth** may become infertile, and one-tenth will go on to have an ectopic pregnancy once they conceive. So the personal and economic costs of untreated chlamydia infection are considerable.

SCREENING
Given the prevalence of chlamydia and the long-term effects of infection, could women be screened for its presence so cases are caught

and treated early before lasting damage has been done?

The first trial of chlamydia screening in women aged 18–34 in the US showed that pelvic inflammatory disease was 56 percent lower in screened and treated women than in those who were unscreened. All women and men with a discharge should therefore be tested for chlamydia. Since this infection is often without symptoms, those who have frequent partner changes should also be tested.

LATEST TESTS FOR CHLAMYDIA
At one time chlamydia was notoriously elusive to track down but tests are becoming more sophisticated with increasing use of **DNA urine check**; there is even talk of a future test being available over the counter. Anyone can request a test at an STD clinic or at their doctor's office.

CHLAMYDIA – THE FERTILITY TIME BOMB
Often neglected by patients and doctors alike, chlamydia infection may not be life threatening but it can be life ruining. It has come to be known as the fertility time bomb, capable of lurking silently for years before causing irreparable damage.

CARRIERS OF CHLAMYDIA
Because chlamydia is virtually symptomless in men, they can carry the disease without knowing. Male carriers can reinfect women and keep a chronic low-grade infection simmering even after a woman has had antibiotics. This means that if chlamydia is found in a woman, her partner(s) must be treated too.

See also:
- Pelvic inflammatory disease p. 251

FOCUS *on* vaginal yeast

Vaginal yeast (thrush) is inflammation of the vagina caused by the candida fungus. Yeast is a very common, not to mention miserable, problem. Three-quarters of all women will get yeast at some stage in their lives. Although the lucky ones only suffer one episode, many get it several times a year.

WHAT EVERY WOMAN SHOULD KNOW

- While yeast isn't life threatening, it can cause a lot of distress – the more you know the less it will worry you.
- As a woman, you're likely to suffer from some form of **genitourinary infection** at some point in your life. The most common infections are **yeast, cystitis,** and **bacterial vaginosis**.
- Men very often reinfect their partners because usually only women seek medical treatment.

HOW CAN I TELL IF I HAVE YEAST?

Do you have any of the following symptoms?
Women
- Itching and/or soreness in and around the entrance to the vagina.
- A thick, whitish discharge that does not smell unpleasant.
- Swelling of the labia.
- Stinging when passing urine.
- Pain during sexual intercourse.

Men
- Irritation, burning or itching under the foreskin or on the tip of the penis.
- Redness or red patches under foreskin or on the tip of the penis.
- A thick, cheesy discharge under the foreskin.
- Difficulty in pulling back the foreskin.
- Slight discharge from the penis.
- Discomfort when passing urine.

If you have any of these symptoms, see your doctor to confirm that you have a yeast infection.

Once your yeast has been diagnosed by your doctor, on future occasions you may treat yourself with an over-the-counter treatment.

The symptoms listed are experienced by some but not all sufferers. They can also be a sign of another type of infection – for example, cystitis, of which pain on passing urine is a common symptom.

HOW TO AVOID YEAST

While there's no simple solution to prevent yeast, there are a number of things you can do to prevent getting it so frequently.

- Avoid wearing pantyhose, underwear not made of cotton, leggings, Lycra shorts, and tight jeans or pants.
- Wash and wipe the genital area from front to back. You can wet a couple of clean cotton balls in water and use to wipe once and then throw them away.
- If possible, don't scratch because the fungus can be spread by hand. Any constant scratching can cause thickening of the skin and proneness to infection.
- Use sanitary pads rather than tampons during a period.
- Avoid perfumed soaps, genital sprays, and deodorants and any other irritants such as disinfectants.
- If prescribed an antibiotic, remind your doctor that you tend to get yeast.
- Yeast can sometimes be passed on through sex. Even though you might be treated, you could be getting it right back again if your sexual partner isn't getting treatment as well. While you're on any treatment for yeast, it's not advisable to have sex until given the all-clear.
- Since the fungus likes warm, moist conditions, folds of fat around the groin may be the reason for recurrent infections. If you're overweight it might help to shed some of those extra pounds.
- Although any man can carry yeast, all uncircumcized men should clean under their foreskins as part of their daily routine.

> **See also:**
> • Bacterial vaginosis p. 283 • Candidiasis p. 450 • Cystitis p. 378

Common myths

THE MYTH: Yeast is a sexually transmitted disease that affects women who have poor personal hygiene or who are promiscuous. **The facts:** Vaginal yeast is NOT necessarily a sexually transmitted disease – it results from an imbalance of bacteria and yeasts in the vagina. The imbalance can allow one type of yeast, *Candida albicans,* to breed faster than usual and this can cause yeast. The imbalance that can lead to yeast can be caused by many things, such as hormonal changes experienced during menstruation, in pregnancy and at menopause. Other common triggers are **antibiotics** and **poorly controlled diabetes, disinfectant** in the bath, and **vaginal deodorants**. Being a yeast sufferer does not mean you're "dirty" – in fact being overzealous with douching can upset the natural balance in the vagina and start an episode of yeast. Men can get yeast as well.

THE MYTH: Yeast has to be treated by a doctor and requires an internal examination and questions about your sex life. **The facts:** If this is your first bout of yeast, you should visit your doctor to confirm that yeast is the problem. Your doctor may take samples from the vagina to check for infection. If you're getting recurrent episodes of yeast, your doctor may test you for diabetes and HIV. If you've had yeast before, had a diagnosis from a doctor and recognize the symptoms, you may find it easier and more convenient to use an over-the-counter treatment.

THE MYTH: All yeast treatments involve either suppositories or creams, which have to be inserted into the vagina. **The facts:** Treatment can be by insertion of a **suppository** or **cream** into the vagina, but oral treatments have been available from the doctor for more than eight years and this form of treatment is preferred by many women. Home remedies such as **live yogurt** applied to the vagina are NOT proven cures for yeast. If any treatment causes soreness, stop using it immediately.

Safe sex

- Safe sex helps protect you from STDs and HIV/AIDS.
- Safe sex means being responsible about sex.
- Always practice safe sex; nothing less will do.

Condoms and STDs

In order for sex to be safe from STDs, you should always use a condom for vaginal and anal sex – for oral sex too if you're worried about HIV (but HIV infection from oral sex is rare). Make sure that you know how to use one properly, and never use condoms from expired packages. Practice safe sex; think carefully about your sexual behavior.

Your rights

Demanding safe sex is your right. If your partner resents this, he or she is not thinking about you, and you should question your relationship. If your partner won't use a condom, refuse to have sex, and consider ending the relationship. By acting irresponsibly he or she puts you in danger.

Preventing pregnancy too

While condoms are great for safe sex, don't rely on them alone to prevent pregnancy. Semen can leak if you haven't managed to use the condom correctly, or if you've used an expired one. It's best for women to either be on the pill or to use a diaphragm as well.

Getting help...

Your doctor or family planning clinic will gladly give you information on condoms. A whole variety of condoms is available, and some of them have been designed to make sex a little more interesting! Condoms are available from retail outlets, supermarkets, pharmacies, and even public bathrooms. You can get advice on safe sex practices from AIDS organizations, hospitals, and gay helplines (see Useful addresses, p. 567).

Next time...

Don't drop your guard for a second; always practice safe sex. You want to be able to relax when you have sex; you don't want to have to worry about pregnancy and STDs.

Dos and Don'ts

Carry a condom

Do carry a condom with you at all times, women as well as men.

Practice first

Do make sure you know how to use a condom before you have sex with someone.

Condoms every time

Do use a condom until you're absolutely sure there's no risk to or from your partner.

Be frank

Do be open when you start a relationship. Tell your partner about any chronic infections, such as herpes.

Once only

Don't ever try to use a condom more than once.

No casual sex

Don't have sex with someone at a party, or on vacation, whom you hardly know and may never meet again.

How do I protect myself?

Try saying something like this:

1. Talking to a partner:
"My ex has sent me a card...no, not for my birthday – it says he's got something nasty and I might have caught it. So that could include you too. We'd better go to the STD clinic and get this sorted out."

But your partner may not know he or she has an STD so...

2. Going for a checkup:
"Contraception's figured out – but why don't we both get a checkup?"
"Okay. Good idea. Let's call the doctor or clinic."

3. Using a condom for protection:
If he says: "You don't think I'd wear one of those,..." tell him:
"You obviously haven't looked at some of them recently."

A condom will protect you from infection, and the pill will protect you from pregnancy.

Genital herpes

HERPES SIMPLEX IS THE NAME OF A VIRUS THAT CAN CAUSE COLD SORES OR GENITAL SORES, DEPENDING ON WHICHEVER PART OF SKIN IS INFECTED.

Herpes is called a cold sore on the face but you can get it on the genitals or anywhere else. Cold sores are often due to a mother passing on the virus to her children through kissing. In genital herpes the virus is transmitted through infected skin coming into contact with a partner's skin – for example, during sex or from mouth to genitals during oral sex. It's more common in women because their genital areas are warmer and moister than men's.

WHAT ARE THE CAUSES?
■ Genital herpes was originally thought to be caused only by the **herpes simplex virus type 2**, while cold sores on the lips were thought more likely to be due to **herpes simplex type 1**. However, with the increase in oral sex this distinction has become blurred.
■ In Europe, genital herpes infection is the most common cause of genital ulceration and it's increasing among women.

HOW COMMON IS GENITAL HERPES?
Blood tests show that most of us have been exposed to the **herpes simplex** virus by the time we reach middle age. Millions of people are infected with the virus but probably only one-quarter of those infected have symptoms of any kind. Many people have what is called a **subclinical attack** – with no visible signs of infection and no ill effects. These people don't know they've been infected.

WHAT HAPPENS TO THE VIRUS?
Once in the body, the virus can retreat to nerve cells near the base of the spine. If the virus is reactivated, it can return to where it entered the body and cause a recurrence. Not all people have recurrences; some have a few and for some the problem recurs from time to time. Usually the initial outbreak is the most severe.

HOW INFECTIOUS IS IT?
As you'd expect, genital herpes is highly contagious. New research indicates that the

virus can also be transmitted by people who don't have any symptoms. Symptoms appear between three and seven days after sexual contact with an infected partner.

WHAT ARE THE SYMPTOMS?
■ The genital skin feels overly sensitive to the touch.
■ Itching and irritation around the genitals.
■ A general feeling of being unwell.
■ Headache.
■ Muscle aches and joint pains.
■ Abdominal pain.
■ Shooting pain in the lower limbs.
■ Enlarged tender glands in the groin.
■ Pain on passing urine.
■ Blisters appear within a few hours, enlarge, burst, and become painful ulcers within two or three days.
■ The ulcers form scabs and take 14–21 days to heal completely.

WHAT ARE THE TRIGGERS FOR GENITAL HERPES?
Recurrences don't depend on having intercourse with an infected partner. Outbreaks can be triggered by:
● physical and mental stress
● excessive cold or heat, including fever
● irritation of delicate genital tissues
● local genital trauma (e.g. rough sexual intercourse, plucking, or shaving pubic hair)
● general ill health and other infections such as a cold causing fever
● the time of menses.

WHAT IS THE TREATMENT?
■ Genital herpes should always be looked at by a doctor and not treated by yourself at home.
■ See your doctor immediately if you feel numb or sensitive in the genital area or if you've had sexual relations with anyone with the herpes virus.
■ There's no cure for genital herpes but the sooner treatment is given the more likely it will prevent or ameliorate an attack. Antiviral drugs, such as **acyclovir**, taken orally make the ulcers less painful and encourage healing if taken early in the attack.
■ Other remedies include bathing the area with salt solution (a heaping teaspoon of salt to three cups of water).

SELF-HELP
■ Always use a condom to protect yourself from genital herpes.
■ Painful blisters can be relieved by a soak in a lukewarm bath with salt added and cold

NEVER!

Once you have got herpes it's for life, so here are a few nevers:
NEVER have sex if you have symptoms, except with the person from whom you got it (or whom you gave it to). When both partners have the same virus they don't reinfect each other.
NEVER have unprotected sex with a relative stranger.
NEVER have oral-genital sex if you have a cold sore.
NEVER be dishonest about your herpes. It's best to be open about herpes simplex and tell your partner. And you must avoid skin contact when the virus is active. It may be easier to explain that you sometimes get cold sores on your genitals.
NEVER be shy about telling your doctor about possible contacts.

Genital herpes and pregnancy
If you or your partner has had an outbreak of genital herpes, it should be recorded on your medical notes, but you should still tell your doctor if you have or have had herpes. Swabs during the last stage of pregnancy are no longer thought necessary since we now know that the delay in getting the results makes it pointless. cesarean sections are rarely performed except when the mother is experiencing a primary infection. A mother's antibodies protect her baby from becoming infected during birth.

packs (not ice) applied to the infected area.
■ To prevent genital herpes from recurring get plenty of rest and eat a balanced diet with nutritional foodstuffs – fresh fruit and vegetables, whole foods and plenty of liquids.
■ Manage stress by learning relaxation exercises or taking up yoga.
■ Wear loose underwear so air can circulate and keep your genitals cool. Leave the sores exposed to air as much as possible.
■ Keep a record of when you get recurrent outbreaks in an attempt to find a pattern. If, for example, recurrences are related to rough sex, try using a lubricant such as KY jelly.

WARNING:
The herpes virus MAY have a role in indicating cervical cancer, so women who have had genital herpes should have a Pap smear regularly, preferably every year usually performed at annual gynecological checkups.

See also:
• **Herpes simplex p. 336**

Genital warts

GENITAL WARTS, LIKE WARTS ON THE HANDS OR FEET, ARE CAUSED BY A VIRUS,
IN THIS CASE THE HUMAN PAPILLOMA VIRUS (HPV).

Genital warts grow in and around the entrance of the vagina and the anus and on the penis. They can be transmitted sexually or they can just grow in the genital area much as they grow on other parts of the body. Genital warts can be as tiny as pin heads or take on a distinctly cauliflower-like appearance.

A man may not actually know that he has a wart because it may be hidden inside the urethral opening, and a woman can have a wart deep inside the vagina which she doesn't know about. There may be an interval of up to 18 months between infection and the appearance of the warts. You shouldn't automatically assume you have caught them from a recent sexual contact.

Warts are spread through skin-to-skin contact. If you have sex or genital contact with someone who has genital warts you may develop them too. Not everyone who comes into contact with the virus will develop warts. As with all infections, the immune system plays an important role, so if this is depressed in any way (for example during pregnancy, due to HIV, or to generally being run down), the warts can be difficult to treat.

WHAT ARE THE SYMPTOMS?

■ Genital warts may occur singly or in groups; an individual may have dozens of warts or just one or two.
■ They may itch but are usually painless.
■ Often there are no other symptoms and the warts may be difficult to see.
■ In women, warts can develop inside the vagina and on the cervix; warts on the cervix may cause slight bleeding or, very rarely, an

unusual colored vaginal discharge.
■ In men, warts on the scrotum or shaft of the penis usually resemble the ordinary warts that occur on the hands.
■ Under the foreskin and around the anal area, they are usually a shiny pinkish white.
■ A doctor or nurse can usually tell whether you have genital just warts by looking. If warts are suspected but not obvious, the doctor may apply a weak vinegar-like solution to the outside of the genital area. This turns any warts white.

GENITAL WARTS AND CERVICAL CANCER

In women, an association between the human papilloma virus (HPV) and the development of **cancer of the cervix** has been established. Cervical cancer is more common in women who suffer from HPV than in the rest of the population. It is extremely important for any woman who has either suffered from genital warts herself or has had unprotected sex with a man with genital warts to have regular Pap smears.

SAFETY FIRST

■ Go to your doctor or nearest STD clinic for a diagnosis and treatment.
■ Avoid sexual intercourse or use condoms for 12 weeks after the warts have gone.
■ Condoms will only protect against the wart virus if they cover all the affected areas.
■ As with herpes, genital warts can be transmitted through nonpenetrative sex if areas on the outside of the genitals are affected.

WHAT IS THE TREATMENT?

You should never try to treat genital warts yourself. There are a number of different treatments and the choice depends on a number of factors, including the appearance and site of the warts. Not all treatments work all the time and your doctor may need to select an alternative after the first. Many of these treatments kill the cells that are infected with the virus, leaving small sores that eventually heal up.

PODOPHYLLOTOXIN SOLUTION AND PODOPHYLLOTOXIN CREAM (WARTICON)
This treatment can be applied in the doctor's office or at home by the patient. A typical course of treatment lasts up to four weeks.

PODOPHYLLIN SOLUTION
This treatment has to be administered by clinical staff. It must be washed off by the

individual within four hours because it is toxic and can irritate the surrounding skin if left in contact for too long.

TCA (TRICHLOROACETIC ACID)
This is a caustic chemical applied to the warts by the clinic staff.

IMMUNE RESPONSE MODIFIERS (ALDARA)
These enhance the immune system's ability to fight the virus responsible for genital warts.

CRYOTHERAPY
This procedure involves freezing the warts with liquid nitrogen by clinical staff. This kills the cells in the wart and some of the surrounding skin.

CAUTERIZING (HYFRECATION)
This involves burning of the warts by clinical staff with an electrically heated probe, after numbing the area with local anesthetic.

LASER TREATMENT
This may be done under general or local anesthetic at the doctor's office – useful for treating large warty areas. The heat of the laser kills the cells.

SURGERY
Surgical removal of warts may be done under general anesthetic in the hospital.

WHERE CAN YOU GET GENITAL WARTS TREATED?
■ Treatment is available at your doctor's office or at a local STD clinic. These clinics do not require referral from your general practitioner and offer completely confidential treatment. The telephone numbers are available from the Yellow Pages, local hospitals, and on the internet.
■ Some gynecologist may offer facilities for the diagnosis and treatment of visible genital warts.
■ Family planning clinics may also offer advice and treatment.

WORD OF WARNING
■ Don't try to treat warts in the genital area on your own with any of the wart treatments you can buy from the pharmacy. **These are for use on the hands only**.
■ Warts can disappear of their own accord. However, the problem hasn't necessarily disappeared. Since the virus can remain in the skin, warts may reccur.

General advice

Infection with the human papilloma virus is very common. Condoms offer some protection but it is best to seek advice from the clinic.
Since warts are sexually transmitted it is always worth:
• practicing safe sex
• getting a checkup to exclude other sexually transmitted infections
• ensuring that your partner is aware that you have HPV and knows what to look out for in case he/she develops genital warts
• all women ensuring they have routine Pap smears.

Bacterial vaginosis

BACTERIAL VAGINOSIS IS BACTERIAL INFECTION OF THE VAGINA THAT SOMETIMES CAUSES AN
ABNORMAL DISCHARGE. UNPROTECTED SEX WITH MULTIPLE PARTNERS IS A RISK FACTOR.

Bacterial vaginosis is caused by excess growth of some of the bacteria that normally live in the vagina, particularly *Gardnerella vaginalis* and *Mycoplasma hominis*. As a result, the natural balance of organisms in the vagina is altered. The reason for this excess growth is unknown, but the condition is more common in sexually active women and often, but not always, occurs in association with sexually transmitted diseases. Vaginal infections can also be caused by an overgrowth of the **candida fungus** and the protozoan *Trichomonas vaginalis*. Bacterial vaginosis often causes no symptoms.

However, some women may have a grayish-white vaginal discharge with a **fishy or musty odor**, and vaginal or vulval **itching**. Rarely, the disorder leads to **pelvic inflammatory disease**, in which some of the reproductive organs become inflamed. Women should seek treatment for bacterial vaginosis before getting pregnant.

WHAT MIGHT BE DONE?
■ Your doctor may be able to diagnose bacterial vaginosis from your symptoms.
■ Swabs of any discharge may be taken and tested to confirm the diagnosis.

■ Vaginosis is usually treated with antibiotics, either orally or as suppositories.
■ Sexual partners should also be checked for infection and treated if necessary.
■ Vaginosis usually clears up completely within two days of starting treatment, but the condition tends to recur.

See also:
• **Pelvic inflammatory disease p. 251**

Trichomoniasis

TRICHOMONIASIS IS A GENITAL TRACT INFECTION THAT IS OFTEN SYMPTOMLESS
BUT MAY CAUSE A DISCHARGE. IT USUALLY AFFECTS SEXUALLY ACTIVE PEOPLE
OF ANY AGE AND UNPROTECTED SEX IS A RISK FACTOR.

Trichomoniasis is an infection caused by the organism *Trichomonas vaginalis*. In women, the infection may cause inflammation in and around the vagina, which may lead to cystitis. In men, the infection sometimes causes mild inflammation of the urethra with or without a pusslike discharge. In most cases, trichomoniasis is transmitted through sexual intercourse.

WHAT ARE THE SYMPTOMS?
Some women have no symptoms, and the infection is often detected only by a routine Pap smear. If symptoms do occur, they may include:
● profuse, yellow, frothy and **offensive-smelling** discharge from the vagina
● painful inflammation of the vagina
● itching and soreness of the vulva (the skin around the entrance to the vagina)
● burning sensation on urinating
● discomfort during intercourse.
　Men too may not have symptoms, but if present, they may include:
● discomfort on passing urine
● discharge from the penis.
　If you or your partner develops any of these symptoms, consult your doctor or go to a clinic specializing in STDs.

WHAT MIGHT BE DONE?
Swabs will be taken from infected areas and tested for the presence of the organism. You will probably also be tested for other STDs at the same time.
　If you have trichomoniasis, antibiotics will be prescribed by your doctor. Sexual partners should also be tested even if they have no symptoms and should be treated if necessary.

CAN IT BE PREVENTED?
You can reduce your own risk of contracting trichomoniasis by practicing **safe sex**. If you or your partner becomes infected, you should avoid spreading the infection further by abstaining from sexual contact until you have both finished your course of drug treatment and your doctor has confirmed that the infection has completely cleared up. You should also be tested for other STDs.

See also:
• **Pelvic inflammatory disease p. 251**
• **Safe sex p. 280**

Syphilis

Syphilis is a bacterial infection initially affecting the genitals that, left untreated, can damage other parts of the body years later, including the spine and brain. Once diagnosed, syphilis can be treated successfully with antibiotics by a specialist in genitourinary infections at an STD or family planning clinic.

Gonorrhea

Gonorrhea is a bacterial infection that causes genital inflammation and discharge. Once diagnosed it can usually be eradicated by antibiotics but, because strains are becoming resistant to conventional therapy, it's important to seek specialist help at an STD clinic or your doctor's office.

Threats to mental well-being

Image shows a positron emission tomography scan of the brain during hallucination

Miriam's overview

Few people hesitate to seek treatment for a physical illness, but many find it hard to accept they have a mental health problem. That's a great pity because depression, anxiety, and irrational fears are common, well understood, and often treatable.

No one should feel embarrassed about a mental illness or believe that they must deal with it alone. Anxiety disorders, including panic attacks, are among the most common mental health problems in the US. Feeling worried is a natural reaction to problems and stress. But persistent anxiety, often with no obvious cause, needs treatment to prevent it from becoming a long-term problem.

Anxious personalities may be prey to obsessive-compulsive disorder (OCD) and phobias, irrational fears of anything from spiders to confined spaces – which can dominate a person's life. Other anxiety related illnesses include post-traumatic stress disorder, a prolonged reaction to events such as serious accidents and natural disasters.

Depression affects as many as 1 in 3 people at some time in their lives but is quite difficult to understand.

"*harness* stress and *manage it*"

Nonetheless it requires prompt treatment to relieve symptoms and prevent long-term feelings of despair, possibly culminating in suicide.

The two eating disorders anorexia nervosa and bulimia are most common in teenage girls, but they're also being diagnosed at a younger age and in boys too. They have been falsely attributed to the desire to be slim but that's to misunderstand what's going on. Anorexia is the expression of profound psychological disturbance and the desire to exert some control over life with the only tool at the anorexic person's disposal – a refusal to eat. Losing weight is a consequence, not a cause, of anorexia.

A new syndrome in men is related to anorexia where there's a similar obsession with shape and weight, but it's to do with muscular development rather than thinness. Men spend hours in the gym "purging" themselves on the treadmill rather than with laxatives.

Stress is ever present and virtually unavoidable in modern life. But that doesn't mean we have to succumb to it. A better strategy, if you can do it, is to harness stress and manage it so that stress leads to greater, not less,

productivity. Learn to do that and you'll be able to defuse stressful situations – you may even find you thrive on a bit of stress every now and then.

A phenomenon of the new millennium seems to be a preoccupation with appearance to the point where feelings of ugliness may become obsessive. This disturbance of the way we see our bodies is called body dysmorphic disorder but it goes way beyond the common belief that our thighs are on the wide side or our faces are asymmetrical.

Few people hesitate to seek treatment for a physical illness, but many find it hard to accept they have a mental health problem. That's a great pity because depression, anxiety, and irrational fears are common, well understood, and often treatable.

No one should feel embarrassed about a mental illness or believe that they must deal with it alone. Anxiety disorders, including panic attacks, are among the most common mental health problems in the US. Feeling worried is a natural reaction to problems and stress. But persistent anxiety, often with no obvious cause, needs treatment to prevent it from becoming a long-term problem.

Anxious personalities may be prey to obsessive-compulsive disorder (OCD) and phobias, irrational fears of anything from spiders to confined spaces – which can dominate a person's life. Other anxiety related illnesses include post-traumatic stress disorder, a prolonged reaction to events such as serious accidents and natural disasters.

Depression affects as many as 1 in 3 people at some time in their lives but is quite difficult to understand.

"*harness* stress and *manage it*"

Nonetheless it requires prompt treatment to relieve symptoms and prevent long-term feelings of despair, possibly culminating in suicide.

The two eating disorders anorexia nervosa and bulimia are most common in teenage girls, but they're also being diagnosed at a younger age and in boys too. They have been falsely attributed to the desire to be slim but that's to misunderstand what's going on. Anorexia is the expression of profound psychological disturbance and the desire to exert some control over life with the only tool at the anorexic person's disposal – a refusal to eat. Losing weight is a consequence, not a cause, of anorexia.

A new syndrome in men is related to anorexia where there's a similar obsession with shape and weight, but it's to do with muscular development rather than thinness. Men spend hours in the gym "purging" themselves on the treadmill rather than with laxatives.

Stress is ever present and virtually unavoidable in modern life. But that doesn't mean we have to succumb to it. A better strategy, if you can do it, is to harness stress and manage it so that stress leads to greater, not less, productivity. Learn to do that and you'll be able to defuse stressful situations – you may even find you thrive on a bit of stress every now and then.

A phenomenon of the new millennium seems to be a preoccupation with appearance to the point where feelings of ugliness may become obsessive. This disturbance of the way we see our bodies is called body dysmorphic disorder but it goes way beyond the common belief that our thighs are on the wide side or our faces are asymmetrical.

PSYCHOLOGICAL THERAPIES

Counseling

In days gone by, when faced with an emotional crisis we might have gone to a local priest, family doctor, or village "wise woman." Nowadays a therapist can fill that role. Trained to listen while you talk through your personal problems, a therapist can support you through a bad patch and help you see the overall picture. Friends can be wonderful but they can't give the same kind of concentrated time and objectivity.

Counseling is gentle and supportive, relying on trust. The goal is to help you develop your own insights into what's gone wrong so you can approach the problem in a fresh way. That should mean you feel less like the victim of circumstances and have more control over your life. In the course of counseling you can reassess your coping skills – how you deal with problems, challenges, relationships, work – and learn new ways that would be more effective. It can also help to make you clearer and more direct when communicating with others – saying what you mean and asking for what you want, being assertive without being aggressive.

Short-term counseling for a specific difficulty may only take a few weekly sessions while more complex deep-rooted problems will need longer, perhaps an hour every week for several months.

Some family practices now have a counselor as a member of their primary care team. Community counseling services exist in many areas and there's almost certainly an individual practitioner within traveling distance of your home. Many therapists try to offer a sliding scale of fees that takes your ability to pay into account.

Support groups have branches in most parts of the country and you should find the address you need in your local telephone directory. If you don't feel comfortable with one group's approach, try another group – support styles vary although most will do their best to help. It's sometimes possible to find a group that meets in the daytime. Many groups though, will conveniently meet in the evenings or on weekends.

If you're between 16 and 25 you might prefer to see a counselor who specializes in helping young people. Look in the telephone directory to see if there's a youth counseling and center in your area or see Useful addresses (p. 567) for further information.

Counseling is about trust so it's important that you feel comfortable with a therapist. The more open you can be, the more you gain from the experience. Most professionals recommend that you "shop around" by talking to two or three practitioners before deciding which one is the right therapist for you.

Cognitive therapy

Cognitive therapy is based on the idea that some psychological problems stem from inappropriate ways of thinking. It helps people recognize and understand their current thought patterns and shows them ways to consciously change the way they think. Cognitive therapy does not look into past events and is often used in conjunction with behavior therapy.

Psychoanalysis

Psychoanalysis in its purest form is inevitably lengthy and therefore expensive. It is not uncommon for a course of therapy to demand daily attendance at the analyst's office for several years. An acceptable minimum might still involve two or three visits a week for more than a year.

One of the reasons why psychoanalysis is so protracted is that the analyst and the patient join in a contract to explore every aspect of the patient's feelings in a close, intimate way in order to understand all facets of the patient's life as far back as the patient can remember. During the therapy, the analyst will attempt to interpret the patient's personality, motivations, inadequacies, and symptoms and relate them to family, personal, social, and professional

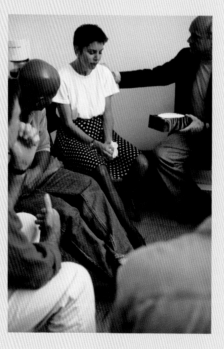

relationships. Such a complex exploration is necessarily long.

The goal of psychoanalysis – and every other form of psychological treatment – is to help people to have insight into themselves. In doing so, it attempts to explain the underlying reasons for psychological disturbance and symptoms. Once explained, the technique then builds in a positive way to provide support while patients face their difficulties and deal with them.

Short-term psychotherapy

Psychotherapy is an important form of treatment because it doesn't require hospital admission and can be fit into daily life. So a mother can stay at home, and an employed woman doesn't have to miss work.

As with most other forms of psychological treatment, psychotherapy must cover all aspects of the patient's life. It is useless to embark on a course of psychotherapy if you are not prepared to explore your feelings candidly and accept the involvement of your psychotherapist in the intimate details of your problems and in forming a treatment plan.

In the broadest sense, psychotherapy is useful for managing any illness that has a psychological component, the most common being an inability to adjust to stress. Since just being alive in the 21st century is stressful, most of us would probably be better off for having psychotherapy.

Group therapy

There are many forms of group therapy but all rely on one basic premise: they set out to help individuals to take well-defined steps toward being able to deal with their problems alone. There are usually four steps:

1. to discover what the real problems are
2. to rationalize them
3. to adjust to them
4. to cope with them.

Whatever the form of group therapy, this step-by-step progress is facilitated by the presence of others. It may be possible to identify with another group member and share experiences. It may be possible to assess behavior in others as irrational even though it's difficult to recognize and admit to the same thing in oneself when alone.

In group therapy, members use the group as a crutch, a cathartic, and an instrument to work through their own difficulties. With successful group therapy, however, the patient ceases to be dependent on the group and has the confidence to face life alone.

Anxiety

TEMPORARY FEELINGS OF NERVOUSNESS OR WORRY IN STRESSFUL SITUATIONS ARE NATURAL AND APPROPRIATE. HOWEVER, WHEN ANXIETY BECOMES A GENERAL RESPONSE TO MANY ORDINARY SITUATIONS AND CAUSES PROBLEMS IN COPING WITH EVERYDAY LIFE IT IS DIAGNOSED AS ABNORMAL.

Anxiety disorders occur in a number of different forms, the most common being generalized, persistent background anxiety that is difficult to control.

Any type of anxiety can escalate to **panic**, in which there are recurrent attacks of intense frightening anxiety and alarming unpleasant physical symptoms (see box, below). These attacks occur unpredictably and usually have no obvious cause.

In another type of anxiety disorder, known as a **phobia**, severe anxiety is provoked by an irrational fear of a situation, creature, or an object, such as fear of enclosed spaces (claustrophobia) and fear of spiders (arachnophobia).

Generalized anxiety disorder affects about 1 in 15 people and it can occur in childhood, adolescence, or at any age with women more commonly affectd than men. This kind of anxiety may respond well to a variety of medications, therapy,, relaxation exercises, and other self-help treatments.

WHAT ARE THE CAUSES?

An increased susceptibility to anxiety disorders may be inherited or may be due to childhood experiences. For example, poor bonding between a parent and child and abrupt separation of a child from a parent have been shown to play a part in some anxiety disorders. Generalized anxiety disorder may develop after a stressful life event, such as the death of a close relative. However, the anxiety frequently has no particular cause. Similarly, panic attacks often develop for no obvious reason.

WHAT ARE THE SYMPTOMS?

People with generalized anxiety disorder and panic attacks experience both psychological and physical symptoms. However, in someone with generalized anxiety disorder, psychological symptoms tend to persist while physical symptoms are intermittent. In panic attacks, both psychological and physical symptoms come on together suddenly and unpredictably. The psychological symptoms of anxiety include:
- a sense of nameless foreboding with no obvious reason or cause

- being on edge and unable to relax
- impaired concentration
- repetitive worrying thoughts
- disturbed sleep and sometimes nightmares.

In addition, you may have symptoms of depression, such as early waking or a general sense of hopelessness. **Physical symptoms** of the disorder, which occur intermittently, include:
- headache
- abdominal cramps, sometimes with diarrhea and vomiting
- frequent urination
- sweating, flushing and tremor
- a feeling of something being stuck in the throat.

Psychological and physical symptoms of **panic attacks** include the following:
- shortness of breath
- sweating, trembling, and nausea
- palpitations (awareness of an abnormally rapid heartbeat)
- dizziness and fainting
- fear of choking or of imminent death

continued on page 292

Panic attacks

A panic attack is a short burst of overwhelming anxiety. It occurs without warning and unpredictably and tends to happen in public places such as a crowded supermarket or a cramped elevator. The symptoms begin suddenly with a sense of breathing difficulty, chest pains, palpitations, feeling light-headed and dizzy, sweating, trembling and faintness, fast, shallow breathing, and pins and needles. Although very unpleasant and frightening, panic attacks usually last for only a few minutes, cause no physical harm, and are rarely associated with a serious physical illness.

How to help yourself:
- **Exercise** can be very helpful by diverting the mind and alleviating mental stress. It also increases blood flow to the brain. Studies have shown that **jogging** for 30 minutes three times a week is as effective as psychotherapy in treating depression and will work just as well for you. So, if you can, establish a **routine of regular exercise** – walking, swimming, or whatever appeals to you. Start gradually, building up to a more energetic pace as you progress.
- **Avoid junk food and sugar** and increase your intake of whole grain cereal, vegetables, fruit, lean meats, low-fat dairy products, and fish. The

amino acid tryptophan has been found to relieve anxiety and natural sources include turkey, chicken, fish, peas, nuts, and peanut butter; when possible you should eat them with a carbohydrate such as potatoes, pasta, or rice, which facilitates the brain's uptake of tryptophan.
- You might also find it helpful to use **essential oil of clary sage** (available from health food stores and pharmacies). This is both a powerful relaxant and mentally uplifting. It eases mental fatigue and depression and helps bring good sleep. Put two to three drops into a bowl of steaming water and inhale or add a little to your bath water. You could also place four to six drops on a tissue when you're going out and inhale whenever you feel particularly tense.
- **Passion flower** and **valerian root** taken as a tea or tincture have a calming effect. Some people have also found **ginger, cayenne pepper, dandelion root,** and **Siberian ginseng** to have helpful, calming properties.
- **Instant help during a panic attack:** You also need to have a way of relaxing **instantly** when you are in public if you feel a panic attack coming on and you'll be able to do that once you have got used to practicing relaxation techniques in your own time at home. Try the following exercise

when you are out. (I think it is a particularly good one to try when you are waiting in a line.)
1. Stand as comfortably and as relaxed as you can.
2. Take a deep breath to the count of five, and then breathe slowly out.
3. Mentally tell all your muscles to relax.
4. Repeat this two or three times until you're feeling relaxed.
5. Imagine yourself in a pleasant situation such as walking along a beach, or sitting in a beautiful garden.

If you find yourself hyperventilating (breathing rapidly and shallowly) cover your mouth and nose with a **small paper bag** and breathe into it for a few minutes. You will soon feel much calmer. During an attack **concentrate as hard as you can** on something you can see, such as the pattern on the rug or a picture on the wall. Stay calm. Try to continue with what you were doing but take it slowly.
- **More help:** Panic attacks may be a symptom of a more deep-seated problem that may be helped by **counseling** (see Psychological therapies, opposite). This could be a way of finding your own inner resources – resources you may have forgotten you possess because of your present anxiety.

FOCUS *on* stress

Many people need some stress to optimize their performance and, up to a point, stress can help us get the job done. However, too much stress, particularly if it is continuous, can cause serious health problems.

Although many people still think of stress as wholly negative, it can, in fact, be either positive or negative. Stress is energy that's generated by change and can range from something as minor as getting out of bed in the morning to a major life event such as giving birth or bereavement.

WHAT MAKES US STRESSED?
The short answer is potentially anything. In general the greater the number of events that happen to us in a given time, say a year, and the higher the combined rating (see below), the more likely we are to suffer a physical or emotional stress response.

And, of course, a stress-related illness such as indigestion, heart pain, or irritable bowel syndrome will add to the pressure.

PHYSICAL EFFECTS OF STRESS
The stress reaction is a natural response to fear. It prepares the body for **fight** or **flight**.

It follows that if we're in a constant state of fear, we're in a constant state of stress. And that can make us ill. This is called **stress-related illness**.

When faced with a stressful situation, the brain and then the body respond by increasing production of certain hormones such as cortisol and adrenaline. These hormones lead to changes in heart rate, blood pressure, metabolism, and physical activity designed to improve overall performance.

We all recognize the physical effects of adrenaline:
● Our hearts begin to pound so that the maximum amount of blood is being pumped around our bodies to make them ready for action.

● The rate at which we breathe increases so that our blood carries the maximum amount of oxygen to our muscles to make them work efficiently.
● Our blood pressure increases so that our essential organs are well supplied with blood.
● Blood vessels in our skin and internal organs constrict, diverting blood to our muscles, making us ready to run.
● Our pupils enlarge so that we can see both what's frightening us and a clear path to get away from it.
● The blood sugar rises steeply, providing the large amount of energy we'll need if we have to fight with, or flee from, an adversary.

A certain amount of stress isn't all bad since it helps us to meet challenges and stay motivated. But when stress levels rocket, our ability to cope is disrupted. Fewer than 20 percent of people are effective in the face of crises such as fires or floods.

WHY STRESS MAKES US ILL
Living in the 21st century means that we feel more stress than any member of the human race has ever felt. We live in a success oriented society where it's impossible to escape from competitiveness and the desire to succeed.

We suffer from stress because we've evolved a long way from the time when stressful situations could be resolved by fighting or fleeing. Yet adrenaline is being pumped into our bodies and makes us ready to do both. Our bodies are switched on, but our instincts to run or face the enemy are repressed.

The resulting tension and frustration promotes further stress, and a vicious circle is set up that may develop into physical and mental illness.

STRESS-RELATED ILLNESSES
Continued exposure to stress (fear) often leads to stress-related illnesses such as depression, headaches, indigestion, palpitations, and muscular aches and pains.

Constriction of the blood vessels due to long-term stress can give you **high blood pressure** too. If blood pressure remains elevated for any length of time, it leads to damage to the arteries and possibly to a heart attack.

Migraine headaches, **skin conditions** such as **eczema** (dermatitis) and **itching** (pruritis), and **digestive problems** such as **IBS, dyspepsia,** and **peptic ulcer** may also result.

The high stress league

EVENT	STRESS RATING	EVENT	STRESS RATING
Death of spouse	100	Large mortgage/loan	31
Divorce	73	New responsibilities at work	29
Marital separation	65	Children leaving home	29
Prison term	63	In-law trouble	29
Death in the family	63	Outstanding personal achievement	28
Personal injury or illness	63	Spouse begins or stops work	26
Marriage	50	School or college ends or begins	26
Losing job	47	Living conditions change	25
Marital reconciliation	45	Personal habits change	24
Retirement	45	Trouble with boss	23
Illness of family member	44	Change in working conditions	20
Pregnancy	40	Change in residence	20
Sex problems	39	Change in school or college	20
New baby	39	Change in social activities	18
Business readjustment	39	Change in sleeping habits	16
Change in financial circumstances	38	Change in eating habits	15
Death of a close friend	37	Vacation	13
Change in work	36	Christmas	12
Increased marital argument	35	Minor law violation	11

There are other major diseases that may be aggravated by stress, such as **arthritis**, **asthma**, and **diabetes**. Research has shown that when we're under stress we're more **susceptible to infection**, particularly from viruses.

Certain stress-related problems specific to women include **menstrual disorders**, **pelvic pain**, **sexual difficulties**, **premenstrual tension**, **unwanted hair growth**, and disturbance of **ovarian function** leading to a failure to ovulate.

The stress of modern living isn't going to go away so our only hope is to change our attitude to it.

In other words, we have to manage stress or, even better, harness it and use it as energy.

In order to live with stress, we need to decide what's causing it and if our responses to stress are sensible. If they're not, they'll prevent us from coping and taking control.

Some people are more susceptible to stress than others but with some training and practice most of us can learn to handle it.

LIFESTYLE AND STRESS

To help pinpoint the source of your stress, begin by asking yourself whether there are any social, physical, or emotional factors affecting you:
- Are you smoking heavily as a response to stress?
- Is stress making you drink too much?
- Do you exercise or are you a couch potato?
- Could you be ill?
- Is there some new element of challenge in your life?
- Has there been any change in your general circumstances?
- Have long-standing problems recently become worse?
- Is someone close to you facing difficulties that affect you?

OVERCOMING STRESS

Often the hardest thing about stress is recognizing it.

If you're feeling stressed there's every reason to be optimistic that you'll be able to overcome it.

There are several simple and effective things you can try to reduce and overcome stress.

It's a very satisfying feeling to handle stress confidently and once you've done it you'll feel stronger and more confident that you'll be able to do it next time.

TOO MUCH TO DO?

It doesn't have to be this way. Learn to prioritize and make lists.
- What **must** I do?
- What **should** I do?
- What can **"wait"**?
- What **don't I have to** I do?

Only tackle the first two, let the rest wait.

GAIN CONTROL OF YOUR LIFESTYLE – MANAGING STRESS

- Plan a daily or weekly timetable of things you love doing and include one of them in each day.
- Plan for the future and don't dwell on past mistakes or disappointments.
- Reward your successes and challenge your critics – don't accept criticism at face value.
- Find time every day for rest and relaxation, even if it's just a soak in the bath or 10 minutes with your feet up in a comfy chair reading a magazine.
- Involve your family – especially your kids – and friends in helping you to change your lifestyle. Children will force you to relax or put your feet up.

DIET

How well we handle stress can be helped by how well we eat.

People who eat a diet high in whole grain breads and cereals, fruit, and vegetables, and low in refined carbohydrates, sugar, caffeine, and fat, show greater ability to manage stress.

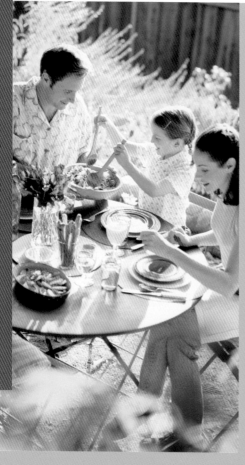

THE ANTISTRESS DIET
Every day have:
- **An orange**, fresh vegetables, and dark green leaves for vitamin C, folic cacid, selenium, antioxidants.
- **Fish**, such as tuna, herring, salmon, and salad oil on your salads for vitamins A, D, and E, essential fatty acids for your brain, zinc and manganese for your immune system.
- **Two to three cups of skim milk** or two low-fat yogurts for calcium.
- **Unrefined carbohydrates**, like whole grain bread, brown rice, oatmeal – eat three portions, to keep brain serotonin levels up, provide mood regulating B vitamins and make you feel optimistic and positive.
- **Onions, broccoli, and tomatoes** and **drink tea** for flavonoids – potent antioxidants that may help prevent cell death (aging) and cancer.

In addition:
- **Don't eat your largest meal** after 8 p.m. – it may interfere with a good night's sleep
- **Drink something hot and sweet** (diet cocoa will do) in bed and go to sleep listening to music or read a book.
- **If you can cuddle up close** to someone – it's the best antidote to stress and anxiety.

LOSS OF APPETITE
Stress often decreases your appetite. So:
- Eat small portions of food that you particularly like.
- Take your time eating.
- Temporarily avoid situations that put you under pressure to finish eating.
- Drink plenty of fluids, especially water, fruit juices, and skim milk.

Weight loss may be an important indicator of the extent of stress, so if you continue to lose weight seek help from your doctor.

LOSS OF SEX DRIVE
Waning sexual interest is frequently a feature of stress and a cause of much distress – and as a consequence more stress.

It won't last forever, so stay calm but in the meantime try to enjoy those parts of your sexual relationship that are still a pleasure. Cuddling, caressing, and kissing always are.

DEFUSING STRESS
In my book, anything that helps you defuse stress is good for you. Here are a few suggestions.

EXERCISE
Exercise is what the body instinctively wants to do under stress – fight or flight – and it's extremely beneficial in relaxing the mind and body.

Regular running, walking, bicycling, swimming or any other aerobic exercise, ideally done for at least 20 minutes three times a week, can make a big difference.

Even a walk around the block can help blow off steam and ease stress. Choose an exercise that you find pleasurable.
- Warm up for two or three minutes before by stretching before starting exercising vigorously.
- Build up slowly and don't overextend yourself. Always exercise within the limits of comfort, letting your breathing be your guide. If it hurts, stop.
- If you feel tired, stop and rest.
- When stopping exercise, cool down gradually and slowly to avoid stiffness.
- Exercising at a pace that keeps you moderately winded but not gasping for breath is best for stimulating both your muscles and circulation and for burning calories.
- Keep an eye on your heart rate; if you're a medically fit person (check with your doctor) your heart rate shouldn't exceed 110 beats per minute during warm-up, and during vigorous

Aromatherapy to help stress

- Keep some essential oil of lavender by you – it has been shown in studies to reduce stress.
- Use five or six drops in a bath or on a handkerchief. If you have sensitive skin, it's advisable to test a little of the diluted essential oil on a small area.
- You should avoid contact with the eyes and always close them when inhaling. Smells are interpreted by the inner core of the brain, the area that is concerned with emotions. Scents therefore tend to have powerful effects on mood and health.
- Concentrated essences, such as those used by aromatherapists, are a complex mixture of chemicals. Different essences have specific properties.

Oil	Effect
Bergamot	Antidepressant
Camomile	Tranquilizer
Clary sage	Stimulant
Geranium	Antidepressant
Jasmine	Antidepressant
Lavender	Tranquilizer
Marjoram	Sedative
Neroli	Sedative
Rose	Sedative

Warning: Aromatherapy oils should never be taken internally. Except for bergamot, rose, and neroli, the oils in this chart should be avoided in pregnancy, although lavender and camomile need to be avoided only for the first three months.

exercise it shouldn't exceed 130 beats per minute.
● If you're prepared to exercise for 30 minutes, your own endorphins kick in and they're wonderful. They suppress your appetite, give you an amazing high, cure headaches, and make you sleep well.

RELAXATION
Yogic breathing:
Kneel on the floor, place one hand on your stomach and the other on your chest. Inhale for about two seconds, allowing your stomach to bulge out, then slowly exhale for about four to eight seconds, feeling your stomach deflate. Then place your hand on your chest and repeat the procedure, allowing your chest to bulge and deflate. Repeat this pattern for several minutes.

Attending a yoga class and practicing it and meditation at home will divert your mind from stress, relax muscle tension through stretching, and teach you to breathe more completely. If you'd rather give yoga a pass, the following relaxation routine might help.

1. Lie on a firm surface, close your eyes, and become aware of how your body feels.
2. Imagine a calm scene. Blue is a relaxing color, so try a clear blue sky and calm sea.
3. Focus your attention on each part of your body, starting with the tips of the toes and finishing with your face and eyes.
4. Consciously try to relax every part of your body in turn.
5. The whole procedure should take at least 10 minutes and you should do it at least once a day to benefit. If you prefer, buy a relaxation tape or borrow one from the library.

THE IMPORTANCE OF TOUCH
Touch is essential for health. People can become depressed and irritable if they aren't touched enough.

In addition, touch lowers blood pressure. Massage not only relaxes and soothes, it also stimulates the circulatory and lymphatic systems – both are important in preventing swelling of the face, hands, and feet from developing.

If necessary, touch, stroke, and massage yourself – you'll feel your stress ebbing away.

People with pets live longer than people without them and this is thought to be due to the calming effect of stroking.

BE POSITIVE
● Make a list of your three best attributes. Do people describe you, for example, as generous, affectionate, and trustworthy? Carry the list with you and read it to yourself whenever you find yourself thinking unpleasant thoughts.
● Keep a daily diary of all the small, unpleasant events that happen and talk about them with your partner or a friend each day. Write down what you did for enjoyment or fun. Look back at your diary every week to see what progress you have made and to make plans for what you intend to achieve next week.
● Recall pleasant occasions in the past and plan pleasant ones for the future.
● Avoid talking about your unpleasant feelings.
● Keep your mind occupied by planning and doing constructive tasks – avoid sitting or lying around daydreaming or doing nothing.
● Keep a list of affirmations to say to yourself when under stress. It's amazing – chanting simple phrases such as "I really can handle this" can divert the stress response.

WAYS TO COPE
● Be reasonable with yourself.
● Avoid perfectionism.
● Figure out what really matters in your life.
● Think ahead and try to anticipate how to get around problems.
● Share your worries with family or friends.
● Exercise regularly.
● Give yourself treats and rewards for positive actions, attitudes, and thoughts.
● Relax every day.
● Make small, regular changes to your lifestyle.
● Learn to delegate.
● Take short rests throughout the day.
● Take real breaks for meals.
● Make time for yourself every day and every week.
● Know your limits and try to work within them.

TOP TIP
The secret of dealing with stress is similar to handling with a child who's having a tantrum – yes, honestly. Take control and use distraction tactics. Then stress is what it should be – a sudden brief reaction to a threatening situation, not a long, drawn out state of affairs.

continued from page 287

● a sense of unreality and fears about loss of sanity.

Many of these symptoms can be misinterpreted as signs of a serious physical illness, and this may increase your level of anxiety. Over time, fear of having a panic attack in public may lead you to avoid situations such as eating out in restaurants or being in crowds.

WHAT MIGHT BE DONE?

■ You may be able to find your own ways of reducing anxiety levels, including **relaxation exercises** (see box, below). If you are unable to deal with or identify a specific cause for your anxiety, you should consult your doctor.

■ It is important to see a doctor as soon as possible after the first panic attack.

■ If you are dealing with a particularly stressful period in your life or a difficult event, your doctor may prescribe a **benzodiazepine**, but these drugs are usually prescribed for only a short period of time, i.e. 3–4 weeks, because there is a danger of dependence.

■ You may be prescribed **beta blocker drugs** to treat symptoms of anxiety; actors find them useful to overcome stage fright.

■ If you have symptoms of depression, you may be given **antidepressant drugs**, some of which are also useful in treating panic attacks, particularly the newer SSRIs (selective serotonin reuptake inhibitors).

■ In most cases, the earlier anxiety is treated, the quicker its effects can be controlled. Without treatment, an anxiety disorder may develop into a lifelong condition.

SELF-HELP

There are several measures you can try to help control a panic attack, such as the simple expedient of **breathing into a bag**. For any anxiety disorder, your doctor may suggest **counseling** to help you manage stress. You may also be offered **cognitive therapy** or **behavior therapy** to help you control anxiety. A support group may also be useful.

See also:
● **Phobias p. 293**
● **Psychological therapies p. 286**

Relaxation

Practice the following relaxation exercises for at least 20 minutes a day in a warm, comfortable, and private room. Don't be surprised if it takes several weeks to notice a difference, but once you've mastered these techniques you will find that you will be able to face stressful situations with less anxiety.

Head Sit in a chair with arms, shoulders, and head supported. Clench fists, hold tension, and relax. Repeat until hands feel relaxed. With mouth open, take a deep breath, hold it for five seconds,

and let the air out. Repeat six times. You will feel calmer and more relaxed.

Legs Stretch both legs out, holding them in the air. Point toes away from yourself, holding the tension. Pull toes to point toward yourself and tense muscles. Relax, letting legs flop onto the floor. Repeat until legs feel loose and relaxed.

Stomach Contract stomach muscles and take a deep breath and hold the tension. Relax, letting breath out. Repeat five times.

Arms Clench fists, hold tension, and relax. Stretch arms up (as if to touch the ceiling) and tense

muscles, reaching as high in the air as possible. Relax, letting arms drop to sides. Repeat until your arms feel very loose and relaxed.

Shoulders Shrug shoulders so that they touch your ears. Then let them drop and relax. Repeat five times. Push shoulders forward and inward to meet each other, making a "hump" in your back (pushing arms forward). Push shoulders backward and inward, arching your back. Hold the tension and then relax, falling back into the chair. Repeat five times.

Neck Move head to left, hold tension. Turn head to right and hold tension. Push head forward with your chin on your chest and tense back of neck. Relax, allowing head to fall back onto chair. Repeat five times.

Head and face Raise eyebrows, tense, and then frown and tense. Repeat until scalp and forehead are relaxed. Close eyes very tightly. Tense up eyes and hold tension. Relax, letting eyelids drop to close eyes. Clench teeth, feel the tension and then relax, letting jaw drop slightly. Tense mouth into a whistling shape or "O," then tense lips as if to make an "E" sound. Relax mouth.

Concentrate on breathing deeply and regularly, letting breath out when breathing in. **Pick your favorite** relaxing scene and fill your mind with it (visualization). **Let yourself sink**, relaxed, into a chair. Remain like this for about 10 minutes – and let yourself enjoy it.

Breathing

Proper deep breathing is the key to all relaxation routines. Most of us breathe incorrectly, using no more than one-third of our lung capacity. You can test this for yourself by standing in front of a mirror with no clothes on. Your abdomen should move when you breathe in, but most of us only use the upper part of the chest. Try to change your shallow breathing to deep, slow breathing. Besides improving the function of your lungs and the muscles of your abdomen, it will relax your whole body.

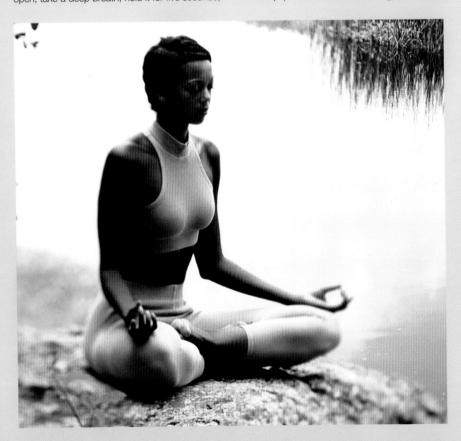

Obsessive-compulsive disorder

A PERSON WITH OBSESSIVE-COMPULSIVE DISORDER IS COMPLETELY NORMAL OTHER THAN BEING DOMINATED BY UNWANTED THOUGHTS THAT ENTER THE MIND REPEATEDLY.

These persistent thoughts (called obsessions) cause the affected person to perform repetitive, pointless actions (called compulsions). In obsessive-compulsive disorder (OCD), obsessive thoughts are frequently accompanied by a form of a compulsive but pointless **ritual**, in which a behavior or action, such as checking that your keys are still in your pocket, is repeated again and again. The person affected does not want to perform these actions but feels driven to do so. Thoughts may be concerns about hygiene, personal safety, security, or possessions. Alternatively, there may be violent and obscene thoughts that are completely out of character.

Examples of common compulsions include **hand washing**, **checking that windows and doors are locked,** and **arranging objects** on a desk in **precise patterns**. Carrying out the ritual reinforces a sense of control and brings short-lived relief, but, in severe cases, the ritual is done hundreds of times a day and interferes with work and social life.

If it's any comfort about **3 in 100** people experience OCD at some time in their lives. It sometimes runs in families and stressful life events may trigger the condition.

Many famous people have suffered from OCD. For example, it's well documented that the tycoon Howard Hughes was obsessed about hygiene. It's rumored that the pop star Michael Jackson is similarly obsessive about hygiene. The condition is partly inherited but environmental factors also play a part. Personality traits of orderliness and cleanliness are said to be related.

It's important for your family and friends to understand that while you do regard these thoughts and compulsions as senseless you are unable to ignore or resist them. That's because, once the disorder has developed, a chemical imbalance occurs in the brain that's been identified as changes in **serotonin** levels, which is why selective serotonin reuptake inhibitor (SSRI) drugs are helpful.

WHAT ARE THE SYMPTOMS?
- Intrusive, irrational mental images.
- Repeated attempts to resist thoughts.
- Repetitive behavior.

The person may be aware that the behavior is irrational and be distressed by it but cannot control the compulsions.

GETTING HELP
Deeply established, severe OCD needs professional help.

Psychotherapy and counseling are "talking treatments" that provide the opportunity to discuss difficulties with someone who will listen and accept what you say without ridicule and who will offer support in your attempts to overcome your compulsion. Talking treatments boost self-esteem and increase confidence because it's therapeutic to express feelings and feel understood.

Cognitive therapy is a behavior therapy that helps us to change our mood by changing the way we think. In other words it teaches us to challenge self-defeating beliefs and develop positive ones.

Behavior therapy is a treatment that has been used successfully to treat phobias and compulsive disorders for many years. The focus is placed on practical forms of treatment that work to modify behavior and overcome fears. The major tool is exposure treatment which means confronting whatever frightens you until you get used to it.

Drugs for OCD have proven helpful. There are several types available, all within the category of antidepressants though the newer ones such as SSRIs have many other actions. Drugs for OCD have a specific antiphobic action on the brain, and some of the most successful are SSRIs, which include Prozac and Paxil. They work by increasing levels of serotonin in the brain.

> See also:
> • **Psychological therapies p. 286**

Phobias

MANY PEOPLE HAVE A PARTICULAR FEAR, SUCH AS A FEAR OF DOGS OR HEIGHTS, THAT IS OCCASIONALLY UPSETTING. HOWEVER, A PHOBIA GOES MUCH FURTHER THAN THIS, BEING A PERSISTENT FEAR OR ANXIETY THAT DISRUPTS NORMAL LIFE.

A phobia is a fear or anxiety that has been carried to extremes – we and the sufferer recognize that it is irrational. A person with a phobia has such a compelling desire to avoid contact with a feared object or situation that it interferes with normal life. About 1 in 20 people has a phobia. Most phobias have their roots in childhood and the problem usually develops in late childhood, adolescence, or early adult life.

Being exposed to the subject of the phobia causes a **panic reaction** with crippling **anxiety**, **sweating,** and a **rapid heartbeat**. Even though aware that this intense fear is irrational, a person with a phobia still feels anxiety that can be alleviated only by avoiding the feared object or situation. The need to do this may disrupt routines and limit the person's capacity to take part in day-to-day activities.

WHAT ARE THE TYPES?
Phobias take many different forms, but they can be broadly divided into two types: **simple** and **complex** phobias.

SIMPLE PHOBIAS
Phobias that are specific to a single object, situation or activity, such as a fear of spiders, heights, or air travel, are called simple phobias. For example, **claustrophobia**, a fear of enclosed spaces, is a simple phobia. Another example is a fear of blood, which is a common simple phobia that affects more men than women.

COMPLEX PHOBIAS
These phobias are more complicated and have a number of component fears. **Agoraphobia** is an example of a complex phobia that involves multiple anxieties. These fears may include being alone in an open space or being trapped in a public area with no exit to safety. The kind of situations that provoke agoraphobic anxiety include riding on public transportation, using elevators, and visiting crowded stores. Tactics to avoid these situations may disrupt work and social life, and a person with severe agoraphobia may eventually become housebound. Agoraphobia may occasionally develop in middle age and is more common in women.

Social phobias, such as excessive shyness, are also classified as complex phobias. People with social phobias have an overwhelming fear of embarrassing themselves or of being humiliated in front of other people in social situations, such as when they are eating or speaking in public.

WHAT ARE THE CAUSES?

Often, no explanation can be found for a phobia. However, occasionally a simple phobia may be traced to an experience earlier in life. For example, being trapped temporarily in a confined enclosed space during childhood may lead to claustrophobia in later life. Simple phobias appear to run in families, but this is thought to be because children often learn their fears from a family member with a similar phobia.

Complex phobias, such as agoraphobia, sometimes develop after an unexplained panic attack. Some people recall a stressful situation as the trigger for their symptoms and then become conditioned to be anxious in these circumstances. Most social phobias also begin with a sudden episode of intense anxiety in a social situation, which then becomes the main focus of the phobia. A person who is lacking in self-esteem is also more likely to develop agoraphobia or a social phobia.

WHAT ARE THE SYMPTOMS?

Exposure to or simply thinking about the object, creature, or situation that generates the phobia leads to intense anxiety accompanied by:

- dizziness and feeling faint
- palpitations (awareness of an abnormally rapid heartbeat)
- sweating, trembling, and nausea
- shortness of breath.

A factor that is common to every phobia is **avoidance**. Activities may become so limited because of fear of unexpectedly encountering the subject of the phobia that sufferers become housebound and depressed. Sometimes, a person with a phobia attempts to relieve fear by drinking too much or abusing drugs.

WHAT MIGHT BE DONE?

If you have a phobia that interferes with your life, you should seek treatment. Many simple phobias can be treated effectively using a form of behavior therapy, such as desensitization. During treatment, a therapist gives support while you are safely and gradually exposed to the object or situation that you fear. Inevitably, you will experience some anxiety, but exposure is always kept within bearable limits.

Members of your family may be given guidance on how to help you handle your phobic behavior. If you have symptoms of depression, your doctor may prescribe antidepressant drugs.

SELF-HELP

Some research has shown that people who suffer phobias experience similar symptoms to people with **low blood sugar**. Ensuring blood sugar levels remain stable may help prevent attacks.

- Have many small meals over the day.
- Eat complex carbohydrates (potatoes, whole grain breads and cereals, rice, and pasta); avoid simple carbohydrates (sugar, candy, cakes, and cookies).
- Keep a snack with you at all times – nuts and fresh or dried fruit are best.

WHAT IS THE OUTLOOK?

A simple phobia often resolves itself as a person gets older. However, complex phobias, such as social phobias and agoraphobia, tend to persist unless they are treated. More than 9 in 10 people with agoraphobia are treated successfully with **desensitization** therapy.

Types of phobia

Acrophobia – fear of heights

Agoraphobia – fear of open spaces

Ailurophobia – fear of cats

Anthrophobia – fear of people

Aquaphobia – fear of water

Arachnophobia – fear of spiders

Brontophobia – fear of thunder

Claustrophobia – fear of enclosure

Cynophobia – fear of dogs

Equinophobia – fear of horses

Microphobia – fear of germs

Murophobia – fear of mice

Mysophobia – fear of dirt

Ophidiophobia – fear of snakes

Pterophobia – fear of flying

Pyrophobia – fear of fire

Thanatophobia – fear of death

Triskaidekaphobia – fear of number 13

Xenophobia – fear of strangers

Zoophobia – fear of animals

Shyness and social phobia

No matter how confident we seem, most of us know what it is to feel shy. For some, the feeling is temporary while for others it's a permanent, disabling condition that involves feeling desperately uncomfortable in certain situations. The basic cause is always the same: lack of confidence. The symptoms can vary from strong physical reactions such as palpitations, diarrhea, sickness, panic attacks, butterflies, and sweaty palms, to tension, flushing, and being tongue-tied. This is one area where positive thinking won't work. Telling yourself you feel confident when you don't won't stop the uncomfortable sensations and may make you feel even worse the next time around. The solution is to decide how you want to feel and when you want to feel it, then figure it out. First, think about the situations you dread most. What do they have in common? Does a certain kind of person make you feel uncomfortable? Then decide how you would like to behave when you are in these situations with these people. Next, decide what you are good at. Be honest. Then look at what other people see – the image you are projecting. Is it really who you are? It's very hard to project something you're not. People will see through it eventually, if not immediately. Be genuine and people will warm to your honesty. Once you feel they like what they see, you can relax, and you won't feel shy any more. The first step is to **focus outward**.

How to focus outward

■ There are some tried and tested ways to shift the emphasis from your feelings onto what's going on around you. The first and most important trick is to learn to listen to others.

You'll quickly find yourself so caught up in what people have to say you'll forget how you're feeling. If you're truly responsive – which means concentrating on what's being said instead of examining yourself for excuses to go home – people will respond to you.

■ Learn to smile – it automatically relaxes you and others.

■ Learn a relaxation technique and use it before you go into difficult situations. One of the best is to tense and then release each part of the body in turn, moving from your toes to your head. Another is to breathe in and out deeply and slowly.

■ Learn how to start a conversation. Talking about the weather is fine. If you're watching a football game or a TV program, use it as a starting point. Ask the other person's opinion. Ask leading questions that require a full answer. If you say "isn't it hot?", the short answer will be yes or no. Ideally, questions should seek opinions; for example if you say "What do you think of Mel Gibson?" or "What's your opinion of the stock market?" or "How do you spend your weekends?"– you should get positive answers and can keep the conversation going.

■ Move onto interests and hobbies – you may have something in common. Keep it light and cheerful and don't moan or be dreary. People don't like to be sucked into other people's problems – at least not when first meeting. If you're asked something painful, try to be honest. Don't be embarrassed and don't feel the need to talk more if there's a lull in the conversation. Some lulls can be quite comfortable if you are relaxed.

■ Remember, there's nothing wrong with

feeling shy. It's normal. It's quite all right if you're at a party with no one to talk to, to say something like "I'm afraid I get a bit nervous on these occasions. Do you?" The other person then has to say, "No," in which case they'll talk to prove it, or "Yes," in which case they'll be glad to have someone to talk to. If you're feeling lonely in a new town, own up. Choose a friendly face and say, "I'm new here. Are there any good playgroups/fitness clubs/mothers' groups to join?" Remember that most people want to be accepted and part of a group. And they'll understand that need in others.

■ Finally, a great way to deal with situations for which preparation is impossible is to think of the worst that can possibly happen. If you're giving a speech and you lose the thread of what you're saying, if you're meeting the president and you simply dry up when he asks you something, it's not going to kill you, is it? No one ever actually died of embarrassment. Don't take yourself too seriously. A lot of human failings are quite funny if you think about them. It would be much better for you to laugh afterward than to go over things again and again until your confidence is lowered further.

Social phobia

There is a kind of shyness that is so severe it's crippling and just about prevents normal life: it's called social phobia. Paxil, belonging to the latest generation of antidepressants (SSRIs), has been shown to help greatly. Your doctor can prescribe it but since all antidepressants are powerful drugs it should be reserved for people who are seriously afflicted with shyness.

Fear of flying

If you're terrified of flying you are in good company. Many famous show business personalities and sports figures, including David Bowie, Whitney Houston, Dina Carroll, Billy Bob Thornton, Aretha Franklin, Mr. T of the *A Team*, Cher, and Muhammad Ali, all know what it's like to run a mile rather than take to the air. Many thousands of people suffer from pterophobia, fear of flying. It's been estimated that 20 percent of the population are too scared to fly. It can affect anyone, from young children to seniors, at any time. Most people's biggest anxiety is losing control of them-selves and running up and down the aisle screaming. Turbulence and the plane crashing are other major worries. It's no

laughing matter suffering the discomfort and embarrassment of palpitations, gastric disturbance, uncontrollable shaking, and profuse sweating.

Self-help

Here are some useful tips to ease your fears.

■ Don't hesitate to let the cabin crew know you find flying difficult. They are likely to make an extra effort to make you feel comfortable and generally look after you.

■ Concentrate on getting through the next 10 minutes rather than worrying all through the flight.

■ Wear loose clothing in layers so you can adjust easily to hotter or colder temperatures.

■ Breathe slowly and steadily.

■ Don't drink alcohol since this makes anxiety worse.

■ Last but not least, keep thinking that it's all normal and not that you're doing something strange.

There may also be fear of flying courses available in which a senior pilot explains the mechanics of flying, dealing with safety procedures, preflight checks, and what the different bumps and noises mean. After all the theory, you are taken on a 45-minute to one-hour flight with the senior pilot talking you through it. A psychologist is on hand to help you cope with any remaining anxiety or fear. One organization that arranges these courses claims a 95 percent success rate.

Posttraumatic stress disorder

POSTTRAUMATIC STRESS DISORDER (PTSD) IS A CONDITION IN WHICH INTENSE EMOTIONS PERSIST FOR A CONSIDERABLE TIME AFTER BEING FIRST TRIGGERED BY A TRAUMATIC EVENT. ABOUT 1 IN 10 PEOPLE HAS PTSD AT SOME TIME IN LIFE.

Firsthand experience of a stressful event that threatens life and personal safety, or in some cases simply witnessing such an event, can trigger posttraumatic stress disorder in some people. The kind of events that result in PTSD include natural disasters, accidents, being assaulted, and war experiences.

Children and elderly people are more susceptible to PTSD, as are people who lack family support or who have a history of anxiety disorders. The cause of PTSD isn't known, but psychological, genetic, physical, and social factors all contribute to it. In studies of Vietnam War veterans, those with strong family support were less likely to develop PTSD than those without it.

WHAT ARE THE SYMPTOMS?

The symptoms of PTSD occur soon after the event or develop weeks, months or, rarely, years later. They may include:
- involuntary thoughts about the experience
- daytime flashbacks of the event – a sense of reliving the event
- panic attacks with symptoms such as shortness of breath and fainting
- avoidance of reminders of the event and refusal to discuss it
- sleep disturbance and nightmares
- poor concentration
- irritability.

A person with PTSD may feel emotionally numb, detached from events, and estranged from family and friends. He or she may also lose interest in normal day-to-day activities. Other psychological disorders, such as depression or anxiety, may coexist with PTSD. Occasionally it leads to alcohol or drug abuse.

WHAT MIGHT BE DONE?

The goal of treatment is to encourage sufferers to express grief and complete the mourning process. Support groups are good at providing a setting where people who have similar experiences can share their feelings and weep openly.
- **Counseling** may encourage the person to talk about his or her experiences, and support

for the individual and family members is often an important part of treatment.
- **Behavior therapy** can be used to help the person "reenter" the real world and leave behind harrowing memories. Behavior techniques include graded exposure and flooding (frequent exposure to an object that triggers symptoms).
- Drugs such as **antidepressants** may be used with counseling, and this approach often produces an improvement within eight weeks. Newer antidepressants, such as Prozac, Paxil, and Zoloft, can really improve mood and help sufferers face the future calmly. Drugs may need to be taken for at least a year. PTSD often disappears after a few months of treatment but some symptoms may persist. In some cases, PTSD may last for years. In susceptible people, the disorder may recur after other traumatic events.

See also:
• Psychological therapies p. 286

Insomnia

INSOMNIA IS A VERY COMMON PROBLEM, AFFECTING AS MANY AS 1 IN 3 ADULTS AT SOME TIME IN THEIR LIVES. SUFFERERS MAY HAVE DIFFICULTY FALLING ASLEEP OR MAY COMPLAIN OF LACK OF SLEEP DUE TO FREQUENT WAKING.

Sleep enemies

STRESS: When we're stressed out, the production of adrenaline increases, heightening alertness and making sleep difficult.

DEPRESSION: Feeling low affects hormone levels and the sleep cycles of Non-Rapid Eye Movement (NREM) and Rapid Eye Movement (REM) sleep are often unbalanced.

RESENTMENT: Bearing a grudge or plotting revenge can prevent sleep completely. Save formulating a smart reply to your critical boss until daylight hours.

CAFFEINE: Coffee has an accumulative effect in the system and there is hidden caffeine in things like carbonated drinks and chocolate.

BAD HABITS: Smoking and heavy drinking cause insomnia and reduce sleep quality. It

has been shown that smokers sleep less deeply than nonsmokers. Cigarettes raise the heart rate, blood pressure, and adrenaline levels, hindering sleep. Alcohol wreaks havoc with the hormones controlling sleep.

MEDICAL CONDITIONS: Sleep apnea causes people to have loose muscles at the back of the throat, which lead to snoring and blocking of the airways as air is sucked in. People with this condition appear to choke and even though they may not completely wake up, the sleep pattern is disturbed.

An **overactive thyroid gland** produces too much hormone (thyroxine), the symptoms of which can include insomnia. Foods that help regulate thyroid activity include brussels sprouts, cauliflower, broccoli, and kale.

Investigations at sleep research laboratories have blown away the myth that everyone needs eight hours' sleep a night. In fact, the amount of sleep needed by individual people varies enormously. The older we get, the less we need. British Prime Minister Margaret Thatcher is said to have managed with four or five hours and there have been other famous brief sleepers, including Winston Churchill and Napoleon.

Studies have shown that many people with insomnia sleep much more than they think they do. However, they also tend to wake more frequently than normal sleepers. It is the quality rather than the quantity of sleep that is often the problem in insomnia.

Sleep researchers believe the really essential part of sleep consists of **slow wave sleep**. This is the only time when the brain is totally at rest and it occurs largely during the first half of a night's sleep. While that's encouraging, it doesn't get away from the reality that there is nothing more dispiriting than lying in bed exhausted unable to get to sleep.

Promoting sleep

■ Take a fresh look at your bedroom. It should be a peaceful sanctuary for sleeping. If there's a TV, move it somewhere else. Clutter can have an unsettling effect so pay special attention to keeping the bedroom tidy and free of clutter. Invest in a pair of heavy curtains to keep out the light. Also, the air shouldn't be too stuffy. Your bed should be firm and if it's past its best, put plywood under the mattress.

■ Eat well during the day. Carbohydrates such as whole grain bread, whole grain cereals, and pasta are important for good sleep. There is an established link between high-carbohydrate foods and the body's ability to sleep. Carbohydrates help produce serotonin, a calming hormone that regulates sugar in the body. A low blood sugar level can lead to poor sleep.

■ Make sure the last meal of the day is satisfying. Lettuce, banana, and avocado are good late night snacks because they contain tryptophan, which is a natural sleep-inducing chemical.

■ Fit in some form of exercise in the day, even if it is just a walk. Inactivity is a major cause of insomnia, because the unused energy stops us from sleeping. It also means that toxins that are released by moving around build up in the body and make people feel uncomfortable and achy.

■ Read or watch something relaxing the last hour before bed to help unwind. Have a relaxing bath with essential oil of lavender added. While you're in there, drink a warm glass of milk with a little honey. Milk also contains tryptophan and honey is an ancient remedy for insomnia. If milk doesn't work for you, try an herbal tea such as camomile or valerian.

■ Prepare the bedroom by dimming the lights and putting a few drops of a calming essential oil such as jasmine in an incense burner.

■ Turn the alarm clock to the wall so you

Keeping your bedroom well ordered and free from clutter helps to promote a peaceful atmosphere, which helps you relax and fall asleep.

can't worry about not being asleep. This in itself causes insomnia.

■ Bedtime is often the only time couples have alone but don't try to discuss difficult issues because adrenaline will be released, guaranteeing poor sleep.

■ Sleep will come more easily if your pulse rate is slow and your blood pressure is down. This can be helped by lying fairly still and controlling your movements by taking deep, slow breaths and concentrating on the process of breathing; the closer you are to sleep the slower your pulse rate will be. To help you do this you can concentrate on

relaxing various parts of your body. Start with your forehead and relax any frown. Then relax the muscles of the jaw, chin, and neck. Make your arms feel limp. Become aware of the pressure of your body lying on the bed and then gradually relax the muscles down your legs until they are completely relaxed, including your toes. Many people find this process so soporific that they are asleep before they get to their feet.

■ Another trick is to empty your mind and think about a favorite thing. Mine is black velvet. Every time another thought creeps in, concentrate on the favorite thing again.

WHAT ARE THE CAUSES?

The most common cause of insomnia is worry about a problem, but other causes include physical disorders such as **sleep apnea**, **restless legs**, and environmental factors such as noise and light. Insomnia can also be a symptom of a psychological illness. For example, people with anxiety or depression may find it difficult to fall asleep. However, some sleep experts believe that anger and resentment are more frequent causes of insomnia.

WHAT IS THE TREATMENT?

An obvious physical or psychological cause for insomnia will be treated.

■ For long-term insomnia with no obvious cause, **electroencephalograms** (recordings of brain wave patterns, also called EEGs) and an **assessment of breathing**, **muscle activity**, and other bodily functions during sleep may be useful in discovering the extent and pattern of the problem.

■ Keeping a **log** of sleep patterns may also be

helpful. Sleep clinics for insomniacs are an option and you could ask your doctor to make enquiries for you.

■ **Sleeping pills** or **tranquilizers** may be prescribed as a short-term measure, but only for severe cases and generally as a last resort.

See also:
• **Restless legs p. 437** • **Snoring p. 480**

Depression

DEPRESSION IS THE MOST COMMON SERIOUS PSYCHIATRIC ILLNESS,
AND IT BECOMES MORE COMMON WITH AGE. WOMEN ARE PARTICULARLY
VULNERABLE BECAUSE OF THEIR HORMONES.

Plummeting hormone levels can trigger depression when menstruation stops at menopause, after the birth of a child, and after a miscarriage or termination. About 1 in 6 women seek help for depression at some time in their lives, as opposed to only 1 in 9 men. Most depressed people find they feel slightly better as the day progresses.

RISK FACTORS
■ Depression in the past or a family history of depression.
■ Poor health (such as a stroke or heart attack).
■ Widowhood and widowerhood.
■ Loss of a partner.
■ Personality problems.
■ Isolation.
■ Lack of confidence.
■ With elderly people, alterations in health and circumstances, such as giving up the family home.

WHAT ARE THE CAUSES?
The cause of depression is complex but is probably related to a reduction in the level of certain chemicals in the brain, called **neurotransmitters**, which keep us in a good mood by stimulating brain cells. The best known of these mood elevators is **serotonin**.

WHAT ARE THE SYMPTOMS?
■ Fatigue.
■ Sleep problems.
■ Worry.
■ Weepiness.
■ Sadness, despair, misery, gloom, and blackness.
■ Loss of affection toward oneself and others.
■ A sense of failure, unworthiness, even self-loathing.
■ Loss of interest in life.
■ Loss of sex drive.
■ Loss of self-esteem and confidence.
■ Altered appetite (usually a loss of appetite).
■ Lethargy, slovenliness, and apathy.
■ Insomnia or sleeping for long periods as a means of escape.
■ Early morning waking – typically between 2 a.m. and 4 a.m.
■ A conviction that the world is against you, paranoia, recurrent thoughts of death, even suicide.

WHAT IS THE TREATMENT?
Try to see your doctor at once if you feel depressed. Don't wait and hope your mood will pass. In the case of weepiness after the birth of a baby, see your doctor if you're still depressed after two weeks. The longer postpartum depression stays untreated the harder it is to cure.
■ **Psychotherapy**, whether individual or in a group, is most useful for those whose personality and life experiences are the main causes of their illness. The goal of one of the most successful treatments, **cognitive therapy**, is to change the way you think about problems and therefore be able to deal with them.
■ **Drug treatment** is used for people with more **severe** symptoms. There are two main groups of antidepressants: **tricyclics**, introduced in the 1950s with well-known side effects, and **selective serotonin reuptake inhibitors** (SSRIs), which appeared mainly in the 1990s. The newer antidepressants, such as SSRIs, are costly but have fewer side effects than the older drugs and patients seem to like them. Yet large studies show tricyclics work equally well to cure depression if you can tolerate them. Antidepressant drugs are effective in more than two-thirds of patients, provided the drugs are taken in a sufficient dosage over a long enough period of time. They take between two and three weeks to work. Patient compliance is high – important because halting medication too early is a big factor in depression returning.
■ **Antidepressants and psychotherapy in combination.** Patients who stop drug therapy before six months will relapse. But maintenance therapy with either drugs or psychotherapy will halve the relapse rate. What's more, **cognitive therapy** continues to work after it's stopped, its effectiveness being the same as maintenance drug therapy – something to remember if you don't like taking drugs for long periods.

GETTING HELP
Don't try to handle it alone. Lean on people. Join a support group and get help dealing with your everyday problems. Avoid being alone and make a point of being with people you like. Don't be afraid to approach organizations that can help.

SELF-HELP

For mild depression

WORK: If work distracts you, increase your workload.
KEEPING ACTIVE: Any kind of activity helps reduce sadness and will bring the pleasure of achievement. Completing a task gives you a sense of self-worth, which itself is an antidote to depression.
SEX: Good, wholesome sex makes all aspects of life seem brighter, so if your libido isn't depressed, keep sexually active.
DIET: Avoid junk food and sugar and increase your intake of whole grain cereals, vegetables, fruit, lean meats, low-fat dairy products, and fish.

The amino acid **tryptophan** has been found to relieve depression and natural sources include turkey, chicken, fish, peas, nuts, and peanut butter. Where possible eat them with carbohydrates, such as potatoes, pasta, and rice, which facilitate the brain's uptake of tryptophan. Cut out or cut down on caffeine and alcohol.
EXERCISE: Exercise alleviates all kinds of mental stress. It also increases blood flow to the brain. Jogging for 30 minutes three times a week can be as effective as psychotherapy in treating depression. So, a regular routine of exercise – walking, swimming, or whatever appeals to you – is good for your mood.
AROMATHERAPY: Essential oil of clary sage is both a powerful relaxant and mentally uplifting. It can ease mental fatigue and promote sound sleep. Put two to three drops into a bowl of steaming water and inhale or inhale four to six drops from a tissue.
RELAXATION: Relaxation techniques to reduce stress, such as massage, yoga, aromatherapy, and meditation, are helpful in alleviating the anxiety that is common with depression.

See also:
• **Psychological therapies p. 286**

Depression in children and teenagers

GOOD PARENTS ENCOURAGE THEIR CHILDREN TO TALK ABOUT THEIR WORRIES FROM A VERY EARLY AGE, ALWAYS LISTEN AND OFFER HELP. CHILDREN CAN QUICKLY FEEL ISOLATED, MISUNDERSTOOD, AND IGNORED IF PARENTS ARE PREOCCUPIED WITH THEIR OWN PROBLEMS.

It's difficult to pin down why children become depressed and often it's a combination of factors. But some classical situations seriously affect children and precipitate depression, such as:

- death in the family
- bullying
- exam anxiety
- feeling ugly
- unsympathetic parents
- girls/boys don't like me
- parental illness
- parental discord.

TELLTALE SIGNS FOR PARENTS

Parents often wonder what's wrong with a child who seems out of sorts a lot of the time. Here's a guide to what to look out for.

BABIES AND TODDLERS

They can't tell us if they're sad, so they express themselves through their behavior and:

- become unresponsive
- are clingy but can't accept comfort
- refuse to eat
- can't settle down to sleep.

PRESCHOOLERS MIGHT:

- be tearful all the time
- stop eating
- wake up during the night
- have frequent nightmares and night terrors
- become very demanding and naughty
- bully, hit, and bite other children
- start telling lies
- behave destructively
- have frequent unexplained physical complaints.

A few children can put their sad feelings into words – I well remember one of my sons, normally outgoing and happy, saying "the world doesn't feel right, Mom." Children quickly blame themselves if things go wrong and think they're worthless. Then their behavior seems to ask for punishment – lying, stealing, or playing hooky from school. Remember – a naughty, depressed child isn't an innately bad child.

SCHOOL AGE CHILDREN

If they are depressed they may:

- find it hard to concentrate and lose interest in schoolwork and play
- become loners
- refuse to go to school
- complain of feeling bored all the time
- say they're lonely
- lose confidence

- become difficult to control
- become slovenly.

ADOLESCENTS

Almost without exception, adolescents go through periods of being moody and antisocial and it can be difficult to spot the difference between what's normal and what's depression. Look out for these signs of depression – one or two signs could be a passing phase but three, four, or more mean you should see your doctor:

- being much more moody and irritable than normal
- becoming withdrawn, giving up on friends and hobbies
- losing interest in or not doing well at school
- taking no interest in hair, clothes, music
- not eating enough, even anorexia, or eating too much, even bulimia
- having low self-esteem
- not being able to get out of bed until midday
- getting into bad habits and bad company
- taking drugs

- getting drunk
- becoming preoccupied with thoughts of death
- harming themselves by cutting their skin.

WHAT IS THE TREATMENT?

Getting professional help early from your doctor for any child whose unhappiness is more than a passing phase can often prevent long-term depression. The mainstay of treating childhood depression is what's called talk therapy, sessions with a **psychotherapist**, **clinical psychologist,** or **family therapist**, where the child can vent their anger, frustration, fear, and hopelessness. Loving, caring attention is very powerful medicine for every depressed child.

HOW CAN ADULTS HELP?

By themselves, children simply can't make sense of feeling depressed; they feel helpless. Depressed children need a caring adult to take a loving interest in them and show understanding. Then they can help them deal with their feelings over time.

FOCUS *on* eating disorders

Anorexia and bulimia are abnormal ways of controlling weight but neither one is just a form of chronic dieting. Both are expressions of deep inner turmoil, of psychological problems that are too difficult for the person to deal with in any other way.

Dieting is easy to be good at – you just have to starve yourself. But it's possible for an ANOREXIC to believe it's the only thing she's good at, so thinness becomes an obsession. Anorexics judge themselves only according to how much they've eaten – the less they eat the more successful they judge themselves to be. All their self-worth becomes wound up in not eating and so starving becomes very difficult to give up.

Anorexics hate food and crave love. They remember the time when they felt secure in being loved and didn't have to take on any adult responsibilities, so they may subconsciously try to remain a child. As a child they didn't have to perform and they didn't have to excel. By starving they fight against their developing body – they lose or don't develop breasts and they don't menstruate.

BULIMICS go for several days with very little food and then become crazed with an uncontrollable desire to eat so that they gorge on almost anything in sight that is edible. This may mean eating extraordinary mixtures of raw and cooked food, sweet and savory mixed in huge quantities. Some women have died after a binge because their stomachs have ruptured under the strain. Some women eat normally but then force themselves to vomit immediately afterward or take huge quantities of laxatives to induce purging. This pattern of starving, bingeing, vomiting, and purging is very hard to break. It's also much more common than people think, but treatment can help.

WHAT ARE THE CAUSES?

Desire for control: Dieting can be very satisfying, especially for girls in their teens who feel that weight is the only part of their lives over which they have control. Not eating becomes an end in itself.

Social pressure: In societies that don't value thinness, eating disorders are very rare. In surroundings such as ballet schools, where people value thinness highly, they're common.

Cultural pressure: Generally in Western culture "thin is beautiful." Television, newspapers and magazines are full of pictures of slim, attractive young men and women and there's huge pressure to conform.

Family: Some children and teenagers find saying no to food is the only way they can make their feelings felt and have influence in the family. Eating becomes an important social tool with which to exert pressure on parents.

Not growing up: A girl with anorexia may lose or not develop some of the physical traits of an adult woman, such as pubic hair, breasts and monthly periods. As a result, she may look very young for her age. Not eating can therefore be seen as a way of putting off some of the demands of growing up, particularly the sexual ones.

Depression: Many bulimics are depressed and binges may start off as a way of dealing with unhappiness. A third of people with eating disorders are depressed and can be helped with the new generation of antidepressants.

Upsets: For some people, anorexia and bulimia seem to be triggered by an upsetting event, such as the breakup of a relationship. Sometimes it doesn't even have to be a bad event, just an important one, such as marriage or leaving home.

CONSEQUENCES OF ANOREXIA AND BULIMIA

Starvation leads to broken sleep, constipation, difficulty in concentrating or thinking straight, depression, sensitivity to the cold, brittle bones that break easily (osteoporosis), muscles becoming weaker – it becomes an effort to do anything, menstruation failing to start or stopping, inability to have a baby, death.

Vomiting stomach acid dissolves the enamel on teeth and leads to a puffy face (due to swollen salivary glands), irregular heartbeat, muscle weakness, eventually to kidney damage, and even epileptic fits.

Laxative use causes persistent stomach pain, swollen fingers, and damage to bowel muscles that may lead to long-term constipation.

Bladder problems become common. New research shows that women with anorexia are far more likely to have bladder problems than other women. Nearly two-thirds of women with anorexia, at least three times more than nonsufferers, had symptoms suggestive of an **unstable bladder**, with a sudden and overwhelming desire to go to the bathroom eight times or more in 24 hours, and sometimes actual incontinence. These symptoms usually start about a year after anorexia began.

Symptoms of anorexia and bulimia

Anorexia symptoms:
- Severe weight loss.
- Distorted ideas about body size and weight.
- Excessive exercising.
- Vomiting or purging.
- Social isolation.
- Emotional and irritable behavior.
- Difficulty sleeping.
- Loss of menstrual periods.
- Perfectionism.
- Feeling cold, poor circulation.
- Growth of downy body hair.

Bulimia symptoms:
- Normal weight.
- Binge eating large amounts of food.
- Vomiting or purging after eating.
- Going to the bathroom after meals.
- Secretive and ritual behavior.
- Feeling helpless and lonely.
- Erratic menstrual periods.
- Sore throat and tooth decay caused by vomiting.
- Dehydration and poor skin condition.
- Social isolation.
- Swollen salivary glands.

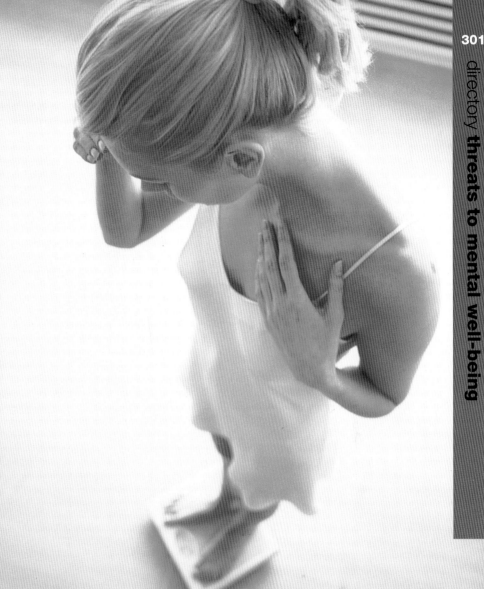

GETTING HELP

As with alcohol or drug dependence, the sooner you admit to having an eating disorder and accept help, the better the chance of a cure. Left untreated, anorexia has one of the highest death rates of all psychiatric illnesses, though deaths can be prevented by proper treatment.

No one form of treatment is 100 percent effective; what's effective for one person may not be effective for you. And despite best efforts, some people only partly recover. But there are a lot of avenues to explore.

YOUR DOCTOR

To help yourself, you have to be open and honest with your family doctor. Don't be ashamed of being anorexic or bulimic or reluctant to admit you have a problem.

Don't be frightened of the consequences of admitting you have an eating disorder. You're entitled to complete confidentiality; this means that your parents don't have to know.

It's your right to be referred for assessment by a specialist who has training in eating disorders; you should be seen as soon as possible so that delays can be avoided. You may get worse if you wait too long and then need inpatient rather than outpatient treatment.

SELF-HELP

Support groups can be a useful addition to treatment but they aren't an alternative. They're very helpful in getting patients and families to understand they aren't alone with the illness.

GENERAL TREATMENT

Treatment must address the psychological aspects of anorexia and bulimia nervosa as well as the abnormal eating. All these treatments work so don't be afraid to try them.
- Counseling.
- Psychotherapy.
- Cognitive therapy.
- Group therapy.
- Family therapy.
- Outpatient hospital programs.
- Inpatient treatment.
- Dietetic advice.
- Drugs can be of help in the short term, particularly to bulimics who are depressed.
- Refeeding is a last resort but may be necessary to save life. Alone, however, it's only successful in short-term weight restoration, but usually isn't effective in the long run.

COUNSELING

For anorexia, counseling is more effective during the early stages (when less than 25 percent of body weight has been lost). Research shows that cognitive behavior therapy is especially effective for people with bulimia.

SPECIALIZED TREATMENT

You should be involved as much as possible in your treatment program and care plan, so you should be able to see your case notes and be involved in setting target weights. Therapy should not be conditional on weight gain, and vegetarian menus and appropriate food for minority groups should be available.

HOSPITAL TREATMENT

Some severely underweight people with anorexia nervosa can be treated successfully as **outpatients** rather than as inpatients.

If you need inpatient treatment, you require:
- a quiet and safe environment
- continuity of care from staff with an understanding of eating disorders
- support during and after your meals
- appropriate food
- ongoing counseling or psychotherapy
- follow-up and support after inpatient care.

COMPULSORY ADMISSION

Out of people who had been admitted or detained against their wishes, 50 percent said they thought it had been "a good thing" in retrospect.

So, in extreme circumstances and when all other alternatives have failed, a parent or guardian may have their child hospitalized to save their life.

TEAMWORK

Good treatment demands selfless teamwork with families, carergivers, and friends all working together. The impact on the family of someone with an eating disorder can be enormous. Families also need support. They need advice on what they should and shouldn't do to help a person's recovery.

WOMEN AND MENTAL HEALTH

In this section, I cover a group of topics that have a direct effect on the mental health of a great many women, as well as an indirect but often considerable effect on women's partners, family members, friends, and colleagues. All women are prey to their hormones, variations which affect them throughout their lives, not least once a month through the menstrual cycle. **Premenstrual syndrome** (PMS) can be a problem throughout a woman's fertile years. After childbirth, changes in female hormone levels may cause the "baby blues" or the more serious condition known as **postpartum depression** (PPD). Then, later in life, women may experience depression and other emotional problems due to hormonal adjustments in **menopause**. I also look at the effects on mental and physical well-being that may follow a **sexual assault**.

Premenstrual syndrome

PREMENSTRUAL SYNDROME, OR PMS, IS A COLLECTION OF UNCOMFORTABLE, PAINFUL, AND ANNOYING SYMPTOMS THAT AFFECT SOME WOMEN BEFORE THEIR PERIODS. ROUGHLY 50 PERCENT OF WOMEN SUFFER FROM PREMENSTRUAL SYNDROME.

Half of those suffer very badly, quite a number so badly that they have to take time off school or work. But what exactly is premenstrual syndrome?

WHAT ARE THE SYMPTOMS?

The symptoms that we associate with PMS vary but include **tension**, **irritability**, **depression**, **headaches**, and an **inability to concentrate**.

They also consist of **breast tenderness, swollen ankles**, **palpitations**, **a change in sexual interest**, **faintness, dizziness, changes in eating habits, an inability to get to sleep at night, indigestion**, and either **diarrhea** or **constipation**.

In addition:

■ All stress-related illnesses – such as **migraines**, **asthma**, and **eczema** – may get worse before a menstrual period.
■ The effects of alcohol are worse just before a period, so a woman may find herself in a dilemma: she drinks to relieve her symptoms of PMS but the effects of drinking are much worse than usual.
■ The severity of symptoms can also vary each month. In addition to the symptoms already mentioned some women complain of **bloating, weight gain, skin problems, mood swings**, and **depression, aggression, fatigue, tearfulness, feeling irrational, difficulty with decision making**, and the **feeling of being misunderstood**.
■ No woman experiences all of these symptoms and the most important factor is their timing. The symptoms are present at some time in the second half of the cycle. Then they disappear or significantly improve either on the first day of your period or the day after the flow is heaviest. You should then be symptom-free.

Simple self-help measures, such as a hot bath and time to relax, can help ease premenstrual symptoms.

NOTE: If you have symptoms after these few days, it's unlikely that you're suffering from PMS and you should see your doctor so that a cause can be found and the appropriate treatment given.

Before blaming symptoms on PMS, it's important to confirm that there's a connection between symptoms and menstrual cycle. The way to do this is to keep a **diary**. Start filling in a daily chart showing exactly when symptoms appear, when they get worse, and when they go away. When symptoms don't disappear or improve after a period, they're unlikely to have anything to do with PMS.

WHAT CAUSES PMS?

Premenstrual syndrome is now widely accepted as a true medical condition that affects women during their fertile years.
■ It's related to menstrual hormones and it can cause **physical** and **psychological** symptoms. There are more than 150 symptoms associated with PMS and the number and type vary from person to person.
■ PMS usually increases in severity when there are **alterations in hormone levels** such as after **pregnancy**, after a **miscarriage**, or **termination**, when starting or **stopping the contraceptive pill**, or even occasionally **after a hysterectomy**.

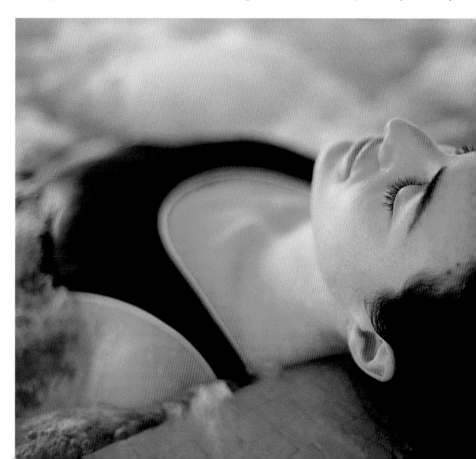

■ If you've suffered from postpartum depression, you are also more likely to suffer from PMS.

■ We used to think that PMS was brought on by the lack of one of our sex hormones, progesterone, in the week prior to menstruation. But, in fact, progesterone levels are quite high until just before a period starts. Our other sex hormone, estrogen, however, is very low seven days before menstruation and experts agree that it's a **shortage of estrogen** that causes symptoms of PMS.

■ PMS can get worse as we get older and after each baby. By the time I was in my 40s, PMS felt like a mini menopause each month and I dreaded having to do a TV show that week.

■ PMS sometimes seems to run in families, but a genetic link has not been established. If you feel able to talk to other family members about PMS, you may find that they also suffer and have found some treatment that has helped them and may help you too.

PMS can wreak havoc in families when a normally lovely wife and mom becomes a shrew. All you have to do is warn your loved ones of your PMS and ask them to understand. Tell your children sooner rather than later.

WHAT CAN I DO?
There are many theories about the best ways to treat PMS but here are several things you can try.

■ Oil of evening primrose may bring relief.

■ If you retain fluid and swell up before a period (fluid sometimes collects in the breasts, sometimes around the waist, and sometimes around the ankles, hands, fingers, and face), try restricting your salt intake for a week to ten days before your period starts.

■ If your breasts swell and become especially tender try experimenting with different bras until you find one that's comfortable with plenty of support; you may find it a help to wear a bra in bed, too, and you may need one cup bigger for your premenstrual week.

■ Don't add salt at the table, cook with less salt (use seasonings such as pepper and garlic instead) and limit salt-rich foods such as hard cheese, prepared meals, bacon, and fish, salted peanuts, potato chips, etc. Look at the labels to find out which other foods contain salt. The recommended limit for women is 5g of salt per day.

■ Try cutting down on your consumption of caffeine too (that means going easy on coffee, tea, and cola drinks); there is thought to be a link between caffeine and menstrual cramps, breast tenderness, and other symptoms. If you find that cutting down on caffeine helps, do so all the time – not just before a period.

■ Keep up your blood sugar levels by eating regular small meals rather than irregular large meals; some experts feel that low blood sugar levels can worsen irritability and aggressiveness.

■ If you suffer from constipation then try a high-fiber diet by simply increasing your intake of green vegetables, fresh fruit, and whole grain bread; or you can try a teaspoon of psyllium husk each morning (you can get it from a health food store).

■ Of the many over-the-counter remedies for PMS, aspirin and acetaminophen are still the best painkillers you can buy.

■ Many women find exercise helps PMS, even if it's only taking the dog for a walk or walking upstairs rather than taking the elevator. If you go to the gym regularly don't stop during the PMS week. Exercise such as swimming and walking, deep breathing, and relaxation techniques can all be helpful in bringing relief from tension and insomnia.

■ Help your PMS with diet (see box, right).

■ Herbs such as black cohosh may help.

WHAT IS THE TREATMENT?
DIET
Not all women require medical help with PMS and often your symptoms will be sufficiently controlled by changes to diet and lifestyle.

There's quite a lot of evidence that a healthy diet, particularly one low in fat and high in fruit, vegetables, and whole grains, can go a long way to relieving PMS.

What's really helpful is to eat starchy food every two to three hours to keep your blood-sugar level up. You can do this by having three main meals and three smaller snacks each day. Eating this way is particularly important in the second half of your cycle when your PMS is likely to occur. On the face of it, it seems to be a lot of food, but try to eat small meals so that you can manage the snacks.

WHAT YOUR DOCTOR MIGHT PRESCRIBE
Progestogen
No matter what you read, there's no evidence that taking progestogen in whatever form – not even progesterone cream – will help to relieve symptoms of PMS, and there may also be unpleasant side effects such as breast tenderness, water retention and loss of sex drive.

Estrogen
■ Estrogen is known to exert a profound effect on mood and mental state. Rapidly falling levels of estrogen run parallel with PMS, postpartum depression and postmenopausal depression.

■ Doctors at Chelsea and Westminster Hospital in London have developed a treatment for PMS based on giving natural estrogen by means of skin patches. This has the effect of suppressing ovulation and eliminating fluctuations in the menstrual cycle. The patches are like sticky plastic wrap and women can swim, bathe, or shower as usual. Estrogen skin patches are one of the few treatments proven scientifically to be highly effective for PMS.

Helping PMS with diet

Try to eat LESS:
■ Saturated fat
■ Sugar
■ Salt
■ Caffeine
■ Alcohol

Try to eat MORE:
■ Starchy foods
■ Fiber
■ Vegetables
■ Fruit
■ Nuts and seeds

Snack ideas
■ Bowl of unsweetened cereal (with low-fat milk).
■ Sandwich with low-fat filling.
■ Fruit, low-fat yogurt or rice pudding.
■ A plain cracker, for example, a digestive, or rich tea.
■ Any of the following with a thin layer of spread: crispbread, crackers, rice cakes, oatcakes, bread, English muffins, whole grain toast, muffins, scones, or buns.

Antidepressants
Until recently, I was against the use of tranquillizers and antidepressants for PMS, but a new generation of antidepressants has been developed called **selective serotonin reuptake inhibitors** (SSRIs), which will bring relief to some PMS sufferers. It is worth discussing these with your doctor.

Fortunately, the new antidepressants, which include fluoxetine and paroxetine, are not addictive. They work to increase levels of serotonin in the brain and restore emotional balance. Studies have shown that SSRIs work faster in PMS than in depression (three weeks).

BREATHING TECHNIQUES
The way you breathe is closely related to the way you feel. If you're angry or upset, breathing is fast, shallow and irregular. When you're calm and relaxed, your breathing is slow and deep. You can consciously affect the way you feel by altering your breathing. Here are two ways to make yourself calmer.

■ **Breath awareness:** close your eyes and just be aware of your breathing. You don't have to change your breathing in any way, just notice your breath as it flows in and out.

■ **Alternate nostril breathing:** there's a greater flow of air through one nostril than through the other. You can activate the relaxation response by blocking the right nostril or by lying on your right side. This allows the right side of the brain to be associated with the relaxation response – to become dominant.

Depression after childbirth

CHANGES IN HORMONE LEVELS AFTER CHILDBIRTH CAN PROFOUNDLY AFFECT THE EMOTIONS. IN MOST WOMEN, EMOTIONAL SWINGS – THE "BABY BLUES" – LAST ONLY A FEW DAYS, BUT IN OTHERS THEY LEAD TO THE MORE PROLONGED, SERIOUS CONDITION CALLED POSTPARTUM DEPRESSION.

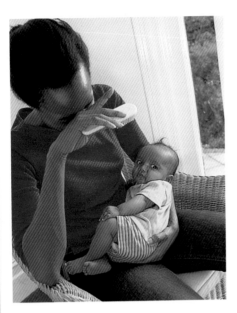

It's certainly true that nothing can prepare you for caring for a new baby. The physical and emotional upheaval is bound to have an impact; quite often when most mothers think they're going to be happiest, they feel very low – the "baby blues." In most instances this only lasts a few days but, sadly, in others, these feelings can continue for months due to a condition known as postpartum depression. It's important for a father to be aware of the symptoms and recognize the difference between the normal "blues" and real depression so that he knows how to help and when to seek medical advice.

BABY BLUES

The "baby blues" are mood swings caused by hormonal changes. In all likelihood this period of feeling low one minute and euphoric the next won't last beyond the first week but you'll still need a lot of support to get you through it. Maybe the "baby blues" are a natural sign to those around you that you need time and space to come to terms with being a mother. That's certainly how a concerned partner, relative, or friend should deal with it, although you'll find that because your hormones are all over the place, you'll also cry when someone's nice to you!

WHY DO YOU GET THE BLUES?

Your hormones, progesterone and estrogen, have been high during pregnancy. After you have had your baby, these hormone levels drop and your body may find it difficult to adjust. This can have a marked effect on your emotions.

With this, and the fact that you're probably completely exhausted from the labor and lack of sleep, it's not at all surprising that you may not be feeling on top of the world.

WHAT CAN YOU DO TO HELP YOURSELF?
■ Give yourself time: accept that you'll feel like this for a short time and that what you're going through is incredibly common.
■ Accept offers of help and don't try to do everything yourself.
■ Try to talk about your feelings and have a good cry if it helps.
■ Tell your partner you need a lot of love and affection, but remember this is a time of upheaval and change for him too.

DO FATHERS GET THE BLUES?
Most fathers feel an anticlimax after the birth. There are the extra responsibilities and sudden changes in lifestyle. If your partner is feeling low, you'll be called on to be a tower of strength, which can be a huge strain. Try to think of the first few months as a period of rapid change that is testing for both of you; when you come through it, you'll emerge closer than you were before. If you get really unhappy,

talk things over with your doctor or a relative or close friend.

POSTPARTUM DEPRESSION (PPD)
If symptoms that started out as the common "baby blues" don't go away and, in fact, start to become worse, you could be suffering from **postpartum depression**. This is a temporary and treatable condition that varies from woman to woman. It can develop slowly and not become obvious until several weeks after the baby's birth, but if it's diagnosed and addressed early enough, there's a good chance of a fast cure. Doctors should recognize the symptoms, and treatment ranges from something as simple as talking to a friend, family member, or doctor about how you feel, to taking medication, such as antidepressants, for more severe cases.

WHY POSTPARTUM DEPRESSION HAPPENS
There are many reasons why postpartum depression occurs. It depends on you as a person, your personal circumstances and the way your baby behaves. Research shows that the following risk factors may make you more susceptible to postpartum depression.

SELF-HELP

Overcoming postpartum depression

If you are feeling low, there are a number of things you can do to help yourself.

Believe in recovery Convince yourself that **you will get better**, no matter how much time that takes.

Correct potassium deficiency Severe exhaustion, another possible problem after giving birth, may be made worse by a lack of potassium in your body. **Low potassium** levels are easily corrected by eating plenty of potassium-rich foods such as bananas or tomatoes.

Rest as much as possible Being tired definitely makes depression worse and harder to deal with. Catnap during the day and, if possible, get someone to help with night feedings.

Maintain a proper diet Eat plenty of fruit and raw vegetables; don't snack or binge on chocolate, candy, and cookies. Eat little and often. Do not go on a strict diet.

Get gentle exercise Give yourself a rest from being indoors or taking care of the baby. A brisk walk in the fresh air can lift your spirits.

Avoid major upheavals Don't start a new job, move to a new home or redecorate.

Try not to worry unduly Aches and pains are common after childbirth, and more so if you are depressed. Try to take them in stride; they will almost certainly fade away as soon as you can relax.

Be kind to yourself Don't force yourself to do things you don't want to do or that might upset you. Don't worry about not keeping the house spotless or letting household chores lapse. Concern yourself with small, undemanding tasks and reward yourself when you finish them.

Talk about your feelings Don't bottle up your concerns; this can make matters worse. Talk to others, particularly your partner.

- If you enjoyed a senior position at work or high-powered career before the birth, it can be difficult to adjust to the status change.
- If you already have difficulties in your relationship, the baby may make them worse; this in itself may lead to disillusionment and low self-esteem.
- If you had an unexpectedly difficult birth experience, you could easily feel demoralized and feel that you've failed in some way.
- If you've had depression in the past, you may be more prone to PPD now.
- A very demanding, sleepless baby can trigger postpartum depression from sheer exhaustion.
- If you have particularly difficult living conditions and no support network, this can exacerbate postpartum depression.
- If you've bottled up your emotions and not sought help early on, PPD may develop.

SEEKING HELP

Many women are too embarrassed to admit how they feel, fearing that it will appear that they have somehow failed. Talking about how you feel is the most important thing you can do; once you accept that you're not "crazy" and that there are things you can do to help yourself, you are on the road to recovery. Once you seek help you'll be guided to:
- understand how you feel and learn to express this
- learn to prioritize and go with the flow
- devote more time to yourself and find ways to relax
- visit the doctor more regularly and seek support
- begin taking medication if your postpartum depression is very extreme.

WHAT FATHERS CAN DO

As a father, you may feel helpless because you don't understand PPD. Remember, it's temporary and treatable, so try to be patient. You can be a huge help if you make an effort to understand and do the following:
- Talk and listen to your partner. Never tell her to pull herself together – she can't. Don't assume she'll snap out of it – she won't.
- Mother the mother: encourage her to rest and eat and drink properly.
- Encourage her to be with the baby as much as she wants, so she can take things slowly and gradually figure out how the baby will fit in.
- Make sure she's not alone too much.
- See the doctor first for advice; your partner may refuse to accept she's ill. The doctor may arrange to visit her informally at home.

Menopausal depression

FEELINGS SUCH AS TENSION, ANXIETY, DEPRESSION, LISTLESSNESS, IRRITABILITY, TEARFULNESS AND MOOD SWINGS CAN OCCUR AT ANY AGE, BUT THEY RARELY OCCUR TOGETHER OR AS FREQUENTLY AS THEY DO DURING MENOPAUSE.

If you are experiencing several negative feelings simultaneously, it may be helpful to know that menopause is the reason.

For many women, menopausal mood changes resemble a roller coaster ride. Women describe subtle sensations such as trembling, fluttering, unease, and discomfort. More severe feelings of anxiety or panic can arise with little provocation. Tasks that you used to be able to tackle can leave you in total disarray. Mood swings from elation to despondency are common. Your patience is easily exhausted. The future may look hopeless, your loss of self-esteem is precipitous, and you may feel truly depressed.

WHAT ARE THE CAUSES?

- The centers in the brain that control a sense of well-being, a positive state of mind, and a feeling of control and tranquility are affected by the absence of estrogen. Taking estrogen supplements as hormone replacement therapy (HRT) can cause a dramatic return to normalcy.
- For some women, the emotional troubles they experience around menopause may mainly be due to the fact that their sleep is being interrupted by night sweats. People who are tired are often irritable and anxious. If you're experiencing this problem, try the self-help tips for promoting sleep on p.297.
- A major depression, although rare, can descend upon you during your menopausal years, and this is distinct from other emotional symptoms that you may experience, such as tearfulness and anxiety. These are possible predictors of depression during menopause:

- a past or recent history of stressful events, such as divorce or bereavement
- a surgically induced menopause
- having negative expectations of menopause
- severe hot flashes or night sweats
- a family history of depressive illness
- "empty nest" syndrome.

Depression can be a debilitating illness that can last for weeks, months or even years if left untreated. It affects your body, your mood, your thoughts, and severely interferes with normal life. As a woman, you're more likely to experience depression than a man is.

Consult your doctor if you have experienced four of these symptoms for at least two weeks:
- any extreme eating patterns, such as bingeing or loss of appetite
- unusual sleeping patterns, such as sleeping all the time or insomnia
- being exceptionally lethargic or restless
- an inability to enjoy a once pleasurable activity, including a loss of sex drive
- debilitating fatigue or loss of energy
- feelings of worthlessness and self-reproach
- difficulty concentrating, remembering, and making decisions
- thoughts of death or suicide, or suicide attempts (seek help right away).

COMPLEMENTARY THERAPIES

Herbs that may have a calming effect are **passion flower** and **valerian root**, taken as a tea or a tincture. Passion flower helps insomnia, and elevates the levels of serotonin in the blood, which creates a feeling of well-being. A herbal bath can also be therapeutic.

SELF-HELP

Managing depression

- Severe mood swings and irritability can distance you from your partner and occasionally can jeopardize a relationship. However, if you share your feelings you may find your partner is very supportive. Several studies show that partners are eager to understand menopausal symptoms and would prefer to have insight into potential problems before the onset of menopause.
- Women who go to support groups may be better able to deal with depression. Think about joining such a group or starting one yourself.
- 20–30 minutes of strenuous exercise results in the release of endorphins, which are brain opioids similar to morphine. This can lift mood and produce an "exercise high" that lasts up to eight hours. Exercise can also reduce hot flashes and night sweats, which is helpful if these are the root cause of your depression.
- Yoga, relaxation techniques, and meditation all promote tranquillity and combat anxiety and tension.

Some women find that menopausal depression and stress may be alleviated by **ginger**, **cayenne pepper**, **dandelion root,** and **Siberian ginseng**. These may work because they contain essential nutrients; for instance:

- dandelion root contains magnesium, potassium, and vitamin E
- cayenne pepper contains a high level of magnesium and bioflavonoids
- ginseng contains estrogenic compounds,

and Siberian ginseng and licorice root, which have been important medicines in the Far East for thousands of years, are said to combat lassitude and depression.

MEDICAL TREATMENT
A mainstay of treatment for emotional symptoms is HRT. Studies from all over the world show that after a short period (between two weeks and two months) HRT can bring

about a significant decline in anxiety and depression. Estrogen even lifts the mood in nondepressed, healthy young women. It acts through several well-known antidepressive mechanisms in the brain, on which other antidepressant drugs also act. The tranquilizing effect of estrogen is considerable. Many women describe getting their "bottle" back, feeling more stable, and enjoying sound sleep once again.

Sexual assault

THE PHYSICAL AND PSYCHOLOGICAL AFTEREFFECTS OF BEING SEXUALLY ASSAULTED CAN
BE DEVASTATING. HERE I INCLUDE ADVICE ON REDUCING THE RISKS OF BEING RAPED
AND ON WHAT TO DO BOTH DURING AN ATTACK AND AFTERWARD.

Although the incidence of rape remains alarmingly high, rape rates in the US have generally declined since 1991 but remained the same between 2000 and 2001. Although it is a fact not often recognized, adult men may also be victims of rape. Most cases of rape occur between people who know each other, making it difficult for the victim to prove that rape has taken place. Moreover, it often occurs in circumstances where the victim is unlikely to tell anyone about it or where she is not likely to be believed since there are no witnesses.

This last situation, which says a lot about prevailing double standards in society, has further repercussions for rape victims. Even if the ordeal of rape is bad, going to the police and courts can be worse. Most rape victims find insensitivity and callousness, if not downright obstructiveness and disbelief, at all levels of the legal process – from police questioning, to the gynecological examination, to the questioning of the prosecutor and lawyer. It is a brave woman who follows up a rape charge to the end; most women do not want every detail of their daily lives laid bare in court or to deal with innuendos or implications about their sexual behavior. The present rape laws are designed to protect men from women, and quite innocent behavior on the part of women can be misinterpreted in a very sinister way against them.

THE POTENTIAL RAPIST
While it is impossible to generalize about the kind of man who rapes women, certain characteristics occur too frequently to be coincidental. Rapists very often dislike women and find their desire to intimidate and humiliate them difficult to control. Frequently they are described as immature and are often known to be violent. Usually they believe that the only way they can achieve sexual satisfaction is through violence, and many have sexual problems such as impotence

or an inability to reach orgasm. Very often rapists have been subjected to humiliation at some time in their lives and they feel they have to get rid of their resentment by attacking other human beings.

Alcohol is frequently connected with rape. One study revealed that 50 percent of rapists had used alcohol before the rape, and 35 percent of them were actually alcoholics.

AVOIDING RAPE
There are certain things that you can do to reduce your risk of being raped.

ON THE STREET
- Don't venture alone into areas where you know there has been trouble and where there are street gangs.
- If you suspect that someone is following you, walk out into the middle of the street where there are cars, and run.
- If you feel that you may be about to be attacked, run into the middle of the street and start screaming. It is quite likely (though not certain) that if a potential attacker is faced with a crowd, he will not attack you.

BY YOUR CAR
- Never leave your parked car unlocked.
- Park by a streetlight at night, if possible.
- Before you get into your parked car, look at the backseat.

AT HOME
- Have strong locks on your windows and doors.
- Install and use a peephole.
- Never open your front door to a man who has come to do a job in your house without checking his identity.

ONCE ATTACKED
- If you find yourself in a situation where you are being sexually assaulted, scream as loudly

as you can and fight as hard as you can. Try to get a finger in the man's eye or pull your knee up sharply into his groin.
- On the other hand, if your assailant is armed, lack of resistance on your part may be necessary to save your life.

BEING RAPED
Once you determine that resistance is useless or is likely to lead to more violence against yourself, do the following things.
- Stay calm. Talk quietly and carefully to your attacker to remind him that you are human.
- Don't excite him further by answering leading questions about your feelings during rape – reply with a calm, factual statement about something else, for example, "You're hurting my back."
- Concentrate on his features and clothing and on any regional accent or speech patterns, or other identifying factors.
- Think about something concrete and routine – like what you are going to do about notifying the authorities once you're free.
- Try not to show any pain or weakness as it will only make him more violent.

INFORMING THE AUTHORITIES
When you have to report the case to the police it is almost certain to be embarrassing, so ask to be in a private room, and with a female officer if there is one at that police station. If at any time you think that your investigator is becoming offensive, don't be afraid to say so. Always have a second person with you while your statement is being taken.

If your case goes to trial, you will find it at the least embarrassing and, possibly, psychologically traumatic. However, all the questions that you can be asked either for the police report or in court must, by law, be confined to the rape incident, and questions into your private sex life are not permitted. Many women's groups have volunteers on call who will accompany rape victims to court. If you cannot get one of these women to accompany you, take a friend.

The legal definition of rape is contact between a penis and the vagina against the will of the victim. One of the most difficult things to prove is that there was force, particularly if there is no bodily injury. This is why you should contact your doctor as soon as you can after rape, so that he or she can perform a careful medical examination; the testimony may count in your favor in court.

Also by legal definition, fear of bodily injury is considered force, and you will have to prove that in court too. In other words, you must prove you did not willingly engage in sexual activities.

THE MEDICAL EXAMINATION

The presence of sperm or semen in your vagina is considered to be very strong corroborative evidence of rape. However, it is possible that your rapist did not ejaculate – 1 in 3 don't – and therefore the medical examination becomes crucial to see if there is any evidence of injury. It is very important for you to tell the doctor and the police if you think that the man didn't ejaculate.

■ You will first have a general examination of your whole body, so that the doctor can describe bruises, redness, cuts, pain, and tenderness.

■ Then you will have an internal pelvic examination, partly to look for evidence of injury and partly to take a sample of the vaginal secretions. Examination of these secretions will show if there are any sperm present. It will also identify a chemical called **acid phosphitase**, which is found in seminal fluid and will be present in your vagina if the man ejaculated but had no sperm.

■ It is possible that your mouth and anus will be examined to see if the attacker has harmed these areas.

■ Blood samples will be taken to check for HIV infection and syphilis. If there is a risk of developing HIV infection, you may be prescribed a course of antiviral drugs to reduce this risk.

■ The doctor will probably prescribe antibiotics to prevent STDs, such as syphilis and gonorrhea. You will be offered emergency contraception if there is a risk of pregnancy. Doctors are familiar with the use of the morning-after pill to prevent conception. You can discuss this possibility with the doctor, and if you find that your period is delayed, discuss with the doctor the possibility of having a menstrual extraction.

■ Don't let the doctor put you off by saying that the chances of you having caught an STD or being pregnant are very small. Assert yourself and your rights.

■ Never leave the emergency room without getting a name, address, and telephone number, so that you can phone the hospital

Checklist for post-rape action

1. If there is no one in the house, telephone a friend or relative who can get to you fairly quickly, so that they can give you support. Try to keep them with you all the time.

2. Report the crime to the police: if you feel you cannot do this, tell your nearest and dearest friend immediately, who may be able to persuade you to report the incident.

3. Contact your doctor and ask to see him or her as soon as possible or go to hospital if your doctor is not immediately available.

4. Do not take a bath. Take off the clothing you were wearing. Do not wash or change it, as doctors and police may want to examine it.

5. Try to remember every detail you can about the man who assaulted you. Keep a notepad by you and write down everything you can remember: not just physical features, but perhaps a regional accent or peculiar words that the rapist used.

6. After you have made your report to the police, don't go home alone. Don't stay at home by yourself. Try always to have a friend with you or if that is not possible, go and stay with friends or relatives.

7. There are rape crisis centers in many areas, or local women's groups that will give you advice. Contact one of them quickly.

back if any problems arise, and say that you will do so.

■ Subsequent visits may be necessary after six weeks to test for syphilis and gonorrhea and at three and six months for repeat HIV and hepatitis B and C testing.

Your state of mind after being raped makes it quite difficult for you to think calmly and coolly about all the things that you should be doing and asking. Indeed, you may be so shocked that you cannot think straight or say anything. This is one of the reasons why it is very important to have a friend with you so that she can act as your advocate to ensure that nothing is forgotten and that everything is done.

COPING WITH RAPE

The after effects of rape are both physical and psychological. You may discover a vaginal discharge and you may have itching of the perineum – this could be due to an infection of candidiasis (yeast) or trichomoniasis. Quite often bruises, swelling, and tenderness appear several hours after the rape. If they do, go back to the same doctor who examined you to make sure that they are recorded. It is possible for slight tears to occur in the lining of the rectum if your assailant involved this area. Sometimes they may bleed when you move your bowels. Make sure that you report this also to the doctor who examined you, even if some time has elapsed.

No woman who is raped does not suffer some sort of psychological aftereffect, though it differs greatly. Some women are completely stunned, and others are quite calm. However, it is quite normal to suffer some anxiety, which may go as far as hysterical behavior. It is also

perfectly normal to be afraid of being left alone, even for a few minutes; it is normal not to be able to sleep, and it is normal to want to run away and hide yourself. With the help of family and friends, these feelings will pass more quickly than if you stay alone. When choosing a friend that you want to stay with, choose the one that cares most about you and not about the fact that you were raped. This is because many people have conflicting ideas about rape and they may give more attention to the incident than to your particular needs.

One of the best ways to help yourself is through women's groups and through rape crisis centers; this is because they are experienced in dealing with all the various reactions that a woman can feel after being raped. They will counsel you and give you comfort. They will seek legal advice on your behalf and they will help to get you through your serious psychological upsets. One of the most important things is that you get help and support from friends and sympathetic groups as soon as possible. This way you are giving yourself the best chance of coming through your rape experience without long-term psychological trauma.

Women's rape crisis centers say that one of the most helpful emotions for you to express after rape is rage, so get angry if you feel like it. They also point out that the least helpful emotion is guilt. Sympathetic and understanding friends, and qualified counselors from rape crisis centers, can help you to come to terms with both of these emotions.

Body dysmorphic disorder

PEOPLE WITH BODY DYSMORPHIC DISORDER (BDD) HAVE A DISTORTED PERCEPTION
OF THEIR OWN BODY SHAPE, BECOMING PREOCCUPIED WITH AN IMAGINED DEFECT
OR SHOWING EXCESSIVE CONCERN ABOUT SOME MINOR ANOMALY.

These are normal adolescent anxieties blown up to monstrous proportions, so that eventually you may believe that if anyone even looks at you in the street they're condemning you for living. Like one man with BDD said, "The only place you feel comfortable is in book stores looking at pictures of people with horrible deformities."

Self-loathing can be so intense that you repeatedly mutilate yourself. Life may become one complex ritual. You check your face in the mirror hundreds of times a day and it can take you five hours to get ready to go out.

Just why someone tumbles into the BDD pit of self-loathing no one knows. There's speculation about triggering events in childhood. Researchers at a hospital in England have shown that anorexics have reduced blood flow to the part of their brain that controls vision, which might be linked with the distortion of their body image.

Brain scans have revealed that several areas in the brain malfunction in cases of obsessive-compulsive disorder. Is something similar going on with BDD? No one knows yet. However, about 60 percent of those affected recover with therapy.

What's so fascinating about BDD is that, although it involves a level of obsession and isolation that most of us can barely imagine, we can all dimly empathize with it. We all feel our noses could be smaller or that we could be shorter or taller or fatter or thinner, and we wish we had perfect skin, longer legs, or more or less hair.

In our body-beautiful and celebrity-obsessed culture, the BDD sufferer is like the rest of us, only more so.

Body dysmorphic disorder (BDD sufferers typically try to hide their "affliction." We have known for some time that anorexics have a distorted perception of their bodies: no matter how thin they are they still see themselves as the Michelin man. And it's not restricted to women – men are increasingly perceiving themselves as too thin and becoming obsessive about weight training and body building, even to the extent of taking anabolic steroids. In the most severe cases people go to extraordinary lengths to rid themselves of their ugly feature, in some cases amputating an unwanted limb.

WHAT ARE THE CAUSES?

Body dysmorphic disorder shares features with several other psychiatric conditions, including anorexia and obsessive-compulsive disorder (OCD). Like anorexics, BDD sufferers see their body in a distorted way, but while anorexics flaunt their thinness and are proud of it, people with BDD regard their affliction as a terrible secret.

Preoccupation with an imagined defect in appearance is the basis of this disorder. If a slight physical anomaly is present, the person's concern is markedly excessive.

BDD quite often starts in adolescence when teenagers are plagued with insecurity and shyness. It wouldn't be uncommon to feel that everything about you was wrong, the size of your head, your hands, your height, your thinness, your fatness, your acne. You may resort to all sorts of remedies – Charles Atlas to build you up, cream to stop your hair from falling out, powerful skin treatments because you're convinced your skin looks like the lunar surface.

WHAT IS THE TREATMENT?

The recommended treatment for BDD is cognitive therapy. This involves being exposed to more and more challenging situations until you can begin to function in society again. Selective serotonin reuptake inhibitor (SSRI) drugs can help too. Also, support groups give help and advice.

See also:
• **Psychological therapies p. 286**

Allergies and the Immune System

Image shows a colored scanning electron micrograph of white blood cells and platelets

Miriam's overview

The immune system makes us immune – immune to infections, foreign proteins, and to cancer. It brings together a complex array of interacting genes, cells, enzymes, and chemicals, so complex that much of it still remains a mystery.

We've managed to make sense of a few small corners but are still miles away from making sense of the whole.

I'd be the first to admit that anything I have to say merely scratches the surface. My aim is to throw light on some common conditions involving the immune system so that you'll have a better understanding of what's going on and how to deal with them.

"Boosting your immune system" is a phrase bandied about by manufacturers in the hope that you'll buy their product for which this claim is made. I wish I understood what the phrase means, I'd probably be seduced into buying the product too. But I don't.

I don't know of anything that boosts the immune system, certainly not by a supplement of any vitamin or mineral. The immune system doesn't work like that. The only way that I know of giving the immune system a boost is a dose of an infection. Then the whole defense system swings into action, the T cells get busy and antibodies start pumping.

That's why immunization works so well and why childhood vaccinations are so important. They put our immune systems through their paces. Vaccinations do this so efficiently that they may make us immune for life.

An allergy is simply an expression of an immune system that's out of hand – it's become too sensitive – it tries to protect us from things that most immune systems don't even bother about – pollen, dust, dust mites, mold spores, even foods.

Now it's possible to retrain that trigger-happy immune system with desensitizing injections, but most of the time doctors simply have to numb it with antiallergic medicines, as we do in most cases of asthma.

Sometimes the immune system can get out of hand and start protecting the body against itself. When it does, the resulting condition is called an autoimmune disorder. Rheumatoid arthritis is an example, when the body turns on its own joints.

> "it's possible *to retrain* that trigger-happy *immune system* with desensitizing injections"

And if the immune system falls down on its protective job we can be in an awful lot of trouble. AIDS is one instance of that, where the virus, HIV, systematically dismantles the fundamental elements of the immune system, making us vunerable to opportunistic infections and cancers, often fatally (see p. 338).

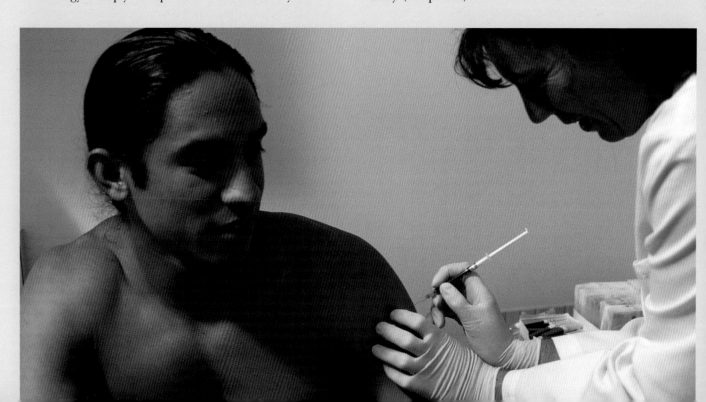

INSIDE
your immune system

The body has many barriers to infection and various types of **immune responses** to invading organisms and cancerous cells. For example, **sebum** and **sweat**, excreted by the skin, are mildly antiseptic. **Tears** contain a more powerful antiseptic. **Mucus**, secreted by the lining of the respiratory tract and the stomach, protects the body by trapping harmful organisms. In the **antibody immune response**, white blood cells known as **B lymphocytes** or **B cells** attack and destroy invading bacteria. In the **cellular immune** response, white blood cells known as **T lymphocytes** or T cells attack and destroy viruses, parasites, and cancer cells.

In an **allergic reaction**, the immune system becomes sensitized to a substance that is normally harmless, such as pollen. Subsequent exposure to the substance causes **mast cells**, which are located in the skin and nasal lining as well as in other tissues, to release **histamine**. Histamine causes an **inflammatory response** and brings on the symptoms of allergy.

the body's defenses

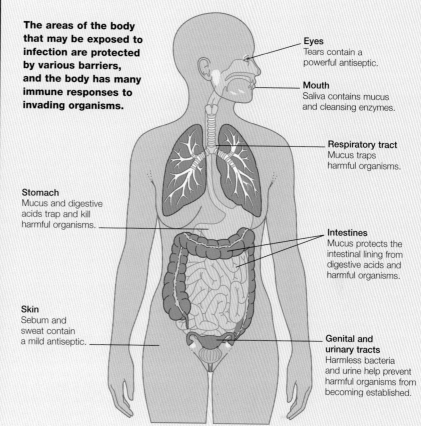

The areas of the body that may be exposed to infection are protected by various barriers, and the body has many immune responses to invading organisms.

Eyes
Tears contain a powerful antiseptic.

Mouth
Saliva contains mucus and cleansing enzymes.

Respiratory tract
Mucus traps harmful organisms.

Stomach
Mucus and digestive acids trap and kill harmful organisms.

Intestines
Mucus protects the intestinal lining from digestive acids and harmful organisms.

Skin
Sebum and sweat contain a mild antiseptic.

Genital and urinary tracts
Harmless bacteria and urine help prevent harmful organisms from becoming established.

THE ATOPIC FAMILY OF CONDITIONS

I'd like to tell you about a particular and common form of allergy. What is atopy? The word "atopic" means that a person is born with a predisposition to develop an extra sensitivity to certain things, usually invisible proteins called allergens, in the environment. The most common triggers or allergens in these people are the house dust mite (more accurately the droppings of the dust mite), grass, tree, and weed pollen, proteins in cat and dog dander and saliva, feather, and occasionally foods, such as egg, milk, or nuts.

Atopic people have a hypersensitivity of their immune system and produce too much of the IgE allergy antibody. They have no other problem with their immune system, but this sensitivity leads to ATOPY. A gene is responsible and the gene can be passed down through a family. Family members show up this atopic gene in any or all of several different ways.

So if you belong to an "atopic" family you can track your "atopic" gene showing up as any of these conditions:

• childhood eczema
• dermatitis
• asthma
• hay fever
• allergies
• migraines (I describe this with other headaches, see p. 407).

At first glance these conditions don't seem to be closely related, but they're all expressions of the atopic gene so I describe them here as a family of conditions.

Eczema

ECZEMA DESCRIBES AN ITCHY, INFLAMED SKIN RASH. THE TERM ECZEMA COMES FROM A GREEK WORD MEANING TO "BOIL OVER" AND IS USED INTERCHANGEABLY WITH ANOTHER TERM, DERMATITIS. THERE ARE SEVERAL DIFFERENT TYPES, INCLUDING ATOPIC OR ALLERGIC ECZEMA.

The most common type of eczema is atopic eczema, sometimes referred to as "allergic eczema." If someone is atopic they carry a gene that makes their skin react to stress (a virus infection, an irritant in contact with the skin, psychological disturbances) with patches of eczema. Once you have eczema or dermatitis you will **always** have the tendency to develop it, so episodes may return throughout your life.

Atopic eczema sufferers may also develop asthma or hay fever or may have relatives who have those conditions. The gene for atopy tends to run in families but may express itself differently in family members, for example migraine in one, hay fever in another, allergies in another, asthma, etc. All these conditions are close relatives of eczema (dermatitis) and all run in my atopic family.

Though the tendency to develop eczema is undoubtedly genetic, certain foods (most commonly dairy products, eggs, and wheat) and skin irritants (such as pet dander, wool, or laundry detergents) can act as triggers, especially in children.

WHAT ARE THE SYMPTOMS?

■ Dry, red, scaly rash, which is extremely itchy, occurring on the face, neck, and hands, and in the creases of the limbs.
■ The rash usually starts off as minute pearly blisters beneath the skin's surface.
■ When very severe, the rash may weep.
■ Sleeplessness may result if the itchiness is very bad.

AGGRAVATING FACTORS

Symptoms vary from mild to severe and can be made worse by:
● climate changes, especially if exposed to cold winds or excessive heat
● water, especially hard water
● soaps, detergents, cleansers, bubble bath, cosmetics, perfume
● pollen, pet hair, animal dander, dust
● stress and anxiety
● synthetic or wool fibers
● certain chemicals: acids, alkalis, oxidizing or reducing agents, oils, solvents
● colds, flu, infections of any kind.

LIFESTYLE

■ People with eczema should avoid contact with soap, detergents, and other irritants and immersing hands in water. This means wearing rubber gloves for household wet work, or cotton gloves for cleaning.
■ They should avoid jobs or occupations that expose their skin to irritants, such as in hairdressing, catering, mechanics, and perhaps nursing, especially if the eczema affects the hands.
■ Reduce the population of dust mites in the home by regular dusting and vacuuming of carpets. Dust mite bedcovers have benefited some eczema patients, and frequent airing and changing of bed linen should reduce the dust mite population in bedding.
■ Bed linens should be washed at 50°C (122°F) or more to kill dust mites.
■ Old mattresses are more likely to harbor large populations of dust mites, and furry toys are another source of exposure.
■ Shaking soft toys vigorously or placing them into a plastic bag in the freezer for a few hours helps.
■ Some atopic people are sensitive to cat or dog dander and it makes sense to avoid having these animals as pets when a family member suffers from atopic eczema.
■ The use of makeup can irritate facial skin in a person with eczema, and these preparations should be used with care.
■ It is best to keep the heat turned as low as is comfortable since it has a tendency to dry out the skin.
■ Cotton clothes are less irritating on eczema skin than polyester or wool.
■ Bathing and showering are safe, provided that a soap substitute such as water-based cream is used, or a bath oil is added.
■ Bubble bath should be avoided, since it is a detergent. The moisturizer that the person uses should be applied after the skin has been patted dry.
■ Vacations in a warm environment are beneficial since the skin's moisture is improved and, of course, the person is more relaxed.
■ Although sunlight is usually helpful, atopic eczema may make the skin more sun-sensitive and covering up with cotton clothes and using a sunscreen are advised in hot climates to avoid burning.
■ People with eczema can **go swimming**. Putting an emollient ointment or cream on the skin before and after swimming reduces irritation.

IS DIET IMPORTANT?

■ In very young children, atopic eczema may be worsened by **cow milk formulas** and so infants with eczema are often put on soy milk, or low-allergy milk formulas. This problem generally settles in the second year of life and cow milk may then be tolerated in slowly increasing amounts.

■ **Eggs** may worsen eczema, although they may be tolerated in highly processed form, such as in cakes.

■ Families may feel that other food items are important and if several foods are suspected or you decide to put your child on a restricted diet, then it is wise to discuss this with a nutritionist or allergist to make sure your child is getting enough protein, calcium, and calories.

■ Fortunately, most apparent food allergies get better during childhood.

■ One food item that continues to cause problems in a few atopic individuals is **peanuts**.

■ **Tomato sauce** and **citrus fruits** seem to worsen facial eczema because they irritate broken skin and can produce welts around the mouth.

CHINESE HERBAL TREATMENTS

Chinese herbal treatments have fallen into disrepute since herbal creams were found to contain anti-inflammatory steroids.

WHAT MIGHT THE DOCTOR DO?

■ Your doctor will question you on your family's medical history, particularly whether anyone has ever suffered from eczema or related conditions such as asthma and hay fever.

■ The doctor will ask you about any changes in diet, whether you have recently changed your laundry detergent, whether you have just brought a pet into the house, and whether natural or synthetic fibers are worn next to the skin.

■ If your baby has eczema and you've just started weaning him from the breast or bottle, your doctor may recommend that you avoid dairy products and continue breast-feeding or use formula milk. If you don't want to do this, your doctor may recommend that you wean your baby onto soy milk instead.

■ Your doctor may prescribe an anti-inflammatory skin cream to reduce redness, scaliness, and itchiness. In severe cases, very weak steroid creams may be prescribed. These creams should be used very sparingly, especially on a child's skin.

■ If the itching is causing sleepless nights, your doctor may prescribe antihistamine medicine to improve sleep.

■ If the skin has become infected through scratching, your doctor may prescribe an antiseptic cream or antibiotics.

■ Your doctor will advise you to add bath oil

to bath water and to stop using soap. Soap can be an irritant to the already sensitive skin; the oil will help to keep the skin supple and less dry.

WHAT'S THE OUTLOOK?

Many children outgrow eczema (and asthma) around the age of seven. They will, however, retain a life-long tendency to develop transient eczema if the body is under stress and may pass on this tendency to their children.

In adult life, dermatitis isn't the same as that in a child. The eczema looks different, it's in different places and it may come and go. It may take the form of seborrheic, contact or photo-dermatitis (caused by light).

Eczema in babies and children

Baby eczema, also called infantile eczema, is common and usually develops when a baby is about 2–3 months old, or at 4–5 months when solid foods are introduced. Most children grow out of eczema by the age of three or, if not, by seven.

Some important points

■ **Baby** eczema is less common in breast-fed babies than those fed by bottle.

■ **Baby** eczema isn't caused by an allergy and allergy tests don't help.

■ **Children** with eczema don't benefit from a special diet.

What should I do first?

■ If your baby is scratching, look at his neck and scalp, his face, his hands, and the creases of his elbows, knees, and groin, classic sites for baby dermatitis.

■ Keep his fingernails short to minimize the possibility of breaking the skin. If the skin becomes broken, put mittens on him to prevent infection.

■ If you've just started weaning your breast-fed child, return to breast-feeding until you've seen your doctor. If you've been using formula, return to that.

■ Apply oily calamine lotion to ease irritation and soothe the skin.

■ Soap should be avoided as it de-fats the skin and makes it drier, more scaly and irritable.

■ Avoid woollen or hairy garments; use cotton or linen instead.

What else can I do?

■ Use an emollient cream whenever your child washes. This will keep his skin soft, prevent it from drying out, and damp down the itchiness.

■ Underplay the condition in front of

your child. Your anxiety can make the condition worse.

■ Keep your child's fingernails short so that scratching doesn't cause the skin to break and give rise to infection.

■ Make sure all your child's clothes, and anything that comes next to his skin, are rinsed thoroughly to remove all traces of powders and conditioners.

■ If the eczema is found to be made worse by pet fur, you may need to consider giving your family pet away.

■ Use a water-based cream from your pharmacy as a soap substitute.

■ Use a bath emollient (available from your pharmacist) dissolved in bath water to put a protective layer over your child's skin.

■ Think about installing a home water softener.

■ Dress your child with cotton next to his skin at all times.

■ Don't eliminate any foods from your child's diet without your doctor's supervision.

■ Remove as many irritants from your child's environment as possible. For example, feather and down pillows can be a source of irritation.

Vaccinations

It is generally safe to vaccinate children with eczema in the usual way. However, if a child has a proven egg allergy, their MMR (measles, mumps, and rubella) vaccination should be given in a hospital setting in case there are problems, although this is very rare in practice.

Contact dermatitis

THE NAME CONTACT DERMATITIS IS USED TO DESCRIBE AN ITCHY, INFLAMED SKIN RASH THAT
DEVELOPS WHEN SOMETHING IN THE OUTSIDE WORLD COMES INTO CONTACT WITH THE SKIN.
OCCUPATIONAL DERMATITIS IS A TYPE OF CONTACT DERMATITIS.

Contact dermatitis may develop if an offending substance is touched directly or sometimes if there is contact with particles of the substance carried in the air. If all further contact with this substance is avoided the dermatitis should get better.

There are two main types of contact dermatitis: **irritant** and **allergic**.

Irritant contact dermatitis is a very common skin problem that affects many people at some stage of their life. It is caused by contact with substances that damage the outer layers of the skin and typically affects the hands. One of the most common situations giving rise to irritant contact dermatitis is repeated contact with mildly irritant substances such as water and detergents (dish washing liquid, soaps, etc.). Other irritant substances include solvents, for example gasoline, cleaning chemicals, oils, and metalworking fluids used in industry. The skin problem often starts as chapping, soreness, and redness, and if untreated leads to a stubborn dermatitis. Once damaged, the skin is no longer a barrier against the outside world and can easily be irritated further. This sets up a vicious circle that can be difficult to break.

Allergic contact dermatitis is less common than irritant contact dermatitis and you're born with the tendency to get it. It happens because the body's immune system reacts against a specific substance or "allergen," making the skin hypersensitive. The tendency to allergic response, or "atopy," is genetic, and you and your relatives may have other atopic conditions such as eczema, asthma, hay fever and migraine. People are not born with this type of allergy, but develop it later, usually in adulthood.

Allergic contact dermatitis usually affects only a minority of people who come into contact with the allergen. What makes an allergy develop at a certain time is unknown, and why one person gets affected while others don't is also unclear. **The most common cause of**

allergic contact dermatitis in women is nickel, which is found in metallic jewellery. About 1 in 10 women has this type of allergy and typically develops itchy, sore, red patches on the ear lobes after wearing inexpensive earrings. Other things that commonly cause allergic contact dermatitis include perfumes, rubber, additives, leather additives, and preservatives in creams and cosmetics. Allergies can also develop to medicated creams and ointments, and sunscreens.

A person can actually suffer from more than one type of dermatitis. For example, someone with atopic eczema (i.e. constitutional eczema) who works as a hairdresser could get skin irritation on their hands from frequent shampooing (i.e. irritant contact dermatitis).

OCCUPATIONAL DERMATITIS
In some cases a person's dermatitis is caused primarily by substances to which they are exposed at work. These may be irritants or allergens depending on the nature of the job. Patch tests should be carried out if the work involves exposure to substances that can cause allergy.

PREVENTING FURTHER DERMATITIS
■ Minimize contact with all irritant substances at work and at home.
■ Avoid skin contact with the substances you are allergic to.
■ Take general skin care measures to keep the skin strong and healthy.

ACTIVE TREATMENT
Treat the dermatitis with frequent application of moisturizers and regular use of steroid creams or ointments once or twice a day. If the dermatitis has become additionally infected, a course of antibiotic cream may be necessary.

GENERAL HAND CARE
The hands are one of the most common parts of the body to be affected with dermatitis. Because they are so important for carrying out the tasks of daily life, skin problems here can be especially troublesome. Good general skin care measures can help to look after the skin and are a major part of the treatment of hand dermatitis.
■ Avoid frequent contact with water and use protective gloves where possible.
■ Use gloves and emollient creams if provided at work.
■ Avoid direct contact with other harsh substances such as the juices from fruit and vegetables, detergents, and cleaning agents.
■ Use a gentle skin cleanser instead of soap for washing with warm water, and dry the hands thoroughly afterward to prevent chapping.
■ Use plenty of moisturizers and reapply them frequently (e.g. during tea and coffee breaks, while watching television and before going to sleep at night).

It can take several months for the skin to recover completely from an episode of dermatitis, so even when it looks apparently normal it is still vulnerable. Try to find the time to take care of your skin and treat it with respect – it has to last you a lifetime!

See also:
• The atopic family of conditions p. 311

Common causes of allergic contact dermatitis

Substance	Where is it often found
Nickel	Cheap jewelry, studs on jeans, metal objects including coins
Fragrance	Perfumes, toiletries, cosmetics
Chromate	Leather items, wet cement
Preservatives	Cosmetics, especially creams (cleansers, moisturizers, etc.)
Rubber additives	Rubber gloves, shoes

Seborrheic dermatitis

THE TERM SEBORRHEIC DERMATITIS DESCRIBES PATCHES OF RED, SCALY, ITCHY
SKIN THAT OCCUR MAINLY ON OILY PARTS OF THE SKIN SUCH AS THE SIDES OF THE NOSE,
SCALP, FACE, AND CHEST. STRESS IS OFTEN A TRIGGER.

Some people are born with the tendency to get seborrheic dermatitis and may get recurrent episodes throughout their life. Seborrheic dermatitis is not an allergy, rather it is a skin rash that commonly occurs in infants and adults. In infants, either the scalp (cradle cap) or the diaper area (diaper rash) may be affected. In adults, the rash tends to occur on the central part of the face, the eyebrows, and the scalp, where it often leads to flaking of the skin. Sometimes seborrheic dermatitis also develops in the armpits, the groin, or the middle of the chest and back. In men, the condition may develop in the beard area.

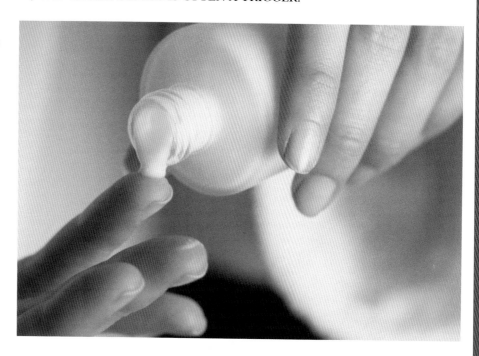

WHAT IS THE TREATMENT?
- Use soap and water.
- Use moisturizing emollient creams.
- Use a weak steroid preparation, such as 1 percent hydrocortisone cream, sparingly and only under medical supervision.
- Avoid stress as much as possible.

ALLERGIES

Some people become ill when they come into contact with a substance that may have no effect on other people. Their illness is due to an allergy – an abnormal response by the immune system to a foreign invader. When a person's immune system reacts abnormally to a substance that has no effect on most people, we say that the affected person has an "allergy" to the substance and that they are suffering from an allergic reaction.

An allergic reaction can show itself in different ways, such as sneezing, an itching or runny nose, breathing problems, swelling of the face (angioedema), and the most serious form, anaphylaxis.

The substance that causes such a reaction is known as an allergen. Common examples of allergens that affect the lungs include pollens from grass and trees, dust mites, and animal fur.

Some people – between a quarter and a third of us – are more likely than others to have allergies of one kind or another. This tendency runs in families and is called "atopy." However, not all the people who have this tendency will actually get allergy problems.

HOW THE BODY RESPONDS TO ALLERGENS
Allergens, usually proteins, are seen by the body as "foreign" and the body's natural response to anything foreign is to repel it.

The body makes antibodies to neutralize and repel the allergen. If you make the allergic type of antibodies (IgE), when allergens and antibodies meet up inside the body there's quite an explosion, with the release of many chemicals that can irritate tissues and even cause disease and illness. An example would be

histamine, which narrows the bronchial tubes and causes wheezing as in asthma.

The symptoms of an allergic disease simply depend on where this explosion happens. So if it's in the skin, you'll get a rash; if it's in the nose, you'll get itching and sneezing; if it's in the lungs, you'll get wheezing.

Very rarely, and for reasons we don't understand, the body may see part of itself as the allergen and attack the thyroid gland or the joints or the pancreas and we then get thyroid disease, arthritis, and diabetes respectively, which are called "autoimmune diseases."

THE MOST COMMON ALLERGIES
1. Some allergies can cause problems all through the year; others only affect us at certain times. The most common cause of year-round allergy is the **dust mite**. These tiny mites,

continued on page 318

FOCUS *on* asthma in children

More cases of asthma are being reported than ever before. Is this because we're all more allergic than we were? Is it because, in towns at least, there's more pollution? Or is it because we don't understand what we have to do to prevent asthma? There's quite a lot of evidence that it is the latter.

Studies from Europe show that children raised on farms and in touch with livestock are two-thirds less likely to develop asthma. The same has been shown in Italian soldiers.

The suggestion is that contact with common or garden bacteria at a young age gives protection.

One theory for the sharp increase in asthma is that children today are so protected against dirt and everyday infections that their immune systems fail to develop normally and are prone to become hypersensitive and then vunerable to allergies.

WHAT IS ASTHMA?

In children, asthma is primarily an allergic disease that affects air passages (bronchi) that are extra sensitive to triggers.

When the allergic reaction takes place, the bronchi constrict and become clogged with mucus, making breathing difficult. The muscle around the walls of the airways tightens so that inhaled air can't be forced out. An asthma attack can be very frightening for a child because the feeling of suffocation can cause panic, making breathing even more labored.

The initial cause of the allergic reaction, the **allergen**, is usually airborne – pollen, house dust, or dust mite for example. Once asthma is established, emotional stress or a mild infection such as a cold can also bring on an attack.

Asthma doesn't usually begin until a child is about two years old. The condition tends to run in families and may, unfortunately, be accompanied by other allergic diseases, such as eczema, hay fever, and penicillin sensitivity.

However, the good news is that most children get better as they get older.

WHEEZING IN BABIES

Many babies under one year wheeze if they suffer from bronchiolitis, when their small air passages become inflamed. These babies aren't necessarily suffering from asthma; as they grow, their air passages widen and the wheezing will stop. Infection, not an allergic reaction, is the usual cause of this kind of wheezing.

IS IT SERIOUS?

Asthma attacks can be frightening but, with medication and advice from your doctor, your child should suffer no serious complications. If inadequately treated, however, patients may die from asthma.

POSSIBLE SYMPTOMS

● Labored breathing: breathing out becomes difficult and the abdomen may be drawn inward with the effort of breathing in.
● Sensation of suffocation.
● Wheezing.
● Persistent cough, particularly at night.
● Getting short of breath – a child doesn't run around as much as usual.
● Blueness around the lips (cyanosis) because of lack of oxygen.

WHAT SHOULD I DO FIRST?

1. Consult your doctor immediately if your child is having any kind of difficulty with breathing.
2. If the attack occurs when your child is in bed, sit him up, propped up with pillows. Otherwise, sit him on a chair with his arms braced against the back to take the weight off his chest; this allows the chest muscles to force air out of the lungs more efficiently.
3. Stay calm; a show of anxiety would only make your child more fearful.
4. While waiting for the doctor, try to take your child's mind off the asthma attack. Sing to him, for example, to try to help him forget about the wheezing.
5. Put a humidifier in the room to ease his sensitive air passages.
6. Give him a lot of reassuring cuddling.

CONSULTING YOUR DOCTOR

The mainstays of treatment are **reliever** drugs to relieve an attack of asthma and **preventer** drugs to stop an attack from happening. Preventer drugs must be taken all the time to keep a child free of asthma symptoms.
● Your doctor will treat the attack with a reliever drug, usually a bronchodilator, which opens up the bronchi by relaxing muscles in the lining of the air passages. This drug is inhaled directly into the bronchi and gets right to the site of the obstruction. A severe attack may need treatment in a hospital, where bigger doses of bronchodilator drugs may be given by inhalation or by intravenous drip.

- If there's evidence of a chest infection, your doctor will prescribe antibiotics.
- Your doctor will want to prevent further attacks. He may, for instance, try to determine the allergen, so that your child can avoid it, probably by performing skin tests for the most likely allergens, such as pollen and house dust.
- He'll give you a supply of a bronchodilator drug, usually as an inhaler used with a "spacer" that is easy for children to use, to be taken as soon as an attack begins.
- Your doctor will ask you to inform him if your child has a severe attack, or if an attack doesn't respond to two doses of the bronchodilator.
- Your doctor may prescribe a steroid drug if other simple measures don't stop more attacks. Don't be afraid, steroids for asthma are nearly always inhaled into the deepest parts of the lungs, and are quite safe. A small dose of steroid may be inhaled daily.

WHAT CAN I DO TO HELP?

- If your doctor has not pinpointed the allergen, try to track it down yourself. Notice when the attacks occur and at what time of the day or year. Avoid obvious allergens such as feather pillows and keep the dust down in your house by damp dusting and vacuuming floors rather than sweeping them.
- Many asthmatics are allergic to animals – their hair, fur and saliva. If you have a pet, ask a friend to care for it for two weeks and see if your child's attacks reduce in frequency.
- Make sure your child has the prescribed drugs nearby at all times.
- Inform his school about the possibility of attacks occurring.
- It's vital your child takes his preventer medicine continuously and does not stop just because he's feeling fine. Never stop a preventer without consulting your doctor.
- Ask to be referred to a respiratory therapist so your child can learn breathing exercises to help him to relax during an attack.
- Encourage your child to stand and sit up straight so that his lungs have more space. Don't let him get overweight, since this will put an extra burden on his lungs.
- Moderate exercise can help his breathing, but too much can bring on an asthma attack. Swimming, however, can be especially helpful for children with asthma.

continued from page 315

found in every home, feed off human skin scales, which we all shed naturally. Dust mites are especially common in bedding, such as pillows and mattresses.

2. Another common cause of year-round allergy is **skin and fur from cats and dogs**, horses, and other animals.

3. Some people suffer from allergy because of substances at their **place of work**, such as certain kinds of dust.

4. Allergens that cause problems only at certain times of the year include **pollen** from trees (springtime), from grass (midsummer), or from weeds (late summer). Some fungi produce mold spores that may cause allergy in late summer and autumn.

SOME ALLERGIC ILLNESSES

■ By far the most common allergic illness in the US is summer **hay fever** from grass pollen. Hay fever usually causes itching, sneezing, and a runny or blocked nose. Other problems can include sore eyes, an itchy palate (the roof of the mouth), and breathing problems.

■ Allergy can often cause **asthma**, a common lung disease which can make breathing out difficult, and gives a tight feeling in the chest. Asthma affects people of any age, although it is most often found in the young and middle-aged. Asthma may be set off by a year-round allergen such as dust mites, or by a seasonal one such as pollen.

■ Some **skin conditions** are allergic in origin, e.g. contact dermatitis and drug rashes.

■ The **autoimmune** group of allergic diseases is huge, affecting every organ in the body.

HOW DO I KNOW IF I HAVE AN ALLERGY?

Never **assume** you have an allergy and take unilateral action, such as embarking on an exclusion diet or putting your child on one – that can be dangerous.

Your family doctor may be able to tell right away if you have an allergy. However, some allergies are easier to diagnose than others. For example, if you have hay fever or asthma that gets worse in June and July, it is very likely that you are allergic to grass pollen.

With other allergies, such as dust mite or animal fur, you may have to have special tests before the doctor can be sure what the problem is. If she thinks you might have a lung allergy, she may refer you an allergist or a lung specialist.

CAN I TAKE AVOIDING ACTION?

■ It is difficult to avoid **pollens**, the most common cause of allergic illness. It may help to wear sunglasses and to keep windows shut, especially when in cars and tall buildings. Avoid open grassy spaces, particularly during the evening or at night, when there is more pollen at ground level. A vacation by the sea or abroad

during the peak pollen season may help.

■ If a bad allergic problem is caused by **cats or dogs**, then it is better not to keep such pets. Of course, most people would not want to get rid of a family friend, but when the time comes, you should think carefully before replacing your pet.

■ In the meantime, it will help if the animal stays outdoors as much as possible and the house is kept very clean. **Washing your cat or dog once a week** is also an effective way of reducing allergen levels in the home, although it won't make you very popular with your pet!

You can reduce dust mite problems by using special covers for mattresses, pillows, and duvets. Clean the house often, as carefully as you can, and allow plenty of air in – this will help to reduce the dampness that house dust mites like. It will help if you have a good vacuum cleaner that's equipped with a small pore-size filter.

TESTS FOR ALLERGY

A skin prick test or patch test are the **only true tests** for an allergy. If you don't have these tests done you can never be sure you actually have an allergy. Both are simple and painless procedures to find out if you're allergic to anything.

1. **In a skin prick test**, dilute solutions are made from extracts of allergens, such as pollen, dust, dander, and food, that commonly cause allergic reactions. A drop of each solution is placed on the skin, which is then pricked with a needle. The skin is observed for a reaction, which usually occurs within 30 minutes of applying the solution. Antihistamines should not be taken on the day of the test because they may prevent any reaction.

NB An exclusion diet shouldn't be undertaken unless you've had a skin prick test done first by a board-certified allergist.

TEST

Patch testing

Patch testing is performed by a dermatologist to find out which substances provoke a reaction in people suspected of having allergies. Possible allergens (substances that can cause an allergic reaction) are diluted and placed on small strips or disks. The test strips are then applied to the skin using inert

(nonallergenic) tape. After 48 hours, the strips are removed and the skin underneath is examined. A red, inflamed area of skin where the strip was indicates a positive reaction to the allergen. The tested area is examined again two days later to check for delayed reactions. Patch tests are for skin allergies only.

Minute quantities of diluted test substances are placed on small strips. The strips are then stuck with inert tape to an inconspicuous area of the skin, usually on the back. After 48 hours, the strips are removed and the skin underneath is examined. A reddened area of skin indicates an allergic reaction to the substance.

2. **Patch testing** (see box, above) is performed on people with contact dermatitis. The test is done by a dermatologist to find out which substances provoke an allergic reaction in the skin. Possible allergens (substances that can cause an allergic reaction) are diluted and placed on small strips or disks. The test patches are then stuck to the skin using inert (nonallergenic) tape. After 48 hours, the patches are removed and the skin underneath them is examined. A red, inflamed area indicates a positive reaction to an allergen. The tested area is examined again two days later to check for delayed reactions.

WHAT IS THE TREATMENT?

■ Nasal sprays containing steroids can be used and are taken daily.

■ Nasal sprays containing decongestants can relieve symptoms but should not be used regularly.

■ Oral antihistamines are often combined with decongestants to relieve inflammation and itching.

■ Eyedrops may help relieve eye symptoms.

■ Rarely, if symptoms are severe, your doctor may prescribe an oral corticosteroid.

■ The most specific treatment is immunotherapy, in which you are injected with gradually increasing doses of allergen to desensitize the immune system. The treatment can take up to four years and is not always successful.

See also:
• **The atopic family of conditions** p. 311
• **Autoimmune disorders** p. 323
• **Contact dermatitis** p. 314
• **Drug allergy** p. 322

Hay fever

HAY FEVER, ALSO CALLED ALLERGIC RHINITIS, IS DUE TO INFLAMMATION OF THE MEMBRANE LINING THE NOSE, THROAT, AND EYES. THIS INFLAMMATION IS THE RESULT OF AN ALLERGIC REACTION TO SPECIFIC AIRBORNE SUBSTANCES KNOWN AS ALLERGENS.

Magnified pollen grains from an acacia tree (Robinia pseudoacacia)

Allergic rhinitis may occur only during the spring and summer, in which case it is known as **seasonal allergic rhinitis** or hay fever and is due to **inhaled pollen**. If it occurs all year round it's called **perennial rhinitis** and is most commonly due to an allergy to **house dust** or **dust mites**. Allergic rhinitis is more common in people who have other allergic disorders, such as asthma, eczema, or migraines; that is, they have atopy.

WHAT ARE THE CAUSES?
Seasonal allergic rhinitis is usually due to grass, tree, flower, or weed pollens; it occurs mostly in the spring and summer when pollen counts are high. The most common allergens that provoke perennial allergic rhinitis include house dust and dust mites, animal fur and dander, feathers, and mold spores.

WHAT ARE THE SYMPTOMS?
The symptoms of both forms of allergic rhinitis usually appear soon after contact with the allergen but tend to be more severe in hay fever. They include:
- itchy sensation in the nose
- frequent sneezing
- blocked, runny nose
- itchy, red, watery eyes.

Some people may develop a headache. If the lining of the nose is severely inflamed, nosebleeds may occur.

WHAT MIGHT BE DONE?
■ Your doctor may recognize allergic rhinitis from your symptoms, particularly if you can identify the substance that triggers a reaction.
■ A skin prick test may be performed in order to identify the allergen that causes the allergic rhinitis. In some cases, the allergen cannot be found.

■ If you can avoid the allergens that affect you, your symptoms will subside.
■ Oral antihistamines are often combined with decongestants to relieve inflammation and itching.
■ Many antiallergy drugs are available over the counter or by prescription. For example, allergies can be blocked by nasal sprays that contain cromolyn sodium.
■ Alternatively, nasal corticosteroids in the form of a spray are effective for hay fever but may take a few days to work.
■ Nasal sprays containing decongestants can relieve symptoms but should not be used regularly.
■ Eyedrops may help relieve eye symptoms.
■ Rarely, if symptoms are severe, your doctor may prescribe an oral corticosteroid.

The most specific treatment for allergic rhinitis is **immunotherapy**, in which you are injected with gradually increasing doses of allergen with the aim of **desensitizing** the immune system. This treatment, which typically takes as long as 3–4 years, is not always successful.

Hay fever calendar

If you suffer from seasonal allergic rhinitis, this list may help you identify the cause.

January–April	Alder
February–March	Hazel
February–April	Elm
February–April	Willow
April–May	Birch
May–August	Grasses
May	Horse chestnut
June–July	Lime
June–August	Mugwort
July–September	Nettles
July–October	Dock

See also:
• **Allergies p. 315**
• **The atopic family of conditions p. 311**

SELF-HELP
Dealing with hay fever (allergic rhinitis)

Perennial allergic rhinitis
The measures listed below are all aimed at maintaining an allergen-free environment in your home in order to prevent perennial allergic rhinitis.
■ Avoid keeping furry animals as pets if you are allergic to them.
■ Replace pillows and quilts containing animal materials such as duck feathers with those containing synthetic stuffing.
■ Cover mattresses with plastic.
■ Remove dust collecting items such as upholstered furniture and curtains if possible.

Hay fever
To help prevent the symptoms of hay fever, the following measures may be effective.
■ Avoid areas with long grass or where grass is being cut.
■ In summer, keep doors and windows closed and spend as much time as possible in air-conditioned buildings.

■ Try to stay inside during late morning and early evening when the pollen count is highest.
■ Keep car windows shut while driving.
■ Make sure your car is equipped with an effective pollen filter.
■ When outside, wear sunglasses to help prevent eye irritation; sunglasses can help stop the pollen from entering eyes.
■ Shower and change when you get home.
■ Eat health-building foods such as fruit and vegetables.

Alternative remedies have never been proven to work but some people find herbal pills helpful. **Homeopathic preparations** are seen by users as preventatives. **Aromatic tissues** impregnated with vapors help dry up mucus. **Eye glasses** now exist that can filter the air around the eyes. **Supplements** such as zinc that are said to boost the immune system are taken for hay fever.

Food allergy

MANY PEOPLE CONFUSE FOOD ALLERGY AND FOOD INTOLERANCE BUT THE TWO ARE QUITE DIFFERENT. FOOD ALLERGY INVOLVES AN ABNORMAL REACTION BY THE IMMUNE SYSTEM AND CAN BE VERY SERIOUS. FOOD INTOLERANCE NEVER INVOLVES THE IMMUNE SYSTEM.

Let's clear up a common misunderstanding.
■ Food INTOLERANCE is common.
■ Food ALLERGY is relatively rare.
The two must not be confused.
■ An easy way to distinguish them is that an intolerance makes you feel uncomfortable; a food "doesn't agree with you" but you can still eat it. You're NOT allergic to it.
■ If you're allergic to a food, you can't eat it at all. The minutest amount, even on a knife, can cause very severe symptoms like angioedema.
■ Food allergy causes serious illness; intolerance NEVER does.

Food allergy is an uncommon condition in which the immune system reacts in an inappropriate or an exaggerated way to a specific food or foods, causing development of various symptoms such as an itchy rash. In contrast, food intolerance, which often causes abdominal discomfort and indigestion, does not involve the immune system in any way.

WHAT ARE THE CAUSES?
■ Food allergy is more common in **atopic** people with other allergy-related conditions such as asthma, eczema, or hay fever. There is a greater risk of developing a food allergy if a close relative is allergic to a particular food.
■ Although allergic reactions can occur with any food, nuts (especially peanuts) are probably the most common cause.
■ Other relatively common causes of food allergy include seafood, strawberries, and eggs.
■ Though often blamed in the media and by wishful parents, food colorings and preservatives **rarely** cause allergic reactions, but **intolerance** to the food additive monosodium glutamate (MSG) is common.
■ Wheat (gluten) allergy may cause a condition known as **celiac disease**.
■ An allergic reaction to the protein in cow milk is especially common in infants and young children.
■ Both of these conditions differ from immediate sensitivity to nuts or other foods in that they are more chronic conditions.

WHAT ARE THE SYMPTOMS?
Symptoms may appear almost immediately after eating the food or develop over a few hours. They may include:
● an itchy, red rash anywhere on the body (urticaria)
● nausea, vomiting, and diarrhea
● difficulty in swallowing (a medical emergency)

● itching and swelling affecting the face, lips, mouth, and throat (angioedema)
● shortness of breath or wheezing – **anaphylaxis**, a **life threatening** allergic response that causes sudden difficulty in breathing and collapse. If you develop the symptoms of a severe reaction, call an ambulance immediately.

WHAT MIGHT BE DONE?
1. You may be able to diagnose food allergy yourself if the symptoms occur soon after you eat a particular food. However, you should consult your doctor. If he or she is unsure what is responsible for the reaction, you may have a **skin prick test**.
2. Your doctor may also recommend an **exclusion diet** (don't embark on one yourself). By eating a restricted diet for one or two weeks, you may avoid the foods that cause your symptoms. If your symptoms improve substantially while on the diet, you may have one or more food allergies. You can gradually add other foods to your diet, but if symptoms recur when a particular food is eaten, you should avoid it in the future. You should NEVER embark on an exclusion diet without first consulting your doctor. Nor should you follow a nutritionally restricted diet for more than two weeks. Interpreting the results of an exclusion diet is often difficult.

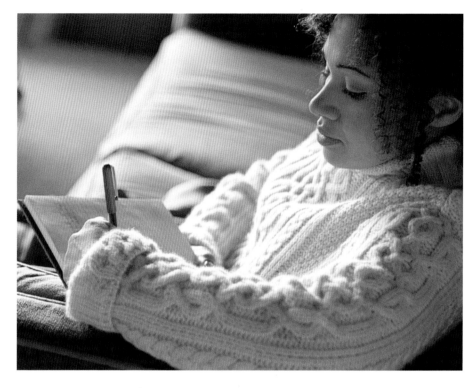

Keeping a food diary can help you identify particular foods to which you may be allergic.

SELF-HELP
■ Keep a food diary and note symptoms. Show it to your doctor.
■ Avoiding the problem food is the only effective treatment.
■ Always ask about ingredients when eating out, and check labels on packaged foods.
■ Consult a nutritionist if you need to exclude a food that is a major part of a normal diet, such as wheat.
■ If a major permanent dietary change is needed, be sure to maintain a balanced diet.

WHAT IS THE OUTLOOK?
Many food allergies, particularly nut allergies, are permanent, and people must avoid the relevant foods throughout their lives. Some food allergies may disappear. Children under age 4 who completely avoid problem foods such as wheat for two years have an excellent chance of outgrowing their allergy.

See also:
● Anaphylaxis p. 321 ● Angioedema p. 321
● Malabsorption p. 365 ● The atopic family of conditions p. 311 ● Urticaria p. 322

Angioedema

ANGIOEDEMA IS AN ALLERGIC CONDITION THAT TYPICALLY AFFECTS THE LIPS, MOUTH, THROAT, AIR PASSAGES, AND EYES, CAUSING SUDDEN AND SOMETIMES SEVERE SWELLING. BECAUSE THE SWELLING CAN INTERFERE WITH BREATHING, IT SHOULD BE TREATED AS AN EMERGENCY.

In angioedema, the mucous membranes and tissues under the skin suddenly become swollen due to an allergic reaction. In some cases, swelling of the mouth, throat, and air passages is severe enough to prevent swallowing, even breathing. For this reason, angioedema requires emergency medical treatment.

WARNING:

■ Any severe allergy may develop at some time into an attack of angioedema. The swelling may affect the larynx (voice box) and can be life-threatening if the airway becomes blocked. Angioedema may occur at the same time as ANAPHYLAXIS, a potentially fatal allergic reaction that requires urgent medical attention.

■ If you develop the symptoms of angioedema or experience difficulty breathing, you should call an ambulance immediately.

WHAT ARE THE CAUSES?

■ The most common cause of angioedema is an allergic reaction to a type of **food**, such as seafood, nuts, or strawberries.

■ Less commonly, the condition may result from an allergic reaction to **drugs**, most often to **antibiotics**.

■ Angioedema may also develop after an **insect bite or sting**.

■ Rarely, a person may inherit a tendency to develop angioedema that is unrelated to an allergy. In such cases, episodes of unexplained angioedema may begin in childhood and may be triggered by **stressful events**, such as an injury or a dental extraction.

■ It is not unusual for people to have only a single episode of angioedema, for which no cause can be determined.

WHAT ARE THE SYMPTOMS?

Swelling usually develops within a few minutes and is often asymmetrical; for example, only one side of a lip may be affected. The main symptoms are:

● swelling of any part of the body, especially the face, lips, tongue, throat, and genitals

● sudden difficulty breathing, speaking, or swallowing due to swelling of the tongue, mouth, and airways

● in about half of all cases, an itchy rash (urticaria) affecting areas that are not swollen.

WHAT MIGHT BE DONE?
EMERGENCY!

■ Severe angioedema requires an urgent injection with **adrenaline**, followed by observation in the hospital. In milder cases, a **corticosteroid** or an **antihistamine** may be prescribed to reduce the swelling; this may take hours or days to subside.

■ Your doctor may perform tests to determine the cause. If a food allergy is suspected, a **skin prick test** may identify the substances to which you are allergic. If you suffer from severe angioedema, your doctor may teach you how to self-inject adrenaline.

See also:
● **Drug allergy p. 322**
● **Food allergy p. 320**
● **Urticaria p. 322**

Anaphylaxis

ALSO CALLED ANAPHYLACTIC SHOCK, ANAPHYLAXIS IS A RARE BUT POTENTIALLY FATAL CONDITION. IT IS A SEVERE ALLERGIC REACTION THAT SPREADS THROUGHOUT THE BODY, CAUSING SHOCK WITH A SUDDEN DROP IN BLOOD PRESSURE AND NARROWING OF THE AIRWAYS.

Anaphylaxis occurs in people who have developed an extreme sensitivity to a specific substance (allergen). The allergic reaction is so severe that it can be fatal unless immediate treatment is available.

WHAT ARE THE CAUSES?
Anaphylaxis is most commonly triggered by **insect stings** or certain **drugs** such as **penicillin**. Foods such as **nuts** or **strawberries** may also trigger this serious form of allergic reaction.

WHAT ARE THE SYMPTOMS?
If you have an extreme sensitivity to a substance, you may experience some or all of the following symptoms as soon as you are exposed to it:

● sudden feeling of extreme anxiety
● swollen face, lips, and tongue
● wheezing and difficulty breathing
● in some cases, an itchy, red rash (urticaria) and flushing of the skin

● lightheadedness or, in some cases, loss of consciousness.

If either you or anyone you are with develops these symptoms, you should call an ambulance immediately.

WHAT IS THE TREATMENT?
EMERGENCY!

■ Emergency treatment for anaphylaxis is an **immediate injection of adrenaline**. Injections of **antihistamines** or **corticosteroids**, together with **intravenous fluids**, are also given.

■ You should avoid any substance to which you are sensitive, especially if you have had a previous anaphylactic reaction. You may be given **adrenaline to self-inject** (an Epi-Pen).

■ You will also be advised to carry an **emergency card** or **bracelet** to alert others to your allergy.

See also:
● **Drug allergy p. 322** ● **Food allergy p. 320**
● **Urticaria p. 322**

Emergency aid for anaphylaxis

If you have previously experienced anaphylaxis or severe angioedema, your doctor may provide you with syringes of injectable adrenaline, often called Epi-Pens (keep one at home and one at work and carry one with you at all times). In the event of an episode of anaphylaxis, inject adrenaline immediately, then call for an ambulance.

Drug allergy

TREATMENT WITH VARIOUS DRUGS CAN RESULT IN A RANGE OF DIFFERENT SIDE EFFECTS.
THE REACTION IS CAUSED BY AN ALLERGIC RESPONSE TO THE DRUG OR TO SUBSTANCES
FORMED WHEN THE DRUG IS BROKEN DOWN BY THE BODY.

Rashes are a common side effect of drug treatment. Antibiotics and aspirin, for example, commonly cause urticaria (also called hives or nettle rash; see below). There may be other, more dramatic, effects such as nausea, diarrhea, wheezing, swelling of the face and tongue (**angioedema**), and collapse. People with severe reactions need hospital treatment. Repeated exposure to a drug that causes a rash or angioedema can precipitate **anaphylaxis**.

The drugs that most often produce rashes are antibiotics, such as **penicillin**, but almost all drug treatments can cause an allergic reaction if a person becomes sensitive to them. Drug induced rashes usually develop within the first few days of starting treatment but they can also occur after a course of treatment has finished.

Sensitivity can only develop after at least one previous exposure to a drug. It is usual for people to take a certain drug for the first time without experiencing any allergic reaction and then to develop a rash when the drug is taken in a subsequent course of treatment.

WHAT MIGHT BE DONE?

■ If you develop a rash while you are taking a drug, you should consult your doctor before the next dose is due. .

■ Most drug induced rashes disappear when the drug responsible is stopped.

■ If itching is a problem, your doctor may advise that you apply a topical corticosteroid or take an oral antihistamine, but something simple like calamine lotion can bring relief.

■ Once you know you are allergic to a drug, you should make sure you notify any doctor who treats you in the future.

■ If you have had a severe reaction to a particular drug, you should consider wearing a **medic alert** tag or bracelet.

See also:
• **Anaphylaxis p. 321**
• **Angioedema p. 321**

Urticaria (hives)

URTICARIA, ALSO KNOWN AS HIVES OR NETTLE RASH, IS AN INTENSELY ITCHY RASH THAT MAY
AFFECT THE WHOLE BODY OR JUST A SMALL AREA OF SKIN. IT IS AN ALLERGIC REACTION TO
VARIOUS SUBSTANCES, INCLUDING FOODS, DRUGS, AND STINGS.

The rash consists of raised, red areas and, sometimes, white lumps. The inflamed areas usually vary in size and may merge to involve very large areas of skin. Urticaria comes and goes. Typically it lasts for only a few minutes or hours and there may be only one or two attacks. But sometimes it recurs for several months (chronic urticaria) and we rarely find a cause. Sometimes urticaria occurs at the same time as the more serious condition affecting the face called **angioedema**. Urticaria is sometimes an early symptom of **anaphylaxis**, a severe and potentially fatal allergic reaction to something.

WHAT ARE THE CAUSES?

■ The tendency to develop urticaria may run in families – atopic families.

■ Urticaria can occur as a result of an allergic reaction to a particular food, such as shellfish, fruits, and nuts – peanuts having received publicity.

■ The condition may also be due to a **drug allergy** (see above).

■ It may be due to an allergy to plants.

■ It may develop after an insect bite or sting.

■ However, when urticaria occurs for the first time in an adult, it is often difficult to identify the cause.

WHAT MIGHT BE DONE?

A one-time bout of urticaria generally disappears with treatment within a few hours.

The chronic form of the condition may take several weeks or months to clear up. Over-the-counter products such as calamine lotion and daily oral antihistamines may help relieve itching.

If your symptoms persist or recur and the cause of the problem is not obvious, you should consult your doctor. A skin prick test will identify the substances to which you are allergic (allergens). When the substance causing your urticaria has been identified, you should take all possible steps to avoid coming into contact with it in future in order to prevent a recurrence of the condition.

Never again eat a food to which you've been proven to be allergic. Avoid dishes and cutlery that may have touched the food.

See also:
• **Anaphylaxis p. 321** • **Angioedema p. 321**
• **Food allergy p. 320**
• **The atopic family of conditions p. 311**

AUTOIMMUNE DISORDERS

If someone has an autoimmune disorder, their immune system mistakenly interprets their body's own tissues as **foreign**. As a result, antibodies are formed that attack the tissues and try to destroy them.

In general terms an autoimmune disease shows up in those tissues that are attacked by a particular antibody; for instance, the kidneys in glomerulonephritis and the joints in rheumatoid arthritis.

WHAT ARE THE TYPES?

1. In some autoimmune disorders, the tissues of a **single organ** are damaged, preventing normal function. Here are some examples of organs that may be affected:
- the **thyroid** gland in Hashimoto's disease
- the **pancreas** in diabetes mellitus
- the **adrenal glands** in Addison's disease.

2. A second group of autoimmune disorders affects **connective tissue**, the "glue" that holds together the structures of the body, e.g. **scleroderma** and **lupus**. In these disorders, the immune system may react against connective tissues **anywhere and everywhere** in the body, resulting in many and varied symptoms.

WHAT MIGHT BE DONE?

If your doctor suspects an autoimmune disorder, you'll have blood tests to assess your immune function and look for evidence of tissue inflammation.

The **treatment** of autoimmune disorders depends on which organs are affected. In Hashimoto's thyroiditis or Addison's disease, damage to the affected organs leads to a deficiency in the hormones they normally produce. However, replacement can often restore health. In other cases the goal of treatment is to block antibody production in the first place with drugs such as **immunosuppressants** and **corticosteroids** or limit the effects of antibodies. **Non-steroidal**

anti-inflammatory drugs (NSAIDs) can treat symptoms such as pain and stiffness.

WHAT IS THE OUTLOOK?

The outlook for people who have autoimmune disorders depends on the amount of damage to the body's tissues and organs. Autoimmune disorders are nearly always chronic, but the symptoms can often be controlled with drugs. In some cases, serious complications such as kidney failure may develop. Quite often, though, the disease eventually "burns out" in middle age and symptoms subside.

Acquired immune deficiency

IMMUNE DEFICIENCY IS THE COMPLETE OR PARTIAL FAILURE OF THE IMMUNE SYSTEM, THE BODY'S NATURAL DEFENSE SYSTEM AGAINST DISEASE. IF THE IMMUNE SYSTEM FAILS AT SOME POINT DURING LIFE, THE CONDITION IS KNOWN AS "ACQUIRED" IMMUNE DEFICIENCY.

WHAT ARE THE CAUSES?

■ In the most infamous form of this condition, acquired immune deficiency syndrome (AIDS), the **human immune deficiency virus** (HIV) destroys a particular type of white blood cell, the T cell, and this causes progressive weakness and vulnerability of the immune system.

■ Infections such as **measles** or **flu** damage the body's ability to fight infection. They do this partly by reducing the number of white blood cells involved in fighting the infection. Usually, this type of immune deficiency is mild, and the immune system returns to normal once the infection is overcome.

■ A mild form of immune deficiency may develop in some chronic disorders, including **diabetes mellitus** and **rheumatoid arthritis**. This may occur partly because these diseases stress on the immune system, reducing its ability to resist other diseases.

■ Certain types of **cancer**, particularly tumors of the lymphatic system (lymphomas), may cause a more severe form of immune deficiency by damaging the cells of the immune system and by reducing production of normal white blood cells.

■ The long-term use of **corticosteroids** suppresses the immune system and has the inevitable effect of causing immune deficiency.

■ **Immunosuppressant drugs**, which may be given to prevent the rejection of an organ following transplant surgery, also produce immune deficiency and affect the body's ability to fight infections.

■ **Chemotherapy** can damage the bone marrow, where the majority of blood cells are made, and may also lead to the development of acquired immune deficiency.

■ Immune deficiency may also develop **after removal of the spleen**, an organ in which some of the white blood cells are produced.

WHAT MIGHT BE DONE?

Your doctor may suggest continual low doses of **antibiotics**, **antiviral drugs** and/or **antifungal drugs** and various **immunizations**, such as the pneumococcus vaccine, to protect against pneumococcal pneumonia.

The effects of immune deficiency can usually be controlled by treatment, although immune deficiency due to HIV infection tends to worsen over time.

FOCUS *on* lupus

Lupus (sometimes known as systemic lupus erythematosis or SLE) is an autoimmune disease that can attack many different parts of the body and produces a great variety of different symptoms. Because the effects of lupus are so variable, this disorder can be very difficult to diagnose.

Although few people have heard of lupus, worldwide it's far more common than leukemia, muscular dystrophy, and multiple sclerosis, which, after extensive publicity, have become household names.

Lupus mainly attacks women during their childbearing years, but sometimes men and even young children are affected. It's estimated that 1,400,000 Americans have a form of lupus and, for reasons we don't understand, it is more common in some races than in others. For example, the frequency in white women is 1 in 1000 compared with that in black women of 1 in 250.

WHAT ARE THE SYMPTOMS?

Because lupus can attack so many parts of the body, it can show up in a bewildering number of ways, even to the extent of mimicking other diseases such as rheumatoid arthritis, multiple sclerosis, or chronic fatigue syndrome (ME). So lupus can be difficult to diagnose and it can be overlooked, often for years.

Lupus is a disease that can present many different facets. Rarely do two people have exactly the same symptoms, and they can vary from just one to many:
- joint and muscle aches and pains
- permanent rash, which may be raised and

scaly, over the nose and cheeks
- extreme fatigue and weakness
- rashes from sunlight
- recurring flulike symptoms and/or night sweats
- poor blood circulation causing the tips of the fingers and toes to turn white then blue on exposure to cold – Raynaud's phenomenon
- anemia
- headaches, migraines
- increased risk of miscarriage
- kidney problems
- oral ulcers
- hair loss
- depression
- low platelet count.

Some drugs, such as certain antihypertensive drugs, may cause similar symptoms.

THE TREATMENT OF LUPUS

Currently, there's no cure for lupus, but it can be controlled with special treatment so that most patients are able to live a normal life span. The majority of lupus patients should be in the ongoing care of their specialist.

If you have a lupuslike condition that has been triggered by a particular drug, your doctor may be able to prescribe an alternative drug. Symptoms should then disappear gradually over a period of weeks or months.

WHAT CAN I EXPECT AT THE DOCTOR'S OFFICE?

- You'll have your urine tested for protein, blood and glucose to check on your kidneys and for diabetes.

Lupus triggers

Lupus can be triggered:
- at puberty
- after childbirth
- through sunlight
- by some medications
- during menopause
- after a viral infection
- as a result of injury.

The typical rash of lupus is butterfly-shaped and spreads across the nose and cheeks.

- You'll be weighed at each visit as some treatments, such as steroids, can cause water retention.
- You'll have a blood test to check for anemia.
- An MRI scan, X-rays and nerve conduction tests may be done.
- Eye checkups will be done before starting some treatments.
- When you start new medication, you'll be given information to help you understand how your treatment works.
- You may need a lot of support and understanding in coming to terms with lupus. You may have gone undiagnosed for several years, and feel frustrated that no one understands what you're going through. If there's a nurse counselor attached to the doctor's office, get her help.

WHAT KIND OF TREATMENT WILL I GET?

Lupus is usually treated with four main groups of drugs, depending on the severity of the disease.

Aspirin and nonsteroidals: Nonsteroidal anti-inflammatory drugs (NSAIDs) are used for patients with mainly joint and muscle pain. In the case of patients with sticky blood, aspirin in low dosage, 75–150mg daily, is used to thin the blood.

Antimalarials: These drugs are of help in patients with skin and joint disease. They may be sufficient for patients with moderately active lupus to avoid using steroids. Hydroxychloroquine and mepacrine are most commonly used.

Steroids: Drugs such as prednisone have been vital in the improvement in lupus and for some people can be lifesaving. They have a profound effect on inflammation and can suppress the disease. Once lupus is under control, you can be weaned off steroids gradually under your doctor's supervision.

Immunosuppressants: These drugs are used in more severe disease. The most commonly used are azathioprine, methotrexate and cyclophosphamide. You'll have regular blood tests to check on your bone marrow and liver.

You may also have physical therapy to help improve mobility in affected joints. It's important to remain as physically active as the condition will allow, so try to get moderate exercise regularly.

With treatment, most people with lupus are able to lead normal, active lives.

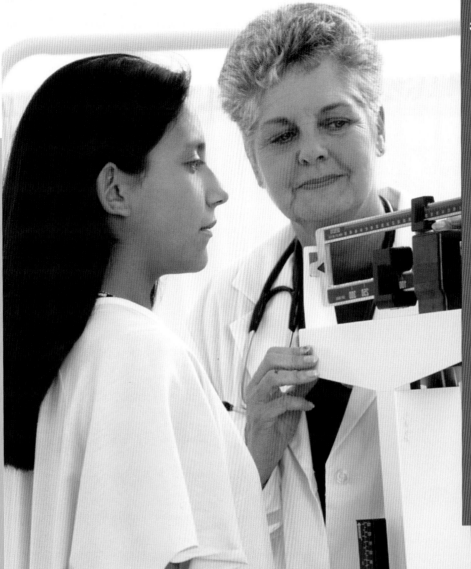

Self-help

- Become well educated on lupus.
- Try to prepare for the up and down nature of the disease. Plan for alternatives. Allow for rest when the disease is active but try to maintain general fitness.
- Reduce fatigue by developing priorities and learning to pace yourself. Break down big, long-term goals into small, manageable steps that can be easily accomplished.
- Be open with family and friends about the unpredictable pattern of lupus, and how the disease affects you.
- By listening to your pain, you can begin to control it.
- Try to accept the things you cannot change, rather than feeling constantly

frustrated and upset over situations beyond your control.
- Remember that stress, depression, and pain are all closely connected and each affects the other. Reduce one and you reduce them all.
- Approximately one-third of lupus patients are sensitive to light, so avoid direct and prolonged sun exposure and ultraviolet light from artificial sources (such as fluorescent lights). Wear broad-brimmed hats and cover other exposed parts of the body when out in sunlight and use sunscreen.
- Ask for help. Family, friends, health-care professionals, and The Lupus Foundation (see Useful addresses, p. 567), are all sources of support.

Polymyositis and dermatomyositis

THE NAME POLYMYOSITIS MEANS INFLAMMATION OF MANY MUSCLES. THE DISEASE MAY AFFECT BOTH SKELETAL MUSCLES AND MUSCLES ELSEWHERE IN THE BODY SUCH AS IN THE THROAT OR HEART. IN DERMATOMYOSITIS, THE SYMPTOMS OF POLYMYOSITIS ARE ACCOMPANIED BY A RASH.

WHAT ARE THE SYMPTOMS?

Polymyositis results in the following symptoms:
- weakness of affected muscles, leading to, for example, difficulty raising the arms or getting up from a sitting or squatting position
- painful, swollen joints
- fatigue
- difficulty swallowing if the muscles of the throat are affected
- shortness of breath if the heart or chest muscles are involved.

In cases of dermatomyositis, the symptoms outlined above may be preceded, accompanied, or followed by the following additional symptoms:
- a red rash, often on the face, chest, or backs of the hands over the knuckles
- swollen, reddish-purple eyelids.

WHAT IS THE TREATMENT?

This condition must always be treated by a specialist. Usually, high-dose steroids are given along with analgesics for symptomatic relief.

Scleroderma

SCLERODERMA IS THICKENING AND HARDENING OF THE CONNECTIVE TISSUES IN THE SKIN, JOINTS, ARTERIES, AND INTERNAL ORGANS. IT IS A RARE AUTOIMMUNE CONDITION THAT IS TWICE AS COMMON IN WOMEN AS IN MEN AND USUALLY DEVELOPS BETWEEN THE AGES OF 40 AND 60.

WHAT ARE THE SYMPTOMS?

These include:
- fingers or toes that are sensitive to the cold, becoming white and painful (Raynaud's phenomenon)
- small, hardened areas that appear on the fingers and may go on to ulcerate
- swollen fingers or hands
- pain in the joints, especially the joints in the hands
- thickening and tightening of the skin, which is most severe on the limbs but may affect the trunk and face
- muscle weakness
- difficulty swallowing due to stiffening of the tissues of the esophagus (the tube that runs from the mouth to the stomach).

If the lungs are affected, shortness of breath may develop. Sometimes it causes high blood pressure and, rarely, eventual kidney failure.

WHAT IS THE TREATMENT?

- Immunosuppressant drugs or drugs that interfere with collagen production may be given.
- Support and education are important.

See also:
- **High blood pressure p. 226** • **Acute, chronic and end-stage kidney failure p. 380**
- **Raynaud's phenomenon p. 232**

LYMPHATIC SYSTEM

The lymphatic system is quite difficult to get your mind around because it's distributed around the body with no real shape. There are some main features, however. Firstly, the lymphatic channels are vague, shapeless spaces between muscles, under the skin, and around joints through which the lymph flows, always in a direction toward the heart. At certain points the channels join up in a group of glands – you find them in the groin, neck, and armpit. From there they run into one large lymph tube that joins the main vein of the heart. But the lymphatic system extends further than

that. Its main cell is called a lymphocyte and it's made in the liver and the bone marrow. So it's useful to think of the liver and bone marrow as connected with the lymphatic system. Then there's the spleen, lying under the left ribcage, whose job it is to break down old red blood cells. So add the spleen to the lymphatic family. The lymph, the colorless fluid that's slowly flowing around this system, seeps out from cells, from blood vessels and from veins. It then circulates back to the heart. So there is a true lymphatic "circulation," not that different from the circulation of the blood.

Swollen glands

SWOLLEN GLANDS (ENLARGED LYMPH NODES) ARE A COMMON SYMPTOM OF MANY CONDITIONS, MOST OF THEM NO CAUSE FOR CONCERN. HOWEVER, THEY MAY ALSO INDICATE THE SPREAD OF CANCER, SUCH AS FROM THE BREAST TO NODES IN THE ARMPIT.

Swollen glands, known medically as lymphadenopathy, are really enlarged lymph nodes. They usually develop in response to a **bacterial or viral infection**, and are most likely to be noticed in the neck, groin, or armpit, because the nodes in these places lie closest to the skin. Infection anywhere can spread to the glands. So, for example, an infection spreading from an ingrown toenail can give you swollen glands in your groin.

Swollen lymph nodes in the neck are usual with a **throat infection** and can be tender. Swollen glands **at the back of the head** usually indicate German measles (rubella). If swollen glands are due to an infection, the swelling subsides when the infection clears up.

A SPECIAL NOTE ON THE SPREAD OF BREAST CANCER

The glands, also called nodes, in the armpit swell up and can be felt when breast cancer spreads.

Treatment for breast cancer involves surgery as a first step then further treatment with radiation therapy, hormones, and chemotherapy to contain the tumor and catch any cancer cells that are spreading.

To help doctors decide what will be the best regimen for each individual woman, they have to know how far her cancer has spread.

The simplest way to do this is to **sample or remove** the glands in the armpit. The surgeon will hope that he can take a deeper and deeper sample until he reaches a gland that's completely clear. Then he will have a good idea of how far the tumor's spread and be able to come up with a plan for radiation therapy, hormones, or chemotherapy tailor made to give the best chance of recovery.

There are several surgical operations to remove a breast tumor, such as lumpectomy (only the lump) and partial and simple mastectomy, but in all of them the surgeon will aim to take away the smallest part of the breast that will get rid of the cancer. At the same time the glands in the armpit will be sampled and may be removed to reduce the risk of cancer spread to other parts of the body.

See also:
• **Breast cancer p. 261**
• **Chemotherapy p. 257**
• **German measles (chart) p. 544**
• **Lumpectomy p. 262**

Lymphedema

LYMPHEDEMA IS A LOCALIZED ACCUMULATION OF FLUID IN THE LYMPHATIC VESSELS, CAUSING PAINLESS SWELLING OF A LIMB. IT RESULTS FROM DISRUPTION OF THE NORMAL DRAINAGE OF LYMPH DUE TO LOCAL BLOCKAGE, DAMAGE, OR REMOVAL OF LYMPH VESSELS.

Most commonly, lymphedema is caused by damage to the lymphatic vessels following **surgery** or **radiation therapy**, for example in **the arm** in the treatment of **breast cancer** and in **the leg** after treatment of **ovarian cancer**.

The skin over the affected limb often becomes rough and thickened. You should contact your doctor immediately if you injure a limb affected by lymphedema, even if it only seems trivial, because lymphangitis (see box, right) may ensue. However, it is also a condition where often there is no known cause and, for reasons we still do not understand, it affects twice as many women as men.

See also:
• **Breast cancer p. 261**
• **Cancer of the ovary p. 260**
• **Lumpectomy p. 262**
• **Radiation therapy p. 395**

WHAT IS THE TREATMENT?
■ In most cases, lymphedema is a lifelong disorder and treatment is directed at relieving symptoms. You can reduce swelling by keeping the affected limb elevated. Wearing an elastic stocking or sleeve can prevent further swelling.
■ There is no cure as such and treatment consists of taking diuretic drugs, massage, wearing an elastic bandage or compression sleeve, and performing exercises with the affected limb elevated. Surgery is possible in the most severe cases and this involves removing the swollen tissues and some of the overlying skin.
■ **Lymphatic drainage** can bring relief in some cases although, again, this is not a cure and will only bring temporary respite. It's done through massage, which encourages the tissues to expel the excess fluid back into the blood vessels and so out of the body. Qualified practitioners will do this massage for you and some aromatherapists are trained to do lymphatic drainage.

Lymphangitis

Lymphangitis develops when bacteria spread into lymphatic vessels close to the site of an infection, possibly as a result of an injury. The condition usually affects lymphatic vessels in an arm or leg. The infected vessels become inflamed and tender, and hot, red streaks may appear on the skin over the inflamed vessels. Lymph nodes near to the affected area sometimes become swollen. If you develop any of these symptoms following an injury, you should consult your doctor immediately. You'll need antibiotic treatment to prevent further spread.

Lymphoma

THE WORD LYMPHOMA STRIKES FEAR INTO MANY PEOPLE BECAUSE IT'S ILL-UNDERSTOOD. LYMPHOMAS ARE CANCERS OF THE GLANDS (LYMPH GLANDS OR LYMPH NODES) AFFECTING BOTH ADULTS AND CHILDREN, BUT THE OUTLOOK FOR CANCERS OF THIS TYPE IS BETTER THAN MOST.

Cancers are simply cells whose growth has gotten out of hand; they invade healthy organs with differing degrees of aggressiveness according to how malignant they are.

There are two types of lymphoma – Hodgkin's disease (HD) and non-Hodgkin's lymphoma (NHL), which differ in their behavior and treatment.

The first symptom may be a painless lump in the neck, armpits, or groin. Fatigue, weight loss, fever, night sweats, and itching can be prominent symptoms too.

HOW IS LYMPHOMA DIAGNOSED?
Your doctor will ask you many questions and examine you to see if the glands in your neck, armpits, and abdomen are enlarged.

After a small operation (biopsy) to remove one of the glands, the gland will be examined under a microscope.

This enables an accurate diagnosis to be made and with the results of other tests (X-rays, blood tests, scans) helps to decide the best form of treatment.

WHAT IS THE TREATMENT?
Some low-grade (nonaggressive) lymphomas

need no treatment but most require treatment with radiation, chemotherapy, or a combination of both.

Radiation therapy uses powerful X-rays that kill cancer cells. Chemotherapy uses powerful chemicals in the form of pills, injections, or an IV drip to do the same thing.

CHEMOTHERAPY
Lymphomas are one of the most sensitive cancers to chemotherapy. The overall goal of chemotherapy is to give drugs that have maximum cancer fighting effect, but with the least possible damage to the body's normal cells.

Chemotherapy drugs interrupt cell growth so they end up killing large numbers of cells.

However, many "normal" body cells (such as the bone marrow and the lining of the intestine and the mouth) divide rapidly and are vulnerable to cancer drugs, giving rise to many of the side effects caused by chemotherapy.

WHICH CHEMOTHERAPY?
The type of chemotherapy you'll get depends on the type of lymphoma, and the extent to which it may have spread.

Although some chemotherapy drugs are given as pills, most people with lymphoma are treated with intravenous chemotherapy.

Several drugs are usually given in combination to help stop cancer cells becoming resistant to any one drug.

There are several combinations in routine use, and new ones are being tried all the time. If you're asked to take part in a clinical trial, don't be afraid – trials usually compare a standard treatment with one that's judged to be better.

HOW IT IS GIVEN
Method
Most chemotherapy is given as outpatient treatment, either as a short injection into a vein, or as an intravenous drip over an hour or so. It rarely involves staying in hospital overnight.

Timing
■ Chemotherapy is given once every 3–4 weeks.
■ You'll receive 6–8 courses of treatment.
■ Treatment usually lasts around 5–6 months.
■ Some treatments may be given on a weekly basis.

Questions you may want to ask

About your diagnosis
- What kind of lymphoma do I have?
- What is the spread of the lymphoma?
- If it's non-Hodgkin's lymphoma, is it high- or low-grade? What's the difference?
- Where is it? Is there any doubt?
- What do these tests I'm having tell you? What are they for?

At the hospital
- Does the hospital have modern radiation equipment, specialists in radiation therapy and chemotherapy, hormone therapy, and surgery?
- Does it have supportive care and counseling?

About the treatment
- What kind of treatment will I have – radiation, chemotherapy, or none?
- Is it aimed at curing the disease or relieving the symptoms?
- Are there any other options?
- How will the drugs be given?
- Are there any special instructions about taking the pills at home?
- How do these pills help?
- When will the treatment start and how often will it be given?
- Are there things I should or shouldn't do during treatment?
- What are the possible side effects?

- Will the treatment affect the possibility of having children?
- Do I contact the hospital or my doctor if I'm unwell at home?
- Can I drive during and after treatment?
- May I drink alcohol and take medicines for other complaints?
- Are there foods I should or shouldn't eat during the treatment?
- When will I know if the treatment has worked?

Coping with chemotherapy

SIDE EFFECTS
You may well have no, or very few, side effects. However, it's preferable to know something about possible consequences so that you can let your medical team know if you get them.

Nausea and vomiting
Chemotherapy drugs can cause nausea and vomiting. However, this can largely be controlled by new antinausea medications, given as injections or pills. You may be given them before chemotherapy to avoid sickness in the first place.

Fatigue
Fatigue is one of the most common side effects of chemotherapy, though we don't know exactly why. If the cause is anemia then a simple blood transfusion may correct the problem.

Hair loss (alopecia)
Hair loss is an effect of the chemotherapy on the rapidly dividing cells of the hair follicle but many patients have no hair loss at all. If it does occur, it will only be temporary

and your hair will grow back when the chemotherapy is over.

Many people find that a wig is helpful and it is worth arranging one sooner rather than later, so that your hair can be matched. Scalp cooling slows blood flow to the scalp and can stop the chemotherapy from reaching hair follicles. Ask your medical team about it.

LONG-TERM SIDE EFFECTS
Sterility
Chemotherapy agents can affect fertility, though it's usually temporary. Women may stop having periods. Rarely, chemotherapy has been known to cause permanent sterility.

Low white blood cell count
If your white cell count drops (neutropenia) – a fairly common side effect of chemotherapy – you'll have an increased risk of infection. Look out for signs of infection and let your doctor know if you have any of the following symptoms:
- Fever, with temperature above 100°F (38°C).

- Chills and sweating.
- Mouth sores and ulcers.
- Coughs and sore throat.
- Redness or swelling around sores on the skin.
- Loose stools/diarrhea.
- Cystitis or burning sensation during urination.
- Unusual vaginal discharge or itching.

Questions to ask
- What are the possible side effects?
- Will the treatment affect my ability to have children?
- Should I contact the hospital or my own doctor if I'm unwell?
- Will I be able to drive during and after treatment?
- Can I drink alcohol and take medicines for other complaints during treatment?
- Are there foods I should or shouldn't eat during the treatment?
- When will I know if the treatment has been successful?

Infections

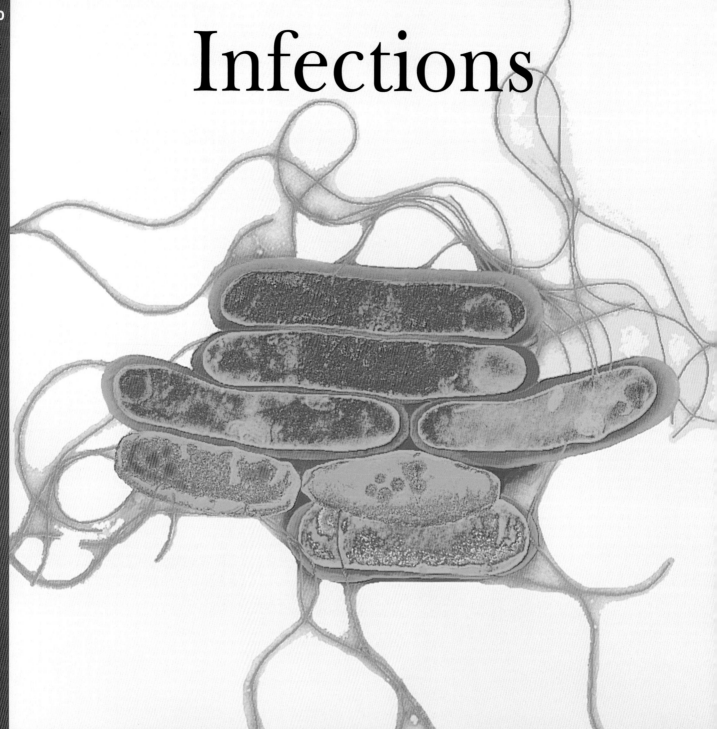

Image shows a colored transmission electron micrograph of Legionella pneumophilia *bacteria*

Miriam's overview

I'm making the distinction in this book between infections and "infectious diseases," which are historically confined to childhood and usually to those under age five and school children.

So you'll find diseases such as measles and whooping cough in the chapter on children's conditions.

You won't find sexually transmitted diseases here either. Gonorrhea, yeast, and the like are all together with STDs in the chapter on sexuality, though infection with the HIV virus and AIDS are in this chapter.

By and large, few infections are serious and very few indeed are life threatening. On these grounds most need not be a cause for concern and don't even require the attentions of a doctor. All that's required is symptomatic relief with over-the-counter medicines you can buy from the pharmacy.

By the same token, antibiotics are rarely required since most infections are self-limiting, meaning your healthy body will fight the infection, limit its effect, and cure you of it without outside help.

As an extension of such a principle you can see that I'd be an advocate of only the most judicious use of antibiotics. I'd define judicious as meaning strictly when needed, and except in the case of emergencies, when it's

known which bacterium is to be treated. The reasons for this caution are compelling, the most persuasive being the increasing numbers of resistant bacteria, a problem caused by abuse of antibiotics in the past. This abuse took the form of unnecessary overuse that actually encouraged bacteria to breed forms that could survive the presence of antibiotics rather than succumbing to them.

> ## "*antibiotics are rarely required* since most infections are *self-limiting*"

As a result we are now left with monster forms of bacteria and few antibiotics to curb their growth. The most notorious is methicillin-resistant *Staphylococcus aureus* (MRSA), usually picked up in hospitals, where the use of antibiotics has been traditionally concentrated.

continued on p. 332

Miriam's overview *continued from p. 331*

Thousands of people in the US die in the hospital from opportunistic infections, not necessarily related to MRSA, every year.

"we're infected by *very few* organisms"

Researchers are constantly pursuing a new super-antibiotic to cope with this new breed of super bug, but such is the speed of bacterial mutation there's the chance that our best research efforts will likely be outstripped by nature's ingenuity.

Besides bacteria, viruses, fungi, and parasites we've become aware of a new and potent infecting agent – the PRION – a small, subviral particle that enters cells and

destroys DNA, the cell's reproductive code. These prions cause BSE in cattle, scrapie in sheep, and new variant CJD in human beings.

At first it was thought that prions were species specific, meaning they could not escape from one species (cattle, for instance) to another (man). Given the new variant of CJD only recently described it would appear that our assumptions were wrong.

The truth is that we're infected by very few organisms be they bacteria, viruses, fungi, or parasites despite there being many millions of potential invaders out there.

In trying to decide what I could possibly cover for you here I've been guided by what's most common, what infections you're likely to meet, and what's serious enough to have the potential to make us very ill or kill us. So, for instance, I consider it very important to tell you how to spot the early signs of meningitis, always very serious, so that you can take rapid action to safeguard the well-being of your family.

INSIDE
infections and infestations

There are a number of organisms and microorganisms that cause infection and infestation, including lice and mites, worms, fungi, protozoa, bacteria, and viruses. **Lice** and **scabies mites** are easily transmitted and infestations are common in children. **Worms** may be microscopic or several feet in length. Two types, **flatworms** and **roundworms**, may infest humans. **Fungi**, broadly divided into the filamentous type (which grow threads) and the single-celled yeasts, are responsible for many infections in humans, such as candida. The single-celled organisms known as **protozoa** are responsible for diseases such as malaria and toxoplasmosis. **Bacteria** form a large group of single-celled organisms, of which relatively few types cause disease. **Viruses** are the smallest infectious agents, much smaller than a single human cell. A virus can only reproduce by invading a host cell and copying its own genetic material using substances from the host cell, which it then usually destroys.

how infections invade the body

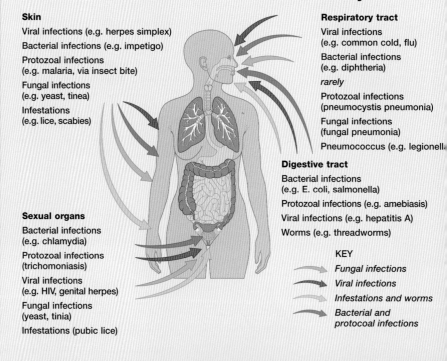

Skin
Viral infections (e.g. herpes simplex)
Bacterial infections (e.g. impetigo)
Protozoal infections (e.g. malaria, via insect bite)
Fungal infections (e.g. yeast, tinea)
Infestations (e.g. lice, scabies)

Sexual organs
Bacterial infections (e.g. chlamydia)
Protozoal infections (trichomoniasis)
Viral infections (e.g. HIV, genital herpes)
Fungal infections (yeast, tinia)
Infestations (pubic lice)

Respiratory tract
Viral infections (e.g. common cold, flu)
Bacterial infections (e.g. diphtheria)
rarely
Protozoal infections (pneumocystis pneumonia)
Fungal infections (fungal pneumonia)
Pneumococcus (e.g. legionell

Digestive tract
Bacterial infections (e.g. E. coli, salmonella)
Protozoal infections (e.g. amebiasis)
Viral infections (e.g. hepatitis A)
Worms (e.g. threadworms)

KEY
Fungal infections
Viral infections
Infestations and worms
Bacterial and protocoal infections

Common cold

A COMMON COLD IS AN INFECTION OF THE NOSE AND THROAT CAUSED BY ANY OF A GROUP OF VIRUSES. THERE ARE AT LEAST 200 HIGHLY CONTAGIOUS VIRUSES THAT CAN CAUSE THE COMMON COLD.

The viruses that cause colds are easily transmitted in minute airborne droplets from the coughs or sneezes of infected people. However, the most common route of spread is by hand-to-hand contact with an infected person or by way of things that are contaminated with the virus, such as a cup or towel. In itself, the common cold is not serious, but it can lead to a chest infection in a vulnerable person with, say, chronic obstructive pulmonary disease, or in a baby.

Colds can occur at any time of the year, although infections are more frequent in the autumn and winter. About half the population of the US and Europe develops at least one cold each year. Children are more susceptible to colds than adults because they have not yet developed immunity to the most common viruses and also because viruses spread very quickly in communities such as daycare centers and schools.

WHAT ARE THE SYMPTOMS?

The initial symptoms of a cold generally develop between 12 hours and 3 days after infection. Symptoms usually intensify over 24–48 hours, unlike those of influenza, which worsen rapidly over a few hours. Symptoms include:

- frequent sneezing
- runny nose with a clear, watery discharge that later becomes thick and green-colored
- mild fever and headache
- sore throat and sometimes a cough
- aching muscles
- irritability
- mucus.

In some people, a common cold may be complicated by a bacterial infection of the chest (bronchitis or pneumonia), or of the sinuses (sinusitis). Bacterial ear infections, which may cause earache, are a common complication of colds.

WHAT CAN I DO?

Most people recognize their symptoms as those of a common cold and do not seek medical help.

Despite a great deal of scientific research there is no cure for the common cold but over-the-counter drugs might help to relieve symptoms.

- **Certain pain medications** will relieve a headache and reduce a fever.
- **Decongestants** will clear a stuffy nose.

- **Cough remedies** may soothe a tickling throat.
- It is important to drink plenty of fluids, particularly if you have a fever.

Many people mistakenly take large quantities of vitamin C to prevent infection and treat the common cold, but the latest research shows this remedy to be without value, indeed dangerous, because megadoses of vitamin C could lead to heart disease.

If your symptoms do not improve in a week, or your child is no better in two days, you should consult a doctor.

If you have a bacterial infection, your doctor may prescribe **antibiotics, although they are ineffective against cold viruses**.

The common cold usually clears up with or without treatment within two weeks, but a cough may last longer.

See also:
- **Bronchitis p. 390**
- **Fever in children p. 540**
- **Sinusitis p. 481**

Influenza

INFLUENZA IS A VIRAL INFECTION OF THE UPPER RESPIRATORY TRACT (AIRWAYS),
COMMONLY KNOWN AS FLU. INFLUENZA IS A HIGHLY CONTAGIOUS VIRAL DISEASE
THAT TENDS TO OCCUR IN EPIDEMICS DURING THE WINTER.

Influenza mainly affects the upper airways and can be transmitted easily in airborne droplets from the coughs and sneezes of infected people. However, the influenza virus is usually transmitted from person to person through direct contact.

Many different viral infections can result in mild fllike symptoms, but true influenza is caused by two principal types of influenza virus, A and B. **The type A virus**, in particular, frequently changes its structure (mutates) and produces new strains to which few people have immunity.

The number of influenza cases varies from year to year, but particularly virulent strains have spread worldwide and caused millions of deaths. Such major outbreaks, called pandemics, occurred in 1918 with Spanish flu, in 1957 with Asian flu, in 1968 with Hong Kong flu, and in 1977 with Russian flu.

WHAT ARE THE SYMPTOMS?
The symptoms of influenza develop 24–48 hours after infection. Many people think they have influenza when they have only a common cold, but the symptoms of influenza are far more severe than those of a cold, and develop much faster. The first symptom may be **slight**

chills. Other symptoms, which develop later and worsen rapidly in just a few hours, may include the following:
- high fever, sweating, and shivering
- aching muscles, especially in the back
- severe exhaustion
- frequent sneezing, stuffy or runny nose, sore throat, and cough.

Following a bout of flu, **fatigue** and **depression** are often experienced after other symptoms have disappeared.

The most common complications are bacterial infections of the **airways** (bronchitis) and **lungs** (pneumonia). Such infections can be life threatening in babies, elderly people, those with **chronic heart** or **lung disease**, and people with reduced immunity, such as those with AIDS or **diabetes mellitus**.

WHAT MIGHT BE DONE?
■ For most normally healthy people, the best way to relieve the symptoms of influenza is to rest in bed, drink plenty of cool fluids and follow the advice for bringing down a fever.
■ Painkillers, such as **acetaminophen**, and other over-the-counter remedies may help ease aching muscles and other symptoms.
■ If self-help measures are ineffective, you

may be prescribed **antiviral drugs**, such as **amantadine** or **rimantadine**, which are effective against influenza viruses only ift they are given within 24 hours of the onset of symptoms.
■ You should see your doctor immediately if you have difficulty breathing or if your fever lasts longer than two days. You may be given a chest X-ray to rule out a chest infection such as pneumonia.
■ If a bacterial infection is found, your doctor will prescribe antibiotics. **However, these drugs have no effect on the influenza virus itself**.
■ Vulnerable people, such as babies, young children, the elderly, those with chronic heart or lung conditions, and people with reduced immunity, are at increased risk of serious complications. A doctor should be consulted immediately when anyone in a vulnerable group gets flu.

WHAT IS THE OUTLOOK?
■ If there are no complications, most of the symptoms of influenza usually disappear after 6–7 days, although a cough may persist over two weeks.
■ Fatigue and depression may last even longer.
■ However, for anyone who is in one of the high-risk groups, the complications of influenza may be life threatening and in epidemics, deaths from associated pneumonia are very common.
■ **Immunization** is effective protection. It is highly recommended for people in high-risk groups (excluding babies) and people who are particularly likely to be exposed to the virus, such as healthcare workers or carers or elderly people.

Immunization prevents infections in about two-thirds of people who are vaccinated annually. However, the vaccine can never be completely effective because the viruses frequently mutate, and different strains are responsible for outbreaks each year. The World Health Organization recommends the types of vaccines issued each autumn, depending on which strains are expected to be most prevalent in a particular region. However, if a virus mutates substantially, protection from the vaccine will be minimal and epidemics may occur.

See also:
- **Diabetes mellitus p. 504**
- **Fever in children p. 540**
- **HIV infection and AIDS p. 338**
- **Pneumonia p. 392**

Chickenpox

CHICKENPOX IS AN INFECTION THAT CAUSES A FEVER AND WIDESPREAD CROPS
OF BLISTERS. THE INFECTION IS CAUSED BY THE VARICELLA ZOSTER VIRUS,
WHICH ALSO CAUSES SHINGLES (HERPES ZOSTER).

The chickenpox virus is transmitted in airborne droplets from the coughs and sneezes of infected people or by direct contact with the blisters.

The illness is usually mild in children, but symptoms are more severe in young babies, older adolescents, and adults. Chickenpox can also be more serious in people with reduced immunity, such as those with AIDS.

WHAT ARE THE SYMPTOMS?

The symptoms of chickenpox appear 1–3 weeks after infection. In children, the illness often starts with a mild fever or headache; in adults, there may be more pronounced flulike symptoms. As infection with the virus progresses, the following symptoms usually become apparent.

■ Rash in the form of crops of tiny red spots that rapidly turn into itchy, fluid-filled blisters; within 24 hours the blisters dry out, forming scabs; successive crops occur for 1–6 days. The rash may be widespread or consist of only a few spots, and it can occur anywhere on the head or body.

■ Sometimes, discomfort during eating

caused by spots in the mouth that have developed into ulcers.

A person is contagious from about two days before the rash first appears until it fully crusts over in about 10–14 days.

The most common complication of chickenpox is bacterial infection of the blisters due to scratching. Other complications include **pneumonia**, which is more common in adults, and, rarely, inflammation of the brain (encephalitis). Newborn babies and people with reduced immunity are at high risk of complications. Very rarely, if a woman gets chickenpox in early pregnancy, the infection may result in fetal abnormalities.

WHAT MIGHT BE DONE?

Chickenpox can usually be diagnosed from the appearance of the rash. Children with mild infections do not need to see a doctor, and rest and simple measures to reduce fever are all that are needed for full recovery. Calamine lotion may help relieve itching. To prevent skin infections, keep fingernails short and avoid scratching.

People at risk of severe attacks, such as

babies, older adolescents, adults, and people with reduced immunity, should see their doctor immediately. An antiviral drug may be given to limit the effects of the infection, but it must be taken in the early stages of the illness in order to be effective.

Children who are otherwise healthy usually recover within 10–14 days from the onset of the rash, but they may have permanent scars where blisters have become infected with bacteria. Adolescents, adults, and people with reduced immunity take longer to recover.

CAN IT BE PREVENTED?

One attack of chickenpox gives **lifelong immunity** to the disease. However, the varicella zoster virus remains dormant within nerve cells and may reactivate years later, causing shingles (see below). There is a childhood vaccine, though, that is highly effective in preventing chickenpox.

See also:
- **Fever in children p. 540**
- **Influenza p. 334**
- **Pneumonia p. 392**

Shingles

SHINGLES IS AN INFECTION THAT CAUSES A PAINFUL RASH OF BLISTERS FOLLOWING THE PATH
OF A NERVE, SOMETIMES ON THE FACE, AND OCCASIONALLY AFFECTING THE EYE, WHEN
TREATMENT MUST BE ONGOING TO PREVENT INFECTION.

Shingles is most common between the ages of 50 and 70. People with reduced immunity, such as those with AIDS or those undergoing chemotherapy, are also especially susceptible to this infection. People with AIDS are particularly likely to have severe outbreaks of shingles.

The shingles rash commonly occurs on only one side of the body and usually affects the skin on the chest, abdomen, or face. In older people, discomfort may continue for months after the rash has disappeared. This prolonged pain is called **postherpetic neuralgia**.

Shingles is caused by the same virus that causes chickenpox, which remains dormant in nerve cells. When it is reactivated later in life, it causes shingles. The reason for reactivation is unknown but shingles often occurs at times of stress or ill health.

The virus is spread by direct contact with a

blister and will cause chickenpox in someone who has not already had it.

WHAT ARE THE SYMPTOMS?

Initially, you may experience tingling, itching, and a sharp pain in part of your skin. After a few days, the following symptoms may develop:
- painful rash of fluid-filled blisters
- fever
- headache and fatigue.

Within 3–4 days blisters form scabs. The scabs heal in 10 days but may leave scars. If a nerve that supplies the eye is affected, blisters may cause inflammation of the cornea. Rarely, infection of a facial nerve causes paralysis of one side of the face.

WHAT MIGHT BE DONE?

■ Shingles can be difficult to diagnose until the rash appears, and severe pain following the

line of the ribs (where nerves run around the body) can be mistaken for the chest pain of angina.

■ Your doctor may prescribe antiviral drugs to reduce the severity of the symptoms and the risk of postherpetic neuralgia.

■ Immediate treatment with antiviral drugs is important if your eyes are affected or if you have reduced immunity.

■ Painkillers may help relieve discomfort, and **carbamazepine** may help relieve the prolonged pain of postherpetic neuralgia.

■ Most people who develop shingles recover within 2–6 weeks, but up to half of people over the age of 50 develop post-herpetic neuralgia.

See also:
- **Postherpetic neuralgia p. 408**
- **Facial palsy p. 417**

FOCUS *on* herpes simplex

Herpes simplex is the name given to a virus that can cause cold sores (usually herpes simplex type 1) or genital herpes (usually herpes simplex type 2). The sores appear on whichever part of your skin is infected.

In either type of herpes the virus is transmitted mainly through infected skin coming into contact with another person's skin, for example through kissing, during sex, or from mouth to genitals during oral sex. However, the disease can also be spread by contact with other parts of the body, especially the fingers if a sore has been touched, and herpes may be spread to the eyes in this way. A cold sore that develops near the eye is potentially dangerous and should be seen by a doctor as soon as symptoms, such as tingling or itching, begin.

Originally it was thought that cold sores on the lips were only due to herpes simplex type 1 (HSV1) and genital herpes only due to the herpes simplex virus type 2 (HSV2). This distinction has become blurred, however, with the increased practice of oral sex. In Europe, genital herpes infection is the most common cause of genital ulceration and it is increasing among women. Genital herpes infection is more common in women than in men because their genital area is warmer and moister than a man's.

HOW COMMON IS HERPES?

Blood tests show that most people have been exposed to herpes simplex type 1 by the time we reach middle age. This means that millions of people are infected with the virus, but probably only a quarter of those infected have symptoms of any kind.

Many people have what is called a **subclinical** attack, with no visible signs of infection and no ill effects. These people are then naturally immune to further infection but don't know they've been infected.

WHAT HAPPENS TO THE VIRUS?

Once in the body, the virus can retreat to nerve cells in the face in the case of HSV1, or near the base of the spine in the case of HSV2. If the virus is reactivated, it can return to where it entered the body and cause a recurrence. Not all people have recurrences; some have a few and for some herpes recurs regularly. Normally the initial outbreak is the most severe. Recurrences don't depend on having contact with an infected person. Irritation of affected skin from other causes is

known to trigger outbreaks. If you have genital herpes, you mustn't have sex if the virus is active, i.e. if you have genital blisters or tingling or soreness, and you should always avoid oral sex if a cold sore is present.

As you'd expect, herpes is highly contagious. There is a 90 percent chance of catching it if either partner has an active blister, although new research confirms that **the virus can also be transmitted by people who don't have any symptoms**. Symptoms appear between three and 20 days after contact with an infected person.

WHAT ARE THE SYMPTOMS OF HERPES?

- The **skin** feels overly sensitive to touch.
- Itching and irritation around the affected area of skin.
- **Enlarged** tender lymph glands in the neck or groin.
- A general feeling of being unwell.
- Headache.
- Muscle aches and joint pains.
- Blisters that appear within a few hours of the itching and soreness; these enlarge, burst and become painful ulcers after two to three days.
- Ulcers that form scabs and take 14–21 days to heal completely.
- In genital herpes, shooting pain in the lower limbs.
- In genital herpes, pain on passing urine.

WHAT ARE THE TRIGGERS FOR HERPES?

- Physical and mental stress.
- Excessive cold or heat, including fever.
- For herpes infections of the face, exposure to strong sunlight.
- Local trauma to the skin (e.g. in genital herpes, rough sexual intercourse, plucking or shaving pubic hair).
- General ill health and other infections, such as a cold.

WHAT IS THE TREATMENT?

Cold sores caused by HSV1 can be treated at home using **acyclovir cream**, which is available over the counter from pharmacies. Genital herpes should always be looked at by a doctor and not treated at home. See your doctor immediately if you feel numb or sensitive in the genital area or if you've had sexual relations with anyone with the herpes virus.

There's no cure for genital herpes but the

Family of herpes infections

Type of virus	Condition it causes	Description
Herpes simplex type 1 (HSV1)	Cold sores	Infections of the **lips**, **mouth**, and **face**
Herpes simplex type 2 (HSV2)	Genital herpes	Infections of the **genitals**
Herpes zoster	Chickenpox	Infection causing **blisters**
	Shingles	Infection causing **blisters** along the path of a nerve; only occurs in those who have previously had chickenpox

sooner treatment is given the more likely it will prevent or ameliorate an attack. Antiviral drugs, such as **acyclovir**, taken as pills make the ulcers less painful and encourage healing. Over-the-counter acyclovir cream shouldn't be used to treat genital herpes.

SELF-HELP
● Keep separate towels and face cloths for each member of your household. This helps prevent the virus being spread from one person to another.
● To help prevent herpes from recurring get plenty of rest and eat a balanced diet with nutritional foodstuffs – fresh fruit and vegetables, **whole foods,** and plenty of liquids.
● Manage stress by learning relaxation exercises or taking up yoga.
● For cold sores, wear high SPF sunscreen on your lips and any other affected parts of the face when in bright sunlight.

● Keep a record of when your outbreaks recur in an attempt to find a pattern. If, for example, recurrences of genital herpes are related to rough sex, try using a lubricant jelly.
● Try a cream containing lemon balm, daily or when symptoms start.
● Always use a condom to protect yourself from genital herpes.
● For genital herpes, wear loose underwear so air can circulate and keep your genitals cool. Leave the sores exposed to air as much as possible.
● Painful blisters in the genital area can be relieved by a soak in a lukewarm bath and with cold packs (not ice) applied to the infected area.

WARNING:

The herpes virus may have a role in the development of cervical cancer and women who have had herpes should have a Pap smear regularly, preferably every year.

See also:
● Chickenpox p. 335 ● Cold sores p. 338
● Genital herpes p. 281 ● Shingles p. 335

Cold sores

COLD SORES ARE TINY BLISTERS THAT FORM MOSTLY AROUND THE NOSTRILS AND LIPS
BUT SOMETIMES ALSO ELSEWHERE ON THE FACE. THE BLISTERS BREAK OPEN
AND WEEP BEFORE THEY CRUST OVER AND DISAPPEAR.

Cold sores are caused by the herpes simplex virus, of which there are two types: type 1, which causes most cases of facial cold sores, and type 2, which causes about 70–80 percent of cases of genital herpes. A rise in skin temperature – perhaps caused by a cold, or by going out in the sun – activates the virus. The first outbreak may take the form of painful mouth ulcers. Subsequent outbreaks take the form of skin blisters. Most cold sores last about 10–14 days.

Cold sores are not serious unless they occur near the eye, where they may rarely cause an ulcer to form on the front of the eyeball.

WHAT ARE THE SYMPTOMS?
■ Raised red area, usually around the nostrils and lips, which tingles and feels itchy. Tiny blisters then form on the spot.
■ Weeping blisters, which then crust over.

WHAT SHOULD I DO FIRST?
■ Once blisters have formed, don't touch them.
■ Rubbing alcohol dabbed on the cold sores will dry them up (be careful, it may sting). I'm more in favor of a soothing cream, such as petroleum jelly, to keep them moist while the virus runs its course.

SHOULD I CONSULT THE DOCTOR?
Consult your doctor as soon as possible if the cold sores become redder and develop pus-filled centers, as they may be infected with bacteria. Also, consult your doctor as soon as possible if a cold sore is near your eye. Ask your doctor's advice if you suffer from recurrent cold sores.

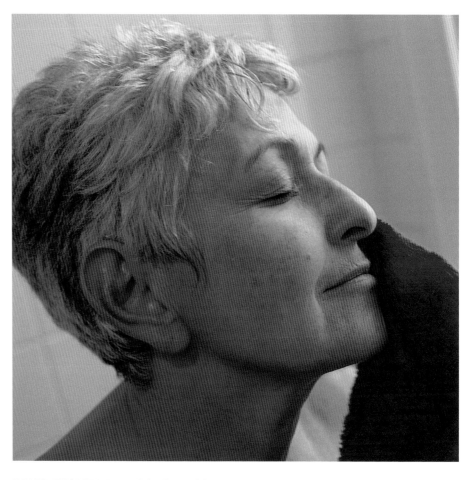

WHAT MIGHT THE DOCTOR DO?
■ If the cold sores are infected, your doctor may prescribe an antibiotic ointment that lubricates the area and treats the infection.
■ Your doctor may prescribe an antiviral cream to spread over the affected area regularly to contain the attack. He may also give you antiviral pills if outbreaks are frequent.

WHAT CAN I DO TO HELP?
■ Make sure that you have a personal towel and face cloth.
■ Don't kiss anyone. The virus can be transmitted this way.
■ If you tend to develop cold sores after exposure to sunlight, smear a sunscreen on your lips or nose when you go out in the sun.

HIV infection and AIDS

HIV IS A CHRONIC VIRAL INFECTION THAT, LEFT UNTREATED, RESULTS IN REDUCED
IMMUNITY TO OTHER INFECTIONS AND CANCERS (PARTICULARLY KAPOSI'S SARCOMA),
WHICH MAY RESULT IN DEATH.

Infection with the **human immunodeficiency virus** (HIV), which in many cases leads to acquired immune deficiency syndrome (AIDS), has been the most written about, most researched and most feared infection of the past two decades. Despite the development of highly effective drugs to control the disease there is

still no vaccine against the virus, and the number of people with HIV infection continues to rise, especially in developing countries.

HIV is believed to have originated in Africa, where a similar virus is carried by some species of primates. The virus is thought to have spread from monkeys to humans through saliva in

bites, then around the world from person to person in body fluids. The first recognized cases of AIDS in the US occurred in 1981, when there was an outbreak of unusual cases of pneumonia and skin cancer in young homosexual men in Los Angeles. Two years later, the virus was isolated and identified as HIV.

HIV infects and gradually destroys cells in the immune system, weakening the body's response to infections and cancers. People infected with HIV may have no symptoms for many years, or they may experience frequent or prolonged mild infections, but they **all** develop **antibodies** to the virus, which can be detected by a **blood test**; they're said to be **HIV positive**. When the immune system becomes severely weakened, an infected person is said to have AIDS. A person with AIDS develops serious infections caused by organisms that are normally harmless to healthy people and is also susceptible to certain cancers.

WHO IS AFFECTED?

There are an estimated 800,000 to 900,000 people currently living with HIV in the US, with about 40,000 new infections each year. Worldwide, over 33 million people are thought to be infected, 9 out of 10 of whom are unaware that they have the condition; the number is rising. As a result of developments in drug treatment, deaths due to AIDS have fallen dramatically in the developed world since 1995. The problem of AIDS is much greater in developing countries, where most people with HIV infection live and where the new drugs are unavailable or unaffordable.

HOW IS HIV TRANSMITTED?

The HIV virus is not the common cold – it's not contagious. HIV is carried in body fluids including blood, semen, vaginal secretions, saliva and breast milk, although not to the same degree. All body fluids do not therefore have the same potential for infection. Saliva from an infected person contains the HIV virus but in such a small quantity that it would be exceedingly difficult to be infected by saliva. HIV is most commonly transmitted sexually – by vaginal, anal and, more rarely, oral intercourse. **You are more susceptible to HIV infection and more likely to pass on the virus if you have another sexually transmitted disease.**

You are also at increased risk of HIV infection if you use **intravenous drugs and share or reuse needles** contaminated with the virus. Medical workers are also at risk from contaminated needles or from contact with infected body fluids, but the risk is very low.

HIV infection can be passed from an infected woman to the fetus or to the baby at birth or by breast-feeding. The virus can also be transmitted through organ transplants or blood transfusions. However, in developed countries screening of blood, organs, and tissues for HIV is now routine, making the risk of infection extremely low.

HIV infection cannot be transmitted by everyday human contact, such as shaking hands or by coughs or sneezes, and there is no risk to your health from working or living with someone who is infected with the virus.

WHAT IS THE CAUSE?

HIV enters the bloodstream and infects cells that have a special structure, known as the **CD4 receptor**, on their surfaces. The infected cells include a type of **white blood cell**, known as a **CD4 lymphocyte**, which is responsible for fighting infection. The virus reproduces rapidly within the cells and destroys them in the process.

At first, for most infected patients, the immune system is able to function normally despite the infection, and symptoms may not develop for years. However, especially if the infection is untreated, the number of CD4 lymphocytes eventually begins to fall, causing increased susceptibility to other infections and some types of cancer.

WHAT ARE THE SYMPTOMS?

The first symptoms of acute HIV infection usually appear within 6 weeks of infection. Some people experience a flulike illness that may include some or all of the following symptoms:
- swollen lymph glands
- fever
- fatigue
- rash
- aching muscles
- sore throat.

These symptoms usually clear up after a few weeks, and many people with HIV infection feel completely healthy. However, in some people, any of the following minor disorders may develop:
- persistent, swollen lymph glands
- mouth infections, such as thrush
- gum disease
- severe, persistent herpes simplex infections, such as cold sores
- extensive genital warts
- itchy, flaky skin (seborrheic dermatitis)
- weight loss
- neurological symptoms similar to dementia.

The time between infection with HIV and the onset of AIDS varies from person to person, but it can be anywhere between 1 and more than 14 years. Often people are totally unaware for years that they are infected with HIV until they develop one or more serious infections or cancers, known as "**AIDS-defining illnesses.**"

ARE THERE COMPLICATIONS?

The single most dramatic complication of HIV infection is the development of AIDS. A person infected with HIV is said to have developed AIDS if the CD4 lymphocyte count falls below a certain level or if he or she develops a particular AIDS-defining illness.

These illnesses include opportunistic infections (infections that occur only in people who have reduced immunity and certain other infections such as TB), certain cancers and problems with the nervous system that may result in dementia, confusion, behavior changes, and memory loss.

OPPORTUNISTIC INFECTIONS

These infections may be caused by protozoa, fungi, viruses, or bacteria, and they can often be life threatening.
- One of the most common illnesses in people with AIDS is a severe infection of the lungs (pneumonia) by the parasite *Pneumocystis carinii.*
- Other common diseases are protozoal, such as **toxoplasmosis**, which can affect the brain.
- *Candida albicans* is a fungus that causes mild superficial infections in healthy people but may produce much more serious infections in people who have AIDS.
- The cryptococcus fungus may cause fever, headaches, and lung infections.
- People with AIDS suffer from severe bacterial and viral infections. Bacterial infections include **tuberculosis** and **salmonella**, which may lead to **blood poisoning** (septicemia). Viral infections include those caused by the **herpes viruses**. Herpes simplex

Diagnosing HIV and AIDS

If you suspect that you may have been exposed to HIV infection, you should have a blood test to check for antibodies against the virus. The blood test may also be performed if you have symptoms that suggest HIV infection. Consent is always obtained before the test, and counseling is given both before and afterward to discuss the implications of a positive result.

If your HIV test result is negative, you may be advised to have another test in three months because antibodies can take time to develop. HIV infection can also be difficult to diagnose in the baby of an infected woman because the mother's antibodies may remain in the baby's blood for up to 18 months.

AIDS is diagnosed when an AIDS-defining illness, such as pneumocystis infection or Kaposi's sarcoma, develops or when a blood test shows that the CD4 lymphocyte count has dropped below a certain level.

Myths about HIV infection

Because HIV/AIDS is a very frightening subject, many myths and half-truths have grown up about how the infection can be transmitted. It should be stressed that HIV is quite difficult to catch. In an infected person, there are large numbers of the virus in blood and semen, but small numbers in saliva and vaginal fluid.

Knowing the truth about HIV helps you to act responsibly.

You won't get HIV
- from swimming in the same pool as an HIV-positive person
- if you kiss an infected person on the mouth, although there is a slight risk if the person has inflamed or bleeding gums
- from drinking from a glass or eating from a plate that's been used by an HIV-positive person
- by going to school or college with an HIV-positive person
- by visiting someone with HIV at their home or in the hospital
- by hugging, shaking hands, or dancing with someone who's HIV positive
- by sitting on a toilet seat that's been used by an infected person
- by standing next to an infected person who is sneezing; the virus doesn't travel through the air
- if you're bitten by an insect
- if you give blood at a blood donation center.

knowing. Men are just as worried about AIDS as women so they're usually grateful if a woman raises the subject as long as it's done in a tactful way.

■ Both partners might think about having an **HIV test before** having unprotected sex in a new relationship.

■ Specific groups also need to take special precautions. For example, if you inject drugs intravenously, you must use a clean needle every time.

■ People who are HIV positive need to take special care to prevent others from coming into contact with their blood or body fluids and should always inform dental or medical staff that they are HIV positive.

■ If you are HIV positive and pregnant, antiviral drugs will be given to reduce the risk of transmission to the fetus. You may also be advised to have a cesarean section.

■ Avoid breast-feeding if you are HIV positive to reduce the risk of transmitting the virus to your baby.

Medical professionals take many steps to prevent transmission of HIV, including screening all blood products and tissues for transplant and using disposable or carefully sterilized equipment.

Extensive research is being carried out either to develop a **vaccine** against HIV or to prevent the development of AIDS. However, although researchers are optimistic they will succeed, there will inevitably be millions more deaths worldwide before an affordable cure is found and made available to everyone.

infections can also affect the brain, causing meningitis and viral encephalitis.
■ **Cytomegalovirus** infection may cause a number of severe conditions, especially a type of eye inflammation that can result in blindness.

However, people with AIDS are no more susceptible to common infections such as colds.

CANCERS
The most common cancer that affects people with AIDS is **Kaposi's sarcoma,** a type of skin cancer that can also affect the inside of the mouth and internal organs. Other cancers that commonly develop in people with AIDS include **lymphomas,** such as non-Hodgkin's lymphoma. **Cancer of the cervix** is an AIDS-defining illness in women infected with HIV.

WHAT IS THE TREATMENT?
If your HIV test result is positive, you will probably be referred to a specialist where you will receive monitoring, treatment, and advice from a team of healthcare professionals.

Drug treatment may be started when you are diagnosed with HIV infection or when CD4 lymphocyte levels start to fall. Advances in the use of combinations of specific antiviral drugs, called antiretroviral drugs, that prevent HIV from replicating have made it possible to prevent progression of HIV infection to AIDS and to suppress the viral infection to undetectable levels in many people.

There are three main groups of antiretroviral drugs used in the treatment of HIV infection and AIDS.

Once AIDS has developed, opportunistic infections are dealt with as they occur, usually

by treatment with antibiotic drugs. There are also be long-term preventive treatment against the most common infections.

Emotional support and practical advice can be obtained from the many groups and nonprofit organizations that help people with HIV infection and AIDS.

WHAT IS THE OUTLOOK?
There is no cure for HIV infection, but the drug treatments available in the developed world have made it possible to regard the condition as a chronic illness rather than as a rapidly fatal one. In the two years following the introduction of antiviral drug combination therapies in 1995, deaths from AIDS in the developed world fell dramatically. However, for most of the people with HIV who live in the developing world, the prognosis is bleak. Few have access to up-to-date treatment, and left untreated, half of all people infected with the virus develop AIDS within 10 years and die.

CAN IT BE PREVENTED?
HIV infection can be prevented by teaching everyone about the risks of infection from an early age.

■ The two main precautions that everyone can take to avoid sexual transmission are to **use a condom during sexual intercourse** and to **avoid sex with multiple partners**. No matter how much you like someone, never give in to the temptation to have sex with a partner you barely know. Talk to him or her before you do anything you might regret. Talk about the risk; if he or she gets angry or resentful, you should ask yourself whether this person is really worth

See also:
- **Blood poisoning p. 345**
- **Cold sores p. 338**
- **Genital warts p. 282**
- **Herpes simplex p. 336**
- **Pneumocystis infection p. 396**
- **Safe sex p. 280**
- **Seborrheic dermatitis p. 315**
- **Toxoplasmosis p. 344**

Hepatitis

HEPATITIS IS A USUALLY SUDDEN, SHORT-TERM INFLAMMATION OF THE LIVER
DUE TO A VARIETY OF CAUSES, THE MOST COMMON BEING THE HEPATITIS
VIRUSES A, B, AND C; C IS THE MOST SERIOUS.

About 1 in 1000 people in the US carry the virus for hepatitis at any one time, although not all of them will necessarily go on to develop the disease. The condition has various causes and has a sudden onset. Most people with acute hepatitis recover within a month or two. However, in some cases inflammation of the liver persists for many months or may even persist for years (**chronic hepatitis**) and may progress to liver failure.

WHAT ARE THE CAUSES?

Worldwide, the most common cause of acute hepatitis is infection with any one of the several types of **hepatitis viruses**. Until the late 1980s, there were only two known hepatitis viruses, **hepatitis A and B**. Additional hepatitis viruses have now been identified, including **hepatitis C, D, and E**. Other hepatitis viruses are almost certainly yet to be discovered. The known viruses can all cause acute hepatitis, and they have many features in common, although the way in which they are transmitted and their long-term effects may differ.

Infections with some types of bacteria, other nonhepatitis viruses and some parasites can also lead to acute hepatitis. In addition, the condition may be caused by noninfectious agents, such as some **drugs** and **toxins**, including **alcohol**.

OTHER INFECTIOUS CAUSES

Acute hepatitis may also be caused by other viral infections, such as cytomegalovirus and the Epstein–Barr virus (the cause of mononucleosis). Some bacterial infections, such as Legionnaires' disease, can cause hepatitis. Parasitic infections that may also result in acute hepatitis include infection with plasmodium, the cause of malaria.

NONINFECTIOUS CAUSES

In developed countries, **excessive alcohol consumption** is one of the most common causes of acute hepatitis. The condition can also be caused by other toxins, such as those found in poisonous fungi. Acute hepatitis can also be caused by certain drugs, such as some **anticonvulsants**, the **anesthetic gas halothane,** and an overdose of acetaminophen.

WHAT ARE THE SYMPTOMS?

Some people infected with a hepatitis virus have no symptoms, or symptoms that are so mild they are not noticed. In other cases, the disorder may be life threatening. If hepatitis is due to a viral infection, the time from infection to appearance of symptoms can vary from up to six weeks for hepatitis A to six months for hepatitis B. Some people who have no symptoms may become carriers of the virus. If symptoms do develop, they may initially include:

- fatigue and a feeling of ill health
- poor appetite
- nausea and vomiting
- fever
- discomfort in the upper right side of the abdomen.

Several days after the initial symptoms develop, the whites of the eyes and the skin may take on a yellow tinge (**jaundice**). Often, the initial symptoms improve once jaundice appears. At this time, the feces may become paler than usual, and **widespread itching** may be present. Acute hepatitis caused by the hepatitis B virus may also cause **joint pains**.

Severe acute hepatitis may result in **liver failure**, causing mental confusion, seizures, and sometimes coma. Liver failure is relatively common following an overdose with the painkiller **acetaminophen**, but it is less common with some types of hepatitis, such as those due to the hepatitis A virus.

HOW IS IT DIAGNOSED?

If your doctor suspects that you have hepatitis, he or she may order blood tests to evaluate your liver function and to look for possible causes of the hepatitis. Blood tests will probably be repeated in order to help monitor your recovery. If the diagnosis is unclear, you may also have an ultrasound scan and, in some cases, a liver biopsy, in which a small piece of liver is removed and examined under a microscope.

WHAT IS THE TREATMENT?

There is no specific treatment for most cases of acute hepatitis, and people are usually advised to rest.

■ **Consult your doctor before taking any medicines,** such as painkillers, because there is a risk of side effects.

■ If you have viral hepatitis, you will need to take precautions to prevent the spread of the disease, including **practicing safe sex**.

■ You should **avoid drinking alcohol** during the illness and for a minimum of three months after you have recovered. However, if the cause was alcohol-related, you will be advised to give up drinking alcohol permanently.

WHAT IS THE OUTLOOK?

■ Most people with acute hepatitis feel better after 4–6 weeks and recover after three months.

■ However, for some people with **hepatitis C,**

Hepatitis viruses

Hepatitis A virus

The hepatitis A virus is the most common cause of acute viral hepatitis in the West. Often, the virus does not produce symptoms, or symptoms are so mild that the infection passes unrecognized. The hepatitis A virus can be detected in the urine and feces of infected people, and it can be transmitted to other people in **contaminated food or water**.

Hepatitis B virus

It is estimated that each year about one million people in Europe become infected with the hepatitis B virus. The virus is spread by contact with an infected person's body fluids. For example, the virus can be spread by **sexual intercourse** or by sharing contaminated needles used for taking drugs intravenously. In developing countries, the infection is most commonly transmitted from mother to baby at birth. Before blood banks routinely screened blood for the virus, blood transfusions used to be a source of hepatitis B infection, and many people with hemophilia contracted hepatitis. All blood used for transfusions is now screened for the hepatitis B virus.

Hepatitis C virus

About 3 percent of people worldwide are infected with the hepatitis C virus each year. The virus is most commonly transmitted by blood, often by sharing contaminated needles used for taking drugs intravenously. All blood used for transfusions in the US is now screened for the hepatitis C virus. It is also spread by **sexual intercourse**.

Hepatitis D and E viruses

Infection with hepatitis D occurs only in people who already have hepatitis B infection. It is spread by contact with infected body fluids. The hepatitis E virus is a rare cause of hepatitis in the developed world. The virus is excreted in the feces of infected people and is spread in much the same way as the hepatitis A virus.

recovery is followed by a **series of relapses** over several months.

■ About 3 out of 4 people with hepatitis C, and 1 out of 20 with hepatitis B and D **develop chronic hepatitis.**

■ People with acute hepatitis caused by an infection other than the hepatitis viruses usually recover completely once the infection clears up.

■ Recovery from acute hepatitis due to excessive alcohol consumption, drugs, or other toxins depends on the extent of the liver damage. The substances causing the acute hepatitis must be avoided in the future.

■ In the rare cases in which hepatitis progresses to liver failure, a liver transplant may be necessary.

CAN IT BE PREVENTED?

■ Infection with hepatitis A and E may be prevented by good personal hygiene.

■ The risk of infection with hepatitis B, C, and D can be reduced by practicing safe sex and by not sharing needles or other objects that might be contaminated with infected body fluids.

■ Immunizations to protect against hepatitis A are given to travelers to certain countries, and others at risk of contracting the infection.

■ Hepatitis B vaccination is recommended for high-risk groups, such as healthcare workers.

■ To avoid the transmission of hepatitis through blood transfusion, blood banks routinely screen all blood for the hepatitis B and hepatitis C viruses.

See also:
• **Alcohol-related liver disease p. 356**
• **Jaundice p. 355**
• **Malaria p. 343**
• **Safe sex p. 280**

Mononucleosis

INFECTIOUS MONONUCLEOSIS, ALSO KNOWN AS GLANDULAR FEVER, IS A VIRAL INFECTION CAUSING SWOLLEN LYMPH NODES AND A SORE THROAT THAT IS COMMON IN ADOLESCENCE AND EARLY ADULTHOOD.

Mononucleosis is known as the "kissing disease" of adolescence and early adulthood because it is mainly transmitted in **saliva**. Its name comes from the symptoms, which include widespread swollen lymph glands and a high temperature. Initially, the illness may be **mistaken for tonsillitis**, but it is more severe and lasts longer.

WHAT IS THE CAUSE?

Infectious mononucleosis is caused by the **Epstein–Barr virus** (EBV), which attacks lymphocytes, the white blood cells that are responsible for fighting infection. EBV infection is very common, and about 9 in 10 people have been infected by the age of 50. More than half of infected people do not develop symptoms and, consequently, are unaware that they have been infected.

WHAT ARE THE SYMPTOMS?

If symptoms of infectious mononucleosis develop, they usually do so 4–6 weeks after infection and appear over several days. Symptoms may include:

● high fever and sweating
● extremely sore throat, causing difficulty swallowing
● swollen tonsils, often covered with a thick grayish-white coating
● enlarged, tender lymph glands in the neck, armpits, and groin
● tender abdomen as the result of an enlarged spleen and liver
● rash.

These distinctive symptoms are often accompanied by poor appetite, weight loss, headache, and fatigue. In some people, the sore throat and fever clear up quickly, and

the other symptoms last less than a month. Other people may be ill longer and may feel lethargic and depressed for months after the infection. Mononucleosis was one of the first virus infections associated with post-viral fatigue syndrome.

WHAT MIGHT BE DONE?

Your doctor will probably diagnose the infection from your enlarged lymph nodes, sore throat and fever. A blood test may be performed to look for antibodies against EBV in order to confirm the diagnosis. A throat swab may also be taken to exclude bacterial infection, which would need to be treated with antibiotics.

There is no specific treatment for infectious mononucleosis, but simple measures may help relieve symptoms.

Drinking plenty of cool fluids, and taking over-the-counter painkillers, such as acetaminophen, may help control the high fever and pain. Contact sports should be avoided while the spleen is enlarged because of the risk of rupture, which causes severe internal bleeding and can be life threatening.

WHAT IS THE OUTLOOK?

Almost everyone who has infectious mononucleosis makes a full recovery eventually. However, in some people, recovery may be slow, and fatigue and depression may last for weeks or even months after the symptoms first appear. One attack of the disease, with or without symptoms, provides lifelong protection.

Typhoid and paratyphoid

TYPHOID AND PARATYPHOID ARE INFECTIONS CAUSED BY SALMONELLA BACTERIA THAT RESULT IN HIGH FEVER FOLLOWED BY A RASH.

Visiting or living in areas where the disease occurs is a risk factor. Typhoid and paratyphoid are almost identical diseases that are caused by the bacteria *Salmonella typhi* and *Salmonella paratyphi*, respectively. The bacteria multiply in the intestines and spread to the blood and to other organs, such as the spleen, gallbladder, and liver. The diseases are transmitted through infected feces and most commonly occur in areas where hygiene and sanitation are poor. Infection is commonly due to food or water contaminated by unwashed hands and consumption of raw and undercooked eggs and contaminated chicken.

WHAT ARE THE SYMPTOMS?
Symptoms of both diseases appear 7–14 days after infection and may include:
- headache and high fever
- dry cough
- abdominal pain and constipation, usually followed by diarrhea
- rash of rose-colored spots appearing on the chest, abdomen and back.

If left untreated, both infections can sometimes lead to serious complications, such as intestinal bleeding and, rarely, perforation of the intestines.

WHAT MIGHT BE DONE?
Typhoid and paratyphoid can be diagnosed by testing blood or feces samples for the bacteria. The diseases are usually treated with antibiotics in hospital. Symptoms usually subside 2–3 days after treatment has begun, and most people fully recover in a month.

Even with treatment the bacteria are excreted for about three months after the symptoms have disappeared. Some people may become lifelong **carriers** of the bacteria and transmit the infection to others, although they appear to be healthy.

Good hygiene is the best protection against infection. Several vaccines are available, and if you intend to travel to a developing country, immunization may be advisable. Consult your doctor before traveling because recommendations change.

Malaria

MORE THAN 1 IN EVERY 3 PEOPLE WORLDWIDE IS AFFECTED BY MALARIA, A PARASITIC INFECTION THAT LEADS TO THE DESTRUCTION OF RED BLOOD CELLS. MALARIA IS SPREAD BY INFECTED MOSQUITOES, WHICH PASS THE PARASITE ON THROUGH THEIR BITES.

In tropical countries, about 10 million new cases of malaria and 2 million deaths occur every year. Most of those who die from malaria are children.

WHAT ARE THE SYMPTOMS?
The symptoms of malaria usually begin between 10 days and 6 weeks after being bitten by an infected mosquito. However, in some cases, symptoms may not develop for months or years, especially if preventive drugs were being taken at the time of infection.

If not treated, malaria due to the **plasmodium** parasites – *P. vivax*, *P. ovale*, and *P. malariae* – causes recurrent attacks of symptoms each time the parasites multiply inside red blood cells and destroy them. Each attack usually lasts for 4–8 hours and may occur at intervals of 2–3 days, depending on the species of parasite. Symptoms of an attack include:
- high fever
- shivering and chills
- heavy sweating
- confusion
- fatigue, headaches, and muscle pain
- dark brown urine.

Between each attack, extreme fatigue due to anemia may be the only symptom.

Falciparum malaria (caused by *Plasmodium falciparum*) causes a continuous fever that may be mistaken for influenza. It is more severe than the other types, and attacks may lead to

SELF-HELP

Preventing malaria

If you plan to visit an area where malaria occurs, your doctor will be able to give you up-to-date advice about **antimalarial drugs** for that area. You may need to start taking the drugs several days or weeks before you leave and continue taking them during and after your visit. To protect yourself against mosquito bites, you should:

- Keep your body well covered.
- Sleep under a mosquito net that is impregnated with insect repellent.
- Use insect repellent on clothes and exposed skin.

These measures against mosquito bites are especially important at dusk and dawn, when mosquitoes bite.

loss of consciousness, cerebral malaria, and kidney failure and may be fatal within 48 hours of symptoms appearing if left untreated.

WHAT MIGHT BE DONE?
Your doctor may suspect malaria if you have an unexplained fever within a year of a trip to a region where the infection occurs. Diagnosis is confirmed by identifying the malarial parasite in a blood smear under a microscope.

If you are diagnosed with malaria, you should be given **antimalarial drugs** as early as possible to avoid complications. Treatment depends on the type of malaria, how resistant the parasite is to drugs, and the severity of the symptoms. If you have falciparum malaria, you may be treated **in the hospital** with **oral or intravenous antimalarial drugs**. In severe cases, treatment may also involve a **blood transfusion** to replace destroyed red blood cells or **kidney dialysis** if kidney function is impaired. Other types of malaria are usually treated on an outpatient basis with oral antimalarial drugs.

If treated early, the prognosis is usually good, and most people make a full recovery. Malaria caused by *P. vivax* and *P. ovale* may recur after treatment.

Preventive measures, including taking antimalarial drugs, should always be followed when visiting an area where malaria is known to occur.

Toxoplasmosis

TOXOPLASMOSIS IS A PROTOZOAL INFECTION THAT CAUSES SERIOUS ILLNESS IN THE UNBORN BABY AND IN PEOPLE WHO HAVE REDUCED IMMUNITY, SUCH AS AIDS PATIENTS, WHO MAY DEVELOP ENCEPHALITIS AS A RESULT OF THIS INFECTION.

Cysts of the parasite are excreted in the feces of cats and can be passed to people **by direct contact with cats** or by **handling cat litter.** Another source of infection is **raw or undercooked meat** of animals that have eaten cysts from the feces of infected cats.

In most people, the infection does not cause symptoms because the protozoal cysts are dormant. **If a woman develops toxoplasmosis while she is pregnant, the parasites may infect the fetus and cause numerous serious conditions.**

WHAT MIGHT BE DONE?

Usually, no treatment is necessary, although **pyrimethamine** and antibiotics may be prescribed for people with reduced immunity or pregnant women. People with reduced immunity may need to take the drugs for life, or until their immunity recovers, to prevent reactivation of cysts.

Infection can be prevented by avoiding contact with cats, wearing gloves to handle cat litter and for gardening, and by not eating undercooked or raw meat.

Lyme disease

LYME DISEASE IS AN INFECTION TRANSMITTED BY TICKS THAT CAUSES A RASH AND FLULIKE SYMPTOMS. NAMED AFTER OLD LYME, THE TOWN IN CONNECTICUT WHERE THE DISEASE WAS FIRST RECOGNIZED, LYME DISEASE IS CAUSED BY A BACTERIUM CALLED *BORRELIA BURGDORFERI.*

If a person is bitten by an infected tick that remains embedded in the skin, bacteria can enter the bloodstream and may then spread throughout the body.

Most reports of Lyme disease have been documented in the northeastern coastal states of the US, but it can be picked up wherever ticks thrive and is prevalent in southwestern France. The disease also occurs in northern and western US, in Europe, and in Central Asia. People who go camping or walking in wooded areas during the summer months are most at risk of being bitten by a tick carrying Lyme disease bacteria.

WHAT ARE THE SYMPTOMS?

A bite from an infected tick usually produces a red lump with a scab on the skin, although some people who have been bitten may not notice this initial sign. Within two days to four weeks after the bite, the following symptoms may develop:

- spreading circular rash at the site of the bite that may clear in the center
- fatigue
- flulike chills and fever
- headache and joint pains.

If the infection is left untreated, these symptoms may persist for several weeks. In some people who have Lyme disease dangerous complications may develop up to two years later that may affect the heart, nervous system, and joints.

WHAT MIGHT BE DONE?

■ Your doctor may suspect from your symptoms that you have Lyme disease and may also order a blood test to confirm the diagnosis.

■ You will be given prompt treatment with **antibiotics** – most people make a complete recovery.

■ **Nonsteroidal anti-inflammatory drugs (NSAIDS)** can help relieve joint pain.

■ **Vaccines** are now available that offer 70 percent protection against Lyme disease. For continued protection, vaccination needs to be repeated every two years.

■ In regions known to be tick infested, you should cover your arms and legs to reduce the risk of bites and promptly remove any ticks that you find on your skin.

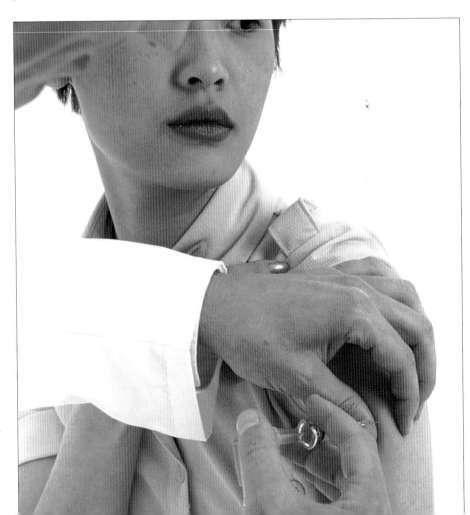

Blood poisoning (septicemia)

BLOOD POISONING, OR SEPTICEMIA, IS A RARE INFECTION IN WHICH BACTERIA
MULTIPLY IN THE BLOODSTREAM. QUITE OFTEN WE HAVE BACTERIA
IN THE BLOOD (BACTEREMIA), BUT THEY DON'T MULTIPLY.

Septicemia nearly always occurs when bacteria escape from a localized infection, such as peritonitis, meningitis, or an abscess, and is more likely to occur in people with a compromised immune system. It is a complication of bacterial meningitis.

WHAT ARE THE SYMPTOMS?
The symptoms of septicemia develop suddenly and include:
- high fever
- chills and violent shivering.

If septicemia is left untreated, the bacteria may produce toxins that damage blood vessels, causing a drop in blood pressure and widespread tissue damage. In this dangerous

condition, called **septic shock**, which is potentially life threatening, symptoms include:
- faintness
- cold, pale hands and feet
- restlessness and irritability
- rapid, shallow breathing
- rash
- jaundice
- in many cases, delirium and eventual loss of consciousness.

In some people, bacteria may lodge on the **heart valves**, especially if the heart has previously been damaged by disease. This serious condition is called **infective endocarditis**. Rarely, septicemia may result in a lack of the blood cells involved in blood clotting

(thrombocytopenia), which increases the risk of bleeding and produces a characteristic **purpuric rash** that doesn't blanch when a glass is pressed on the skin.

WHAT MIGHT BE DONE?
If your doctor suspects that you have septicemia, you will be admitted to the hospital for immediate treatment. **Intravenous antibiotics** are given without delay and blood tests are done to identify the bacterium causing the infection. Once the bacterium has been identified, specific antibiotics are given. With prompt treatment before the onset of septic shock, most people are able to make a complete recovery.

Toxic shock syndrome

TOXIC SHOCK SYNDROME IS A SEPTIC FORM OF BACTERIAL SHOCK, PRODUCED NOT BY BACTERIA
MULTIPLYING IN THE BLOOD BUT BY A TOXIN PRODUCED BY THE COMMON BACTERIUM
STAPHYLOCOCCUS AUREUS AND CERTAIN STREPTOCOCCAL BACTERIA.

When the bacteria multiply, large amounts of the toxin enter the blood and lead to the symptoms of shock.

First described in the 1980s, 7 out of 10 cases were in women using highly absorbent tampons (now taken off the market), but toxic

shock syndrome (TSS) can also arise from skin wounds or infections caused by *S. aureus* elsewhere in the body.

In addition to the symptoms of septicemia, a characteristic reddening of the palms and soles develops, with peeling two weeks later.

Treatment is with antibiotics, sometimes by intravenous infusion.

There seems to be an **individual tendency** to TSS, as it can return to women who've had it. These women, therefore, should avoid using tampons, caps, diaphragms, and so forth.

Tetanus

TETANUS IS A WOUND INFECTION CAUSED BY A POTENT TOXIN THAT IS
PRODUCED BY THE BACTERIUM *CLOSTRIDIUM TETANI*.
THE TOXIN INDUCES SEVERE MUSCLE SPASMS.

Tetanus bacteria live in soil and in the intestines of human beings and other animals. If the bacteria enter a wound, they multiply and release their toxin, which affects the nerves controlling muscle contraction. The condition, also known as lockjaw, is rare in developed countries because most people have been immunized.

The symptoms of tetanus usually appear 5–10 days after infection. Fever, headache, and muscle stiffness in the jaw, arms, neck and back are typical. As the condition progresses, painful muscle spasms may develop. In some people the muscles of the throat or chest wall are affected, leading to breathing difficulties and possible suffocation.

WHAT MIGHT BE DONE?

The disease needs immediate treatment in hospital with **antitoxin** injections, **antibiotics,** and **sedatives** to relieve muscle spasm. **Mechanical ventilation** may be necessary to aid breathing. If given prompt treatment, most people make a complete recovery. If treatment is delayed, tetanus is usually fatal.

CAN IT BE PREVENTED?

Essential precautions against tetanus include the following things.

■ Vaccination against tetanus. This is usually given as part of early childhood immunization; it is highly effective.

■ Booster vaccinations every 10 years.

■ Cleaning wounds thoroughly, especially those contaminated with soil, and treating them with antiseptic. Deep puncture wounds,

which are especially likely to become infected, should be seen by your doctor, who may give you antibiotics to prevent infection.

■ A booster vaccination after any deep wound if your booster vaccinations aren't up to date.

See also:
• **Immunization timetable p. 519**

Listeriosis

LISTERIOSIS IS A RARE INFECTION TRANSMITTED THROUGH CONTAMINATED FOOD. IT MAINLY AFFECTS VULNERABLE PEOPLE SUCH AS INFANTS, THE AGED, PREGNANT WOMEN (IN WHOM IT CAN CAUSE MISCARRIAGE), AND PEOPLE WITH A COMPROMISED IMMUNE SYSTEM.

The bacterium that causes listeriosis, *Listeria monocytogenes*, is widespread in the soil and is present in most animal species. **It can pass to humans through food products, particularly soft cheeses, milk, meat patés, and prepackaged salads.** Storing food incorrectly increases the risk. The bacteria multiply in the intestines and may spread in the blood and affect other organs.

The symptoms of listeriosis vary from one person to another. The infection often goes unnoticed in healthy adults, although some

people may develop flulike symptoms such as fever, sore throat, headache and aching muscles.

WHO IS AT RISK?

In elderly people and people with reduced immunity, such as those with lymphoma or taking immunosuppressant drugs, listeriosis can lead to meningitis, a potentially fatal inflammation of the membranes covering the brain. In pregnant women, infection can pass to the fetus, causing miscarriage or stillbirth.

WHAT MIGHT BE DONE?

Listeriosis is usually diagnosed by a blood test. In otherwise healthy people, mild listeriosis clears up with treatment in a few days. People with serious infection, especially during pregnancy, need urgent treatment in hospital with **intravenous antibiotics**.

Hygienic handling and storage of food reduces the risk of listeriosis.

Rabies

RABIES IS A RARE BUT SERIOUS INFECTION OF THE NERVOUS SYSTEM, USUALLY TRANSMITTED IN SALIVA FROM A BITE BY AN INFECTED, RABID ANIMAL, USUALLY A DOG.

Rabies can be prevented by a vaccine, which is recommended for people working with animals in high-risk areas. All travelers in these areas should avoid contact with stray animals.

WHAT ARE THE SYMPTOMS?

An infected person may develop symptoms within 10 days to 2 months of a bite, although rarely the virus can lie dormant for several years. Rabies usually starts with flulike symptoms that last for about 2–7 days, followed by:

• paralysis of the face and throat muscles
• extreme thirst
• painful throat spasms leading to an inability to drink and a fear of water
• disorientation and agitation
• loss of consciousness
• paralysis of the limbs.

Once symptoms have developed the condition is usually fatal.

WHAT MIGHT BE DONE?

There is no cure once the symptoms have developed. Diagnosis may not be obvious from the symptoms, and blood and saliva tests are usually done to confirm the presence of the virus.

Digestion

Image shows a colored scanning electron micrograph of a section through the duodenum, with microvilli

Miriam's overview

It can be helpful to think of the digestive system as a tube running through the body with an opening at each end, the mouth at the top and the anus at the bottom.

The tube isn't a neat, constant shape throughout its course. It swells into a muscular storage organ at the stomach where the food you swallow is thoroughly mixed with digestive enzymes that start breaking it up into a form that the body can use.

At the exit from the stomach more essential digestive juices are added from the gallbladder and pancreas. Food particles get smaller and smaller until, in the exquisitely adapted small intestine (small only in diameter, not length) the tiniest fragments of nutrients can pass easily though the intestine wall straight into the bloodstream.

We hear a lot about the large intestine (large in diameter) or colon, or more familiar still, the bowel, because it seems to be the focus of many common complaints. Its function in the body is really very simple, it's there to ensure that precious nutrients and water aren't lost. Its main job is to absorb water from its fluid contents. When the stream of digested food leaves the small intestine it's liquid, very runny. When we pass it as a stool it's solid. Its passage through the large intestine has brought about this change, purely through the absorption of water.

The rectum too can absorb water from feces, in fact, it will wring feces dry if they stay in the rectum too long. So if the "call to stool" is ignored for any length of time feces can become stony hard and difficult, even painful, to pass. This form of constipation is often thought of as a fault of the bowel or diet, but it isn't. It's simply due to not emptying the rectum soon enough. And it can be cured by heeding the need to stool as soon as you're aware of it, even though the pressure to ignore it and do something else is strong.

Laxatives aren't necessary to cure this type of constipation, only retraining yourself to heed what your bowel is telling you to do. If you don't, your bowel won't bother to send you the signal and your "constipation" will worsen.

If I were to try to pull out the headlines of what we've discovered over the last decade, two topics would immediately spring to mind, both of them cancer, esophageal cancer and bowel cancer.

The first is referable to heartburn. For decades heartburn has been thought of as nothing more than a mild irritation, a troublesome form of indigestion. In the last five or so years, however, we've come to realize that recurrent heartburn, especially if it's left untreated, can eventually result in malignant change of the lower end of the gullet where it enters the stomach.

It's caused by the chronic irritation from acid gastric contents, which regurgitate into the lower part of the esophagus. Here, the lining has no protection from the burning effect of stomach acid. By contrast the stomach lining is covered with a thick protective layer of mucus, so acid never reaches the delicate walls of the stomach lining.

Rigorous treatment of heartburn can prevent cancerous change, so you must seek advice from your doctor if you have a long-term problem.

> "*we can help* the next generation by making *sure our children* eat the magic number of *five fruits a day*"

We know more and more about bowel cancer. In the US it kills approximately 56,000 people every year and it's almost certainly due to our Western diet of too much fat and too little fiber, and a lifestyle of too little exercise. We can help the next generation by making sure our children eat the magic number of five fruits a day.

There are two cardinal signs of bowel cancer. The first is seeing blood in your stool, though that's a rather late sign. Before that you'll probably have noticed a change in your bowel habits, going more or less often than you used to, a touch of constipation or diarrhea where previously you had none. Or a sudden change in the shape of the stool – narrow where previously it had been round. This change in the bowel habit, in middle age or later, is a sign you must heed and discuss with your doctor. Currently, the best preventive is screening regularly by testing for blood in the stool.

Peptic ulcer now has a new cause. We used to think it was due to too much stomach acid. We now know it's due to an infection, a newly recognized infection, with *Helicobacter pylori*. Treatment has been revolutionized in the last 10 years. Now antibiotics are the lynchpin and, since the bacterium is difficult to eradicate, the course lasts a minimum of two weeks, along with other medicines to increase the effectiveness of the antibiotic. One course of treatment and nearly everyone is cured! Now, that's an advance on the old days.

INSIDE
your digestive system

The digestive tract can be thought of as a single, long, irregular tube and consists of the **mouth** and **throat** (pharynx), **esophagus**, **stomach**, **small** and **large intestines** (bowels), and the **anus**. Other organs that are not part of the digestive tract but are important to digestion are the **salivary glands**, the **liver**, the **pancreas**, and the **gallbladder**.

Food enters the digestive tract at the mouth, where it is mashed by the **teeth** and mixed with **saliva**. It passes down the esophagus to the stomach, where it is mixed with **digestive enzymes** and broken down further into a semi-liquid mixture. This mixture passes into the small intestine, where it is broken down into molecules that are absorbed into the blood. Indigestible material then passes into the large intestine, where some water is reabsorbed before it is excreted as feces. The liver produces the digestive juice **bile**, which is stored in the gallbladder until it is released into the small intestine.

The pancreas also secretes a digestive juice and produces the hormone **insulin**.

the digestive process

KEY

⇨ *Pancreatic fluids and bile*

⤵ *Food*

➡ *Nutrient transfer to liver*

the digestive system

As food passes through the digestive tract it is broken down into nutrients, which are absorbed by the small intestine, and water, which is absorbed by the small and large intestine. Nutrients pass to the liver in the bloodstream. Feces form in the large intestine and collect in the rectum before excretion.

DISORDERS OF THE MOUTH, TONGUE AND ESOPHAGUS

It's difficult to know where to start discussing the digestive tract, which runs from mouth to anus. Should the most common conditions come first, in which case flatulence, indigestion, constipation, and irritable bowel syndrome (IBS) would head the list? Or do we simply start at the top and work down? That's what I've chosen to do. Nonetheless, inclusion

of topics is based on their importance, which itself relies heavily on incidence.

Digestion begins in the mouth, where food is crushed, minced by the teeth and the tongue, and mixed with saliva secreted by the salivary glands. Swallowing forces the food into the esophagus and thence to the stomach by ripples of muscle contractions.

Causes of mouth ulcers

- The cause of mouth ulcers is not known, but they tend to occur in people who are run down or ill.
- They appear before menstruation in women.
- Mouth ulcers are often stress-related.
- Injuries to the lining of the mouth caused by badly fitting dentures, a roughened tooth or by careless tooth brushing can also result in mouth ulcers.
- **Rarely**, recurrent mouth ulcers may be due to **anemia**, a **deficiency** of either vitamin B_{12} or folic acid, an intestinal disorder such as **Crohn's disease** or **celiac disease**, or **Behçet syndrome**, a rare autoimmune disorder.
- Ulcers may also occur as a result of specific infections, such as **herpes simplex infections**.
- Very rarely, an ulcer that **enlarges** slowly and does not heal may be **mouth** cancer.

Mouth ulcers

PAINFUL SORES IN THE LINING OF THE MOUTH, KNOWN AS MOUTH ULCERS OR APHTHOUS ULCERS, CAN BE EXCRUCIATINGLY PAINFUL.

Mouth ulcers are extremely common, especially in young people and during times of stress or illness. They are slightly more common in girls and women and sometimes run in families, suggesting that a genetic factor may be involved.

Mouth ulcers appear as shallow, gray-white pits with a red border and may occur singly or in clusters anywhere in the mouth. They can cause pain, often excruciating for the first few days and particularly when you are chewing spicy, hot, or acidic food.

If they are very painful, mouth ulcers may deter eating and chewing, which in a child can look like loss of appetite. They may recur several times a year but they usually **disappear with or without treatment** within two weeks.

WHAT IS THE TREATMENT?
Mouth ulcers usually heal without treatment. Over-the-counter preparations containing a corticosteroid to reduce the inflammation combined with a local anesthetic are available in lozenge, gel, and paste form, which sticks to most surfaces.

If you have an ulcer that does not heal within three weeks, you should consult a doctor.

See also:
- Anemia p. 236
- Crohn's disease p. 366
- Herpes infections p. 336
- Malabsorption p. 365

Gastroesophageal reflux, hiatus hernia, heartburn

IN GASTROESOPHAGEAL REFLUX, ACIDIC JUICES ARE REGURGITATED INTO THE ESOPHAGUS FROM THE STOMACH. THIS REGURGITATION CAUSES A PAIN OR DISCOMFORT IN THE UPPER ABDOMEN AND CHEST, KNOWN AS HEARTBURN. ONE CAUSE IS A HIATUS HERNIA.

Gastroesophageal reflux (GERD), commonly known as heartburn or acid reflux, is probably the most common cause of **indigestion**. The discomfort is due to acidic juices from the stomach flowing back up into the esophagus (the gullet, the tube leading from the throat to the stomach). The lining of the esophagus does not have adequate defense against the harmful effects of stomach acid, which causes inflammation,

sometimes even ulceration, and a burning pain known as **heartburn.**

Obesity, a high-fat diet, drinking too much coffee or alcohol, smoking, and in some people, eating chocolate or tomatoes are risk factors.

WHAT ARE THE CAUSES?
The stomach contents are prevented from entering the esophagus by a double action valve mechanism: the lower end of the

esophagus has a muscular ring, known as the **lower esophageal sphincter**, which forms one part of the valve mechanism, and the other part consists of the **hiatus**, a narrow opening in the diaphragm muscle. The combination of these two muscular gateways provides an effective one-way valve.

GERD may develop as a result of several factors acting together to make the valve leak. These factors include:

Dangerous heartburn

If heartburn (gastroesophageal reflux) is a daily occurrence it can develop into something far more serious. The irritating acid causes changes in the cells lining the lower end of the esophagus, leading to a serious form of cancer.

The chances of getting cancer of the esophagus is eight times higher in people who have chronic heartburn and it's increasing faster than almost any other cancer. So take your heartburn seriously and talk to your doctor about it. Simply taking antacids doesn't reduce the danger.

Gastroesophageal reflux

KEY

Reflux

Esophagus

Acidic stomach contents

Stomach

In gastroesophageal reflux (GERD), the acidic contents of the stomach are regurgitated up into the esophagus, which lacks the mucus lining of the stomach and becomes irritated.

The esophagus isn't lined like the stomach and so stomach acid irritates the lower esophagus and over time triggers precancerous changes that can progress to cancer.

What's the connection between heartburn and cancer?

Researchers reported recently that having frequent, inadequately treated heartburn increased the risk of esophageal cancer nearly eight-fold. Among those in the study who had particularly severe and long-standing heartburn the risk of cancer rose more than 40 times. The relationship was so strong, researchers concluded that chronic heartburn was likely to be the cause of this cancer.

Precancerous changes in the esophagus develop in 10–15 percent of patients with chronic heartburn, and these patients face a risk of cancer that is 30–40 times greater than the risk in the general population.

Heartburn is obviously a disease that demands more respect than it gets. It's estimated that at least half the people who suffer from chronic heartburn are not getting the kind of medical care that may protect them from the serious consequences found in the study. The overall risk of developing esophageal cancer is very low, but only 5–10 patients out of 100 survive more than five years after getting the disease.

- poor muscle tone in the sphincter
- increased abdominal pressure due to pregnancy or obesity
- a weakness in the hiatus that allows part of the stomach to slide into the chest (a **hiatus hernia**).

Many people develop mild attacks of GERD after eating rapidly or eating certain foods, especially pickles, fried or fatty meals, or drinks, especially carbonated soft drinks, alcohol or coffee. Smoking worsens symptoms too.

WHAT ARE THE SYMPTOMS?

The main symptoms of GERD are usually most noticeable immediately after eating a large meal or when bending over. They include:
- a burning pain or discomfort in the center of the chest behind the breastbone, known as heartburn
- an acidic taste in the mouth due to regurgitation of acidic fluid into the throat or mouth
- erosion of the teeth due to acid
- persistent cough and sometimes asthma at night and sore throat
- hoarseness of the voice
- belching
- streaks of blood in the vomit.

GERD that persists over many years can cause scarring in the esophagus, which may eventually be severe enough to cause stricture (narrowing). A stricture can make swallowing very difficult and may lead to weight loss. Chronic GERD may lead to the esophageal lining replacing the stomach lining, increasing the risk of developing esophageal cancer.

WHAT IS THE TREATMENT?

The good news is that many products and treatments are now available to alleviate chronic heartburn and prevent stomach acid from damaging cells of the esophagus, which have no protection against a frequent bath of acid.
- Acid reflux may also be aggravated by drugs you can take for other conditions, so consult your doctor about the effects of both over-the-

counter and prescription medications you take and ask whether substitutions may be helpful.
- More severe cases that do not respond to diet and lifestyle changes alone require medication, starting with over-the-counter antacids. Histamine blockers such as Tagamet (cimetidine) and Zantac (ranitidine) help, but may not be strong enough to fully control acid reflux. If not, your doctor can prescribe more potent acid suppressors called proton-pump inhibitors, such as Losec. Other potentially useful drugs protect the lining of the esophagus and speed stomach emptying.
- If acid reflux cannot be controlled through diet, habits, and drugs, surgery may be required.
- One of the newest procedures, done through a laparoscope, involves wrapping a defective esophageal sphincter to strengthen it

against reflux.

Experts agree that it's not enough merely to calm all the symptoms of heartburn. Rather, acid reflux must be prevented and any cellular damage that has occurred must be healed.

It isn't enough to treat chronic heartburn sporadically, stopping treatment when symptoms subside. It has to be long-term. To protect the esophagus adequately, treatment must be aggressive, continuous, and indefinite and so involves some major changes to your life.
- If you have heartburn two or more times in a week, see your doctor and perhaps request a consultation with a gastroenterologist.
- If the problem has been long-standing, an examination and biopsy of the esophagus through an endoscope is the only good way to assess what damage has been done, if any. If

there are abnormal cell changes, endoscopic examinations should be done every year or two to check for possible progression toward cancer.

■ Should a precancerous condition develop, the esophagus can be removed and replaced with a piece of intestine or stomach. There are also experimental treatments that use laser or other forms of heat to obliterate the abnormal cells and allow healthy cells to replace them. Sometimes the precancerous changes can occur without much heartburn. If you feel food sticking on the way to your stomach, see your doctor.

See also:
• Endoscopy p. 353
• Indigestion p. 353

See also:
• Endoscopy p. 353
• Indigestion p. 353

SELF-HELP

Easing chronic heartburn

If you have chronic heartburn:

■ Chew food well, and eat slowly.
■ Watch what you eat. Stay away from or limit spicy or fatty foods, as well as chocolate, citrus juice, coffee, tea, and alcohol.
■ Eat five or six small meals rather than two large meals a day.
■ Immediately after a meal, avoid exercising, bending over, or lying down.
■ Lose weight if you need to.
■ You will feel better if there is some food in your stomach, so eat little and often.
■ Raise the head of your bed by about four inches or sleep on at least four pillows.

■ Antacid pills will help to neutralize the acids and protect the esophagus.
■ Give up smoking.
■ Consult your doctor if the problem occurs two or more times a week.

If you have recently developed pain in the center of your chest that seems to be unrelated to mealtimes, you should seek immediate medical help because the heart condition angina may sometimes be mistaken for the pain of severe heartburn.

THE STOMACH AND DUODENUM

When you think about it, the stomach and the duodenum (the short first part of the small intestine) are exposed to quite a few potentially irritating substances, including acid produced by the stomach to help digest food, alcohol, and hot foods such as spices. The stomach and duodenum have a natural defense mechanism that protects against damage, but sometimes the mechanism fails, leading to disease.

The two most common conditions that affect the stomach and duodenum are **indigestion** and **peptic ulcer**. We now know that peptic ulcers (ulcers of the duodenum and the stomach) are caused by a **bacterium** and symptoms are made worse by excess stomach acid. The importance of the *Helicobacter pylori* bacterium was only recognized in the early 1980s and it is now estimated that about half the world's population is infected with *H. pylori*. In most people there are no symptoms but others can develop **gastritis**, which is inflammation of the lining of the stomach, **peptic ulcer,** and **stomach cancer**, a cancer with a rather poor outlook. *H. pylori* infection can usually be treated successfully with drugs.

Indigestion (dyspepsia)

PAIN OR DISCOMFORT IN THE UPPER ABDOMEN BROUGHT ON BY EATING IS COMMONLY KNOWN AS INDIGESTION. THE MEDICAL NAME IS DYSPEPSIA. THERE ARE VARIOUS CAUSES, AND STRESS, BEING OVERWEIGHT, SMOKING, AND CERTAIN DIETARY HABITS ARE RISK FACTORS.

WHAT ARE THE SYMPTOMS?

Indigestion is a grab bag word covering many upper abdominal symptoms related to eating food, including heartburn, fullness, discomfort, pain, nausea, flatulence, and belching.

For most people it's a feeling of discomfort induced by eating too much, too quickly or by eating very rich, spicy, or fatty food.

"Nervous" indigestion can be a reaction to stress and it can be a symptom of peptic ulcer, gallstones, or heartburn.

WHAT IS THE TREATMENT?

■ Eat small meals often or at least regularly three times a day.
■ Avoid foods and situations that bring on indigestion.
■ Take an antacid when symptoms start.
■ See your doctor if you need to take antacids often or if your pain lasts longer than a few hours.
■ Indigestion starting suddenly in middle age must always be investigated to exclude stomach cancer.

See also:
• Gallstones p. 357
• GERD, hiatus hernia, heartburn p. 360
• Peptic ulcer p. 353

Preventing indigestion

Some measures can be taken to prevent or reduce the frequency of episodes of indigestion. You may find some of the following helpful.
■ Eat small portions of food at regular intervals without rushing or overfilling your stomach.
■ Avoid eating in the three hours before going to bed to allow your body enough time to digest food.
■ Reduce or eliminate your intake of alcohol, coffee, and tea.
■ Avoid rich, fatty foods such as butter and fried foods.
■ Keep a food diary to help identify foods that cause indigestion.
■ Learn to overcome stress, which can often trigger episodes of indigestion (see Relaxation, p. 292).
■ Try to lose excess weight and avoid tight-fitting clothing.
■ If possible, avoid medicines that irritate the digestive tract, such as aspirin and non-steroidal anti-inflammatory drugs (NSAIDs).

Peptic ulcer

A PEPTIC ULCER OCCURS WHEN THE TISSUE LINING THE STOMACH OR DUODENUM IS ERODED BY ACIDIC DIGESTIVE JUICES. PEPTIC ULCERS ARE ALSO CALLED STOMACH (OR GASTRIC) ULCERS OR DUODENAL ULCERS, DEPENDING ON THEIR LOCATION.

The lining of the stomach and duodenum (the first part of the small intestine) is normally protected from the effects of acidic digestive juices by a barrier of mucus. If this barrier is damaged, acid may cause inflammation and erosion of the lining. The resulting eroded areas are known as peptic ulcers, and there are two different types: duodenal ulcers and stomach (gastric) ulcers.

Stomach ulcers are more common over age 50. **Duodenal** ulcers have been common in men between the ages of 20 and 45 and now commonly occur in older men and women too. Duodenal ulcers sometimes run in families, and stress, excess alcohol, and smoking are risk factors. About 25 million Americans will develop an ulcer at some time in their lives.

WHAT ARE THE CAUSES?

■ Peptic ulcers are most commonly associated with *Helicobacter pylori* infection. This bacterium releases chemicals that increase gastric acid secretion. Acidic digestive juices are then more likely to erode the lining of the stomach or the duodenum, which allows peptic ulcers to develop.
■ Peptic ulcers may sometimes result from the long-term use of aspirin or nonsteroidal anti-inflammatory drugs (NSAIDs), such as **ibuprofen**, that damage the lining of the stomach.
■ Other factors that may lead to peptic ulcers include smoking and occasionally alcohol.

In some people, there is a strong family history of peptic ulcers, suggesting that a gene may be at work.
■ It is currently thought that psychological stress is probably not one of the primary causes of peptic ulcers; however, it may make an existing ulcer worse.

WHAT ARE THE SYMPTOMS?

Many people with a peptic ulcer do not experience symptoms or dismiss their discomfort as indigestion or heartburn. Those with persistent symptoms may notice:
● pain or discomfort that is felt in the center of the upper abdomen, often just under the tip of the breastbone
● pain going through to the back
● loss of appetite and weight loss
● a feeling of fullness in the abdomen
● nausea and sometimes vomiting.

Pain comes in attacks and is often present for several weeks and then disappears for months or even years. The pain from a duodenal ulcer can be worse **before** meals

Contrast X-rays

In a contrast X-ray, a substance known as a contrast medium is introduced into the body to help an organ show up better on X-ray film. Contrast media, such as barium, are harmless and are expelled or absorbed by the body after the X-ray has been taken. They are usually given as a drink but may sometimes be given as an injection. A few people may experience a flushing sensation when a contrast medium is injected.

Mass of barium in the digestive tract

Barium solution coating the intestinal lining

when the stomach is empty and can be quickly relieved by eating but usually recurs a few hours afterward. By contrast, pain caused by a gastric ulcer may be worse **after** food.

ARE THERE COMPLICATIONS?

■ The most common complication of peptic ulcer is **bleeding** as the ulcer becomes deeper and erodes into nearby blood vessels.
■ Minor bleeding from the digestive tract may cause no symptoms except those of **anemia**, such as pale skin, fatigue, and faintness.
■ Bleeding from the digestive tract may lead to **vomiting of blood**.
■ Alternatively, blood may pass through the digestive tract, resulting in **black, tarry stools**.
■ In some cases, an ulcer perforates all the layers of the stomach or duodenum, allowing gastric juices to enter the abdomen and causing severe pain and peritonitis. Bleeding from the digestive tract and perforation of the stomach or the duodenum may be life threatening and require immediate medical attention.
■ In rare cases, stomach ulcers may result in narrowing of the stomach outlet into the duodenum, which prevents the stomach from emptying fully. Symptoms may then include bloating after meals, vomiting undigested food hours after eating, and weight loss.

WHAT MIGHT BE DONE?

If your doctor suspects that you have a peptic ulcer, an **endoscopy** will be arranged to view the stomach and duodenum directly. During endoscopy, a sample of the stomach lining will be taken to look for evidence of *H. pylori* infection and exclude stomach cancer, which may cause similar symptoms. In some cases a barium X-ray may be done instead. Your doctor may also arrange for you to have blood tests to detect antibodies against the *H. pylori* bacterium and to check for evidence of anemia.

WHAT IS THE TREATMENT?

Treatment of a peptic ulcer is designed to heal the ulcer and to prevent it from recurring. You will be advised to make some **lifestyle changes**, such as giving up smoking and drinking less alcohol.
■ *H. pylori* is treated with a combination of antibiotics to kill the bacteria and ulcer healing drugs to cut acid production and promote healing. Because three drugs may be involved the combination is often called "triple" therapy. Triple therapy needs to be taken religiously for 1–2 weeks, which usually eradicates *H. pylori* and the condition never recurs. Occasionally, however, it may be necessary to take another course. Ulcer healing drugs are usually given to

maximize the chance of healing even if tests for *H. pylori* prove negative.
■ If long-term treatment with aspirin or a non-steroidal anti-inflammatory drug is the cause, your doctor may prescribe an alternative drug or an additional drug, such as **misoprostol**, to protect the lining of the stomach and duodenum.
■ A bleeding or perforated ulcer is an emergency requiring urgent admission to hospital. If blood loss is severe, a blood transfusion may be necessary. Endoscopy may be done to view the stomach lining; during this, bleeding blood vessels may be treated with diathermy, a technique that uses heat to seal them. Alternatively, an injection of drugs may be given to stop bleeding. If bleeding is severe or the ulcer is perforated, surgery is usually necessary.

With treatment, about 19 in 20 peptic ulcers disappear completely within a few months. However, the ulcer may recur if lifestyle changes are not made or if there is reinfection with *H. pylori*.

See also:
- Anemias p. 236
- GERD, hiatus hernia, heartburn p. 350
- Indigestion p. 352

Stomach cancer

CANCER OF THE STOMACH IS A CANCEROUS TUMOR THAT USUALLY DEVELOPS IN THE LINING OF THE STOMACH WALL AND MAY SPREAD RAPIDLY AROUND THE BODY. CERTAIN FOODS, SMOKING, AND A HIGH ALCOHOL INTAKE ARE RISK FACTORS.

Stomach cancer is more common over the age of 50 and twice as common in males. Oddly enough, it is more common in people with blood group A and sometimes runs in families.

Worldwide, stomach cancer is the **second most common cancer** after lung cancer. Stomach cancer is a particular problem in Japan and China, possibly because of dietary factors. However, in most other countries the disease is now less common, a change thought to be due to less smoked and salted food in the diet. Each year about 24,000 people in the US learn they have stomach cancer.

In most cases, stomach cancer develops in the stomach lining. The cancer may spread rapidly to other parts of the body. Early diagnosis is rare because the symptoms are usually mild or overlooked, and by the time people seek medical help, the cancer has often spread.

WHAT ARE THE CAUSES?

The causes of stomach cancer are not fully understood, but there are a number of factors at work.

■ Chronic gastritis due to infection with the *H. pylori* bacterium increases the risk of stomach cancer.
■ Certain diets may increase the risk, such as a diet with high intake of salt, pickled and smoked foods, and a low intake of fresh fruit and green vegetables.
■ Smoking and high alcohol intake are also risk factors.

WHAT ARE THE SYMPTOMS?

The early symptoms of stomach cancer are mild and vague, and many people ignore them. Any stomach symptom such as **indigestion suddenly starting in middle age** must be investigated. Symptoms include:
- discomfort in the upper abdomen, indigestion, heartburn
- pain in the stomach after eating not relieved by antacids and lasting longer than a few weeks
- loss of appetite and weight loss
- nausea and vomiting
- passage of a black stool.

In many people, **anemia** develops due to chronic minor bleeding from the stomach lining. Later on, swelling may be felt in the upper abdomen.

WHAT IS THE TREATMENT?

■ The only effective treatment for stomach cancer is **early surgery** to remove the tumor. However, this option is only appropriate in about 1 in 2 cases because in others the cancer has already spread too widely to be operable.
■ The operation involves the removal of part or all of the stomach. The surrounding lymph nodes are also removed since they are possible sites of cancerous spread.
■ In cases where the cancer has spread to other parts of the body, surgery may help improve life expectancy, although in some cases the operation may be done to relieve symptoms rather than attempt a cure.
■ Radiation therapy and chemotherapy slow the progress of the disease and relieve pain.
■ Strong painkillers may help relieve severe discomfort.

WHAT IS THE OUTLOOK?

If detected and treated early, stomach cancer has a good cure rate. Some countries in which stomach cancer is common, such as Japan, have efficient screening programs to detect the cancer early. In these countries, about 4 in 5 people treated by surgery are alive five years after diagnosis. However, the outlook worldwide is generally poor, with only about 1 in 5 affected people surviving for five years after diagnosis.

See also:
- Anemias p. 236 • CT scanning p. 401
- Contrast X-rays p. 353
- Peptic ulcer p. 353

Diagnosing stomach cancer

■ Your doctor may arrange for you to have an endoscopy, in which a thin, flexible viewing tube is used to examine the lining of the stomach. Samples of tissue are taken from abnormal areas of the stomach lining during the procedure and tested to look for the presence of cancerous cells.

■ You may also have a barium swallow, in which a liquid barium mixture is swallowed to show the stomach clearly on an X–ray.

■ The doctor may order blood tests for anemia, which may indicate that there has been bleeding from the stomach lining.

■ If a diagnosis of stomach cancer is confirmed, further tests, such as CT scanning and blood tests, may be performed to check whether the cancer has spread to other organs.

THE LIVER, GALLBLADDER, AND PANCREAS

One of the main functions of the liver and pancreas is to manufacture enzymes that digest food. The liver makes the digestive fluid, **bile**, which is stored in the **gallbladder**. The pancreas makes digestive enzymes that break down food into elements that can be absorbed through the intestinal wall and used by the rest of the body. The pancreas also produces a hormone that controls the level of glucose in the blood – **insulin**.

The yellow discoloration of the skin and eyes known as **jaundice** is very often a sign of liver disease, so it seems appropriate to cover it here. In Western countries, the main cause of liver disease is **hepatitis**. "Cancer of the liver" is usually due to the spread of cancer from other organs to the liver (properly called liver metastases). Primary liver cancer is uncommon in the West.

Gallstones frequently don't cause symptoms and need no treatment, but may lead to gallbladder inflammation, called **cholecystitis**, which can be very painful and most certainly needs treatment. Inflammation of the pancreas, an enzyme gland cupped in the curve of the duodenum just below the stomach, is becoming increasingly common because it's probably caused by a viral infection. This **pancreatitis** can be very painful and debilitating so I've included it in this section. Finally, there's **pancreatic cancer**, which is becoming more common in Western countries in parallel with the increase in pancreatitis.

Jaundice

JAUNDICE IS THE NAME FOR YELLOW DISCOLORATION OF THE SKIN AND THE WHITES OF THE EYES. IT IS A SYMPTOM OF MANY DISORDERS OF THE LIVER, GALLBLADDER, AND PANCREAS, AND MAY ALSO BE CAUSED BY SOME BLOOD DISORDERS.

Jaundice results from excessively high blood levels of the pigment **bilirubin**, a breakdown product of red blood cells. Bilirubin is processed by the liver and then excreted as a component of bile. In liver disease the liver cannot process bilirubin, so levels gradually rise in the blood, leading to jaundice. If, for some reason, many millions of red blood cells are being broken down, bilirubin levels rise because even healthy livers become overloaded. A few days after birth, many babies develop a form of jaundice that is usually harmless and disappears quickly.

Jaundice always requires investigation because the underlying disorder may be serious.

WHAT ARE THE CAUSES?

Levels of bilirubin in the blood can increase if the amount of bilirubin produced is too great for the liver to process. Damaged liver cells or obstruction of the bile ducts, which carry bile from the liver to the gallbladder and then to the small intestine, can also lead to high levels of bilirubin in the blood. The following are possible causes of this.

■ **Excess red cell breakdown.** In a healthy person, red blood cells have a lifespan of about 120 days, after which they are removed from the blood and broken down by the spleen to produce bilirubin. The bilirubin then passes to the liver. If the number of red blood cells being broken down is above normal (hemolysis), the liver cannot process the large amounts of bilirubin produced. This is known as **hemolytic jaundice**.

■ **Liver cell damage.** If the liver is damaged, its ability to process bilirubin is reduced.

Liver cell damage may occur for a variety of reasons, including viral infection, alcohol abuse, and an adverse reaction to some drugs. Jaundice due to liver cell damage is sometimes accompanied by nausea, vomiting, pain in the abdomen, and a swollen abdomen.

• **Bile duct obstruction**. An obstruction in the bile ducts, the channels through which bile leaves the liver, may result in jaundice. Obstruction may be due to disorders such as pancreatic cancer or gallstones. If the bile ducts are blocked, bile builds up in the liver, and bilirubin is forced back into the blood. This type of jaundice may be accompanied by itching of the skin, dark-colored urine and lighter than normal stools.

WHAT MIGHT BE DONE?

■ Your doctor may order blood tests to assess liver function and to look for evidence of excess red blood cell destruction, viral hepatitis, or other disorders affecting the liver.

■ To look for signs of inflammation or obstruction, your doctor may use imaging techniques such as computerized tomography (CT) scanning, magnetic resonance imaging (MRI), endoscopy of the pancreas (ERCP), or ultrasound scanning using an endoscope.

■ A sample of liver tissue may be taken – liver biopsy – for microscopic examination to look for underlying liver disease.

WHAT IS THE OUTLOOK?

If the underlying cause of jaundice can be treated, jaundice will disappear. If the cause is not curable, as in the case of pancreatic cancer, treatment may be given to relieve symptoms associated with jaundice, such as itching.

> **See also:**
> • **CT scanning p. 401**
> • **ERCP p. 360**
> • **Gallstones p. 357**
> • **MRI p. 409**
> • **Pancreatic cancer p. 360**
> • **Ultrasound scanning p. 277**

Alcohol-related liver disease

EXCESSIVE ALCOHOL CONSUMPTION CAN CAUSE EITHER SHORT-TERM OR PROGRESSIVE LIVER DAMAGE. ALCOHOL IS A POISON AND IF DRUNK IN EXCESS OVER THE LONG TERM MAY CAUSE THREE TYPES OF LIVER DISEASE: FATTY LIVER, ALCOHOLIC HEPATITIS, AND CIRRHOSIS.

Heavy social drinking over the long term can contribute to alcohol-related liver disease.

Typically, alcoholic liver disease progresses as follows. Over a number of years, most heavy drinkers develop a **fatty liver**, in which fat globules develop within liver cells. If alcohol consumption continues, **hepatitis** or inflammation of the liver develops. With continued drinking, **cirrhosis** or scarring develops. In this condition, liver cells that are damaged by alcohol are replaced by fibrous scar tissue. If cirrhosis has developed, liver damage is **irreversible**.

WHAT ARE THE SYMPTOMS?

In many cases, **fatty liver** does not cause symptoms and often remains undiagnosed. However, in about 1 in 3 affected people, the liver becomes **enlarged**, which may lead to discomfort in the right upper abdomen.

Alcoholic **hepatitis** also may not produce liver symptoms, but after about 10 years of heavy drinking in men, and sooner in women, the first symptoms usually develop. These may include:

• nausea and occasional vomiting
• discomfort in the upper right side of the abdomen
• weight loss or gain
• fever
• yellowing of the skin and the whites of the eyes (jaundice)
• swollen abdomen.

Cirrhosis may often cause no symptoms for a number of years or only mild symptoms, including:

• poor appetite and weight loss
• nausea
• muscle wasting.

In some cases, severe cirrhosis may lead to a serious condition is which there is bleeding into the digestive tract from varicose veins that develop in the wall of the esophagus. Severe alcoholic hepatitis and cirrhosis can lead to **liver failure**, which may result in **coma** and **death**.

WHAT IS THE TREATMENT?

People with alcohol-related liver disease must stop drinking completely and forever. Many people need professional help to achieve this. If drinking continues, the disease will probably progress and may be fatal. If drinking stops, the outcome is likely to improve, except if cirrhosis is well-established.

WHAT IS THE OUTLOOK?

■ Fatty liver often disappears after 3–6 months of abstinence from alcohol. Some people with alcoholic hepatitis who stop drinking recover completely. However, in most cases **damage to the liver is irreversible**, and the condition progresses to cirrhosis. Severe alcoholic cirrhosis can cause a number of serious complications, which in some cases may be fatal.

■ About **half of all people** who have cirrhosis **die from liver failure** within five years if they continue to drink.

■ More than 1 in 10 people with cirrhosis go on to develop liver cancer.

■ People with serious alcohol-related liver disease who have no other serious health problems and have stopped drinking may be candidates for a liver transplant.

■ Many of the symptoms and some of the complications of alcohol-related liver disease can be treated with some success. For example, swelling of the abdomen, which results from fluid accumulation in the abdominal cavity, may be decreased by diuretic drugs and a diet that is low in salt. Nausea can frequently be relieved by antiemetic drugs.

> **See also:**
> • Cirrhosis p. 357   • Jaundice p. 355
> • Liver cancer p. 359

Cirrhosis

CIRRHOSIS IS IRREVERSIBLE SCARRING OF THE LIVER, OCCURRING IN THE LATE STAGES OF VARIOUS LIVER DISORDERS. IN CIRRHOSIS, NORMAL LIVER TISSUE IS DESTROYED AND REPLACED BY FIBROUS SCAR TISSUE. LONG-TERM EXCESSIVE ALCOHOL CONSUMPTION IS A RISK FACTOR.

Cirrhosis may be caused by several different disorders, including **viral infections** and **excessive alcohol consumption**. The liver damage is irreversible and prevents the liver from functioning properly. Some people with cirrhosis may feel well for years despite having severe liver damage. However, with time they may develop complications, such as liver failure and liver cancer.

In developed countries, cirrhosis is the **third most common cause of death** in people aged 45–65, after **coronary artery disease** and **cancer**. In the US, chronic liver disease and cirrhosis are responsible for about 25,000 deaths each year. Cirrhosis is much more common in men than in women.

WHAT ARE THE CAUSES?

There are various causes of cirrhosis.

■ Worldwide, the most common cause is infection with a **hepatitis virus**, particularly the hepatitis B and C viruses.

■ However, in developed countries cirrhosis is most frequently caused by **excessive alcohol consumption.**

■ Cirrhosis may also be caused by **sclerosing cholangitis,** a condition in which the bile ducts inside the liver become inflamed. The cause of this condition is not known although it can be associated with some inflammatory

bowel diseases, such as **ulcerative colitis** and **Crohn's disease**.

■ Cirrhosis may develop as a result of a blockage of the bile ducts by **gallstones**.

■ Cirrhosis may follow **bile duct surgery**.

WHAT ARE THE SYMPTOMS?

Cirrhosis often produces no symptoms and is only detected during a routine examination for another condition. If there are symptoms, they include:

● poor appetite and weight loss
● nausea
● yellowing of the skin and the whites of the eyes (jaundice).

WHAT IS THE OUTLOOK?

In the long term, life threatening complications may arise.

■ Cirrhosis can lead to high blood pressure in veins in the esophagus, which causes them to be fragile and to bleed easily.

■ Malnutrition may also develop from being unable to absorb fats and certain vitamins.

■ Eventually, cirrhosis can lead to liver cancer or liver failure. The symptoms of liver failure include a swollen, fluid-filled abdomen and visible spiderlike blood vessels in the skin, known as spider nevi.

■ A failing liver may also result in abnormal

bleeding and easy bruising. This occurs as a result of reduced production of essential blood clotting factors in the liver.

WHAT MIGHT BE DONE?

■ If your doctor suspects that you have cirrhosis from your symptoms, blood samples will be taken to assess liver function and look for hepatitis viruses.

■ You may also have ultrasound scanning, computerized tomography (CT) scanning, or magnetic resonance imaging (MRI) to assess the liver.

■ To confirm the diagnosis, you may have a liver biopsy, in which a small sample of tissue is removed from your liver for microscopic examination.

Damage to the liver caused by cirrhosis is always irreversible. However, if the underlying cause can be treated further deterioration may be prevented.

> **See also:**
> • **Crohn's disease p. 366**
> • **Jaundice p. 355**
> • **Liver cancer p. 359**
> • **MRI p. 409**
> • **Ultrasound scanning p. 277**

Gallstones

GALLSTONES ARE STONES OF VARIOUS SIZES AND COMPOSITION THAT USUALLY OCCUR IN THE GALLBLADDER.

Gallstones are formed from bile, a digestive liquid produced by the liver and stored in the gallbladder. Most gallstones do not cause symptoms. Gallstones occur in about 1 in 10 people over age 40, with twice as many women as men being affected. The typical patient is described as "female, fair, fat, and forty." Gallstones may run in families, and are more common in Native American and Hispanic people for reasons that are not fully understood.

Bile, the liquid from which gallstones are formed, is made up mainly of the fatty substance cholesterol, pigments, and various salts. A change in the composition of bile may trigger stone formation. Most gallstones are a mixture of cholesterol and pigments. In about

1 in 5 cases stones consist of cholesterol only, and in about 1 in 20 cases stones consist of pigment only. Often, there are many stones, and some can reach the size of a golf ball.

WHAT ARE THE CAUSES?

There is often no obvious cause for gallstones. However, cholesterol stones are more likely in people who are very overweight or who eat a high-fat diet.

Pigment stones may form if there is excessive destruction of red blood cells, as may occur in hemolytic anemia and sickle-cell anemia. Poor emptying of the gallbladder caused by narrowed bile ducts may also increase the risk of gallstones.

WHAT ARE THE SYMPTOMS?

Gallstones often cause no symptoms. However, symptoms may occur if one or more stones **block the cystic duct** (the exit tube from the gallbladder) or the **common bile duct** (the main bile duct from the liver to the duodenum). A stone that partially or completely blocks the flow of bile will cause attacks known as **biliary colic**, which cause symptoms that include:

● very severe upper abdominal pain
● nausea and vomiting.

Episodes are normally brief and typically occur following a fatty meal, which causes the gallbladder to contract.

ARE THERE COMPLICATIONS?

Stones that remain lodged in the bile ducts block the release of bile, causing severe inflammation or infection of the gallbladder and bile ducts. Blocked bile ducts may also cause jaundice, a condition in which the skin and whites of the eyes become yellow. In addition to jaundice, blockage of the common bile duct may cause inflammation of the pancreas (pancreatitis).

HOW ARE THEY DIAGNOSED?

Most people only become aware that they have gallstones by chance when an unrelated condition is being investigated.

■ If your doctor suspects from your symptoms that you have gallstones, you may have blood tests to check your red blood cell count and cholesterol levels.

■ You may also have imaging tests, such as ultrasound scanning.

■ If a bile duct is found to be blocked, the exact position of the gallstones may be located using a specialized imaging procedure called ERCP, in which an endoscope is used to inject a contrast medium into the bile ducts prior to X-rays being taken.

WHAT IS THE TREATMENT?

■ Gallstones that do not cause symptoms need no treatment.

■ If you have mild or infrequent symptoms, adopting a diet that is low in fat may prevent further discomfort.

■ If your symptoms are persistent or become worse, you may have your gallbladder removed by conventional (open) surgery or by endoscopic (keyhole) surgery (see box, left). Removal of the gallbladder usually cures the problem. The absence of a gallbladder does not usually cause any health problems, and the bile simply drains continuously through a duct directly into the intestines.

■ In very rare cases, the stones reform in the **bile duct** and may need to be removed by open surgery or during endoscopic examination.

■ Drugs are available that dissolve gallstones made of pure cholesterol, but it may take months or years for the stones to dissolve completely.

■ Rarely, you may be treated with ultrasonic shock waves (lithotripsy), which shatter the stones into tiny pieces so that they pass painlessly into the small intestine and are excreted in the feces.

Use of drugs or ultrasonic shock waves avoids the need for surgery. However, because the gallbladder is still present there is an ongoing risk that more gallstones will form.

TREATMENT

Endoscopic surgery

Endoscopic surgery is a technique that enables various surgical procedures to be performed without making large incisions in the skin. An endoscope is a tubelike viewing instrument with a light source. Some endoscopes have a built-in miniature camera that relays pictures to a monitor. Endoscopes are inserted either through a natural body opening, such as the anus, or through a small incision, depending on the site to be accessed. Most endoscopic surgery through incisions is performed under general anesthesia; endoscopic surgery through natural openings may require only a local anesthetic.

How it is performed

Endoscopic surgery performed through skin incisions is often called minimally invasive or "keyhole" surgery. Tiny instruments, such as forceps, are passed through small incisions in the skin or through side channels in the endoscope to reach the operating site. These instruments are operated by the surgeon, who is guided by the view through the endoscope or on the monitor.

Since endoscopic surgery may not involve any incisions or only require small ones, the length of stay in hospital and recovery time are shorter than for conventional surgery. However, there is a slightly greater risk of damage to an organ or blood vessel with endoscopic surgery than with conventional surgery because the surgeon has to work in a smaller area. As with all surgery, there is a risk of an adverse reaction to a general anesthetic, which depends on the person's preoperative health, the specific anesthetic used, and the type of operation being done. During the operation, the surgeon may need to access a larger area and perform open surgery. You will be asked for your consent to open surgery before an endoscopic operation.

See also:
• **Acute pancreatitis p. 359** • **Anemias p. 236**
• **ERCP p. 360** • **Jaundice p. 355**

Cholecystitis

THE NAME CHOLECYSTITIS REFERS TO INFLAMMATION OF THE GALLBLADDER WALL, USUALLY ASSOCIATED WITH GALLSTONES BLOCKING THE FLOW OF BILE, A DIGESTIVE FLUID PRODUCED BY THE LIVER.

Cholecystitis usually occurs when the outlet from the gallbladder becomes blocked by a gallstone. Bile becomes trapped in the gallbladder, causing inflammation of its walls. A bacterial infection may then develop in the stagnant bile. In rare cases, cholecystitis occurs when there are no gallstones present.

Anyone who has gallstones is at risk of developing cholecystitis. Risk factors associated with gallstones include **obesity**, **a high-fat diet**, and some **blood disorders** such as sickle-cell anemia.

WHAT ARE THE SYMPTOMS?

The symptoms of cholecystitis can vary in severity. They usually develop over a period of hours and include:

● constant severe pain in the right side of the abdomen, just below the rib cage

● pain in the right shoulder

● nausea and vomiting

● fever and chills.

Sometimes, jaundice causing yellowing of the skin and the whites of the eyes may develop. Symptoms often improve over a few days and disappear after about a week. However, in some cases symptoms become progressively worse and need urgent treatment.

Rarely, bacterial infection may cause the gallbladder to perforate. This allows irritant bile to leak into the abdomen, resulting in **peritonitis**, a serious condition in which there is inflammation of the membrane lining the wall of the abdomen. Cholecystitis may also be accompanied by **acute pancreatitis**, in which there is sudden and painful inflammation of the pancreas.

WHAT MIGHT BE DONE?

Your doctor may suspect cholecystitis from your symptoms and after a physical examination.

If so, ultrasound scanning or ERCP will be done to confirm the diagnosis and to indicate the position of any gallstones.

WHAT IS THE TREATMENT?

■ If your symptoms are mild, you may be treated at home with **antibiotics** and **painkillers**.
■ If your symptoms are severe, you will need treatment in the hospital with intravenous fluids, painkillers, and antibiotics.

■ You may have a tube passed into your stomach in order to remove the contents by suction. This procedure stops acid from entering the duodenum, which would cause the gallbladder to contract.
■ Although cholecystitis often subsides after treatment with antibiotics, surgery to remove the gallbladder is usually recommended to prevent the condition from recurring. Surgery is always necessary if complications such as perforation of the gallbladder arise.

WHAT IS THE OUTLOOK?

Removal of the gallbladder after an attack of cholecystitis prevents recurrences. Absence of the gallbladder has no long-term ill effects on the digestive system.

See also:
- Anemias p. 236 • ERCP p. 360
- Gallstones p. 357
- Ultrasound scanning p. 277

Liver cancer

LIVER CANCER MAY BE PRIMARY, MEANING IT ARISES IN LIVER CELLS, OR SECONDARY, MEANING IT ARISES ELSEWHERE AND THEN SPREADS TO THE LIVER. PRIMARY LIVER CANCER IS RARE IN THE WEST BUT SECONDARY LIVER CANCER IS COMPARATIVELY COMMON.

By far the most common form of liver cancer is secondary cancer (metastases) from elsewhere in the body, commonly cancers of the lung, breast, colon, pancreas, and stomach. Other types of cancer, such as **leukemia** and **lymphoma**, may also spread to the liver. Liver metastases form when cancerous cells separate from the original cancer, circulate in the blood and settle in the liver, where they multiply and enlarge.

WHAT ARE THE SYMPTOMS?

People may already have symptoms due to the original cancer, but sometimes this cancer is not apparent. The symptoms of liver metastases may be the only warning of illness. They include:
- weight loss
- reduced appetite
- fever
- pain in the upper right side of the abdomen
- yellowing of the skin and whites of the eyes (jaundice).

As the disease progresses, the abdomen may become swollen due to enlargement of the liver or fluid accumulation.

WHAT MIGHT BE DONE?

Anyone who has cancer will have tests, such as ultrasound scanning, computerized tomography (CT) scanning, and magnetic resonance imaging (MRI) to find out if the liver is affected. To confirm diagnosis, a piece of liver tissue (biopsy) may be removed for microscopic examination. Treatment aims to maintain liver function and relieve symptoms. You may be offered analgesics for pain and chemotherapy or radiation therapy to reduce the size of metastases. Surgery may be considered if there are localized metastasis.

WHAT IS THE OUTLOOK?

Primary liver cancer is rare in the West, where most cases occur following long-standing cirrhosis due to **long-term alcohol abuse** and from **hepatitis C**. Another cause of liver cancer is contamination of food by carcinogens (cancer causing

agents) such as aflatoxin, a toxin produced by a fungus that grows on stored grain and peanuts. In developing countries, liver cancer is closely linked with viral hepatitis, especially that due to the hepatitis B and C viruses, which account for approximately 7 in 10 cases.

Surgery offers the only chance of a cure. A liver transplant may be considered but is rarely done because in many cases the cancer is likely to recur. More commonly, the aim is to slow the progress of the disease with treatments that include **chemotherapy** and blocking the blood supply to the tumor, causing it to shrink.

The outlook for people with liver cancer is poor. Many people do not respond to treatment and survive less than a year after diagnosis.

See also:
- Chemotherapy p. 257 • CT scanning p. 401
- Hepatitis p. 341
- Jaundice p. 355 • MRI p. 409
- Radiation therapy p. 395 • Tissue tests p. 259

Acute pancreatitis

IN ACUTE PANCREATITIS, THE PANCREAS SUDDENLY BECOMES INFLAMED DUE TO DAMAGE FROM ITS OWN ENZYMES, CAUSING VERY SEVERE UPPER ABDOMINAL PAIN AND OTHER SYMPTOMS.

The condition is serious and can be life threatening if left untreated. Acute pancreatitis almost exclusively affects adults and excessive alcohol consumption is a risk factor.

WHAT ARE THE CAUSES?

Acute pancreatitis may be caused by:
- gallstones
- viruses (mumps, hepatitis)

- injury
- gallbladder surgery
- certain drugs (diuretics, sulphonamides)
- long-term alcohol abuse
- hyperlipidemia.

WHAT ARE THE SYMPTOMS?

Acute pancreatitis causes a range of symptoms that occur suddenly and may be severe, including:

- sudden and very severe upper abdominal pain, often spreading to the back and made worse by movement and relieved by sitting up
- nausea and vomiting
- bruised appearance of the skin around the abdomen or side
- fever.

In severe cases, inflammation affects the whole abdomen, making it rigid and increasing pain. Acute pancreatitis may also lead to shock, a potentially fatal condition in which the blood pressure falls dangerously low.

Blood tests, a computerized tomography (CT) scan, or endoscopy of the pancreas (ERCP; see box, right) may be used to confirm a diagnosis of acute pancreatitis.

WHAT IS THE TREATMENT?

■ Your stomach will be kept empty to prevent the pancreas from being stimulated to produce more enzymes. A tube will be passed through your nose into your stomach to remove its contents by suction.

■ You will be given fluids intravenously. If tests have detected a gallstone, ERCP may locate the stone more precisely and remove it.

■ Rarely, if damaged pancreatic tissue becomes infected, surgical drainage may be needed.

■ If the pancreatitis was caused by gallstones, it may be advisable to have your gallbladder removed once you have recovered.

WHAT IS THE OUTLOOK?

About 9 in 10 people survive an attack of acute pancreatitis, but the gland may be damaged so that it is unable to produce adequate amounts of enzymes and you develop **malabsorption syndrome**. You may then need to take enzyme supplements for the rest of your life.

> **See also:**
> • **CT scanning p. 401** • **Gallstones p. 357**
> • **Inherited hyperlipidemia p. 223**
> • **Shock p. 560**

TEST

ERCP

Endoscopic retrograde cholangio-pancreatography (ERCP) is used to look for problems in the bile ducts and pancreatic duct. A contrast dye is injected into the ducts via an endoscope passed through the mouth and the path of the dye is then tracked on X-ray images. Doctors can also look directly down the endoscope. The procedure is done in a hospital under sedation and takes about an hour.

Pancreatic cancer

PANCREATIC CANCER IS A MALIGNANT TUMOR OF THE MAIN TISSUE OF THE PANCREAS. SMOKING, DIABETES, AND ALCOHOL ABUSE ARE RISK FACTORS.

Pancreatic cancer is more common over age 50 and almost twice as common in men. Cancer of the pancreas is a relatively uncommon cancer, with about 27,000 new cases diagnosed in the US each year. The tumor may be symptomless in its early stages.

WHAT ARE THE SYMPTOMS?

Symptoms often develop gradually over a few months and may include:

● pain in the upper abdomen that radiates to the back

● loss of weight

● reduced appetite.

Many pancreatic tumors cause obstruction of the bile ducts through which the digestive liquid bile leaves the liver. Such blockage leads to **jaundice**, in which the skin and whites of the eyes turn yellow. Jaundice may be accompanied by itching, dark-colored urine and lighter than normal feces.

WHAT IS THE TREATMENT?

Surgery to remove part, or all, of the pancreas offers the only chance of cure. However, the cancer has usually spread by the time it is diagnosed. In such cases, surgery to relieve symptoms may be possible. For example, if the bile duct is obstructed by a tumor, a rigid tube known as a stent may be inserted to keep the duct open. This procedure is usually done during endoscopic examination of the pancreas (ERCP; see box, above) and helps to reduce jaundice. Treatment such as chemotherapy and radiation therapy may be used to slow the progress of the disease.

Pain can often be relieved with analgesics. Severe pain may be treated by a nerve block, a procedure using an injection of a chemical to inactivate the nerves supplying the pancreas.

WHAT IS THE OUTLOOK?

In many cases, pancreatic cancer is not diagnosed until it is far advanced, at which time the outlook is poor. Fewer than 1 in 50 people survives more than five years. Even with surgery, only 1 in 10 people survives more than five years. Most people survive for less than a year.

> **See also:**
> • **Chemotherapy p.257** • **Jaundice p.355**
> • **Radiotherapy p.395**

DISORDERS OF THE INTESTINES, RECTUM, AND ANUS

Irritable bowel syndrome (IBS) is probably the most common bowel condition in the West along with its symptoms of **flatulence** and **bloating**. **Constipation** and **diarrhea** are almost as common, and then **diverticulosis** and **diverticulitis**, which arise as we get older. Malabsorption, such as occurs with **lactose intolerance** and **celiac disease**, can leave the body short of important nutrients. When the bowel becomes inflamed, **Crohn's disease** and **ulcerative colitis** may result. Finally, **colorectal cancer**, a common cause of death in the West, and disorders of the rectum and anus, such as **hemorrhoids** and **anal fissure**, are covered.

Flatulence and bloating

MOST OF US OCCASIONALLY EXPERIENCE THE EMBARRASSMENT OF PASSING GAS (FLATULENCE), BUT FOR SOME IT CAN BE A RECURRING AND DISTRESSING PROBLEM. SWELLING OF THE ABDOMEN DUE TO A BUILDUP OF GAS (BLOATING) MAY ACCOMPANY MENOPAUSE.

FLATULENCE

This is a feature of many gastrointestinal conditions, in particular **indigestion** and **irritable bowel syndrome (IBS)**, which is said to affect at least a fifth of the population. However, there are other symptoms with IBS, including pain, constipation, or diarrhea or a mixture of both, and since these symptoms also occur in more serious bowel conditions it is important to have them checked out by a doctor. There is not usually more actual gas in sufferers of IBS, but a feeling of gas. Self-diagnosis is not a good idea. Flatulence can also be a problem in pregnancy.

WHAT CAN BE DONE TO BRING RELIEF?

Thankfully there is quite a lot we can do to help ourselves. The most common cause of wind is what we eat. So you should look very carefully at your diet. Keep fried food to a minimum since this is not only unhealthy in itself, it is also a frequent cause of gas. Baked beans and peas are notorious for causing gas but there are other foods and drinks that should also be taken in moderation.

■ Eat more fish and skinless white meat instead of red meat.

■ Allow enough time to sit down and have a meal rather than snacking on the go, since gulping food and drink is often responsible for a bad bout of gas.

■ For those who are lactose intolerant, milk can cause excessive gas and replacing dairy foods with calcium fortified soy drinks often helps.

■ As we age, small pockets of tissue may balloon out from the bowel, giving rise to the conditions known as diverticulosis and diverticulitis. Within these small pockets

bacteria may accumulate, ferment carbohydrates, and produce gas.

■ Try to eat foods that can affect fermentation, such as those containing yeast and sugar, only in the early part of the day. A yeast-free alternative to regular bread would be crackers, rice cakes or soda bread.

■ Charcoal pills available from pharmacies can provide immediate relief by absorbing gas.

■ Natural herbs and spices contain substances that calm the bowels and prevent a buildup of gas. These include aniseed, camomile, lemon balm, fennel, dill, cloves, black pepper, marjoram, parsley, peppermint, rosemary, and spearmint. Use them as a garnish on food or as a soothing, herbal tea.

■ Gulping mouthfuls of air can cause or aggravate gas. If you are inclined to do this, try and break yourself of the habit and you may find the flatulence gradually becomes less frequent. Gum chewing, for example, causes us to take in air.

■ Stress is another important factor in flatulence and if you are feeling stressed you need to identify the reason so you can find effective ways of reducing anxiety. However, as a short-term solution studies have shown essential oil of lavender can reduce stress. Use five or six drops of oil in your bath or on a tissue.

■ Exercise can help reduce gas since it tones up our stomach muscles and prevents our intestine from being able to swell up so much that it holds large pockets of gas. Exercise is also very good for relieving stress and even a walk round the block is beneficial, although it isn't sensible to exercise within two hours of eating a meal.

■ For some, an upset in bowel bacteria is a problem. Reducing sugar and yeast, for example in bread, wine, and beer, may help,

along with a supply of beneficial lactobacillus bacteria from a daily container of "live" yogurt.

BLOATING

Bloating with abdominal swelling may be a problem during menopausal years. It is usually due to **gas** in the large intestine, produced by fermentation in the bowel. As we age, small pockets of tissue may balloon out from the bowel, giving rise to the condition called **diverticulosis**. Within these small pockets bacteria may accumulate, ferment carbohydrates and produce large amounts of gas. The intestine may end up coated with food remnants that form small centers of fermentation.

It is quite common to wake in the morning with a flat stomach and for the abdomen to swell as the day progresses so that by bedtime the swelling is noticeable. During the night lack of food and sugar in the intestine allows fermentation to abate. After a breakfast that contains sugars and yeasts, fermentation in the bowel flares up again.

WHAT CAN YOU DO TO EASE THE PROBLEM?

■ Try to eat foods with yeast and sugar in the early part of the day only to see if that helps.

■ Slowly increasing fiber in your diet, drinking, plenty of fluids, and frequent exercise will keep the bowels normal.

■ Try to eat a container of "live" yogurt each day.

■ Reduce carbohydrates in the diet.

See also:
- **Diverticulosis and diverticulitis p. 364**
- **Indigestion p. 352**
- **Irritable bowel syndrome p. 362**
- **Menopause p. 497**

FOCUS
on irritable bowel syndrome

Irritable bowel syndrome, or IBS, is the most common disorder of the intestine. It affects from 10 to 20 percent of the population and is the most common disease diagnosed by gastroenterology specialists. IBS is twice as common in women as in men, usually beginning in early or middle adulthood.

Although symptoms subside and even disappear for a time the condition usually recurs **throughout** life. But on the positive side, it's not life threatening and is unlikely to lead to complications that can cause much distress.

WHAT CAUSES IBS?
● The cause isn't fully understood, but we think there is a basic abnormality in the way muscles contract in the large intestine. For some reason, the bowel becomes sensitized. That means the intestine, including the rectum, is more easily aroused into contracting by food, anxiety, illness, or any other stress. Intestinal activity may verge on excessive, so the intestine may even go into spasm, causing colicky pain.

● In addition, the sensitized intestines signal too frequently to the brain that something is wrong. So the conscious mind becomes aware of uncomfortable and embarrassing symptoms such as pain, bloating, the urge to pass gas or the urge to pass stools more often than usual. It's easy to focus too hard on a twinge and make it into a pain.

● The symptoms of IBS can nonetheless be dramatic and worrying, so much so that many people consulting their doctor about IBS are afraid there's something seriously wrong. They imagine they have cancer, ulcerative colitis, even AIDS. But they shouldn't worry – the symptoms of IBS have a lot of features that point to a functionality problem rather than one due to serious disease.

● For some people, emotional stress and anxiety are the main causative factors, and IBS may be linked to a person's inability to express negative emotions such as anger.

● Excessive gas is quite a common problem for sufferers and again, it's thought that diet plays a part. Much more important, though, is a condition called **diverticulosis**, so common as to be viewed as part of normal aging. In diverticulosis, small pockets may balloon out from the bowel wall and within these pockets bacteria may accumulate, ferment carbohydrates and produce gas. The intestine

Living with IBS

Some people learn to control the symptoms of irritable bowel syndrome by making dietary and lifestyle changes. The symptoms may improve if you follow a diet that is high in fiber and low in fat. You may need to try several different approaches before finding one that helps you. Try the following:
● Keep a food diary; try to eliminate any food or beverage that seems to bring on an attack of irritable bowel syndrome.
● Avoid large meals, spicy, fried, or fatty foods and milk products.
● If constipation is a problem, try gradually increasing your fiber intake.
● Cut out or reduce your intake of tea, coffee, milk, cola, and beer.
● Eat at regular times.
● Stop smoking.
● Try relaxation exercises to alleviate stress, which is often a contributing factor.
● Eliminate dairy foods for 5-7 days and monitor symptoms.
● It often helps to eat more fiber-rich

foods, such as fresh fruit, vegetables, prunes, figs, and whole grain cereals, unless they cause bloating.
● Some people need to change their diet. If particular foods or drinks trigger attacks or worsen symptoms, they should be avoided or limited until the attack is over.
● **Exercise** can help reduce episodes of gas because it tones the stomach muscles and prevents the intestine from swelling up so much that it holds large pockets of gas. Any kind of physical activity is a natural tranquilizer, so incorporating some form of exercise into your routine should help tension and anxiety too.
● **Cut down on sugar**, dairy products, and **alcohol**, especially wine. Grapes should also be avoided. If you must eat foods that cause fermentation, such as those containing yeast and sugar, only do so in the early part of the day.
● A sensible alternative to eating bread would be to switch to rice cakes or crackers.

● Eat more fish and skinless white meat instead of red meat.
● Some people need to lay off coffee because it stimulates the central nervous system, including the part that controls movement of the intestines.
● If emotional stress and anxiety are major triggers for you, try to limit emotional upheaval as much as you can. A daily routine of **mental and physical relaxation exercises** can greatly reduce the effects of both stress and anxiety on the bowel, as well as other organs such as the heart.
● Your doctor may give an antidepression medication in a dose lower than what is used to treat depression.
● Research has shown that five or six drops of **essential oil of lavender** in your bath, or on a tissue, may relieve stress, as can sleeping on a lavender pillow.
● Over-the-counter bulk forming agents are often found useful.

may end up containing many small pockets of fermentation. If the pockets are inflamed, the condition is called **diverticulitis**.

WHAT ARE THE SYMPTOMS?

The symptoms of IBS are:
- abdominal pain
- excessive flatulence
- bloating
- pain with bowel movement
- sense of incomplete evacuation of bowels
- constipation
- diarrhea
- commonly, a mixture of constipation and diarrhea.

HOW IS IT DIAGNOSED?

Your doctor may be able to come to a diagnosis from talking to you and examining you. Doctors also routinely examine the feces, do a barium X-ray and possibly a **sigmoidoscopy** (examination of the colon through a viewing instrument passed via the anus) simply to exclude anything serious, not because they suspect cancer.

WHAT IS THE TREATMENT?

- A high-fiber diet or bulk forming agent, such as **psyllium husk**, **bran**, or **isphagula**, **sterculia**, and **methylcellulose** help everyone.
- Peppermint is worth a try.
- Short courses of **antidiarrheal** drugs (such as **loperamide**) may be given for persistent diarrhea.
- Antispasmodic drugs such as **mebeverine** may be prescribed to relieve muscular spasm and abdominal pain.
- Hypnosis, psychotherapy, and counseling have proved effective for some people. However, most sufferers find treatments relieve the symptoms but don't cure IBS.

Constipation

IF YOUR STOOLS ARE SMALL AND HARD OR IF YOU HAVE TO STRAIN TO PASS THEM, YOU PROBABLY ARE CONSTIPATED.

Most people tend to have a regular routine, and bowels usually function best if allowed to follow a consistent pattern. Constipation is defined medically as the difficult and infrequent passage of small, hard stools. How **frequently you pass stools isn't very important** because healthy people have bowel movements at widely differing intervals. Usually intervals range from **three times a day** to **three times a week**. Harmless bouts of constipation are common, but occasionally there is an underlying disorder that needs to be investigated. You should consult your doctor if you have **recently** developed constipation that is severe or lasts more than two weeks, particularly if it first occurs after the **age of 50**. Persistent constipation may lead to fecal impaction, in which hard feces remain in the rectum. Liquid feces may leak around the partial obstruction, resulting in diarrhea. So if constipation and diarrhea alternate, see your doctor.

WHAT ARE THE CAUSES?

■ A diet that is low in fiber and fluids is the most common cause of constipation.
■ The second most common cause is ignoring the urge to defecate, resulting in drying out of the stools in the rectum, where they can become impacted and difficult to remove.
■ Drinking too many alcoholic drinks or drinks containing caffeine, which may lead to mild dehydration, can also make feces hard and difficult to pass.
■ Other factors that decrease the frequency of bowel movements are doing too little exercise and long periods of immobility.
■ Hypothyroidism and depression may also lead to constipation.

■ Diverticulosis is associated with constipation.
■ People recovering from abdominal surgery and people with anal disorders, such as hemorrhoids, may find it painful to defecate and develop constipation as a result.
■ Certain drugs, including some antidepressants, and antacids containing aluminium and calcium carbonate may cause constipation.
■ Increasing immobility in elderly people makes constipation much more common in this age group.

WHAT MIGHT BE DONE?

■ No bowel can resist five fresh fruits eaten every morning or half a dozen prunes and figs eaten each evening and I distrust anyone who doesn't have regular bowel movements if they follow these suggestions.

A good intake of fluids, such as fruit juice or water, and fiber can help prevent constipation.

SELF-HELP

Preventing constipation

There are some simple steps you can take to prevent or reduce the severity of constipation.
■ Increase your daily fiber intake. Fiber-rich foods include bran, whole grain bread, cereals, fruit, leafy vegetables, potato skins, beans, and dried peas.
■ Reduce your intake of highly refined and processed foods, such as cheese and white bread.
■ Increase your daily fluid intake to at least 6–8 glasses a day, but avoid or at least limit drinks containing caffeine or alcohol.
■ Do not use stimulant laxatives persistently because the bowel will become lazy and won't function without them.
■ Do not ignore the urge to defecate The longer the feces remain in the bowel, the drier and harder they become.
■ Try to have a regular routine in which you go to the bathroom at the same time of day.
■ Build some daily, regular exercise into your routine.

- If constipation is associated with your **lifestyle**, there are several simple measures you can take to relieve it and prevent recurrence.
- If constipation persists despite self-help measures, you should consult your doctor, who will perform tests to look for an underlying cause. Your rectum will be checked by inserting a gloved finger.
- You may be asked for a fecal sample, which will be examined for the presence of blood.

If more tests are necessary, you may have a barium enema to exclude abnormalities.

WHAT IS THE TREATMENT?
- You may have an enema, in which liquid is passed through a tube into the rectum to stimulate bowel movements.
- This treatment should be followed by a change in diet to include more fiber and fluids.
- Constipation linked to a painful anal

disorder may be relieved with a soothing ointment or suppositories.
- If a drug is to blame your doctor may be able to give you an alternative.

See also:
- **Anal fissure p. 370**
- **Diverticulosis and diverticulitis p. 364**
- **Hemorrhoids p. 370**
- **Preventing constipation p. 363**

Diarrhea

DIARRHEA IS THE PRODUCTION OF STOOLS THAT ARE MORE WATERY, MORE FREQUENT, OR GREATER IN VOLUME THAN IS NORMAL FOR YOU. ALTHOUGH NOT A DISEASE ITSELF, DIARRHEA MAY BE A SYMPTOM OF AN UNDERLYING DISORDER.

In some cases, diarrhea is accompanied by abdominal pain, bloating, loss of appetite, and vomiting. Severe diarrhea can lead to dehydration that may be life threatening, particularly in babies and elderly people.

Short episodes of diarrhea, especially if they are associated with vomiting, are often due to **gastroenteritis** or **food poisoning**. Diarrhea that lasts more than 3–4 weeks usually indicates that there is an intestinal disorder and requires medical attention.

WHAT ARE THE CAUSES?
- Diarrhea that starts abruptly in a person who is otherwise healthy is often caused by a change in diet or contaminated food or water and may last a few hours to 10 days. This type of diarrhea often occurs during travel in a foreign country.
- Diarrhea may also be caused by a viral infection that is spread by close personal contact. Such infectious gastroenteritis is the most common cause of diarrhea in babies and young children.
- People taking drugs such as **antibiotics** may develop sudden diarrhea if the drugs disturb the normal balance of bacteria in the colon.
- Persistent diarrhea may be a result of

chronic inflammation of the intestine due to disorders such as **Crohn's disease** or **ulcerative colitis**.
- Diarrhea is a symptom of some conditions, such as **celiac disease**, in which the small intestine cannot absorb nutrients.
- **Lactose intolerance**, a disorder in which lactose (a natural sugar present in milk) cannot be broken down and absorbed, can also cause diarrhea.
- Infection with **parasites,** such as **giardiasis** and **amebiasis**, may lead to chronic diarrhea.
- **Irritable bowel syndrome** may produce abnormal contractions of the intestine, which result in alternating episodes of diarrhea and constipation.

WHAT MIGHT BE DONE?
- In most cases, diarrhea clears up within a day or two.
- Other symptoms that can accompany diarrhea, such as headache, weakness, and lethargy, are most often caused by dehydration. The symptoms of dehydration disappear as soon as the fluids and salts that have been lost are replaced.
- If your diarrhea lasts longer than 3–4 days, you should consult your doctor, who may

request a sample of feces to look for evidence of either infection or unabsorbed nutrients.
- If your diarrhea persists for more than 3–4 weeks or if there is blood in the feces, your doctor will probably arrange for you to have certain investigative procedures, such as contrast X-rays of the intestines or sigmoidoscopy or colonoscopy (endoscopy of the rectum or colon).
- Specific treatments given for diarrhea depend on the underlying cause.
- If you need to curtail your diarrhea quickly, your doctor may prescribe an antidiarrheal drug, such as **loperamide**. However, antidiarrheal drugs should usually be avoided if your diarrhea is due to an infection because they may prolong the infection.
- Antibiotics are only needed to treat persistent diarrhea that has a known bacterial cause.

See also:
- **Crohn's disease p. 366**
- **Irritable bowel syndrome p. 362**
- **Lactose intolerance p. 366**
- **Malabsorption p. 365**
- **Ulcerative colitis p. 367**

Diverticulosis and diverticulitis

THE PRESENCE OF SMALL POUCHES KNOWN AS DIVERTICULA IN THE WALL OF THE COLON IS KNOWN AS DIVERTICULOSIS. INFLAMMATION OF THESE POUCHES IS CALLED DIVERTICULITIS. A LOW-FIBER DIET AND THE CHRONIC USE OF LAXATIVES ARE RISK FACTORS.

In diverticulosis, pea- or grape-sized pouches protrude from the wall of the large intestine, usually from the part of the colon closest to the rectum. The pouches form when parts of the wall of the intestine bulge outward

through weakened areas, often close to an artery. In many cases, the bulging of the intestinal wall is associated with **chronic constipation** and occurs when the pressure inside the intestine increases as the person

strains to defecate or if there is insufficient residue such as fiber. Sometimes, one or more pouches become inflamed, a condition known as **diverticulitis**.

Diverticulosis is rare before age 50 but about

1 in 3 people between the ages of 50 and 70 has diverticulosis, and it becomes progressively more common after age 70. However, most affected people have no symptoms.

Diverticulitis is strongly associated with a low-fiber Western diet, which may cause constipation.

WHAT ARE THE SYMPTOMS?
More than three-quarters of all people with diverticulosis do not know that they have the condition because there are no symptoms. If symptoms are present, they may include the following.
■ Occasional bright red bleeding from the rectum, which may be painless.

In some cases, diverticulosis is difficult to distinguish from **irritable bowel syndrome** (IBS) because both have similar symptoms. such as episodes of abdominal pain, especially in the lower left abdomen, that are relieved by a bowel movement or a release of intestinal gas

and intermittent episodes of constipation and diarrhea.

If diverticulitis develops, the symptoms may become worse, with:
● severe lower abdominal pain and tenderness in the abdomen
● fever
● nausea and vomiting.

If you notice any change in your bowel habits or you have rectal bleeding, you should consult your doctor immediately because these symptoms may indicate a more serious underlying disease, such as **colorectal cancer**.

ARE THERE COMPLICATIONS?
If an inflamed diverticulum bursts, feces and bacteria can spill into the abdominal cavity. As a result an **abscess** may form next to the colon or **peritonitis**, an inflammation of the membrane that lines the abdominal cavity, may develop. Fortunately, both are uncommon.

HOW IS IT DIAGNOSED?
■ If your doctor suspects that you have diverticulosis, a barium enema to highlight the shape of the intestines will be arranged.
■ If your symptoms include rectal bleeding, a colonoscopy may be done to examine the colon and exclude colorectal cancer.

WHAT IS THE TREATMENT?
■ Often, a high-fiber diet with plenty of fluids is the only treatment given for diverticulosis.
■ You may also be given **antispasmodic drugs** to relax the intestine and relieve abdominal pain.
■ If you develop severe diverticulitis, you will be given antibiotics to treat bacterial infection.

See also:
● **Colorectal cancer p. 368**
● **Irritable bowel syndrome p. 362**

Malabsorption

IMPAIRED ABSORPTION OF NUTRIENTS FROM THE SMALL INTESTINE IS
CALLED MALABSORPTION. IT OCCURS WHEN THE SMALL INTESTINE CANNOT
ABSORB NUTRIENTS FROM FOOD PASSING THROUGH IT.

Common symptoms are bulky, pale, foul-smelling, floating feces and weight loss. Malabsorption sometimes runs in families. If left untreated, certain nutritional deficiencies can develop, which may lead to further problems, such as **anemia** or **nerve damage**.

WHAT ARE THE CAUSES?
Malabsorption is due to:
● inadequate breakdown of food during digestion due to lack of essential enzymes
● damage to the lining of the small intestine so that nutrients can't be absorbed.

Various medical conditions can give rise to these factors.
■ In some cases, the small intestine cannot break down food because digestive enzymes or juices are missing or in short supply. For example, **disorders affecting the pancreas**, such as **chronic pancreatitis** and **cystic fibrosis**, may result in the faulty digestion of fatty foods and proteins so that the body is unable to use them. Sometimes, there is a problem in breaking down a specific nutrient. For example, people with **lactose intolerance** lack an enzyme in the intestine needed to break down the sugar, lactose, in milk.
■ Damage to the intestinal lining due to inflammation in **celiac disease**, **Crohn's disease**, and infections such as **giardiasis** will prevent nutrients from crossing the intestinal lining and entering the bloodstream.
■ In the **autoimmune** disorder **scleroderma**,

changes in the structure of the intestinal walls occasionally lead to malabsorption of nutrients.
■ **Diabetes mellitus** may cause malabsorption by damaging the nerves that supply the walls of the intestine and allowing bacteria to accumulate.

WHAT ARE THE SYMPTOMS?
The most common symptoms of malabsorption include:
● bulky, pale, foul-smelling feces that float
● flatulence and abdominal bloating
● weight loss
● abdominal pain with cramps
● fatigue and weakness.

Left untreated, malabsorption can lead to **deficiencies in folic acid, vitamin B_{12} and iron**, which may result in **anemia**, the symptoms of which include pale skin and shortness of breath. A deficiency of **vitamin B_{12}** can also affect the spinal cord and peripheral nerves, causing **numbness and tingling** in the hands and feet.

HOW IS IT DIAGNOSED?
■ Your doctor may order a variety of blood tests to look for anemia, vitamin deficiencies, and other signs of malabsorption.
■ If your doctor suspects that your pancreas is damaged, pancreatic function tests or radiologic studies will be arranged.
■ A test may also be performed to confirm the enzyme deficiency that causes lactose intolerance or carbohydrate malabsorption.

■ You may have a blood test to look for the **antibodies** that are present in celiac disease.
■ A contrast X–ray to highlight the inside of the small intestine may be done to look for damage to the digestive tract caused by Crohn's disease or bacterial overgrowth.
■ You may also require an **endoscopy** to obtain a sample of intestinal tissue for microscopic analysis.

WHAT IS THE TREATMENT?
■ Any underlying cause is treated, if possible.
■ Coeliac disease can be treated with a diet excluding **gluten containing foods**.
■ Crohn's disease usually responds to **corticosteroids, sulphasalazine,** or other treatment.
■ If the cause of malabsorption is giardiasis, antiprotozoal drugs will be prescribed.
■ Specific nutritional deficiencies can be corrected by taking vitamin and mineral supplements.

Malabsorption can usually be treated, and most people recover and live normal lives.

See also:
● **Acute pancreatitis p. 359** ● **Anemias p. 236**
● **Contrast X-rays p. 353**
● **Crohn's disease p. 366**
● **Cystic fibrosis p. 521**
● **Diabetes mellitus p. 504**
● **Malabsorption p. 365**

Lactose intolerance

A PERSON WHO IS LACTOSE INTOLERANT IS UNABLE TO DIGEST LACTOSE, A NATURAL SUGAR FOUND IN MILK AND DAIRY PRODUCTS. EVEN SMALL AMOUNTS OF LACTOSE CAN CAUSE ABDOMINAL PAIN AND DIARRHEA. THE PROBLEM IS DUE TO AN ENZYME DEFICIENCY.

Intolerance to lactose usually develops at any time from adolescence onward. The permanent form rarely affects babies. An inability to digest lactose in the diet is particularly common among Afro-Caribbean, Asian, and Jewish people.

WHAT ARE THE CAUSES?

Normally, the enzyme **lactase** breaks down lactose in the intestines to form the sugars **glucose** and **galactose**, which are easily absorbed through the intestinal wall. If the enzyme is absent, the unabsorbed lactose ferments in the large intestine and produces painful symptoms. Although high levels of lactase are present at birth, in many racial groups the level can drop with increasing age and become very low by adolescence, so that milk can no longer be digested.

In children and babies, lactose intolerance sometimes occurs temporarily following an attack of **gastroenteritis** that causes short-term damage to the lining of the intestine.

WHAT ARE THE SYMPTOMS?

The symptoms of lactose intolerance usually develop a few hours after eating or drinking products containing milk. They may include the following:

- abdominal bloating and cramping
- diarrhea
- vomiting.

The severity of the symptoms depends on the degree of lactase deficiency. One person may experience symptoms only after drinking several glasses of milk, but another may feel discomfort after consuming only a small amount of a dairy product. The symptoms are often initially mild but can become more severe with each subsequent episode.

WHAT MIGHT BE DONE?

■ Your doctor may be able to diagnose lactose intolerance from your medical history and symptoms.
■ You'll be asked to keep a diary of all the foods you eat and the symptoms that occur.
■ You may then have a specialized test to confirm lactose intolerance.
■ Alternatively, your doctor may ask you to eliminate all dairy products from your diet for a few days. If your symptoms improve but return when milk is reintroduced into your diet, the

diagnosis of lactose intolerance is confirmed.
■ Don't exclude dairy products from your diet without consulting your doctor first.

WHAT IS THE OUTLOOK?

Lactose intolerance is usually permanent in adults. However, the symptoms can be completely relieved by eliminating lactose from the diet. Hard cheese, butter, and "live" yogurt contain very little lactose and are tolerated by most people. Milk products that have been specially treated by having lactose broken down are available over the counter. In addition, your doctor may suggest lactase supplements in the form of liquid or capsules.

In **babies** whose lactose intolerance is caused by gastroenteritis, milk may be gradually re-introduced into the diet in a few weeks as the intestine recovers. If you exclude most milk products, you may want to take calcium supplements.

See also:
- **Diarrhea p. 364**

Crohn's disease

CROHN'S DISEASE IS A RARE LONG-TERM INFLAMMATORY DISEASE THAT CAN AFFECT ANY PART OF THE DIGESTIVE TRACT, ESPECIALLY THE ILEUM (PART OF THE SMALL INTESTINE) AND COLON. DIARRHEA, PAIN, FEVER, AND LOSS OF WEIGHT ARE COMMON SYMPTOMS.

The onset of Crohn's disease is most common between the ages of 15 and 30, but may start at any age and it sometimes runs in families, indicating that there is a genetic component. Smoking is a risk factor for increased severity.

WHAT ARE THE SYMPTOMS?

The symptoms of Crohn's disease vary among individuals. The disorder usually recurs at intervals throughout life, typically waxing and waning. Episodes of the disease

may be severe, lasting weeks or several months, before settling down to periods where there are mild symptoms or no symptoms at all. The symptoms include:

- diarrhea
- abdominal pain
- fever
- weight loss
- a general feeling of malaise.

If the colon is affected, symptoms also include the following:

- diarrhea, often containing blood
- bloody discharge from the anus.

About 1 in 10 people also develops other disorders that are associated with Crohn's disease, including a form of arthritis known as **ankylosing spondylitis**, **kidney stones**, **gallstones,** and a classic **rash** known as **erythema nodosum**.

Complications

Crohn's disease sometimes leads to complications.
■ Crohn's disease may include an **anal abscess**, which may develop into an **anal fistula** opening onto the skin.
■ **Intestinal obstruction** caused by thickening of the intestinal walls is a fairly common complication of Crohn's disease.

■ Damage to the small intestine may prevent the absorption of nutrients and thus lead to **malabsorption** with anemia and vitamin deficiencies.
■ Inflammation of the colon over a long period of time may also be associated with an increased risk of developing **colorectal cancer**.

WHAT IS THE TREATMENT?

■ Mild attacks of Crohn's disease may be treated with antidiarrheal drugs and painkillers.

■ For an acute attack, your doctor may prescribe oral corticosteroids. As soon as symptoms subside, the dosage will be reduced to avoid the risk of side effects.

■ If your symptoms are very severe, you may need hospital treatment with intravenous corticosteroids. To avoid the risk of side effects, the dosage will be reduced as soon as symptoms subside.

■ In all cases, once the dosage of corticosteroids has been reduced, your doctor may recommend oral **sulphasalazine** or **mesalamine** to prevent recurrent attacks.

■ An immunosuppressant drug, such as **azathioprine**, is an option.

■ You may need **dietary supplements**, such as vitamins, to counteract malabsorption.

■ During severe attacks, nutrients may have to be given intravenously.

WHAT IS THE OUTLOOK?

Crohn's disease is a recurring disorder. Most affected people learn to live reasonably normal lives, but 7 in 10 people eventually need surgery. Complications and repeated surgery can occasionally reduce life expectancy. Crohn's disease may slightly increase the risk of colorectal cancer, and your doctor may advise regular checkups that include colonoscopy.

See also:
• **Anemias p. 236**
• **Ankylosing spondylitis p. 430**
• **Colorectal cancer p. 368**
• **Gallstones p. 357**
• **Kidney stones p. 377**

Ulcerative colitis

ULCERATIVE COLITIS IS CHARACTERIZED BY CHRONIC INTERMITTENT INFLAMMATION AND ULCERATION OF THE RECTUM AND COLON.

This condition affects 1 in 1000 people, sometimes runs in families and is more common in nonsmokers and ex-smokers. The onset of ulcerative colitis most commonly occurs between the ages of 15 and 35.

WHAT IS THE CAUSE?

The exact cause of ulcerative colitis is unknown. However, there is some evidence that genetic factors are involved, since about 1 in 10 people with ulcerative colitis has a close relative with the disease.

WHAT ARE THE SYMPTOMS?

The symptoms of ulcerative colitis are often episodic, with months or years in which there are few or no symptoms. In a mild episode, symptoms develop gradually, often over a few days, and include the following:

• diarrhea, sometimes with blood and mucus in the stool
• abdominal pain
• fatigue
• loss of appetite
• weight loss.

In a severe attack, the symptoms may begin suddenly, developing over just a few hours. Symptoms in a severe attack include:

• severe bouts of diarrhea, at least six times a day
• passage of blood and mucus with or without feces
• pain and swelling in the abdomen
• fever
• weight loss.

People with ulcerative colitis often have other disorders including **arthritis**, causing **pain in the joints**, and **ankylosing spondylitis**, causing **pain in the spine**, **inflammation in the eye** (uveitis), and the **skin condition erythema nodosum**.

WHAT IS THE TREATMENT?

Ulcerative colitis is usually treated with drugs, but surgery may be necessary if you are experiencing frequent severe attacks or if complications develop.

DRUGS

■ Your doctor may prescribe the anti-inflammatory drug **sulphasalazine** to prevent attacks of ulcerative colitis or treat mild episodes.

■ Alternatively, you may be given **mesalamine**, which has fewer side effects.

■ If the inflammation is confined to the rectum or the lower part of the colon, your doctor may prescribe aminosalicylate drugs for you to self-administer in the form of an **enema** or **suppositories**.

TREATMENT

Colostomy and ileostomy

A colostomy is performed following a colectomy (removal of part of the colon, also called the large intestine). In a colostomy, part of the colon opens onto the skin of the abdominal wall to form an artificial opening called a stoma. Feces are expelled through the stoma into a disposable bag. A temporary colostomy may be done if part of the colon has been removed, allowing the rejoined ends to heal without feces passing through the site. A permanent colostomy is needed when the rectum and anus have been removed with part of the colon. In an ileostomy, the ileum is attached to the anus allowing feces to be expelled in the usual way.

In a colostomy, the rectum and anus are bypassed by bringing part of the colon (large intestine) through the abdominal wall, creating an artificial opening (stoma) on the surface of the skin. An ileostomy is created in a similar way using the small intestine.

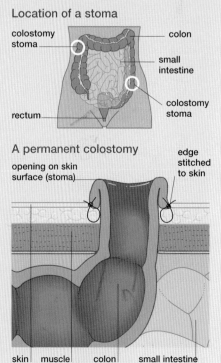

Location of a stoma

colostomy stoma — colon
— small intestine
rectum — colostomy stoma

A permanent colostomy

opening on skin surface (stoma) — edge stitched to skin

skin | muscle | colon | small intestine

■ If the ulcerative colitis has spread farther up the colon, you will be given the drugs orally.
■ If you have severe, sudden attacks of the disorder, your doctor will probably prescribe corticosteroids to be taken orally or as an enema. Long-term use of corticosteroids may cause side effects, such as weight gain and a moon-shaped face. So, the dose will be reduced once your symptoms improve and treatment stopped as soon as possible.
■ Immunosuppressant such as azothiopine may be used.

SURGERY

■ Surgical treatment is usually necessary for people who experience persistent symptoms despite treatment with drugs.
■ Surgery may be recommended for people who have a sudden, severe attack that does not respond to medical treatment.
■ Surgery may be advisable for people with an increased risk of colorectal cancer. Surgery usually involves the removal of the diseased colon and rectum and creation of a stoma, which is an artificial opening in the abdominal wall through which the small intestine can expel feces. This procedure is called ileostomy.
■ A newer procedure called a pouch operation is suitable for some people. In this procedure, part of the small intestine is used to create a pouch that connects the small intestine to the anus. This procedure avoids the need for a stoma, but the pouch may become inflamed and the frequency of bowel movements often increases.

WHAT IS THE OUTLOOK?

Some people have only one attack of ulcerative colitis, but most have recurring episodes. About 1 in 5 people needs to have surgery. Colorectal cancer (see below) is the greatest long-term risk, and it eventually develops in about 1 in 6 people whose entire rectum and colon have been affected for 25 years or more. If you have long-standing, extensive ulcerative colitis but have not had surgery, you will need frequent colonoscopies to detect possible early warning signs of colorectal cancer.

> See also:
> • Ankylosing spondylitis p. 430
> • Arthritis p. 427
> • Colostomy and ileostomy p. 367

Colorectal cancer

COLORECTAL CANCER, SOMETIMES CALLED BOWEL CANCER, IS THE GENERAL TERM FOR CANCEROUS TUMORS OF THE LINING OF THE COLON OR THE RECTUM.

Cancer of the colon (bowel) occurs equally in men and women yet strikes 5-10 years later in women. Colorectal cancer is a disease of middle and late age. A high-fat, low-fiber diet, alcohol abuse, and obesity are risk factors. Getting regular exercise may help to prevent colon cancer.

Colorectal cancer is the **second most common cause of cancer deaths** in the West. It is also one of the few cancers that can be detected at an early stage by screening people thought to be at risk. When it is detected early enough, the disease can often be successfully treated by surgery.

Colorectal cancer is rare under age 40 and most cases occur in people over age 60. Cancer can occur anywhere in the colon or rectum, but about 3 in 5 tumors develop in the half of the colon **nearest the rectum**.

WHAT ARE THE CAUSES?

In less affluent countries, where people traditionally live on a high-fiber diet consisting mainly of cereals and fruit and vegetables, colorectal cancer is rare. However, a typical Western diet, which tends to be high in meat and animal fats and low in fiber, seems to increase the risk of developing colorectal cancer. It is not known how fiber in the diet reduces the risk of the disorder. A possible explanation is that dietary fiber shortens the time that it takes for waste matter to pass through the intestines. As a result, potentially cancer causing substances (known as carcinogens) in food are expelled from the body at a faster rate. Other lifestyle factors, such as **excessive consumption of alcohol, obesity,** and **lack of exercise** may also contribute to the risk of developing colorecteral cancer. Inflammatory disorders affecting the large intestine, such as **ulcerative colitis** or **Crohn's disease**, can also increase the risk of developing colorectal cancer if they are long-standing.

GENETICS

About five percent of cases of colorectal cancer are hereditary. Most of these cases are caused by inheritance of an abnormal gene. People who have this gene are at increased risk of developing a form of cancer known as **hereditary nonpolyposis colorectal cancer** (HNPCC). Rarely, colorectal cancer may be caused by the inherited disorder **familial adenomatous polyposis** (FAP), in which polyps form inside the large intestine. In FAP, there is a 9 in 10 chance that some of the polyps will become cancerous over time. Another gene may cause a **triad of cancers** of **breast, ovary** and **colon** when it runs through a family.

All members of such a family should have regular screening for all three cancers.

WHAT ARE THE SYMPTOMS?

The symptoms of colorectal cancer vary depending on the site of the tumor. They include the following:
• changes in the frequency of bowel movements or in the general consistency of the feces; **any change over the age of 50 should be reported to your doctor**
• abdominal pain
• blood in the feces – always report this to your doctor
• rectal discomfort or a sensation of incomplete emptying of the rectum
• loss of appetite.

The symptoms of colorectal cancer may be mistaken for the symptoms of a less serious disorder, such as **hemorrhoids**. If there is heavy loss of blood from the rectum, iron deficiency anemia may result. As the tumor grows bigger, it may eventually cause intestinal obstruction.

You should consult your doctor without delay if you notice an obvious change in your bowel habits or blood in your feces. Left untreated, colorectal cancer will eventually spread via the bloodstream to the lymph nodes, liver, and other organs in the body.

HOW IS IT DIAGNOSED?

■ Colorectal cancer is often diagnosed during screening before symptoms have developed.
■ If you do have symptoms, your doctor may first feel your abdomen to detect swelling.
■ A rectal examination, in which a gloved

WARNING:
■ People with a family history of colorectal cancer should be screened from age 40.
■ An annual fecal occult blood test is advised for people over age 50 who have a family history of the disease, in addition to sigmoidoscopy (a form of colonoscopy) every 3–5 years or a colonoscopy every 10 years.

Fecal tests

The feces may be examined for small amounts of blood that can't be seen by the naked eye. This blood, known as occult blood because it isn't immediately visible, can indicate a disorder that causes bleeding from the digestive tract, such as a peptic ulcer, polyps in the colon, or bowel cancer. The test is usually repeated several times over a period of several days because blood may not appear in every sample. If blood is found in the feces, other tests may be done to look for the cause, including endoscopy of the digestive tract and contrast X-rays to look for ulcers or tumors.

finger is inserted into the rectum, may also be done to see if a tumor can be felt.
■ A stool sample is tested for the presence of blood.
■ A blood sample may be tested for anemia.
■ The rectum may be examined visually with a viewing instrument inserted through the anus.
■ Your doctor may also order a colonoscopy, in which a flexible viewing instrument is used to examine the entire colon.
■ A biopsy may be taken (in which a small

sample of tissue is removed for microscopic examination) during the procedure.
■ You may also have a contrast X-ray in which a barium enema is used to detect an abnormality of the rectum or colon.

If a cancerous tumor is detected, you will probably need to have computerized tomography (CT) scanning to see if the cancer has spread to the lymph nodes in the abdomen or to the liver.

SCREENING

The goal of all screening is to detect disease before symptoms appear. So it's an early warning system.

Screening for precancerous polyps, which if removed, reduce the death rate from colon cancer. Surgery is also used to remove single metastases and new stool tests are being investigated to increase the early diagnosis of people at risk for colon cancer.

WHAT IS THE TREATMENT?

Treatment for colorectal cancer may involve surgery and/or chemotherapy.

SURGERY

Surgery is the primary treatment for colorectal cancer. If the cancer hasn't spread beyond the wall of the bowel, no further therapy is needed and you'll generally make a full recovery. Unfortunately, cancer is hard to control once it has spread. The search is always going on for more effective ways of treating advanced

disease and preventing cancer from spreading in the first place.

CHEMOTHERAPY

A new technique of giving the cancer fighting drug **5-fluorouracil** (5-FU) directly to the liver after surgery may improve survival in bowel cancer that's spread, and the results of a British trial are due to be released soon.

Another drug, **irinotecan**, has been found to control the spread of colorectal cancer in over 50 percent of patients who had not responded to, or who had relapsed after, conventional treatment with 5-FU.

Trials in America have already shown that the drug **oxaliplatin** could be used as a first line of treatment in cases of advanced colorectal cancer.

Other results suggest that patients may respond better to the traditional treatment with 5-FU if it's given with oxaliplatin. It may be that these drugs given in combination are more effective than either of them given alone.

Studies are underway to identify the best dose and the most effective timing for giving the combination.

See also:
• Anemias p. 236 • CT scanning p. 401
• Crohn's disease p. 366
• Hemorrhoids p. 370
• Ulcerative colitis p. 367

Anal itching (pruritus ani)

ANAL ITCHING, KNOWN MEDICALLY AS PRURITUS ANI, IS A FAIRLY COMMON CONDITION THAT MAY OCCUR EITHER IN OR MORE OFTEN AROUND THE ANUS.

Anal itching is rarely serious, although it may be embarrassing and difficult to treat. It may be either localized around the anus or be part of generalized itching. In postmenopausal women, pruritus ani is often associated with itching around the vagina (pruritus vulvae). The condition may be worse in older people because their skin is drier, less elastic, and more easily irritated.

WHAT ARE THE CAUSES?

The most common cause of anal itching is **candida** (moniliasis, yeast) with redness and scaling of the adjacent skin. Localized itching may also be caused by poor personal hygiene, **hemorrhoids,** or **threadworm infestation**. Generalized itching around the anal area may be a symptom of a skin disease such as

psoriasis or **eczema** or be due to an **allergic reaction** to a substance such as laundry detergent or dish soap. Once the skin has been thickened by chronic scratching (neurodermatitis) it's very difficult to break the itch-scratch-itch cycle.

SELF-HELP

There are several measures you can take to relieve anal itching.
■ It is important to keep the anal area clean by washing and drying carefully (but not excessively) after a bowel movement.
■ Avoid using **soaps** that irritate the skin, and try **not to scratch** because it will worsen the itching.
■ A warm bath or shower before bed may soothe nighttime itching.

■ **Loose underclothes** made of **natural fibers** are less likely than synthetic materials to cause irritation.
■ An over-the-counter cream containing a mild **topical corticosteroid** may give relief.
■ Itching that lasts for longer than three days should be assessed by a doctor.

Your doctor may examine your anus and order tests to look for causes that need treatment. For example, severe hemorrhoids may need to be removed.

See also:
• Candidiasis p. 450 • Eczema p. 312
• Hemorrhoids p. 370 • Psoriasis p. 448
• Worms p. 458

Hemorrhoids

SWOLLEN VEINS INSIDE THE RECTUM AND AROUND THE ANUS ARE KNOWN AS HEMORRHOIDS. THEY ARE MORE COMMON DURING PREGNANCY AND AFTER CHILDBIRTH. BEING OVERWEIGHT AND EATING A LOW-FIBER DIET ARE RISK FACTORS.

Hemorrhoids are a common problem, affecting up to half of all people at some time in their lives. In this disorder, veins in the soft tissues around the anus and inside the lower part of the rectum become swollen. Swellings around the anus are called **external hemorrhoids**, and those within the rectum are called **internal hemorrhoids**. Internal hemorrhoids that protrude outside the anus are known as **prolapsing hemorrhoids** and can be especially painful.

Hemorrhoids often cause bleeding, itching and discomfort. These symptoms are usually intermittent, and the condition is not in itself serious. However, a single so-called sentinel hemorrhoid may be a sign of colorectal cancer.

WHAT ARE THE CAUSES?
■ Hemorrhoids most commonly occur as a result of **constipation** when a person strains to pass stools. Straining in this way increases the pressure inside the abdomen, which in turn causes blood vessels around the rectum to swell.
■ Being overweight also **exerts pressure on blood vessels** and increases the risk of hemorrhoids.
■ During **pregnancy** the growing fetus has the same effect, frequently causing hemorrhoids.

WHAT ARE THE SYMPTOMS?
The symptoms of hemorrhoids commonly develop following constipation. They include:
• fresh blood on toilet paper or in the toilet after a bowel movement
• increasing discomfort on defecation
• discharge of mucus from the anus, sometimes leading to itching
• visible swellings around the anus
• feeling that the bowels have not been fully emptied.

A prolapsing hemorrhoid may protrude through the anus after a bowel movement and may then retract or can be pushed back

inside with a finger. In some cases, a blood clot (thrombus) may form within a prolapsing hemorrhoid, causing severe pain and a visible, tender, blue, grape-sized swelling.

If you have bleeding from the anus consult your doctor without delay, especially if you are over 40, since it may indicate a more serious disorder, such as **colorectal cancer**.

WHAT MIGHT BE DONE?
■ Your doctor will probably examine your rectum by inserting a gloved finger.
■ If there has been bleeding that suggests a serious underlying disease, your doctor may order a colonoscopy.
■ Small hemorrhoids usually do not need treatment.
■ Hemorrhoids due to pregnancy usually disappear soon after the birth.
■ A high-fiber diet helps prevent constipation, and laxatives may help ease defecation.
■ Over-the-counter topical corticosteroids and corticosteroid suppositories can reduce swelling and itching, and anesthetic sprays may

relieve pain. If these measures are not effective within a few days, you should consult your doctor, who may consider surgery.
■ Small internal hemorrhoids may be treated by **sclerotherapy**, in which the affected area is injected with a solution that causes the veins to shrink.
■ Alternatively, the doctor may place a band around the base of an internal hemorrhoid, causing it to shrink and fall off.
■ Persistent, painful bleeding hemorrhoids can be destroyed by electrical, laser, or infrared heat treatment. They can also be removed surgically.

Hemorrhoids may recur, although treatment is usually successful.

See also:
• Colorectal cancer p. 368
• Constipation p. 363

Anal fissure

AN ANAL FISSURE IS A SMALL TEAR IN THE ANUS THAT IS PREVENTED FROM HEALING BECAUSE THE SPHINCTER (ANAL MUSCLE RING) GOES INTO SPASM AND HOLDS IT OPEN. THE PROBLEM IS USUALLY CAUSED BY PASSING A LARGE, DRY STOOL.

I'm including this condition because it causes pain disproportionate to its significance. Anal fissure may be so excruciatingly painful that sufferers suspect the worst and fear they may have colorectal cancer. A visit to the doctor can be entirely reassuring so seek advice and put your mind at rest.

SELF-HELP
■ Use bulk forming agents to soften the stool.
■ Eat a high-fiber diet to overcome constipation.
■ Use a local anesthetic cream to ease pain and promote healing.

Hernias

A HERNIA, COMMONLY CALLED A RUPTURE, IS USUALLY THE PROTRUSION OF A BIT OF THE INTESTINE THROUGH A WEAKENED MUSCLE. OBESITY AND LIFTING HEAVY WEIGHTS MAY BE RISK FACTORS. DIFFERENT TYPES ARE NAMED ACCORDING TO WHERE THEY OCCUR.

Hernias most often occur at sites in the abdomen where there is a weakness in the muscles. If pressure in the abdomen is increased due to causes such as lifting heavy weights, persistent coughing, or straining at defecation, the muscles of the abdomen become stretched at the weak point. A visible bulge can then develop, which may contain fatty tissue or part of the intestine. Abdominal hernias are frequently found in men who have heavy manual jobs.

WHAT ARE THE TYPES?
Hernias are classified according to the site where they occur in the body. Some types occur more often in men; others are more frequently found in women.

INGUINAL HERNIA
This type of hernia occurs when a portion of the intestine pushes through into the inguinal canal, which is a weak spot in the abdominal muscle wall. The hernia causes a visible bulge in the **groin** or **scrotum**. These hernias usually affect men, but sometimes occur in women.

FEMORAL HERNIA
This type of hernia occurs in the part of the groin where the femoral vein and artery pass from the lower abdomen to the thigh. Women who are overweight or who have had several pregnancies are at increased risk of these hernias because their abdominal muscles are weakened.

UMBILICAL HERNIA
Babies may be born with an umbilical hernia, which develops behind the navel due to a weakness in the abdominal wall. Hernias that develop near the navel are known as para-umbilical hernias and are most common in women who are overweight or who have had several pregnancies.

OTHER TYPES OF HERNIA
Epigastric hernias develop in the midline between the navel and the breastbone and are three times more common in men.

Incisional hernias may develop after **abdominal** surgery if there is weakness around the scar. Risk factors include being overweight and having several operations through the same incision.

WHAT MIGHT BE DONE?
Your doctor may be able to feel a hernia by examining the abdomen or groin. Even small hernias eventually need to be repaired because if they are left untreated, they may become strangulated. The type of operation depends largely on the size of the hernia and on your age and general health. Some procedures are done under local anesthesia as outpatient surgery. Umbilical hernias in babies can usually be left untreated since they tend to disappear naturally by the age of five.

Surgery is usually effective. However, a hernia may recur in the same place or elsewhere. After surgery, you may be advised to avoid strenuous activity for a few weeks. You can help prevent a recurrence by losing excess weight, doing gentle exercise, and avoiding constipation.

Types of hernia

INGUINAL HERNIA

FEMORAL HERNIA

UMBILICAL HERNIA

See also:
• Constipation p. 363

Kidneys and Bladder

Image shows a colored X-ray urogram of urine in a healthy human bladder

Miriam's overview

One of the most dramatic scenarios of the whole of modern medicine involves the kidneys – kidney failure, renal dialysis, and organ transplant. Patients who would once have died can now miraculously be pulled back from the brink.

A triumph of modern medicine, yes, but on a much wider scale, more minor conditions bring untold discomfort and social embarrassment. I'm referring to cystitis and incontinence.

More than 13 million people in the US suffer from incontinence. The condition is far more prevelent in women than in men.

I get hundreds of letters from young women embarrassed by incontinence and distressed that they could be looking at another 40 years with this upsetting condition. Few women know that simple Kegel exercises can remedy incontinence, especially if they're done frequently each day. This applies to women of all ages. Research shows that Kegel exercises can make a huge difference even in women as old as 80 years.

Few women are aware that the bladder needs estrogen to keep it healthy and so bladder symptoms arising at menopause are due in great measure to estrogen deficiency. Furthermore they will respond to estrogen used

> *"**Kegel exercises** can make a **huge difference** even in women as old as **80 years**"*

locally (creams and suppositories inserted into the vagina). A woman doesn't have to take HRT by mouth if she doesn't want to in order to clear up her symptoms.

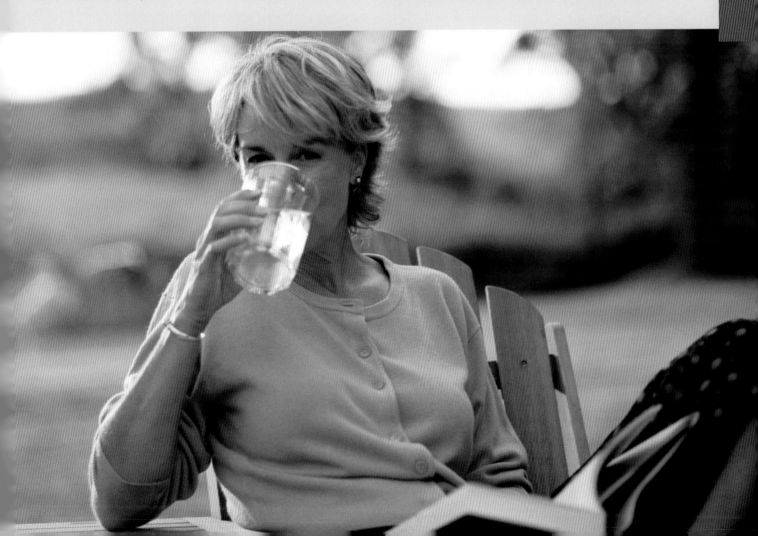

INSIDE
your kidneys and bladder

The kidneys and bladder are the major elements in the **urinary system**, which acts as a **filter** for the blood by removing and excreting waste products and excess water. The urinary system also regulates levels of water in the body and **maintains body fluids** in balance. The kidneys also produce **hormones**, including renin, which is important in the control of blood pressure. The kidneys receive blood from the **aorta**, the main artery connected directly to the heart. Blood passes through filtering units in each kidney, known as **nephrons**, where harmful wastes are removed and the amount of water to remain in the body is regulated. Filtered blood from the kidneys is returned to the heart through the body's largest vein, the **inferior vena cava**. Urine, containing water and waste products, passes through tubes called **ureters** to the **bladder**, where it is temporarily stored until it is emptied through the **urethra** during urination.

the kidney

Each kidney contains about 1 million tiny filtration units (nephrons), which remove waste products from the blood.

Cortex

Nephron

Renal artery

Renal vein

Ureter

Major calyces

Minor calyx

Renal capsule

the urinary tract

Waste products and excess water pass from the kidneys via the ureters to the bladder, where they are stored as urine before being excreted through the urethra.

Inferior vena cava

Aorta

Renal artery

Renal vein

Kidney

Ureter

Peritoneum

Bladder

Prostate gland

Urethra

sexual differences

The male urethra passes through the prostate gland and is about 8in (20cm) long. The female urethra is only about 1½in (4cm) long.

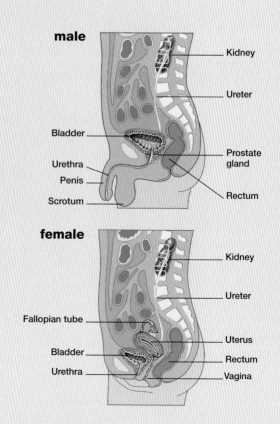

male

Kidney

Ureter

Bladder

Urethra

Penis

Scrotum

Prostate gland

Rectum

female

Kidney

Ureter

Fallopian tube

Uterus

Bladder

Rectum

Urethra

Vagina

Urinary incontinence, including stress incontinence and irritable bladder

ALTHOUGH THERE ARE AN ESTIMATED THIRTEEN MILLION SUFFERERS IN THE US, MOSTLY WOMEN, INCONTINENCE IS A TABOO SUBJECT – NO ONE TALKS ABOUT IT, BUT IT'S IMPORTANT TO BE WELL-INFORMED, BECAUSE IT COULD AFFECT ANY ONE OF US.

There are different types of incontinence, all of which are forms of uncontrollable leakage of urine. Although most older women suffer from it, occasionally incontinence can start surprisingly early in life – many women have occasional bouts of incontinence from their mid-20s onward, particularly if they've had children.

WHAT CAUSES IT?

There are four major causes of incontinence.
■ After pregnancy the pelvic tissues can become so stretched that a slight prolapse of the vaginal wall forms. If even a very small part of the urethra or bladder is trapped in the prolapse, urinary symptoms such as urgency, frequency and pain nearly always follow.
■ After menopause, lack of estrogen weakens the exit valve from the bladder, which may then leak.
■ Urine may also leak when pressure inside the abdomen is increased when we sneeze, cough, strain to open our bowels, or lift a heavy weight. This is called **stress incontinence**.
■ Postmenopausally the muscles of the bladder become oversensitive to the presence of **any** urine in the bladder, and contract spontaneously to empty the bladder even when there's only a small amount of urine there. This is sometimes called an **irritable** or **unstable bladder**.

WHAT ARE THE SYMPTOMS?

■ Inability to prevent your bladder from leaking urine.
■ The urge to pass urine frequently (frequency) even when your bladder isn't full.
■ Urgency (you can't hold on), even when your bladder isn't full.

SHOULD I SEE THE DOCTOR?

Seek help as soon as symptoms appear. The earlier incontinence is treated, the less likely it is that it will become chronic. Both stress incontinence and irritable bladder can be treated successfully.

WHAT WILL THE DOCTOR DO?

■ Your doctor will want to check a midstream urine sample for infection, so take one along when you see her. She may also refer you for a special X-ray of your bladder (cystogram).

■ She will advise you to strengthen your pelvic floor muscles by doing a series of special exercises (see box, below).
■ Since obesity weakens the pelvic floor, you may be advised to reduce your weight.
■ HRT has an almost instant rejuvenating effect on the bladder and urethra. There's no need to take pills; estrogen cream inserted in the vagina each night can be enough.
■ A prolapse can be helped by wearing a special support ring internally during the day, so ask if one is appropriate.
■ If you have a prolapse your doctor may advise you to have an operation to tighten up your pelvic floor muscles – a kind of **pelvic facelift** – called a colporrhaphy.
■ If you are suffering from an irritable bladder, she may suggest a muscle relaxing drug to relax your bladder muscles.
■ If this doesn't work, she may advise a

surgical procedure to "desensitize" your bladder by stretching the urethra.

WHAT CAN I DO?

■ Kegel exercises are most important. All women, whether they have bladder symptoms or not, should do Kegel exercises every time they pass urine.
■ Research has shown that even women as old as 80 years can benefit from a regime of these exercises carried out regularly. Over as short a time as three months, they can regain bladder control and vastly reduce any leaking.
■ Since the pelvic floor muscles contract at orgasm, toning them up can dramatically increase a woman's awareness of vaginal sensation during intercourse, making sex a much more pleasurable experience for her and her partner.
■ Try to avoid smoking, caffeine and alcohol.

Kegel floor exercises

■ The first step is to find the group of muscles that form a figure 8 around the vagina, urethra, and anus. You can do this by stopping the flow several times while you're urinating.
■ Tighten the muscles for five seconds, relax them for five seconds, then tense them again. Make sure you're not just tightening your buttocks and try not to tighten your stomach muscles at the same time. You may not be able to hold the tension for the full five seconds at first, but you are likely to develop this ability as your pelvic muscles grow stronger.
■ The next stage is to tighten and relax the muscles 10 times, as quickly as you can so that they seem to "flutter." You will probably need to practice for a while to control the muscles in this way.
■ Next, contract the muscles long and steadily as though you were trying to

draw an object into your vagina. Hold the contraction for five seconds.
■ The final step is to bear down, as if emptying the bowels, but pushing more through the vagina than the anus. Hold the tension for five seconds.

Gradually build up to 10 contractions, 10 times daily or more, spaced over several hours, and check your progress once or twice a week by stopping the flow when you urinate. After about six weeks of these exercises you should find stopping the flow is much easier than it was in the beginning.

The beauty of Kegel exercises is that, once you've mastered the technique, you can do them anywhere, any time – lying down, standing, watching television, even when you're doing the dishes or vacuuming!

Infection of the kidneys (pyelonephritis)

ONE OF THE MOST COMMON KIDNEY DISORDERS, WHICH PARTICULARLY AFFECTS YOUNG AND MIDDLE-AGED ADULTS, PYELONEPHRITIS IS INFLAMMATION OF ONE OR BOTH KIDNEYS, USUALLY AS A RESULT OF A BACTERIAL INFECTION.

Pyelonephritis is much more common in women and it may be related to sexual activity. In adults, the condition causes intense pain around the kidneys in the back. For this reason it can usually be promptly diagnosed and treated, so it rarely leads to long-term kidney damage. However, in children the symptoms of pyelonephritis may not be so obvious. All they may have are vague symptoms such as a headache and feeling sick. As a result, it may go unnoticed and lead to serious kidney problems, possibly resulting in kidney failure in later life.

WHAT ARE THE CAUSES?

There may be a minor **anatomical abnormality** that predisposes someone to infection and this should always be excluded with special X-rays of the kidneys. Pyelonephritis may be caused by bacteria that enter the urinary tract from the outside through the urethra (the passage from the bladder to the outside of the body). Often, the bacteria migrate upward from an infection in the bladder. Urinary infections, and therefore pyelonephritis, are much more common in women since the female urethra is

Urine test

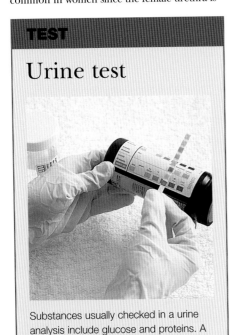

Substances usually checked in a urine analysis include glucose and proteins. A urine sample may also reveal blood cells, bacteria, or other substances that indicate an underlying problem.

shorter than that of the male and its opening is nearer the anus so there's little distance for the bacteria to travel to reach the kidneys. Bacteria from the anal area may enter the urethra during sex or if the area is wiped from back to front after a bowel movement. People with **diabetes mellitus** are more likely to have urinary infections, partly because glucose in the urine may encourage bacterial growth.

In both sexes, pyelonephritis is more likely to develop if there is a **physical obstruction** anywhere in the urinary tract that restricts the normal outflow of urine. Bacteria that have already contaminated the urine are not flushed out as would normally happen, and they multiply in the stagnant urine. An obstruction may be the result of pressure on parts of the urinary tract, such as the **expanding uterus in pregnant women** or an **enlarged prostate gland** in men. Normal urine flow may also be obstructed by **bladder tumors** or **kidney stones**. Kidney stones may harbor bacteria and therefore lead to urinary tract infection. All of these conditions are likely to lead to recurrent episodes of pyelonephritis.

Bacteria may also enter the bladder during bladder **catheterization**, a procedure in which a tube is passed up the urethra into the bladder to drain urine if the bladder can't empty itself. Sometimes bacteria are carried to the kidneys in the bloodstream from infections elsewhere in the body.

WHAT ARE THE SYMPTOMS?

The symptoms of pyelonephritis may appear suddenly, often over a period of a few hours, and include:

● intense pain that begins in the back just above the waist and then moves to the side and groin
● fever over 100.4°F (38°C), resulting in shivering and headache
● painful and frequent urination
● cloudy, blood stained urine
● foul smelling urine
● nausea and vomiting.

If you develop any of these symptoms, consult your doctor immediately.

HOW IS IT DIAGNOSED?

■ If your doctor suspects pyelonephritis, she will probably examine a sample of your urine (see box, left) to find out whether it contains bacteria. If there is evidence of infection, the

urine sample will be sent for laboratory analysis to establish which bacterium is responsible.
■ Further investigations may include a blood test so that the function of the kidneys can be assessed. Imaging tests, such as **ultrasound scanning**, **CT scanning**, or a type of contrast X-ray known as **intravenous urography** may also be performed to check for a blockage and signs of kidney damage or kidney stones.

WHAT IS THE TREATMENT?

■ Pyelonephritis is usually treated with a course of **oral antibiotics** and symptoms often improve within two days of treatment, but the full course MUST be taken to prevent bacterial resistance.
■ When the course of antibiotics is finished, more urine tests may be performed to confirm that the infection has cleared up completely. However, if you are vomiting or in pain, or if you are seriously ill, you may be admitted to the hospital and given **intravenous fluids** and **antibiotics**.
■ If you experience repeated episodes of pyelonephritis, you may be advised to take low-dose antibiotics over a period of six months to two years to reduce the frequency of the attacks. If you have an underlying disorder, such as kidney stones, this may also need to be treated.

WHAT IS THE OUTLOOK?

In most cases, prompt treatment of pyelonephritis is effective, and the condition causes no permanent damage to the kidneys. However, in rare cases, frequent episodes of pyelonephritis may lead to scarring of the kidneys and may result in irreversible damage.

See also:
● **Bladder tumors p. 380**
● **CT scanning p. 401**
● **Diabetes mellitus p. 504**
● **Kidney stones p. 377**
● **Prostate problems p. 266**
● **Ultrasound scanning p. 277**

Glomerulonephritis

THE KIDNEY CONTAINS MANY TINY FILTERING UNITS, THE GLOMERULI, WHICH VERY RARELY BECOME INFLAMED; THE RESULTING DISORDER, GLOMERULONEPHRITIS, CAN COME ON SUDDENLY (ACUTE) OR DEVELOP PROGRESSIVELY OVER A LONG TIME (CHRONIC).

An acute episode of glomerulonephritis is usually followed by complete recovery; however, in severe cases damage to the glomeruli may be permanent. Glomerulonephritis is a serious condition and must be treated in the hospital under the supervision of a renal (kidney) specialist.

WHAT ARE THE CAUSES?

Acute glomerulonephritis may occur as a complication of certain infectious diseases. The antibodies produced by the immune system to fight the infection may attack the glomeruli in the kidneys, causing inflammation and damage. The most common cause, especially in children, is a throat infection due to the streptococcus bacterium. Chronic glomerulonephritis may occur as part of an **autoimmune disorder** such as lupus.

WHAT ARE THE SYMPTOMS?

- Sore throat.
- Fever and shortness of breath.
- Back pain and headache.
- Passing little or no urine.
- Frothy or cloudy urine.
- Blood in the urine.
- Puffiness in the face, with swelling around the eyes in the morning.
- Swollen feet and legs in the evening.
- Loss of appetite.
- Nausea and vomiting.

WHAT IS THE TREATMENT?

- Following a bacterial infection, antibiotics and sometimes corticosteroid drugs may be prescribed.
- If glomerulonephritis is due to an autoimmune disorder it can usually be treated with immunosuppressants and corticosteroids.
- If the blood pressure rises it will be treated at the same time with antihypertensive drugs.
- For chronic glomerulonephritis, a low-salt diet with reduced fluid intake may be recommended to prevent fluid retention in body tissues.

WHAT IS THE OUTLOOK?

In most cases the symptoms of acute glomerulonephritis disappear after 6–8 weeks. In some people, kidney function is impaired but does not deteriorate further. However, other people may develop chronic kidney failure along with irreversible loss of kidney function that may be fatal if not treated promptly.

Kidney stones

NORMALLY, THE WASTE PRODUCTS OF THE BODY'S CHEMICAL PROCESSES PASS OUT OF THE KIDNEYS IN THE URINE. OCCASIONALLY, HOWEVER, THE URINE BECOMES SATURATED WITH WASTE PRODUCTS.

These waste products are able to crystallize into stonelike structures of varying sizes within the kidney – kidney stones. A shortage of chemicals that normally stop crystals from forming can lead to kidney stones, which usually start off as fine gravel and take years to reach a size that causes problems.

WHAT ARE THE CAUSES?

- The most common cause of kidney stones is prolonged **inadequate fluid intake**. People who live in hot climates may be susceptible to kidney stones if they do not drink enough to replace fluid lost in sweat.
- Different types of kidney stones can form, depending on the waste products that crystallize out of the urine; most are made of **calcium salts**.
- Kidney stones may also result from a **long-standing urinary tract infection**. In such cases, the stones can grow into a **staghorn** shape, filling the central cavity of the kidney.
- Rare **disorders of metabolism** may be complicated by kidney stones.

WHAT ARE THE SYMPTOMS?

Very small kidney stones may pass unnoticed in the urine. Larger stones, or small fragments of stones that pass down the **ureter** (the tube from the kidney to the bladder), may cause extremely painful spasms of the ureter wall called **renal colic**. The symptoms usually appear suddenly and include:

- excruciating pain that starts in the back, spreads to the abdomen and groin, and may be felt in the genitals
- frequent, painful urination
- nausea and vomiting
- blood in the urine.

If a kidney stone is passed in the urine the pain will subside rapidly.

WHAT IS THE TREATMENT?

- If the stones are small and remain in the kidney, you may simply be advised to rest, take painkillers to relieve discomfort, and drink plenty of fluids to help flush the stones out of the urine.
- In some instances, kidney stones that have become lodged in the lower part of the ureter can be removed via the bladder. In this procedure, a viewing tube is passed into the bladder and ureter. Instruments are then passed through the tube to crush or remove the stone.
- The most frequently used treatment for kidney stones is **lithotripsy**, in which shock waves are used to break the stones into powder that can be passed easily in the urine.
- The underlying cause needs to be treated to prevent a recurrence of kidney stones.

SELF-HELP

Preventing kidney stones

If you have kidney stones, these dietary precautions may help prevent their recurrence:

- drink at least 3 to 4 quarts (3 liters) of fluids daily to avoid dehydration.
- spread out your fluid intake as evenly as possible throughout the day.
- drink fluids before you sleep to ensure that urine production continues overnight.
- drink more fluids in hot weather, after strenuous exercise, or if you have a fever.
- to prevent oxalate stones (made up of calcium oxalate), avoid rhubarb, spinach, and asparagus, which contain oxalic acid.
- to prevent oxalate stones, a low salt, and low animal protein diet may be helpful.

See also:
- Cystoscopy p. 380

FOCUS *on* cystitis

A very common, annoying, and inconvenient condition, cystitis causes frequent, painful urination as a result of inflammation of the bladder. It hardly ever occurs in men and in women is most often the result of an infection or bruising after athletic or prolonged sex.

Most women have a bout of cystitis at some time in their lives but it doesn't usually endanger health.

WHAT CAUSES IT?

- The most common bacterium to cause cystitis is *E. coli*, which lives without causing problems in the bowel and on the skin around the anus. It only causes infection when it spreads up the urethra into the bladder. Women are more prone to cystitis than men because the female urethra is shorter than the male one and it's therefore a shorter distance for bacteria to travel from the skin.
- Other organisms that cause **sexually transmitted diseases**, such as **herpes** or **trichomonas**, can cause cystitis too.
- The cystitis known as **honeymoon cystitis** is not restricted to honeymooners. It is caused at any time by unusual amounts of frequent, strenuous sexual intercourse, which can cause bruising of the urethra, especially with the man on top position.
- Occasionally, cystitis can be caused by the use of **antiseptics** in bathwater or by over-zealous use of **vaginal deodorants** or **douches** when the normal protective flora in and around the vagina is disturbed.
- As women get older and reach menopause, a shortage of estrogen leads to thinning of all the genital organs, including the bladder and urethra, and this can contribute to **menopausal cystitis**.
- Cystitis can sometimes be a side effect of some cancer treatment. Radiation therapy, particularly if cancer of the cervix or prostate cancer are being treated, may lead to cystitis and chemotherapy has the same effect as the powerful drugs are flushed out with the urine.
- Diabetics often suffer from cystitis because the high sugar content of the urine favors multiplication of bacteria, and people with reduced immunity, for example those with an **autoimmune** disease or HIV infection, are also at greater risk of developing the condition.

WHAT ARE THE SYMPTOMS?

- The frequent and urgent need to urinate, although only a small amount of urine may be passed each time.
- A burning or stinging sensation while urinating.
- A severe knifelike pain when you finish urinating.
- The appearance of blood in the urine, which may be pink, red, or simply streaks.
- A severe dragging-down pain, usually in the front of the abdomen but quite often radiating up the flanks and to the back, or down the front of the thighs.
- Pain and the urge to get up several times at night to empty your bladder, even though there may be very little urine present.
- Fever and shivering attacks.

WHAT CAN I DO?

If the self-help measures listed below don't bring relief, seek help from your doctor as soon as possible:
- Drink large volumes of fluid at the first sign. It's important to get urine flowing fast to flush out the bladder, so try to drink the equivalent of at least a glass of water every **half hour**.
- Drink cranberry juice, which is a urinary antiseptic.
- Make your urine alkaline by drinking milk and adding a little bicarbonate of soda to your drinks. You'll find that making your urine alkaline eases bladder pain quite considerably. However, acidifying the urine helps prevent infection.
- Drink as much bland, nonacidic liquid, such as water, milk, or weak tea, as you can. Try to drink around three quarts a day during the 48-hour treatment.
- Try to avoid alcohol, coffee, strong tea, or fruit juices; they may make matters worse.
- Urinate as often as you feel the need. In this way, you'll produce a flushing-through effect that helps your natural defenses.
- For pain relief, take acetaminophen every four hours. Don't take anything containing aspirin, it makes urine acidic.
- Keep warm. A heating pad or wrapped hot water bottle placed across the stomach can be very comforting.
- Avoid perfumed soaps, deodorants, and bubble baths since these may cause more irritation.

WHAT WILL THE DOCTOR DO?

- Your doctor may take a urine specimen to confirm an infection.
- As soon as the specimen has been taken, he can start you on a course of antibiotics. It's essential that you take the full course of treatment, even if your symptoms subside completely within 24 hours, otherwise organisms may become resistant to antibiotics and your cystitis can become chronic.
- If your cystitis doesn't respond to

Cystitis triggers

- In a sensitive woman not drinking enough water can be enough to cause cystitis.
- Sex, at any time (although not every time) and for the same reason, that is mechanical trauma, horseriding, or riding a bicycle for long periods can induce an attack of cystitis.
- Perfumed soaps, bath foams, or oils, talc and vaginal deodorants can irritate the delicate skin around the vagina and urethra and act as triggers.
- Certain foods and drinks like strong tea, coffee, alcohol, fruit juice, or highly spiced dishes can cause cystitis attacks or make them worse.
- Holding on too long before going to the bathroom, or wearing tight fitting pants, panty hose, or underwear in man-made fibers – creating the warm, moist atmosphere germs love – are also triggers.

treatment, your doctor may recommend a full series of tests to see whether there's any predisposing internal cause.

● If investigation shows no trace of bacteria or any other cause, you may be suffering from an "irritable bladder," in which emotional factors play a part.

CYSTITIS AND PREGNANCY

● Cystitis is fairly common during pregnancy, particularly in the first few months when the urethra relaxes under the influence of the hormone progesterone and infections spread more easily.

● Later on, pressure from the enlarging uterus may cause a small amount of urine to remain in the bladder and become stagnant, encouraging bacteria to multiply, leading to cystitis.

Drinking plenty of fluids, taking acetaminophen, and applying heat to the abdomen can all help ease the symptoms of cystitis.

How to stay clear

● Drink plenty of water at all times.

● Keep cranberry juice in the fridge at all times and start drinking it at the first sign of cystitis.

● At the first symptom, increase your water intake and make your urine alkaline by adding a little bicarbonate of soda to your drinks. (Don't continue this for too long; you could have unpleasant side effects such as gas.)

● **Never** allow yourself to get dehydrated, carry water with you at all times.

● If you're having sex frequently, drink a lot of fluid to keep the urine flowing. Urinate before and after sexual intercourse. Drink cranberry juice before and after.

● If you suspect that wearing a diaphragm is a contributory cause, ask your doctor about another form of contraception.

● Use tampons instead of sanitary pads since they're less likely to allow the bacteria to thrive; some women, however, find that tampons irritate the bladder further.

● Remember to wipe from the front toward the back after bowel motions to avoid spreading bacteria to the urethra.

● **Don't** be obsessive about genital hygiene. However, using a bidet after moving your bowels is a good idea to avoid contamination of the vagina and urethra from the rectum.

● **Don't** use antiseptics in the bath-water, and don't use vaginal douches or deodorants.

● Wear cotton panties or cotton liners.

● Avoid tight clothing, especially if made from synthetic material. Gartered stockings and cotton panties are better than panty hose.

● Keep a diary so that you can spot anything such as alcohol or spicy food that appears to bring on attacks, and avoid it whenever possible.

If you're susceptible to cystitis it's going to be part of your life so you have to learn to "manage" it.

Bladder tumors

GROWTHS THAT OCCUR IN THE BLADDER MAY BE NONCANCEROUS (BENIGN) OR CANCEROUS (MALIGNANT), BUT BOTH TYPES CAUSE BLOOD IN YOUR URINE, WHICH MUST ALWAYS BE REPORTED TO YOUR DOCTOR.

From blood in the urine alone it is impossible for your doctor to tell if the cause is relatively minor or something more serious. A tumor is what your doctor will want to exclude. Tests, including ultrasound and intravenous urography (IVU)

may be arranged and a specialist may want to perform a **cystoscopy** (see box, below) to take a look directly inside your bladder.

Treatment for shallow tumors can often be done during cystoscopy, although

surgery, chemotherapy, and radiation therapy may be used for more serious growths. Shallow cancerous tumors diagnosed early have a high cure rate.

See also:
• Chemotherapy p. 257 • Radiation therapy p. 395 • Ultrasound scanning p. 277

TEST

Cystoscopy

During cystoscopy, a thin, hollow viewing tube, known as a cystoscope, is inserted into the urethra and then into the bladder to look for tumors and other abnormalities. The

cystoscope may be rigid or flexible. Instruments to take tissue samples and destroy or remove tumors and stones can be inserted through the cystoscope as required. Cystoscopy may be carried out under either a local or general anesthetic.

Acute, chronic, and end-stage kidney failure

WHEN BOTH KIDNEYS STOP WORKING NORMALLY, THE CONDITION IS KNOWN AS KIDNEY FAILURE. IT MAY BE SUDDEN (ACUTE) OR GRADUAL AND PROGRESSIVE (CHRONIC).

Chronic kidney failure may lead to irreversible loss of kidney function (end-stage kidney failure), which is life threatening if not treated.

ACUTE KIDNEY FAILURE

■ The kidneys will stop working properly if

their blood supply is suddenly and greatly reduced. This can happen in **surgical shock,** such as after severe bleeding, serious infection, or a heart attack, when there is a profound fall in blood pressure.

■ Kidney failure may result from damage as a

result of **glomerulonephritis**, **pyelonephritis**, **toxic chemicals,** or **drugs**.

WHAT ARE THE SYMPTOMS?
The symptoms of acute kidney failure may appear rapidly, sometimes over a period of

TREATMENT

Transplant surgery

Many organs and tissues can now be transplanted. Kidney transplants have become common, and liver, heart, lung, cornea, and bone marrow transplants are performed routinely. Transplants of the intestines and pancreas are done less often. More than one organ may be transplanted at the same time, as in the case of heart and lung transplants.

Transplants are usually performed only when the tissue types and blood groups of the donor and recipient are similar. This is necessary because the recipient's immune system will attack any organ it identifies as "foreign," a process called rejection. Most transplant organs are taken from donors who

have very recently been declared dead and who are unrelated to the recipient. However, bone marrow and single kidneys can be taken from living donors without damaging their health. Bone marrow is always taken from a living donor. When bone marrow or kidneys are donated by a close, living genetic relative, often a brother or sister, the transplants are far less likely to be rejected by the recipient because the tissue types are likely to match more closely.

Most transplant surgery requires general anesthesia. In an organ transplant, the organ to be transplanted is removed from the donor and chilled in a salt containing solution until it reaches the operating room. This prolongs the time the organ can safely be

deprived of its normal blood supply by a few hours. In most cases, the diseased organ is replaced by the donor organ. However, in kidney transplants the defective organ may be left in place and the new kidney placed in the pelvis, where it is connected to the relevant blood vessels.

After a transplant, you will probably spend several days in an intensive care unit. With all transplants except the cornea, you will need immunosuppressants indefinitely in order to prevent your immune system from rejecting the new organ or tissue. You should be able to leave the hospital after a few weeks if the transplant has been successful. Recovery time for a corneal graft is shorter, and it is usually possible to go home after a few days.

hours only, and may include the following things:

- greatly reduced urine volume
- nausea and vomiting
- drowsiness and headache
- back pain.

If you develop these symptoms, you should call your doctor immediately. Without treatment, acute kidney failure may be fatal within a few days.

WHAT IS THE TREATMENT?

If you have acute kidney failure, you will need immediate hospitalization. You will probably be treated in an intensive care unit.

■ You may have to undergo **dialysis** for a short time so that the excess fluid and waste products can be removed from your bloodstream while the doctors investigate the cause of the kidney failure.

■ If you have lost a large amount of blood, you will need to have a **blood transfusion** to restore your normal blood volume.

■ Any underlying cause will be treated.

■ Finally, if there is a blockage anywhere in your urinary tract, you may need to undergo surgery to have the obstruction removed.

WHAT IS THE OUTLOOK?

If your kidneys have not been damaged irreversibly, there is a good chance that you will make a complete recovery, which may take up to 6 weeks. However, in some cases, the damage resulting from acute kidney failure may not be completely reversible, and in this situation **chronic kidney failure** may develop.

CHRONIC KIDNEY FAILURE

Chronic kidney failure is gradual and progressive loss of function in both kidneys so that eventually the kidneys cannot remove excess water and waste from the blood for excretion as urine. As a result, waste substances start to build up in the body and cause problems. In many cases, kidney function is reduced by over 60 percent before the buildup begins. By this time, often after months or perhaps years, the kidneys may be irreversibly damaged. Dialysis or a kidney transplant may therefore become necessary.

WHAT ARE THE SYMPTOMS?

The initial symptoms of chronic kidney failure appear gradually over several weeks or months and are often vague, such as weakness and loss of appetite. The first obvious symptoms of the condition to appear include:

- frequent urination, particularly during the night
- pale, itchy, and easily bruised skin
- shortness of breath
- persistent hiccups

TREATMENT

Dialysis

Dialysis is used to treat kidney failure by replacing the functions of the kidneys in filtering out waste and excess water from the blood. It can be temporary, as for acute kidney failure, or long-term, as for end-stage kidney failure. There are two forms: **peritoneal dialysis**, in which the peritoneal membrane is used as a filter, and **hemodialysis**, in which a kidney machine filters the blood.

Peritoneal dialysis

In peritoneal dialysis, the peritoneum, the membrane that surrounds the abdominal organs, is used instead of the kidneys to filter the blood. A procedure called an **exchange** is carried out four times a day at home. During an exchange, dialysis fluid that flowed into the abdomen 4–6 hours earlier is drained out of the peritoneum through a catheter in the abdominal wall. The fluid is replaced with fresh solution, then the equipment is disconnected, and you can carry out normal activities.

Hemodialysis

In hemodialysis, blood is pumped by a kidney machine from your body through a filter attached to the side of the machine. Inside the filter, blood flows on one side of a membrane and dialysate fluid flows on the other. Waste products and water pass from the blood across the membrane and into the fluid; the filtered blood returns to the body.

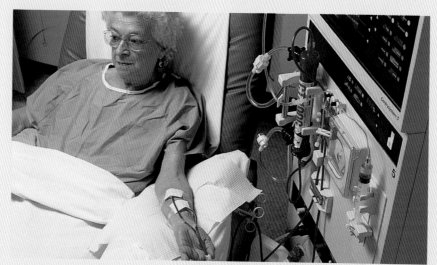

In hemodialysis, a kidney machine filters the blood in place of the kidneys. The procedure takes 3–4 hours and needs to be repeated about three times a week.

- nausea and vomiting
- muscular twitching
- pins and needles
- cramps in the legs.

Chronic kidney failure can lead to a number of complications, such as **high blood pressure** (which may also be a cause of kidney failure), **thinning and weakening of the bones** (osteoporosis), and **anemia**, in which the oxygen-carrying capacity of the blood is reduced.

If chronic kidney failure progresses to **end-stage kidney failure**, with permanent and almost total loss of kidney function, you will need treatment involving **long-term dialysis** (see box, above) or a **kidney transplant** (see box, opposite).

END-STAGE KIDNEY FAILURE

End-stage kidney failure is the irreversible loss of the function of both kidneys, which is often life threatening.

WHAT ARE THE SYMPTOMS?

The main symptoms of end-stage kidney failure usually include:

- greatly reduced volume of urine
- swelling of the face, limbs, and abdomen
- severe lethargy
- weight loss
- headache and vomiting
- furry tongue
- very itchy skin.

Many people who have end-stage kidney failure also have breath that smells of ammonia.

WHAT IS THE TREATMENT?

Long-term renal dialysis or a kidney transplant will be needed.

See also:
- Glomerulonephritis p. 377
- Infection of the kidneys p. 376

Chest and Air Passages

Image shows a colored angiograph of a normal human lung

Miriam's overview

The most dramatic development in this area is the increase in asthma, which some experts liken to an epidemic. I personally don't think the picture is that bleak but certainly there are growing numbers of people developing asthma and at both ends of the age spectrum.

Each is for a different reason. In children asthma is becoming more common because we're too clean. Yes, our modern obsession with all things "antibacterial" is thought to be the primary cause of the increase in childhood asthma. There's much excellent research to support this conclusion. We know, for instance, that children who live on farms and are exposed to countless millions of germs every day hardly ever get asthma. Whereas children brought up in homes where every surface is cleaned with a household cleaner containing antibacterial chemicals are prone to asthma.

"without exposure to an array of *household germs* the immune system is *feeble and weak*"

The reason is that a child's developing immune system needs contact with bacteria to become strong and capable. Without exposure to an array of household germs the immune system is feeble and weak and succumbs to asthma.

We've also recently found out that asthma is not caused by air pollution. Pollution may make asthma worse but it isn't the root of the problem. Asthma is increasing most quickly in the least polluted areas.

At the other end of our lives asthma is largely the consequence of smoking. A lifetime of smoking leaves most people with lung damage. Years of smoking leads to chronic bronchitis which can end up as COPD – chronic obstructive pulmonary disease – a component of which may be asthma.

The treatment of asthma has been revolutionized with the concept of "controllers" and "relievers." These two different kinds of asthma medicines are used in different ways. Controllers are taken every day, even in tip-top health, to prevent an asthma attack from happening and by and large they allow a child to live a normal life, playing sports and swimming.

Relievers are always close at hand, usually in the form of an inhaler for use in an asthma attack should it happen. Between these two regimens most children become unafraid of their asthma and take it in their stride – an essential part of successfully controlling asthma.

Because of the importance of asthma you'll find an article on it in this chapter, as well as a special "Focus on" asthma in the chapter on allergies and the immune system.

INSIDE
your chest and air passages

The function of the lungs is to supply oxygen to the blood and to remove the waste product carbon dioxide from it. This vital exchange of oxygen and carbon dioxide between the air and the blood is known as **respiration**. Air enters the body and leaves it via the respiratory system, which consists of the **mouth, nose, throat** (pharynx), **voice box** (larynx), **windpipe** (trachea), **branching air passages** (bronchi), and the **lungs** themselves. It is the job of the circulatory system, consisting of the heart and blood vessels, to carry oxygenated blood to body tissues and bring deoxygenated blood back to the lungs.

Inhaled air is warmed and moistened by the nose before passing into the lungs, where oxygen from the air passes into the blood via blood vessels. Here, oxygen binds to hemoglobin in red blood cells and travels in the blood back to the heart, which pumps the oxygenated blood around the body. At the same time, the lungs remove carbon dioxide from the fluid part of the blood, known as plasma, and exhale it.

the respiratory system

Adenoids
Nasal cavity
Nostril
Pharynx (throat)
Tonsil
Epiglottis
Vocal cords
Larynx
Trachea
Pulmonary vessels
Bronchus
Lung
Heart
Rib
Intercostal muscle
Pleura
Diaphragm

how breathing works

Decreasing air pressure in the lungs during inhalation causes air to be drawn into the lungs. Air pressure increases in the lungs during exhalation, forcing air out.

Inhaling

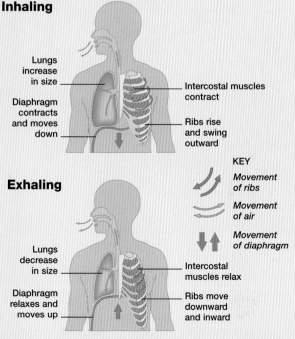

Lungs increase in size
Diaphragm contracts and moves down
Intercostal muscles contract
Ribs rise and swing outward

Exhaling

Lungs decrease in size
Diaphragm relaxes and moves up
Intercostal muscles relax
Ribs move downward and inward

KEY
Movement of ribs
Movement of air
Movement of diaphragm

The lungs receive deoxygenated blood from the body via the heart. The blood is oxygenated through the process of breathing before it is returned to the heart to be pumped around the body.

Cross section of alveoli

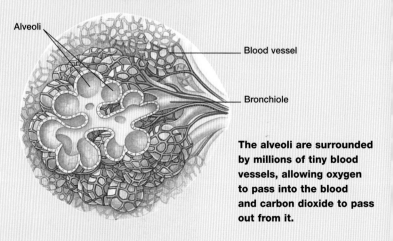

Alveoli
Blood vessel
Bronchiole

The alveoli are surrounded by millions of tiny blood vessels, allowing oxygen to pass into the blood and carbon dioxide to pass out from it.

Asthma

TO UNDERSTAND ASTHMA, AND INDEED ANY PROBLEMS RELATING TO THE CHEST
AND AIR PASSAGES, IT IS NECESSARY TO KNOW WHAT THE LUNGS DO.

When we breathe air in, the lungs remove oxygen from it and pass the oxygen into the blood. The blood then circulates around the body and delivers the oxygen to the tissues. At the same time the blood collects the waste product carbon dioxide, and takes it back to the lungs. The lungs get rid of the carbon dioxide by mixing it with the air that we breathe out. Air gets in and out of the lungs by a series of branching pipes, often called the "bronchial tubes," which get progressively smaller as they penetrate deeper into the lungs.

WHAT IS ASTHMA?

Asthma is caused by an inflammation of the bronchi (large airways) and bronchioles (small airways) that carry air in and out of the lungs. People with asthma have particularly sensitive airways.

These airways can constrict when you have a cold or other viral infection or when you come into contact with an asthma trigger, making breathing much more of an effort.

Asthma is a common condition that affects about 1 in 7 children and 1 in 20 adults. Many people think of asthma as something that starts in childhood, but it can occur for the first time at any age. Asthma may get better or disappear completely during the teenage years, but about half the children with asthma will still have some problems as adults. There is a tendency for asthma to run in families but many sufferers have no relatives with asthma. Asthma cannot, as yet, be cured but it can be kept under control so that asthma attacks are prevented. With proper treatment taken regularly, most people with asthma can lead entirely normal lives, with no time lost from school or work, and enjoy full involvement in sports and other recreations.

WHAT ARE THE SYMPTOMS?

Because it is more difficult to get air in and out of narrowed airways, people with asthma get the following symptoms:
- coughing
- wheezing, or a whistling noise in the chest
- getting short of breath
- a tight feeling in the chest
- coughing up phlegm.

Not everybody will get all of these symptoms. Some people experience them from time to time, perhaps if they get a cold or come into contact with one of their asthma triggers. Others experience the worst symptoms at night, first thing in the morning, or after exercise. A few people may experience symptoms all the time.

HOW DO I AVOID TRIGGERS?
COLDS

Colds are very common triggers of asthma attacks. They are also almost impossible to avoid!
■ Regular use of a controller inhaler reduces the risk of asthma attacks due to colds and infections.
■ Flu shots each autumn are recommended for people with severe asthma.
■ A healthy diet with a lot of fruit and vegetables containing vitamin C may help fight viruses.

PETS

Pets can be great fun and a wonderful source of companionship. Unfortunately, furry animals are also a common allergic trigger of asthma symptoms. The allergens are found in the pet's fur, saliva, dander (minute flakes of dead skin), and urine.
■ If someone in your family has asthma, or if there is a family history of asthma, don't buy a furry or feathered pet.
■ Up to 50 percent of children with asthma have their symptoms triggered by an allergy to cats and/or dogs.
■ The urine from guinea pigs, rabbits, and gerbils can cause problems too.
■ Rarely, even fish can cause problems! Some people have an allergic reaction to the ants' eggs on which tropical fish feed.
■ Bathing cats and dogs once a week can help. Ask your vet for advice on how to do this properly.
■ Always keep pets out of areas such as the living room and bedroom.

POLLEN

There are many different types of pollen grains (from grasses, trees, and plants) that can trigger asthma symptoms in some people.
■ On hot, dry days avoid spending too much time outdoors.
■ Avoid long grass.
■ Keep car windows closed.

SMOKING

■ Give up smoking! Within a few weeks you should start to notice huge benefits to your health – you should feel more physically fit and your risk of smoking-induced illness will rapidly decline. Your airways will start to recover in 3–6 months.
■ If you are planning to have a child, it is very important that neither parent smokes. Studies have shown that children of mothers who smoke are more likely to develop asthma.
■ Inhaling other people's smoke is hazardous for people with asthma too. A British asthma survey showed that cigarette smoke caused an increase in asthma symptoms in 80 percent of respondents.
■ Avoid smoky places. If you are going to be in a smoky room (e.g. at a party or in a bar), remember to take your inhaler with you. Go outside for some fresh air if you start to wheeze.
■ Don't be afraid to tell people how you feel. Ask them to stop smoking if you start to feel wheezy.
■ If you are concerned about smoke in the workplace, speak to your supervisor or coworkers.

The effect of asthma on the airways

NORMAL AIRWAY

thin layer of mucus

relaxed muscle

normal air passage

CONSTRICTED AIRWAY

excess mucus

contracted muscle

inward movement

narrowed air passage

In a normal airway, the muscle is relaxed and only a thin layer of mucus is present, allowing air to flow freely to the lungs.

During an asthma attack, the muscle in the airway contracts and excess mucus is produced, restricting air flow to the lungs.

DUST MITES

Little or no cost measures.

■ Hot wash (at 140°F or 60°C) sheets, duvet covers, and pillow cases at least once a week.

■ Children with asthma who sleep in bunk beds should sleep in the top bunk.

■ Put soft toys in the freezer for 24 hours once every two weeks to kill mites. Then wash at 140°F (60°C) to remove dead mites and their droppings.

■ Vacuum frequently, using a HEPA filter vacuum cleaner.

■ Damp dust all surfaces regularly or use the vacuum attachment.

■ Use cotton or synthetic blankets instead of wool.

■ There is no conclusive evidence that feather pillows are better than synthetic ones (in fact, the opposite may be true). Whichever pillows you choose, use an antiallergen cover and wipe over with a damp cloth once a week.

If the above steps seem to work, you might also like to consider the following measures.

■ Choose short-pile synthetic carpet. It may be better than pure wool carpets, although there is no conclusive proof for this.

■ Replace carpets with linolium, tile, or wood flooring.

■ Plain wooden bed frames are better than upholstered beds or headboards, which tend to collect dust.

■ Wash curtains every 2–3 months. Vertical blinds are often a better choice.

Dust mites love warm, humid environments – the following tips will reduce humidity levels in your home:

■ Keep rooms well aired.

■ Open windows during and after cooking, when you are doing the dishes or using the bathroom.

■ Keep kitchen and bathroom doors closed to prevent dampness from spreading to other parts of the house.

■ Remove damp and mold in the house quickly and avoid condensation.

■ Don't hang wet clothes indoors. It is best to use a tumble dryer that is vented outdoors.

■ A dehumidifier that reduces indoor humidity may be helpful, but the evidence is inconclusive and they can be expensive.

■ Consider using antiallergen covers for your mattress, duvet, and pillow. Make sure all the beds in the room are covered. Covers that completely enclose the mattress are better than ones that just cover the top. Antiallergen covers don't have to be expensive, so shop around for ones that fit your budget.

SELF-HELP

Know your triggers

A trigger is anything that irritates the airways and brings on the symptoms of asthma. There are many different asthma triggers and they vary from person to person. These are some of the common triggers.

Colds, flu, and other viral infections:
A recent survey put viral chest infections as the top trigger of asthma symptoms for both adults and children.

Dust mites:
Many people with asthma are allergic to the droppings of the microscopic dust mites found in our beds and other soft furnishings.

Cigarette smoking (active and passive):
This significantly increases breathlessness and coughing for people with asthma.

Furry or feathery animals:
Fur, feathers, and dander (shed flakes of dead skin) are common allergic triggers of asthma symptoms.

Exercise:
Exercise can make some people's asthma worse, especially when outside on cold, dry days or after a change of weather.

Pollen:
Pollen can trigger asthma attacks in some people.

Air pollutants:
These can include cigarette smoke, car fumes, paint fumes, perfumes, and certain chemicals.

Weather:
A sudden change in temperature, cold air, windy days, poor air quality (often on hot, humid days), thundery weather.

Mold:
Mold spores in wet weather, damp housing or piles of autumn leaves.

Emotion:
Emotional upset, stress, excitement, or even a long fit of laughing.

Drugs:
Some drugs, including aspirin, nonsteroidal anti-inflammatory medication (e.g. ibuprofen), and beta blockers (pills and drops) used for heart disease and glaucoma, can lead to asthma attacks in a small number of people. Always tell your pharmacist that you have asthma.

Hormones:
Some women's asthma varies before a period, during pregnancy or during menopause.

Food:
Although rare, some people have an allergy to specific foods (e.g. dairy products, fish, nuts, or yeast) that can bring on an asthma attack.

Work:
Occupational asthma mainly occurs in people who develop a sensitivity to a chemical in the workplace.

REMEMBER Just avoiding your triggers alone is unlikely to control your asthma. You need to take regular asthma medication as well.

WEATHER

Sudden changes in temperature, cold air, windy days, and poor air quality on dry, still days can all affect your asthma. Thunderstorms can also activate allergens – asthma emergencies rocketed during the summer thunderstorms of 1994, which caused a massive release of pollen into the air.

■ Take a puff of reliever just before going out.

■ Wear a scarf over your face if it's cold and windy. It will help warm the air up before you breathe it in.

■ Try to avoid going out in the middle of the day on hot, smoggy days.

EMOTION

Although it is not true that asthma is "all in the mind," we do know that psychological factors including excitement, stress, or even a long fit of laughing can trigger asthma symptoms. Regular monitoring of your condition and taking your medication regularly should help to minimize these problems.

FOOD

Most people with asthma do not have to follow a special diet. In some cases, however, certain foods can make symptoms worse. Dairy products (including eggs), shellfish, fish, yeast products, and nuts are some of the offenders. Some people can have a severe allergic, or anaphylactic, reaction to these foods. For more information, see Useful addresses (p. 567).

■ If you think you have a food allergy, consult your doctor.

■ Your doctor may ask you to keep a diary of your diet and your symptoms to see if there is a consistent relationship between the two.

■ Your doctor may refer you to a specialist clinic for further tests.

DRUGS

In a few people, certain medications can lead

TREATMENT

Relievers and controllers

Relievers

■ Relievers are bronchodilators; they work by relaxing the muscles in the walls of the airways, which allows the airways to open.

■ Relievers come in differently colored inhalers.

■ Relievers are medicines that you can take immediately when asthma symptoms appear. They quickly relax the muscles surrounding the narrowed airways. This allows the airways to open wider, making it easier to breathe again. However, relievers do not reduce the swelling in the airways.

■ They are essential in treating asthma attacks.

■ If taken before exercise they reduce your chances of getting asthma symptoms.

■ Salbutamol, terbutaline, and albuterol are three examples of relievers. They work almost immediately to relieve the symptoms of asthma. That is why they are sometimes called rescue relievers.

Controllers

■ Most controllers are corticosteroids; they reduce the inflammation in the airways and calm their irritability.

■ Sodium cromoglycate and nedocromil sodium are nonsteroid controllers and must be taken regularly, usually three or four times a day. They are not usually as effective as corticosteroids and are rarely used these days.

■ Leukotriene modifiers are newer types of controller drugs which are taken in pill form and act by blocking the effect of a molecule called leukotrienes.

■ Controllers come in differently colored inhalers.

■ Controllers protect the lining of the airways. They calm down the inflammation in our airways and stop them from being so sensitive. This means that the airways are less likely to react badly when they come across an asthma trigger.

■ They reduce the risk of severe attacks.

■ Their protective effect builds up over a period of time so they need to be taken every day even if you are feeling well.

■ When you first start using them, it may take up to 14 days before you notice any improvement in your symptoms.

Reliever inhalers are used to control an attack of asthma, while controllers should be used regularly to lessen the risk of developing an asthma attack.

■ There are several kinds of inhaled corticosteroids but they all work in the same way. Sometimes a steroid and bronchodilator are combined in the same dose.

---

to asthma attacks. This occurs most often with medicines containing aspirin, nonsteroidal anti-inflammatory pills (e.g. ibuprofen) and beta blockers used for heart disease (as pills), and glaucoma (as eyedrops). Always tell your pharmacist or doctor that you have asthma.

HOW DO I TAKE CARE OF MY ASTHMA?

The best way to take control of your asthma is to follow these golden rules:

● get the best treatment you can and take it regularly

● try to avoid things that trigger your asthma.

Ask your doctor to give you an asthma self-management plan showing you how to alter your own medicine to keep yourself well.

WHAT ARE THE TREATMENTS?

■ Relievers help to relieve breathing difficulties when they happen.

■ Controllers help protect the airways and reduce the chance of getting asthma symptoms.

Both can be inhaled so that the medication reaches the inflamed airways instantly.

WHAT IS A SPACER?

A spacer is a large plastic containe. At one end there is a mouthpiece and at the other a hole for the inhaler to fit into.

There are several different brands of spacer that fit the different inhalers and which are available by prescription. Spacers are very important.

■ They make inhalers easier to use and more effective.

■ You get more medicine into your lungs than you could using just the inhaler on its own.

■ The medicine is trapped inside the spacer so you don't have to worry about pressing the inhaler and breathing in at the same time; this makes spacers particularly useful for children, for whom coordinating breathing and inhaling is almost impossible. For babies and very young children, a mask can be attached so that by breathing normally the drug is inhaled.

■ They help reduce the possibility of side effects from higher doses of inhaled steroids by reducing the concentration of medicine that is swallowed and absorbed into the body.

■ Spacers do need to be used and cleaned correctly and regularly. Ask your doctor or pharmacist for advice on how to do this.

HOW DO I KNOW IF MY ASTHMA'S GETTING WORSE?

A peak flow meter is a simple instrument that determines the maximum rate at which you are able to blow out. If you take peak flow measurements of yourself every day to monitor your asthma you will get an early warning sign – a reduced reading – if your condition is worsening.

Worries about steroids

Many people are anxious about the side effects of steroids used in controller treatment. Here are some points to remember.

■ The steroids used to treat asthma are called corticosteroids and are completely different from the anabolic steroids used by bodybuilders and athletes.

■ Corticosteroids are a copy of chemicals produced naturally in our bodies.

■ Most people use inhaled steroids, which go straight down to the airways, so very little is absorbed into the body.

■ Your doctor will prescribe the lowest possible dose to get your asthma under control.

■ There is a small risk of a mouth infection called yeast and hoarseness of the voice. You can avoid this by using your inhaler before brushing your teeth, and by rinsing out your mouth well afterward. Using a spacer will also help reduce the possibility of yeast.

Swimming is ideal exercise for people with asthma.

Asthma self-management

An asthma self-management plan allows you to adjust your own medication according to guidelines you develop and agree in advance with your doctor.

Self-management involves taking a peak flow reading twice a day and keeping track of the results on a chart. You also use other indicators, such as whether your asthma has disturbed your sleep, to determine how well controlled your asthma is each day. You can then adjust your medication accordingly, using the guidelines set out in your plan.

If you notice any of the following, then you should see your doctor, who can help to bring your asthma back under control.

■ Waking at night with coughing, wheezing, shortness of breath, or a tight chest.

■ Increased shortness of breath when waking up in the morning.

■ Needing more and more reliever treatment or reliever doesn't seem to be working as well as it was.

■ Can't keep up with your usual level of activity or exercise.

ASTHMA AND EXERCISE

Exercise is the best way to keep your body in tip-top condition. It is fun and leaves you feeling good about yourself. However, exercise is also a common asthma trigger. But that doesn't mean you should stop! Exercise is good for everyone, including people with asthma.

● Take a couple of puffs of your reliever inhaler about 15 minutes before you start and keep it close at hand at all times.

● Warm up for 5–10 minutes or so with a few short 30-second sprints.

● If you still get wheezy, it's a sign your asthma might not be properly under control. Go and see your doctor, who will be able to adjust your treatment to help you get back on track.

If your asthma is under control, you should be able to do any sport or exercise that you enjoy. However, you might like to try the following.

■ Swimming is a great form of exercise for people with asthma. This is because the air in the pool is warm and moist – a combination that doesn't seem to irritate sensitive airways so much.

■ Yoga can be extremely good for some people with asthma. It helps relax the body and may improve your breathing.

■ Team games are a good idea too – you can always play in a position that doesn't require so much running around.

■ Long spells of exercise are more likely to bring on asthma symptoms than short bursts. So long-distance running is more likely to be a problem than, say, an exercise class involving short periods of aerobic exercise.

There are some sports and activities you should be careful of. These include scuba diving and sports done at high altitudes such as climbing, hiking, and skiing. Speak to your doctor if you're thinking about doing any of these activities.

CAN COMPLEMENTARY MEDICINE HELP?

Although some people find that complementary therapies, particularly yoga, acupuncture, and homeopathy, seem to improve their asthma symptoms, it is dangerous for a person with asthma to think they can rely on complementary medicines. There is no scientific evidence that complementary treatments used on their own are effective. That is why it is better to regard them as "complementary" rather than "alternative." If you want to try one of the many complementary treatments available, tell your doctor and do not stop taking your normal asthma medication.

What to do in an attack

Sometimes, no matter how careful you are taking medicine and avoiding triggers, you may have an asthma attack. Quite often, a couple of puffs of reliever are all that is needed to get your asthma under control again. At other times, symptoms are more severe and more urgent action is needed. Don't be afraid of making a fuss, even at night.

1. Take two puffs of your reliever right away, preferably using a spacer.

2. Keep calm and try to relax as much as your breathing will let you. Sit down, don't lie down. Rest your hands on your knees to help support yourself. Try to slow your breathing down since this will make you less exhausted.

3. Wait 5–10 minutes.

4. If the symptoms disappear, you should be able to go back to whatever you were doing.

5. If the reliever has no effect, call the doctor or an ambulance.

6. Keep taking your reliever inhaler; use it every few minutes until the ambulance arrives.

7. Take your steroid pills, if your doctor has put them into your self-management plan.

What if my child has asthma?

Is it easy to be sure?

Diagnosing asthma in very young children can be difficult.

■ If your child is under the age of two, it is even more difficult to tell if they have asthma. There are a number of different wheezing illnesses, including acute bronchiolitis and wheezy bronchitis as well as asthma, that can make your baby wheezy.

■ At least 1 child in 7 will have wheezing at some point during their first five years. Many of these children will not go on to have asthma in later childhood, so your doctor may not want to use the term "asthma" at this stage.

■ It is not easy to measure how well a young child's lungs are working. A peak flow meter is used for older children, but is unsuitable for children under the age of six. The pattern of symptoms that develops **over time** shows whether a child has asthma or not. Your doctor may ask you to keep a record of your child's symptoms and when they happen. This will help the doctor get to the bottom of your child's breathing problems.

The typical symptoms of asthma in young children are:

● coughing, particularly at night and after exercise

● wheezing, or a whistling noise in the chest

● getting short of breath – perhaps your child is not running around as much as usual, or needs to be carried a lot.

Can I prevent it?

If you or your partner have asthma, there are steps you can take that could help reduce the chances of your child developing asthma.

■ Breast-feed for at least four months.

■ Don't keep furry or feathery pets. Avoid allergens such as dust mites and pollen during pregnancy and keep your child away from them in the first few months of life.

■ Neither you or your partner should smoke. We know that this increases the likelihood of a child developing asthma. Outdoor air pollution has not been proven to cause asthma although it can make the symptoms of asthma worse.

How will my child manage at school?

Any inhalers that your child needs to take during the school day should be labeled with their name. It is very important that your child can get to their reliever inhaler as soon as they need it. Ideally, children should carry their own reliever inhaler with them at all times. For younger children, their reliever should be kept in a central and accessible place throughout the school day. Make sure that the school knows about your child's asthma.

What about sports?

Exercise is good for everyone, including children with asthma. Nearly all children with asthma become wheezy during exercise. However, if your child takes a few simple precautions, she/he should be able to participate fully in sports at school.

■ Taking a couple of puffs of reliever inhaler 15 minutes before exercise will usually help prevent symptoms.

■ A few short sprints over 5–10 minutes before vigorous games may protect the lungs for an hour or so.

■ If your child takes their reliever inhaler but still gets wheezy after exercising, it's a sign that their asthma might not be properly under control. Go and see your doctor or nurse. They will be able to adjust the treatment to help them get fit and healthy again.

■ And remember – your child should always have their reliever close at hand during exercise.

How do I help?

■ Make sure you tell the school your child has asthma.

■ Tell them about the medication your child requires. Contact the American Lung Association which can provide a free school asthma card to help you do this.

■ Keep the school informed of any changes in your child's medication.

■ Discuss with your teacher any worries you have about your child's asthma.

■ Make sure your child's reliever medication and/or spacer is labeled with his/her name. Make sure the school has a spare inhaler that is also labeled.

■ Make sure your child's medication, and the spare, hasn't exceed its expiration dates.

■ Keep your child at home if he/she is not well enough to attend school.

■ Visit the doctor or nurse regularly to make sure your child's asthma is under good control.

What should the school do?

■ Keep records of children with asthma and the medication they take.

■ Allow children immediate access to their reliever inhaler throughout the school day. That includes during PE, at recess and on school trips.

■ Make sure the school environment is asthma-friendly. For example, do not keep feathery or furry pets in school and adopt a no-smoking policy on school premises.

■ Make sure that pupils take part fully in school life, including PE.

■ Liaise with parents, the school nurse, and make sure your school has an asthma management plan which includes policies on the use of inhalers and medications, actions or emergency procedures, and student asthma action cards.

■ Encourage other children to understand asthma. Schools can contact The American Lung Association to learn about their Open Airways For Schools program, which is now available in English and Spanish.

Bronchitis

WHEN THE LARGE AIRWAYS (BRONCHI) BECOME INFLAMED, MOST OFTEN DUE TO A VIRAL
INFECTION, THE BODY'S RESPONSE IS A PRODUCTIVE COUGH, OFTEN WITH YELLOW OR GREENISH
PHLEGM – THESE ARE THE TYPICAL SYMPTOMS OF BRONCHITIS.

There are two forms of bronchitis: **acute**, which starts suddenly and clears up quickly, and **chronic**, which is long term and recurs each year with cough and phlegm for several months. Chronic bronchitis is one part of chronic obstructive pulmonary disease (COPD; see below) with wheezing, shortness of breath, and eventually serious impairment of lung function due to emphysema. Smoking is undoubtedly a causative factor in COPD.

ACUTE BRONCHITIS
This type of bronchitis is usually a complication of a viral infection such as a cold or flu, when secondary infection by a bacterium supersedes. Attacks usually occur in winter and affect vulnerable people such as smokers, babies, the elderly, and people who already have lung disease.

WHAT ARE THE SYMPTOMS?
Inflammation of the lining of the bronchi causes swelling and congestion leading to a feeling of shortness of breath, with or without wheezing, cough and green/yellow phlegm. There may be a fever and a feeling of soreness behind the breastbone.

WHAT IS THE TREATMENT?
■ Humidify the room or sit in the bathroom with the hot water filling the bath.
■ Inhalations of steam.
■ Acetaminophen, ibuprofen, or aspirin to bring down a fever.
■ Antibiotics if there is a bacterial infection but they are of no use if the cause is viral. However, antibiotics may be given to protect vulnerable people from a secondary bacterial infection.

ARE THERE COMPLICATIONS?
Rarely, acute bronchitis may develop into the following:
● pneumonia, when the lung tissue becomes inflamed and infected
● pleurisy, when the covering of the lungs is inflamed, usually over a patch of pneumonia. You should call the doctor if:
● breathlessness is severe
● there is no improvement after three days
● fever exceeds 101°F (38.3°C)
● there is pre-existing lung disease or you belong to a vulnerable group.

WHAT IS THE OUTLOOK?
If smoking continues, or with preexisting lung disease, there is always the possibility of progression to COPD.
 Once you have continuous production of phlegm for three consecutive months during two consecutive years, you have chronic bronchitis.
 Vulnerable people should have a flu vaccination each autumn.

See also:
• Pleurisy p. 393
• Pneumonia p. 392

Chronic obstructive pulmonary disease

NOWADAYS, PROGRESSIVE DAMAGE TO THE LUNGS – CHRONIC OBSTRUCTIVE PULMONARY DISEASE
(COPD) – IS NEARLY ALWAYS CAUSED BY SMOKING. THE AIRWAYS AND TISSUES OF THE LUNGS BECOME
DAMAGED, EVEN DESTROYED, CAUSING WHEEZING AND INCREASING SHORTNESS OF BREATH.

Some people with COPD eventually become so short of breath that they are seriously disabled and are unable to carry out even simple daily living activities. COPD is rare before age 40 and is twice as common in men, but as more women smoke the prevalence in women is increasing.
 People with COPD usually have separate lung conditions, **chronic bronchitis, airway narrowing, and emphysema**, and any of these conditions may be dominant.
■ In chronic bronchitis, the airways (bronchi) become inflamed, congested, and narrowed, and a cough that produces phlegm is common; in airway narrowing, the flow of air is obstructed.
■ In emphysema, the air sacs (alveoli) within the lungs become enlarged and damaged, making them less efficient in transferring oxygen from the lungs to the bloodstream. The damage to the lungs that is caused by both chronic bronchitis and emphysema is usually irreversible. COPD is extremely common and a leading cause of death, with an estimated 16 million people diagnosed and perhaps as many undiagnosed.

WHAT ARE THE CAUSES?
The main cause of both chronic bronchitis and emphysema, and hence of COPD, is smoking. Occupational exposure to dust, noxious gases, or other lung irritants can worsen existing COPD. So wear protective clothing and ask your employer to install air purification systems. Poorly treated asthma causes a COPD-like disease.
 In chronic bronchitis, the linings of the airways of the lungs respond to smoke irritation by becoming thickened, narrowing the passages that carry air into and out of the lungs. Mucus glands in the bronchial linings multiply so that great quantities of mucus are produced and the normal mechanism for clearing the airways and coughing up excess mucus as phlegm is impaired. As the disease progresses, retained mucus in the airways easily becomes infected, which may lead to further damage and bouts of **pneumonia** and **pleurisy**. Repeated infections may eventually cause the linings of the airways to become permanently thickened and scarred, destroying the normal anatomy of the lungs even further.
 In emphysema, the air sacs eventually lose their elasticity, and the lungs become distended and can't be properly emptied during exhalation. Eventually, the air sacs tear and merge together, reducing their total surface area, and air becomes trapped in the dilated sacs. As a result, the amount of oxygen that enters the blood with each breath is severely reduced.
 People with COPD have restricted lung function, which is evident from lung function tests (see box, opposite).

WHAT ARE THE SYMPTOMS?

Symptoms of COPD may take many years to develop. When they appear, symptoms often include the following:

- shortness of breath on mild exertion, becoming progressively worse so that eventually shortness of breath occurs even when at rest
- coughing in the morning that produces phlegm
- coughing throughout the day
- increasing production of phlegm
- frequent chest infections, especially in winter, producing yellow or green phlegm
- wheezing, especially after coughing.

ARE THERE COMPLICATIONS?

Cold weather and infections, such as flu, cause symptoms to worsen.

■ Some people with emphysema develop a barrel-shaped chest as the lungs become distended.

■ Respiratory failure may develop, in which lack of oxygen causes the lips, tongue, fingers, and toes to turn blue.

■ In addition, swelling of the ankles caused by chronic heart failure may occur.

■ Some people who have COPD unconsciously compensate for their lung problems by breathing rapidly to get more oxygen into their blood, and, as a result, they have a **rosy flush** to their skin, the so-called pink puffers.

■ Other people are unable to compensate in this manner and tend to have a **blue complexion** instead, which is caused by lack of oxygen. These people often have tissue swelling in the feet and legs, which is due to heart failure, the so-called blue bloaters. These patients may experience drowsiness and headaches.

If you are a smoker and notice symptoms that indicate you may have COPD, consult your doctor as soon as possible and consider stopping smoking immediately.

WHAT CAN I DO?

If you develop COPD and you smoke, you should stop! Smoking cessation is the only action that can delay the progress of COPD. Cutting down on the number of cigarettes you smoke will have less effect on the progress of your deterioration.

HOW MIGHT THE DOCTOR TREAT IT?

The damage caused by COPD is largely irreversible, but there are treatments that may ease the symptoms.

■ Your doctor may prescribe an **inhaler** containing a bronchodilator drug.

■ Shortness of breath may also be relieved by continuous **home oxygen therapy**, which also reduces strain on the heart. This therapy concentrates the oxygen available in room air and is used for at least 15 hours a day. It reduces breathlessness, strain on the heart, and the risk of heart failure and increases life expectancy.

TEST

Lung function

Two tests are used to detect air flow problems in the lungs: **spirometry**, which measures how quickly the lungs fill and empty, and the **lung volume test**, which can show how much air the lungs can hold. Other tests not shown here include **gas transfer tests**, which use a small amount of inhaled carbon monoxide to determine how fast a gas is absorbed from the lungs into the blood. Tests to measure blood gases show the level of oxygen and other gases in the blood.

Spirometry

A spirometer is used to measure the volume of air (in liters) that you can inhale and exhale over a period of time. The results show whether the airways are narrowed as a result of lung disorders such as asthma or COPD. Spirometry can also be used to monitor the effectiveness of certain treatments for lung disorders, such as bronchodilator drugs, which widen the airways.

Using the spirometer

You will be asked to inhale and exhale forcefully and fully through a mouthpiece several times. The volume of air inhaled and exhaled is displayed on the monitor.

Lung volume test

This test measures the volume of air (in liters) that can be taken in with a full breath and the volume of air that remains in the lungs when the breath is fully exhaled. The lung volume test is used to help diagnose disorders such as chronic obstructive pulmonary disease that affect the volume of air retained by the lungs after breathing out.

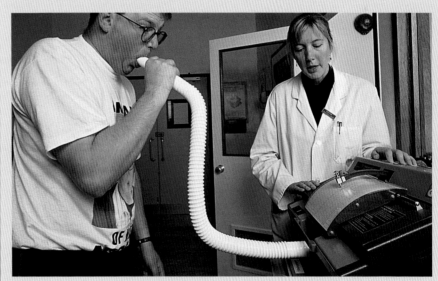

A spirometer is used to measure the volume of air inhaled and exhaled.

■ If you have swollen ankles, your doctor may prescribe **diuretics** to reduce buildup of fluid.

- **Antibiotics** may be prescribed if a chest infection develops.
- You should be **vaccinated against the flu** each autumn and you may also be given another vaccine to protect against infection with the bacterium *Streptococcus pneumoniae*.
- If the lungs are very distended, part of the lung tissue may be removed by **lung volume reduction surgery**. This allows the lungs to inflate and deflate more easily, increasing the amount of oxygen in the blood.
- Pulmonary rehabilitation programs are run by many hospitals. These last 4–6 weeks and teach patients how to breathe most efficiently and how to exercise within their limits.

WHAT IS THE OUTLOOK?

If your COPD is mild and has been diagnosed at an early stage, you may be able to avoid severe, progressive lung damage if you stop smoking at once. However, most people with COPD do not realize they have the condition until it is well advanced. For these people, the outlook is poor. They often need to retire from work early and may become inactive and housebound due to shortness of breath. Although about 3 in 4 people with COPD survive for one year after diagnosis, fewer than 1 in 20 survives longer than 10 years.

See also:
- **Chronic heart failure p. 233**
- **Pleurisy p.393** • **Pneumonia p. 392**

Pneumonia

IN PNEUMONIA, MANY OF THE TINY AIR SACS (ALVEOLI) IN THE LUNGS BECOME
INFLAMED AND FILLED WITH PUS (WHITE BLOOD CELLS) AND FLUID.

When pneumonia develops it is harder for oxygen to pass across the walls of the alveoli into the bloodstream. Usually, only a proportion of one lung is affected, but, in some severe cases, pneumonia affects both lungs ("double" pneumonia) and can be life threatening. Pneumonia is a result of infection but can occur beyond a blockage due to chronic obstructive pulmonary disease or lung cancer, and as a complication of childhood infections such as whooping cough and measles.

WHO IS AT RISK?

■ Infants, elderly people, and people who are already seriously ill or have a chronic disease, such as diabetes mellitus or heart disease, are at greatest risk of developing pneumonia.
■ Other people more likely to develop pneumonia are those who have lowered immunity as a result of a serious disease, such as AIDS. Impaired immunity can also occur during treatment with immunosuppressant drugs or chemotherapy.
■ People who smoke, drink excessive amounts of alcohol, or are malnourished are more likely to develop pneumonia.

WHAT ARE THE CAUSES?

■ Most cases of pneumonia in adults are caused by infection with a **bacterium**, most commonly *Streptococcus pneumoniae.* This type of pneumonia may develop as a **complication** of a viral infection in the upper respiratory tract, such as a cold. Other common causes of bacterial pneumonia in healthy adults include infection with the bacteria *Hemophilus influenzae* and *Mycoplasma pneumoniae.* Viral pneumonia can be caused by the organism that is responsible for **influenza** and **chickenpox**.
■ Pneumonia caused by the bacterium *Staphylococcus aureus* usually affects people who are already in the hospital with another illness, especially very young children and the elderly.
■ The bacterium known as *Legionella pneumophila* causes a form of pneumonia called **Legionnaires' disease**, which can be spread through air-conditioning systems.
■ A rare type of pneumonia, known as **aspiration pneumonia**, may be caused by accidental inhalation of vomit or a food particle as a result of choking.

WHAT ARE THE SYMPTOMS?

Bacterial pneumonia usually has a rapid onset, and severe symptoms generally develop within a few hours. You may experience the following symptoms:
● cough that may produce rust colored or bloody phlegm
● chest pain that becomes worse when inhaling
● shortness of breath at rest
● high fever, delirium, or confusion.
    In infants, children and elderly people, the symptoms associated with all types of pneumonia are often less obvious. Infants may initially vomit and can develop a high fever that may cause a convulsion. Elderly people may not experience respiratory symptoms but often become progressively confused.

ARE THERE COMPLICATIONS?

■ Inflammation may spread from the alveoli in the lungs to the **pleura** (the membrane that separates the lungs from the chest wall) causing **pleurisy**. Fluid may accumulate between the two layers of the pleura, causing a pleural effusion, compressing the underlying

TEST

Chest X-ray

A chest X-ray is often one of the first tests used to investigate lung and heart conditions because it is painless, quick, and safe. To create the image, X-rays are passed through your chest onto photographic film. Dense tissues, such as the bones, absorb X-rays and appear white; soft tissues appear gray; air appears black. Damaged or abnormal lung tissue or excess fluid in the chest shows up as a white area because it does not contain air as it should. Chest X-rays are usually taken from behind, but in some cases side views may also be required.

Having a chest X-ray

You will be asked to raise your arms to move your shoulderblades away from your lungs and to take a deep breath. While the X-ray is being taken, you must remain still to prevent the image from blurring.

The shadows in this X-ray of the lungs show areas of infection due to pneumonia.

lung and making breathing difficult. If pus collects between the layers of the pleura, it is known as an **empyema.** This is a serious complication of pneumonia.

■ In severe cases of pneumonia, the microorganism that initially caused the infection may enter the bloodstream, leading to **blood poisoning** (septicemia).

■ In some vulnerable people, such as young children, elderly people, or those with a weakened immune system, the inflammation may spread and result in **respiratory failure,** which is a life threatening condition. Mechanical ventilation may then be necessary.

WHAT MIGHT BE DONE?

■ Pneumonia can be diagnosed by your doctor examining your chest and listening with a stethoscope.

■ The diagnosis may be confirmed by a chest X-ray (see box, opposite), which will show the extent of infection in the lung.

■ A sample of phlegm may be collected and tested to identify the organism that has caused the infection.

WHAT IS THE TREATMENT?

If you are otherwise healthy and have a mild form of pneumonia, you can probably be treated at home.

■ Acetaminophen, ibuprofen, or aspirin should help reduce your fever and chest pain.

■ If a bacterial infection is the cause of the pneumonia, your doctor will give you antibiotics.

■ Hospital treatment will probably be needed in severe cases of bacterial pneumonia and for infants, children, elderly people, and people whose immune systems are suppressed. Drug treatment is essentially the same as it is for people treated at home.

■ If oxygen levels in your blood are low, you will be given oxygen through a face mask. Less commonly, you may require mechanical ventilation in an intensive care unit.

WHAT IS THE OUTLOOK?

Young people who are in good health are generally able to recover from pneumonia within 2–3 weeks, and there is no permanent damage to the lung tissue. Recovery from bacterial pneumonia usually begins within a few hours of starting treatment with antibiotics. However, some severe types of pneumonia, such as Legionnaires' disease, may be fatal, especially in people whose immune systems are weakened.

See also:
• **Blood poisoning (septicemia) p. 345**
• **Chronic obstructive pulmonary disease p. 390** • **Lung cancer p. 394** • **Pleurisy p. 393**

Pleurisy

THIS IS INFLAMMATION OF THE TWO-LAYERED MEMBRANE (PLEURA) THAT SEPARATES THE LUNGS FROM THE CHEST WALL, OFTEN AS A COMPLICATION OF PNEUMONIA.

Normally, when people breathe, the two layers of the pleura slide over each other, allowing the lungs to inflate and deflate smoothly. In pleurisy, inflammation of the pleura prevents the layers from moving over each other easily; they grate as they rub against each other, causing sharp, severe chest pain when inhaling.

WHAT ARE THE CAUSES?

Pleurisy may be caused by a virus, such as **the flu,** which affects the pleura itself. However, it's often a reaction to damage to the lung just beneath the pleura. The lung damage may be due to **pneumonia** or **pulmonary embolism,** in which the blood supply to part of the lung is blocked by a blood clot. The pleura can also be affected by primary or secondary **lung cancer.**

Occasionally, an autoimmune disorder such as **rheumatoid arthritis** or **lupus,** in which the immune system attacks healthy tissues, affects the pleura and leads to pleurisy.

WHAT ARE THE SYMPTOMS?

If an infection or a pulmonary embolism is the cause of the inflammation, the symptoms usually develop rapidly over 24 hours. In other cases, the symptoms occur gradually. They include:

● sharp chest pain that causes you to catch your breath on inhaling

● feeling that it is difficult to breathe.

The pain is often restricted to the side of the chest affected by the underlying inflamed pleura. In some cases fluid accumulates between the layers of the pleura (**pleural effusion**). This condition may actually lessen the pain because it eases the movements of the pleural layers over each other.

WHAT MIGHT BE DONE?

If you have chest pain when you breathe consult your doctor immediately. The layers of the pleura rubbing can be heard against each other when your doctor listens to your chest with a stethoscope. You may need a chest X-ray to check for a problem in the underlying lung or for the presence of a pleural effusion.

WHAT IS THE TREATMENT?

■ Nonsteroidal anti-inflammatory drugs (NSAIDs) will relieve the pain and inflammation.

■ Holding the affected side while coughing helps relieve the discomfort.

■ If a lung infection is the cause, you will be prescribed a course of antibiotics. If you have a pulmonary embolism, you will be given anticoagulant drugs.

In the majority of people the condition clears up within 7–10 days of the start of treatment.

See also:
• **Lung cancer p. 394** • **Lupus p. 324**
• **Pneumonia p. 392** • **Pulmonary embolism p. 395** • **Rheumatoid arthritis p. 429**

Bronchiectasis

ABNORMAL WIDENING OF THE LARGE AIRWAYS (BRONCHI) IN THE LUNGS THAT CAUSES A PERSISTENT COUGH WITH LARGE AMOUNTS OF PHLEGM IS CALLED BRONCHIECTASIS.

Before mass immunization for childhood infectious diseases, such as **whooping cough** and **measles,** bronchiectasis used to be a common disease. Nowadays, it may still be a complication of pneumonia or occur as part of **cystic fibrosis.** Although bronchiectasis often begins in childhood, the symptoms may not be apparent until after the age of 40.

WHAT ARE THE CAUSES?

■ Childhood infections, such as whooping cough and measles.

■ Repeated lung infections in people with the inherited condition **cystic fibrosis,** in which the mucus produced by the lining of the airways is thicker than normal, blocking the bronchial tubes and collecting in the lungs.

WHAT ARE THE SYMPTOMS?

The symptoms of bronchiectasis gradually worsen over a period of several months or years and include:

● a persistent cough that produces very large quantities of dark green or yellow phlegm and is often worse when lying down

● coughing up blood

- bad breath
- wheezing and shortness of breath
- enlarged fingertips with abnormal fingernails, known as **clubbing**.

Eventually, the effects of long-term infection such as **weight loss** and **anemia** will show. up Bronchiectasis may cause extensive damage to a large area of the lung tissue, and may finally lead to **respiratory failure**.

WHAT MIGHT BE DONE?

- You should not smoke and you should avoid smoke and dust.
- A family member or friend may be taught how to give you chest physiotherapy, which ideally should be carried out on a daily basis.
- Inhaled bronchodilator drugs may be given.
- Any infection will be treated with antibiotics.
- Surgery to remove a single affected area of

the lung may cure the condition, but is very rarely appropriate.

See also:
- Cystic fibrosis p. 521 • Measles (chart) p. 544 • Whooping cough (chart) p. 544

Lung cancer

PRIMARY LUNG CANCER IS NOW THE MOST COMMON TYPE OF CANCER AFTER SKIN CANCER. IT IS THE MOST FREQUENT CAUSE OF CANCER DEATH IN BOTH MEN AND WOMEN. NOT MANY PEOPLE DIAGNOSED WITH PRIMARY LUNG CANCER LIVE LONGER THAN FIVE YEARS.

Lung cancer is a cancerous tumor that develops in the tissue of the lungs; it is most common in men between the ages of 50 and 70, but is rapidly increasing in young women because more people in this group are now smoking.

Smoking is the main cause of lung cancer. The more cigarettes you smoke, the sooner you may develop cancer. For example, if you smoke 20 cigarettes a day you may develop lung cancer 20 years later, if you smoke 40 a day you develop the disease after only 10 years.

WHAT ARE THE TYPES?

Most of these cancers begin in the cells that line the main airways (bronchi) that lead to the lungs. Lung cancer is generally divided into two categories and each has a different outlook:

- small cell carcinoma
- non-small cell carcinoma (including squamous cell carcinoma, Adenocarcinoma, and large cell carcinoma).

The most common cell type for lung cancer is adenocarcinoma, though it is not uncommon to find a combined pattern such as mixed squamous cell and adenocarcinoma. Each type of cancer has a different growth pattern and response to treatment. **Small cell carcinoma** is the most highly malignant type. This type of cancer grows rapidly and spreads very quickly throughout the body. On the other hand, **squamous cell carcinoma** grows more slowly than other types of lung cancer but also spreads to other parts of the body. **Adenocarcinoma** and **large cell carcinoma** both develop at a rate somewhere between small and squamous cell carcinomas.

WHAT ARE THE CAUSES?

About 1 in 7 smokers is likely to develop the disease by the age of 70. The risk is greater for people who have smoked more than 20 cigarettes a day since early adulthood. For people who have never smoked, the risk of

lung cancer is small, but it increases slightly for anyone who may be exposed to **other people's cigarette smoke** on a regular basis.

WHAT ARE THE SYMPTOMS?

The symptoms of lung cancer depend on how far advanced the tumor is, but early symptoms include:

- a new persistent cough or change in a long-standing cough, sometimes with blood-streaked phlegm
- chest pain, which may be felt as a dull ache, or as a sharp pain that is worse when inhaling, and usually a symptom of pleurisy that may overlie the tumor
- shortness of breath
- wheezing, if the tumor is positioned so that it blocks an airway
- abnormal curvature of the fingernails, known as clubbing
- sometimes, hoarseness of the voice can signal lung cancer.

Some lung cancers produce no symptoms until they are advanced, when they may cause shortness of breath.

WHAT MIGHT BE DONE?

- A chest X–ray may be done.
- Samples of phlegm may be taken to look for cancerous cells.
- A bronchoscopy may be performed to examine your airways (see box, right). If a tumor is found, a sample will be removed and examined under the microscope.
- Blood tests, CT (computerized tomography) scanning and MRI (magnetic resonance imaging) of the brain, chest, abdomen, and bones may be order to see if the cancer has spread.

WHAT IS THE TREATMENT?

Treatment of lung cancer depends on the type of cancer and if it has spread to other parts of the body. **Surgery** to remove a tumor in the lung is an option only if the cancer has not spread. Surgery normally involves removal of

the whole lung or a major part of it. However, in over 4 out of 5 cases, the cancer has spread to other organs, and surgery is not an option. Small cell carcinoma is usually treated with **chemotherapy**, and **radiation therapy** is used to treat cancer that cannot be removed surgically, or to reduce symptoms of cancer that has spread from the lungs. Radiation therapy does not destroy all the cancerous cells but slows tumor growth.

TEST

Bronchoscopy

Bronchoscopy is a type of endoscopy that can be used to diagnose or treat various lung disorders, such as lung cancer and tuberculosis. A rigid or flexible instrument called a bronchoscope is used to view the bronchi (airways) directly and take a specimen of the tumor for analysis – a biopsy. The rigid type is passed through the mouth into the lungs under general anesthetic. The flexible type is passed through the nose or mouth into the lungs under local anesthetic. Special instruments can be used to remove tissue samples and if necessary to perform laser surgery.

Before the procedure, you will be asked not to eat or drink anything for at least six hours. You may be given a sedative, and a local anesthetic spray will be used to numb your nose and throat. The length of the procedure depends on what your doctor needs to see and whether or not a biopsy is done.

After a bronchoscopy you may have a sore throat and hoarse voice for the next 48 hours. Over-the-counter throat lozenges may help to relieve discomfort.

WHAT IS THE OUTLOOK?

About 3 in 4 people who have surgery to remove a tumor survive for two years. People with small cell carcinoma usually **survive only 2–10 months after diagnosis.** Although surgery, chemotherapy, and radiation therapy may not always prolong life, they can alleviate symptoms and improve quality of life.

ARE THERE COMPLICATIONS?

■ **Pneumonia** may develop in an area of the lung if an airway is blocked by a tumor.
■ A tumor may also cause **pleural effusion** and **pleurisy.**
■ As the disease progresses, loss of appetite, **weight loss,** and weakness may develop.
■ There may also be symptoms from tumors that have spread from the lungs to other parts of the body. For example, **headaches** may result from cancer that has spread to the **brain.**

SECONDARY LUNG CANCER (LUNG METASTASES)

Cancerous tumors in the lungs that have spread from another part of the body are called secondary lung cancer or lung metastases. These tumors are most common in people between the ages of 50 and 70 and are more common in women than men because breast

cancer may spread to the lungs. Metastases spread to the lungs from other parts of the body via "seedlings" in the bloodstream. The primary cancers that spread most often to the lungs include cancers of the **breast, colon,** and **prostate gland.** By the time lung metastases have been detected, there are usually several tumors present and treatment of both

the primary and secondary cancers is difficult. Relief of symptoms is the best outcome that can usually be achieved.

> **See also:**
> • **CT scanning p. 401** • **MRI p. 409**
> • **Pleurisy p. 393** • **Pneumonia p. 392**

See also:
• **CT scanning p. 401** • **MRI p. 409**
• **Pleurisy p. 393** • **Pneumonia p. 392**

TREATMENT

Radiation therapy

Radiation therapy (exposure of tissue to radiation) destroys or slows the development of cancerous cells. Radiation is usually given after surgery to kill any remaining cancerous cells, but may be used in place of surgery to destroy or reduce the size of certain tumors. Radiation may be external or internal (when radioactive materials are placed in the body).

In external radiation therapy, X-rays, gamma rays, or electron beams are used to target cancerous tumors. The area to be treated is usually outlined with ink.

Pneumothorax

PNEUMOTHORAX, THE PRESENCE OF AIR BETWEEN THE PLEURA (THE TWO-LAYERED MEMBRANE THAT SEPARATES THE LUNGS FROM THE CHEST WALL), MAY OCCUR SPONTANEOUSLY IN HEALTHY YOUNG PEOPLE.

Pneumothorax is thought to be due to the rupture of a congenital blister at the top of the lungs and is rarely serious if treated promptly. It may also result from an injury such as a chest wound or fractured rib or a lung biopsy, or may be a complication of asthma, chronic obstructive pulmonary disease, or chest surgery.

WHAT ARE THE SYMPTOMS?

■ Chest pain, which may be sudden and sharp or cause only slight discomfort.
■ Shortness of breath.
■ Chest tightness.
■ With underlying lung disease, pressure may build up and compress the heart, necessitating emergency relief.

■ The windpipe is moved away from the affected side; this can be felt in the neck.

WHAT MIGHT BE DONE?

■ X-rays clearly show air in the pleural cavity.
■ Air may be removed from the pleural cavity by aspiration with a needle or by insertion of a tube.
■ Surgery may be needed to seal the leak.

Pulmonary embolism

IN PULMONARY EMBOLISM, A PIECE OF A BLOOD CLOT (EMBOLUS) BECOMES LODGED IN AN ARTERY IN THE LUNGS AND PARTIALLY OR COMPLETELY BLOCKS BLOOD FLOW IN THE AFFECTED AREA.

Usually, the clot has broken off from a larger clot (thrombus) in the veins of the legs or the pelvic region (**deep vein thrombosis**) and travelled to the lungs in the bloodstream. Rarely, blockage of a major artery may cause sudden severe symptoms and can be fatal. Pulmonary embolism is more common in

women over 35 who are overweight, smoke, and use oral contraceptives. Being immobile for a long period of time is a risk factor, because blood flow tends to slow down, especially during **pregnancy** and after any **surgery,** when the blood tends to thicken to prevent bleeding.

Pulmonary embolism is most likely to occur in people who have developed deep vein thrombosis as a result of a period of immobility, such as that following childbirth or surgery (especially surgery to repair fractures or pelvic surgery) or, rarely, during a long trip.

A tendency to develop blood clots increases the risk of deep vein thrombosis, as does smoking and taking oral contraceptives.

WHAT ARE THE SYMPTOMS?

A very large embolus that blocks the main pulmonary artery may be fatal. Small clots may cause the following symptoms:

- shortness of breath
- rapid pulse
- low blood pressure and dizziness
- sharp chest pain
- coughing up blood.

WHAT IS THE TREATMENT?

- Anticoagulants to thin the blood and prevent more clots from forming.
- Thrombolytic drugs to dissolve the clot.
- Possibly prophylactic daily low-dose aspirin to prevent clots from forming in vulnerable people.
- Emergency surgery to remove a large clot.
- Possible use of blood thinners.

See also:
- **Deep vein thrombosis p. 235**

Hiccups

THE UNMISTAKABLE SOUND PRODUCED BY HICCUPS IS DUE TO A SPONTANEOUS CONTRACTION OF THE DIAPHRAGM FOLLOWED BY INVOLUNTARY CLOSURE OF THE THROAT.

Hiccups occur even before birth; babies hiccup inside the uterus, possibly in preparation for breathing. Most cases settle after a few minutes.

SELF-HELP

There are a vast number of popular home remedies for hiccups, such as holding your breath or rapidly drinking a glass of water. If your hiccups are persistent and exhausting, your doctor may prescribe a drug, such as **chlorpromazine,** that relaxes your diaphragm. In very rare cases, it may be necessary to paralyze the diaphragm by injecting a drug around the nerves that supply it, or by cutting them.

Pneumocystis infection

ALTHOUGH RARE IN HEALTHY PEOPLE, PNEUMOCYSTIS INFECTION IS A COMMON CAUSE OF PNEUMONIA IN PEOPLE WITH REDUCED IMMUNITY, SUCH AS THOSE WITH AIDS. THIS CONDITION IS CAUSED BY INHALATION OF THE PARASITE *PNEUMOCYSTIS CARINII.*

The symptoms, which are the same as other types of pneumonia, are often more striking because of the inability of the immune system to fight back. In severely debilitated patients, pneumocystis pneumonia may be fatal.

See also:
- **HIV infection and AIDS p. 338**

Brain and Nervous System

Image shows a light micrograph of neurons in the human brain

Miriam's overview

By far the most common conditions affecting the brain are not due to disease of the brain but to disease of the arteries supplying the brain. The arteries get narrower and narrower as we age, not only in "the brain" but around the heart too, leading to stroke on the one hand and heart attacks on the other.

Mini-strokes or transient ischemic attacks (TIAs) share the same cause.

I can remember 10 or so years ago there were many theories, including exposure to aluminium, for the cause of Alzheimer's disease. People went out and replaced their aluminium cooking pans for stainless steel ones – quite unnecessarily as it turned out.

Now we know that there is a genetic background to Alzheimer's, with at least one gene being implicated. Sensitive tests have evolved that allow early diagnosis. Perhaps the best news is that HRT reduces the Alzheimer's risk but must be balanced against the health risk of HRT for some women.

"brain *exercise* is *simply* thinking, concentrating, and *feeling*"

One heartening very new piece of research shows that, contrary to conventional teaching, brain cells retain their ability to regenerate. It was always thought that damaged brain cells had little power to recover or regrow. Now we know that isn't the case. We retain these regenerative powers even into old age. This knowledge has important implications for the rehabilitation of stroke patients and patients who've had treatment for conditions such as brain tumors.

Think of the brain as a muscle that responds – and grows – as the result of exercise. Brain exercise is simply thinking, concentrating, feeling, and we can stimulate cell regeneration by exercising the brain when we think, concentrate and feel.

"We now know that *brain cells* can *regenerate*"

There have been few new treatments for multiple sclerosis (MS) that have stood the test of time but one that seems to help many sufferers, and one which was stumbled on accidentally, is marijuana. The profound symptomatic relief from marijuana makes a powerful argument in favor of allowing its use by prescription.

Opponents of this view, including the government, would prefer the active substance cannabinol to be prescribed in pill form. But many MS users will testify that it isn't as simple as that. There are thousands of active microsubstances in marijuana and they all seem to help. It's marijuana that MS patients need, not pills.

INSIDE
your brain and nervous system

Together, the **brain** and the **spinal cord** form the **central nervous system**. All of the nerves that branch out from the central nervous system and pass through the rest of the body make up the **peripheral nervous system**. The brain and spinal cord process and coordinate the nerve signals that are gathered and transmitted by the peripheral nervous system.

The brain and spinal cord consist of two main types of tissue: **gray matter**, which creates and processes nerve impulses, and **white matter**, which transmits nerve impulses. The brain itself contains structures known as the **cerebrum**, which links to every part of the body; the **cerebellum**, which is involved in balance and movement; the **brain stem**, which relays nerve impulses between the brain and spinal cord and controls heart rate and breathing; and a region that contains the **hypothalamus**, which controls the hormonal system. The spinal cord is actually an extension of the brain stem and travels downward from the base of the skull.

the nervous system

Optic nerve

Cerebrum

Facial nerve

Cerebellum

Vagus nerve

Spinal cord

Spinal nerve

Radial nerve

Ulnar nerve

Median nerve

Femoral nerve

Sciatic nerve

Common peroneal nerve

Tibial nerve

the brain and spinal cord

Subarachnoid space

Cerebral cortex

Meninges

Cerebrum

Choroid plexus

Skull

Thalamus

Pineal gland

Cerebellum

Hypothalamus

Pituitary gland

Brain stem

Spinal cord

Nerve structure

Nerve fiber

Myelin sheath

Blood vessel

The brain and spinal cord coordinate and control the nerve impulses transmitted to and from nerves in the rest of the body.

A nerve contains hundreds of nerve fibers. Larger fibers have a sheath of myelin, a fatty substance.

All of the nerves in the body except for the brain and spinal cord are part of the peripheral nervous system.

ARTERY DISEASE AND THE BRAIN

For most people some degree of blockage of the arteries is inevitable as we grow older. Atheroma, as this narrowing is called, can affect all of our arteries, but the symptoms are most dramatic if the arteries supplying the heart (see Angina, p. 224) and the brain (see Transient ischemic attacks, p. 402 and Stroke, below) are affected, causing the arteries to harden and narrow.

Hardening of the arteries in the brain is exactly the same as hardening of the arteries of the heart and one rarely occurs without the other. Atheroma in any artery interferes with blood supply and leads to blood clots forming. When atheroma affects the arteries supplying the brain, the outcome may be a transient ischemic attack or stroke.

For a doctor, looking at the back of your eyes is like looking through a window at the inside of your body because it's possible to look directly at your arteries on the back of your eye and see if they're becoming blocked up. So when your optometrist or doctor looks at the back of your eyes they aren't just looking to see if your eyes are healthy, they are looking to see if your arteries are healthy too. Your doctor then has a general idea of the condition of all your arteries, including those supplying the heart and the brain.

So a simple eye examination can alert your doctor to the fact that you could be a candidate for a heart attack or stroke in the future, creating the opportunity to advise you appropriately.

Stroke

A STROKE, SOMETIMES CALLED A CEREBROVASCULAR ACCIDENT (CVA), RESULTS FROM DAMAGE TO PART OF THE BRAIN BECAUSE ITS BLOOD SUPPLY IS CUT OFF.

The blood supply to the brain can be compromised by a blockage (thrombosis or embolism) or a leak (hemorrhage) from one of the arteries in the brain. A CVA is more common in people with high blood pressure, diabetes, and high cholesterol levels. People with an irregular heartbeat (atrial fibrillation) are also more susceptible to strokes. After a stroke, part of the brain no longer functions and urgent medical attention is needed.

WHAT HAPPENS?
There is often little or no warning of a stroke. Immediate admission to the hospital for assessment and treatment is essential if there is to be a chance of preventing permanent brain damage. The aftereffects of a stroke vary depending on the location and extent of the damage. They range from mild, temporary symptoms, such as loss of vision, to lifelong disability or, in some people, if the stroke causes extensive brain damage, to coma and death.

If the symptoms disappear within a 24-hour period, the condition is known as a **transient ischemic attack** or **TIA**, which is a warning sign of a possible future stroke.

HOW COMMON IS IT?
Each year about 600,000 people in the US have a stroke and the risk increases with age. The chance of having a stroke more than doubles for each decade of life after age 55. Although the number of deaths from stroke has fallen over the last 50 years, stroke is still the **third most common cause of death** after heart attacks and cancer in the US.

WHAT ARE THE CAUSES?
■ About half of all strokes occur when a **blood clot** forms in an artery in the brain, a process called **cerebral thrombosis**.
■ **Cerebral embolism** occurs when a fragment of a blood clot that has formed elsewhere in the body, such as in the heart or the main arteries of the neck, travels in the blood and lodges in an artery supplying the brain. Just under one-third of all strokes are caused by cerebral embolism.
■ **Cerebral hemorrhage** (bleeding), which causes about one-fifth of all strokes, occurs when an artery supplying the brain ruptures and blood seeps out into the brain itself.

Blood clots that lead to cerebral thrombosis and cerebral embolism are more likely to form in an artery that has been damaged by **atherosclerosis**, a condition in which fatty deposits (atheroma) build up in artery walls. Factors that increase the risk of atherosclerosis are a high-fat diet, smoking, diabetes mellitus, high blood pressure, and high cholesterol levels.

WHAT ARE THE RISKS?
■ The risk of cerebral embolism, thrombosis, or hemorrhage is increased by **high blood pressure**, which should always be assessed and treated promptly.
■ Cerebral embolism may be a complication of some heart conditions such as **heart rhythm disorders**, **heart valve disorders,** and a **recent heart attack**, all of which can cause blood clots to form in the heart.
■ Sickle-cell anemia, an abnormality of the red blood cells, also increases the risk of cerebral thrombosis because abnormal blood cells tend to clump together and block blood vessels.

■ Less commonly, thrombosis is caused by narrowing of the arteries supplying the brain due to the inflammation of an autoimmune disorder, such as **polyarteritis nodosa**, in which the immune system attacks the body's own healthy tissues.

WHAT ARE THE SYMPTOMS?
In most people, the symptoms develop rapidly over a matter of seconds or minutes. The exact symptoms depend on the area of the brain affected. The symptoms may include:
● weakness or inability to move on one side of the body
● numbness on one side of the body
● tremor, clumsiness or loss of control of fine movements
● visual disturbances, such as loss of vision in one eye
● slurred speech
● difficulty in finding words and understanding what others are saying
● vomiting, vertigo, and difficulty in maintaining balance.

With a severe stroke, the affected person may become unconscious and may decline into coma and die.

HOW IS IT DIAGNOSED?
■ If you suspect that a person has had a stroke, take them to the hospital immediately to find the cause and start treatment.
■ Imaging of the brain, such as computerized tomography (CT) scanning or magnetic resonance imaging (MRI), may be done to find out whether the stroke was due to bleeding or a blockage in a vessel.
■ Antihypertensive drugs, which help control

TEST

CT scanning

Computerized tomography (CT) scanning uses X-rays in conjunction with a computer. A series of X-rays is passed through the body at slightly different angles to produce highly detailed cross sectional images (slices) of the body, called tomograms. CT scanning makes it possible to gather detailed information about organs painlessly and so that your exposure to radiation is kept to a minimum.

A CT scanner consists of an X-ray source and an X-ray detector, both of which rotate during the procedure so that they remain opposite each other. CT scanning uses X-rays in a different way from an ordinary X-ray machine to give a higher quality image. A CT scan is able to show details that are impossible to see using ordinary X-rays, including fibrous tissue in solid organs such as the liver.

The information from the X-ray detector is sent to the computer, which builds up cross-sectional images of the body and displays them on a monitor. These resulting images can be stored either as computer files or on conventional X-ray film. More sophisticated computers can produce three-dimensional images from standard CT data. Newer CT scanners use the spiral (or helical) technique, in which the scanner rotates around you as

A CT scan is a painless procedure that may take less than one minute to one hour to perform, depending on the condition being investigated.

the bed moves forward slowly so the X-ray beams follow a spiral course. This type of CT scanning produces three-dimensional images and reduces the time taken for the scans to be completed.

During a CT scan you will lie on a motorized bed that will move you into the scanner. The technician will ask you to lie very still and hold your breath while each scan is taken. The bed moves forward a little more after each scan. If you are very anxious about the procedure you may be given a mild sedative beforehand; you may also be invited to bring a relative or friend with you if you feel you would like moral support. The time it takes to have a CT scan

depends on the nature of the scan and may range from a few seconds to an hour.

CT scans are most often performed on the head and abdomen. However, they are also used for chest, pelvis, and spine and can be used to guide biopsy procedures, in which cells or tissue are taken from internal organs for examination. Like conventional X-rays, CT scanning also produces clear images of bone. Blood vessels and areas of high blood flow, such as the lungs, can also be imaged. These images may be enhanced by using a contrast medium (a substance that makes a hollow or fluid-filled structure visible on the image).

TEST

Carotid Doppler scanning

Carotid Doppler scanning uses ultrasound to look at the flow of blood through blood vessels in the neck. It is generally used to investigate disorders such as transient ischemic attack or stroke. Ultrasound waves from a transducer produce a picture of the blood flow, which can reveal narrowing of the carotid blood vessels in the neck. Scanning takes about 20 minutes and is painless and safe.

In a carotid Doppler scan, the technician places the ultrasound transducer on one of the carotid arteries to look at the flow of blood through it.

high blood pressure, and a daily dose of aspirin, which reduces the risk of blood clot formation, may be prescribed.

■ Smokers should stop smoking immediately.

■ Weakness and loss of movement may be treated with physical therapy.

■ Speech problems can be alleviated with speech therapy.

■ Antidepressant drugs and/or counseling may help treat the depression that can follow a stroke.

WHAT IS THE OUTLOOK?

Treatment of risk factors, such as high blood pressure, will lower the risk of a future, potentially fatal stroke. Clot-busting drugs may be given to dissolve a clot.

TEST

Cerebral angiography

Cerebral angiography uses X-rays to look for abnormalities of the arteries supplying the brain. It is often used to investigate **transient ischemic attack** and **stroke**. Under local anesthesia, a thin, flexible tube called a catheter is inserted into an artery, usually at the groin or elbow, and guided to an artery in the neck. When the catheter is in position, a special dye that shows up on X-rays is injected through it. The outline of the blood flow through the arteries is then seen on the X-ray (angiogram).

See also:
- **Anemias p. 236**
- **Arrhythmias p. 231**
- **Autoimmune disorders p. 323**
- **Diabetes mellitus p. 504**
- **Heart attack (myocardial infarction) p. 230**
- **High blood pressure p. 226**
- **Psychological therapies p. 286**
- **The heart and atherosclerosis p. 222**

Transient ischemic attacks (TIAs)

A TRANSIENT ISCHEMIC ATTACK IS SIMILAR TO A STROKE BUT MUCH LESS SEVERE. IN THE WEST, ABOUT 1 IN 600 PEOPLE HAS A TIA, AND WITHOUT TREATMENT ABOUT 1 IN 5 OF THESE PEOPLE WILL HAVE A STROKE WITHIN A YEAR.

A transient ischemic attack or TIA is like a mini-stroke from which you recover in 24 hours, although usually less. It's due to a reduced blood supply to the brain. Like strokes, TIAs are most common in men and sometimes run in families. Just as with strokes, smoking, high blood pressure, and a high-fat diet are risk factors. A TIA is a warning sign and shouldn't be ignored because there is a strong possibility that it may be followed by a stroke.

WHAT HAPPENS?

In a transient ischemic attack, part of the brain suddenly and briefly fails to function properly because it is temporarily deprived of oxygen by blockage of its blood supply. Transient ischemic attacks can last for anything from a few seconds to one hour and have no aftereffects. However, **if the symptoms persist for longer than 24 hours**, the attack is classified as a stroke.

WHAT ARE THE SYMPTOMS?

The symptoms of a transient ischemic attack usually develop suddenly and are often short-lived, lasting only a few minutes. Symptoms vary depending on which part of the brain is affected and may include the following:

- loss of vision in one eye or blurry vision in both
- slurred speech
- difficulty finding the right words
- problems understanding what other people are saying

- numbness on one side of the body
- weakness or paralysis on one side of the body, affecting one or both limbs
- feeling of unsteadiness and general loss of balance.

Although the symptoms of transient ischemic attacks disappear within an hour, attacks tend to recur. People may have a number of attacks in one day or over several days, and treatment is crucial. Your doctor will probably want to do the same tests as for a stroke. Sometimes, several years may elapse between attacks.

WHAT IS THE TREATMENT?

■ Once a transient ischemic attack has been diagnosed, the goal of treatment is to reduce your risk of having a stroke in the future, so your doctor will prescribe appropriate drugs to treat **high blood pressure** or an **irregular heartbeat** if you have either of these conditions.

■ Treatment after a transient ischemic attack can be as simple as taking a **daily aspirin** to help prevent clots from forming inside blood vessels. Other drugs that help prevent blood clotting, such as **warfarin**, may be prescribed if emboli (clot fragments) originate from clots that have formed in the heart.

■ You will be advised to **reduce the amount of fat in your diet** and, if you **smoke**, you should stop.

■ If you have **diabetes mellitus**, you should make sure your blood glucose levels are well controlled.

■ If your doctor finds that the arteries in your neck are severely narrowed, he or she may recommend a surgical procedure called a **carotid endarterectomy** to clear fatty deposits from the narrowed arteries.

■ Alternatively, you may be referred for a surgical procedure known as a **balloon angioplasty**, in which a small balloon is inserted into the affected artery or arteries. Once in place, the balloon is inflated to open up the narrowed section of artery. Both balloon angioplasty and carotid endarterectomy increase the diameter of the blood vessel and improve the blood supply to the brain.

WHAT IS THE OUTLOOK?

Transient ischemic attacks may occur intermittently over a long period or they may stop spontaneously. Of those people who have a transient ischemic attack, **about 1 in 5 will have a stroke within a year**. The more frequently you have transient ischemic attacks, the higher your risk of having a stroke in the future. However, if you take appropriate steps to change aspects of your **lifestyle**, such as stopping smoking and adopting a low-fat diet, and take the medicines your doctor gives you, you will reduce the risk of having more transient ischemic attacks or a stroke.

See also:
- **Stroke p. 400**

PAIN IN THE HEAD AND FACE

There are many causes of head pain and face pain. The pain varies in severity but in **migraines, cluster headaches, trigeminal neuralgia**, and particularly after shingles, the pain can be very severe and last a long time, making relief difficult to achieve.

Pain that starts out of the blue should always be investigated by your doctor. And pain associated with any other symptom such as nausea, dizziness, and visual disturbance should be discussed with your doctor right away.

In many instances we don't know the exact cause of head and face pain and treatment can only be to relieve the symptoms.

Unusual head or face pain should always have the benefit of a specialist's opinion. You may be referred to a neurologist.

Sadly space only allows me to cover the most common and the most serious causes of head and face pain, that is, **headaches, migraines, meningitis, trigeminal neuralgia,** and **subarachnoid hemorrhage**.

Headache

HEADACHES ARE EXTREMELY COMMON AND MOST OF THEM AREN'T ANY CAUSE FOR ANXIETY. OCCASIONALLY, THOUGH, A HEADACHE IS A SYMPTOM OF A SERIOUS ILLNESS, SUCH AS MENINGITIS OR A BRAIN HEMORRHAGE, AND REQUIRES URGENT MEDICAL ATTENTION.

Headaches are the most common of all head pains and arise for a multitude of reasons. Tension headaches are the most universal.

WHAT ARE THE CAUSES?
There are many possible causes of headache that determine where the pain is and how severe it is.
■ About 3 out of 4 headaches are caused by **tension** in the scalp or neck muscles due to stress. Tension headaches tend to occur frequently and cause moderate pain, particularly

---

WARNING:

If your headache is severe, lasts more than 24 hours or is accompanied by other symptoms, such as fever, problems with your vision, or vomiting and drowsiness, you should seek medical help without delay.

---

at the back and front of the head. It's often described as a tight band encircling the head.
■ Other common causes of headache include a **hangover, irregular meals, long trips, noise,** a **stuffy atmosphere, stormy weather, too much sleep, too much excitement, fever, sinusitis,** and **toothache**.

Reassuringly, very few headaches have a serious underlying cause and all that's required are self-help measures such as painkillers, relaxation exercises, aromatherapy, yoga, or sleep.

HEADACHES REQUIRING URGENT MEDICAL ATTENTION
■ A severe headache with fever, a stiff neck, and rash may be a sign of **meningitis**, a condition in which the membranes covering the brain and spinal cord become inflamed.
■ A sudden headache that feels like a blow to the back of the head could be a **subarachnoid hemorrhage**, in which bleeding occurs between the membranes covering the brain.
■ In elderly people, a headache with tenderness of the scalp or temple may be due

to **temporal arteritis**, in which blood vessels in the head become inflamed.

WHAT MIGHT BE DONE?
If your doctor suspects an underlying condition is causing your headache, you may require tests, such as computerized tomography (CT) scanning or magnetic resonance imaging (MRI) of your brain, and an opinion from a neurologist.

WHAT IS THE TREATMENT?
Treatment depends on the cause of the headache. For example, a tension headache will usually clear up with rest and painkillers. Cluster headaches and migraines (see below) can be treated with drugs such as sumatriptan. Excess painkillers, especially those containing codeine, can actually result in a headache.

See also:
• **Meningitis p. 404**
• **Relaxation p. 292**
• **Subarachnoid hemorrhage p. 408**

Migraines

A MIGRAINE IS ONE OF THE MOST PAINFUL AND DISABLING EXPERIENCES YOU CAN EVER HAVE AND CAN PREVENT NORMAL LIFE WHILE THE HEADACHE LASTS.

Anyone can suffer from migraines regardless of age, race, intelligence, or occupation. At least 10 percent of the population are prone to migraine attacks.

There's quite a lot of evidence that migraine and related conditions, such as asthma, hay

fever, allergies, and eczema, run in families. 1 out of 3 sufferers have a close relative with migraines.

It's not just adults who suffer – migraines typically begin in the teens or early 20s – and even young children can be affected, but for

most people migraines burn out, usually when they are 30–40 years of age.

WHAT ARE THE CAUSES?
The actual cause of migraine is probably a
continued on page 407

FOCUS *on* meningitis

Meningitis is included here because the main symptom is often headache and it affects the membranes over the brain. The headache is so typical that it should alert you to the possibility of meningitis.

Then you should search for other confirmatory signs, and finding even one should be enough for you to seek urgent medical attention. The headache is caused by inflammation of the **meninges**, the membranes that cover the brain and spinal cord, due to an infection by a virus or a bacterium.

WHAT IS IT?

● In meningitis, the membranes that cover the brain and spinal cord, known as the meninges, are inflamed.
● Viral meningitis is more common and usually not as severe as bacterial meningitis.
● While the bacterial form is less common, it can be **life threatening**.
● Both viral and bacterial meningitis can occur at any age but bacterial meningitis occurs predominantly in **children** and viral meningitis is most common in **young adults**.
● There is a form of meningitis now seen in people with **AIDS**.
● In the US, several hundred cases of bacterial meningitis and about 500 cases

of viral meningitis are diagnosed each year, although the true incidence of viral meningitis is thought to be much higher than this.

WHAT ARE THE CAUSES?
Viral:
Many different viruses cause meningitis. Among the most common are **enteroviruses**, such as the **coxsackie virus** that cause sore throats or **diarrhea** too, and more rarely, the virus that causes **mumps**. Viral meningitis tends to occur in **small outbreaks**, most commonly in **summer**.
Bacterial:
Bacterial meningitis usually occurs for no detectable reason in a healthy child or teenager. Less often, bacterial meningitis may occur as a complication of an infection elsewhere in the body that spreads to the **meninges** through the bloodstream.
● The bacterium *Streptococcus pneumoniae*, the most common cause of meningitis in **adults** in the West, can spread from the lungs, where it causes pneumonia, to the meninges.
● The most common cause in unvaccinated

children is *Haemophilus influenzae* type B.
● Another bacterium, called *Neisseria meningitidis*, causes **meningococcal** meningitis. There are three types of these bacteria. Type B is the most common in the US, while type C causes 40 percent of cases in Great Britain. Many people carry the meningitis bug in the back of their throats, but for unknown reasons only a tiny fraction of them develop meningitis.
● The bacterium that causes **tuberculosis** can also infect the meninges.
     Bacterial meningitis usually occurs as **single cases only**. However, there may be small outbreaks, especially in institutions such as **schools** and **colleges**. This form of meningitis is most common during the **winter**.
     People who have a weakened immune system as a result of an existing illness or a particular treatment, such as people with HIV infection or those having chemotherapy, are at increased risk of developing meningitis.

HOW DOES MENINGITIS START?
● Initially, meningitis may produce vague **flulike symptoms**, such as **mild fever** and **aches and pains**, which worsen.
● Symptoms are the most severe in bacterial meningitis and may develop rapidly, often within a few hours.
● The symptoms of viral meningitis may take a few days to develop.

Differences between viral and bacterial meningitis

Meningitis type	Who is at risk?	Symptoms	Diagnosis	Treatment
VIRAL	● Anyone, but more common in **young adults** ● Occurs in small outbreaks ● Most common in summer	Symptoms may develop **quite slowly** over a few days. Severe headache, fever, stiff neck, dislike of bright light	By lumbar puncture; CT scan or MRI to exclude brain swelling	Once a lumbar puncture has excluded bacterial meningitis, **no treatment** is **usually needed** beyond analgesics for pain relief.
BACTERIAL	● Anyone, but more common in **children** ● Usually single cases ● Most common in winter	Symptoms may develop **rapidly**, over the course of a few hours. Severe headache, fever, stiff neck, dislike of bright light, **rash that does not fade when pressed**	By lumbar puncture; CT scan or MRI to exclude raised pressure in brain	If confirmed by lumbar puncture, **antibiotics are continued and patients may be monitored in an intensive care unit**. Anticonvulsant and other drugs may be given as necessary.

TEST

How to recognize the meningitis rash

The meningitis rash on white skin

The meningitis rash on black skin

The rash of meningitis is caused by blood leaking from broken blood vessels beneath the skin and, unlike other rashes, **it does not fade when pressed**. The rash is usually dark red or purple and can appear anywhere on the body.

The best way to check a rash that you suspect may indicate meningitis is to press a clear drinking glass against it; if the rash is still visible through the glass, you should seek medical advice immediately.

Pressing a glass against the rash allows you to see clearly whether it fades.

● In tuberculosis meningitis, symptoms develop slowly and may take several weeks to become pronounced.

WHAT ARE THE MAIN SYMPTOMS?
Symptoms include:
● **severe** headache
● **fever**
● **stiff** neck
● **dislike** of bright light
● in **meningococcal** meningitis, a rash of flat, reddish purple spots, varying in size from **pinheads** to large patches, which **do not fade when pressed by a glass**.

Unless prompt treatment is given, bacterial meningitis may lead to:
● **seizures**, drowsiness and coma
● the collection of pus to form a brain abscess, resulting in compression of nearby tissue.

WHAT MIGHT BE DONE?
If meningitis is suspected, immediate medical attention and admission to a hospital is necessary. The first priority is to start intravenous antibiotics and then to find out which type of meningitis, if any, is present.
● A sample of fluid will be removed from around the spinal cord (lumbar puncture)

and tested for evidence of infection.
● Antibiotics, given intravenously, are started immediately.
● CT scanning or MRI may also be done to look for a brain abscess.
● If the tests exclude bacterial meningitis, people are usually allowed to go home providing they are well enough. There is no specific treatment for viral meningitis, but drugs may be given to relieve symptoms, such as painkillers for headache.
● If bacterial meningitis is confirmed by lumbar puncture results, antibiotics are continued for at least a week.
● If meningitis is found to be caused by tuberculosis bacteria, **antituberculous** drugs will be given.
● In cases of bacterial meningitis, continuous monitoring in an intensive care unit is often needed.
● Intravenous fluids, anticonvulsant drugs, and drugs to reduce inflammation in the brain, such as **corticosteroids**, may be given.

WHAT IS THE OUTLOOK?
Recovery from viral meningitis is usually complete within 1–2 weeks. It may take weeks or months to make a complete recovery from

bacterial meningitis. Occasionally, long-term problems may occur, such as impaired hearing or memory impairment due to damage to part of the brain. About 1 in 10 people with bacterial meningitis dies despite treatment. Deaths most commonly occur in infants and elderly people.

CAN IT BE PREVENTED?
People in close contact with someone with **meningococcal** meningitis, such as family members, are usually given antibiotics for two days as a precaution. This treatment kills the **meningococcal** bacteria that may be present at the back of the throat and prevents their spread to other people.

Children are now routinely vaccinated against *H. influenzae* type b, an important cause of meningitis in childhood, and against *N. meningitidis* type C (meningitis C).

People traveling to high-risk areas, such as Africa, may need to be vaccinated against other types of **meningococcal bacteria**, so consult your doctor.

THE MENINGITIS C VACCINE

This is a vaccine against group C **meningococcal** meningitis and **septicemia** which gives long lasting protection to babies as young as two months old.

HOW EFFECTIVE IS IT?

Scientists say that the new vaccine is at least 95 percent effective against group C meningococcal meningitis and septicemia, but it gives absolutely no protection against group B. About 40 percent of cases in Great Britain, for example, are caused by group C, but group B causes most of the rest. **There is no vaccine to prevent group B disease, so it is still very important to be aware of the signs and symptoms of meningitis and septicemia.**

WHEN SHOULD I BE ON THE LOOK OUT FOR MENINGITIS?

Cases of meningitis and septicemia increase enormously every winter. The goal of the vaccination program is to prevent deaths from the disease by protecting as many of those people who are most at risk as possible before winter comes.

WHO IS AT RISK OF MENINGITIS?

Babies and teenagers in the age groups have the highest risk.

HOW DO PEOPLE GET THE MENINGITIS C VACCINE?

● Babies and toddlers receive the vaccine along with their other routine immunizations. Anyone who hasn't had the vaccine and feels that they should have it should contact their doctor.

IS THE MENINGITIS C VACCINE SAFE?

● The meningitis C vaccine has been tested on over 6,000 people in Great Britain and in 21,000 people elsewhere and has been shown to be safe and to give long-term immunity.
● No serious side effects occurred during safety testing. Some babies and children have had a slight temperature, an unsettled night, or redness and swelling of the skin where they were injected, but the chance of having these mild reactions is no greater than with other childhood vaccines. Older children and teenagers sometimes complain of headache. Vomiting has been reported in some babies, but this is more likely due to other vaccines

that have been given at the same time.
● The vaccine is not "live" and cannot cause even a mild form of meningitis or septicemia.
● There are no new ingredients in the vaccine. All the ingredients of the new vaccine have already been given to millions of children over many years as components of other vaccines, without causing any harm.

ARE THERE ANY PEOPLE WHO SHOULDN'T HAVE THE VACCINE?

● People who have had a severe reaction to the plain **meningococcal** vaccine or **Hib** or **diphtheria** vaccines should not have the vaccine.
● Vaccination should be postponed in anyone who is ill with a high fever.
● It has not been tested in pregnant women, and although there is no reason to suggest it is not safe during pregnancy, women who think they might be pregnant should speak to their doctor or nurse about it.

IS THERE A PROBLEM WITH "MULTIPLE" VACCINES?

Some parents might be worried that having

DTP, Hib, polio, and the new vaccine together will overload babies' immature immune systems.
● There is no danger in having these vaccines at the same time. During trials of the new vaccine, scientists showed that the vaccines could not interact in any way that could harm babies and children.
● These vaccines do not "overload" the immune system. **Vaccines work by arousing a response from the immune system, but getting all the routine vaccinations and the new C-strain vaccine at the same time is less of a challenge to the immune system than everyday events like a baby getting a throat infection or a toddler falling and scraping a knee.**
● Routine vaccinations are timed to protect babies when they need it most.

See also:
● Chemotherapy p. 257
● HIV infection and AIDS p. 338
● Mumps (chart) p. 544
● Immunization timetable p. 519
● Thrombocytopenia p. 239

Preventing a migraine and avoiding the triggers

You should try to be aware of your migraine triggers and avoid them as much as possible. You'll be able to spot warning signs and therefore control the migraine attack better. You can very often abort a migraine attack if you take some form of treatment as soon as you sense the aura, then the headache may never appear. If an attack starts, try to treat it as quickly as possible with a pain medication such as acetaminophen, the soluble form if possible.

Many factors are known to trigger a migraine. You need to identify the ones that affect you. Avoiding these factors may help reduce the frequency and severity of attacks.

■ Keep a diary for a few weeks to help pinpoint trigger factors.

■ Avoid any food you find brings on an attack. Common dietary triggers of migraines include red wine, cheese (especially aged cheese), and chocolate.

■ Eat regularly, because missing a meal may trigger an attack.

■ Follow a regular sleep pattern if possible, because changing it may trigger an attack.

■ If stress is a trigger, you may find it helpful to try relaxation exercises.

continued from page 403
change in brain hormones, resulting first in constriction of blood vessels (causing the flashing lights) then dilatation (causing the thumping headache). There are many well-known triggers that change these brain hormones, the best known of which is **serotonin.**

HOW LONG DO MIGRAINE ATTACKS LAST?
Migraines can vary in severity from being a throbbing headache, usually on one side, which lasts an hour or so, to one that's so excruciating you have to lie immobile in a darkened room for two or more days.

WHAT ARE THE SYMPTOMS?
Migraine symptoms can take a variety of forms.

VISION PROBLEMS
About half an hour prior to the start of the headache you may notice flashing lights or that lights have a halo around them. Part of your visual field may go dark. These symptoms can occur on their own **without a headache,** in which case it's called an **optical migraine.**

HEADACHE
Migraine is a headache plus. The throbbing or knifelike headache, usually above one eye, is followed by nausea (feeling sick), vomiting (being sick), and an aversion to light, sound, and movement of any kind. More than one of these symptoms has to be present to be considered a migraine, but not all.

PARALYSIS
Sometimes sensation and movement on one side of the body are affected – like a mini-stroke – and return to normal when the headache goes. This is called a **hemiplegic migraine.**

ABDOMINAL PROBLEMS
A migraine where there are mainly abdominal symptoms, such as vomiting and stomach pain, is called **abdominal migraine** and is common in children.

WHAT'S AN AURA?
An aura precedes the headache and can be anything from distorted vision to "pins and needles," or simply an odd feeling.

MIGRAINE IN WOMEN
Many women find that migraine forms a part of the **premenstrual syndrome (PMS)** due to the hormonal changes that take place each month.

Women's hormone levels change constantly throughout their reproductive lives, and this could be why more women suffer from migraines than men. There's also **menopausal migraine** that occurs when hormonal levels sink as menstruation stops.

MIGRAINE IN CHILDREN
Between the ages of 5 and 15, **1 child in 9** suffers from migraine attacks. Until puberty, boys and girls suffer equally.

Childhood migraine can differ quite dramatically from the adult form. Attacks tend to be shorter (sometimes only an hour) with the emphasis on abdominal pain, nausea, and vomiting; the headache can be mild, even absent.

Young children are often unable to describe the symptoms of a migraine and may describe the way they feel as a "sick headache" or "a headache in my tummy." As children get older, abdominal symptoms usually subside and the headache becomes prominent.

The differentiation from **appendicitis** can be difficult and children have been opened up unnecessarily.

CAN CERTAIN FOODS BE A TRIGGER?
Certain foods such as chocolate, cheese, fortified wine like sherry and port, and caffeine may trigger an attack. Missing meals, causing a **drop in blood sugar,** can precipitate a migraine attack.

CAN STRESS CAUSE MIGRAINE?
A period of stress is often followed by a migraine – usually when you're beginning to unwind. If you have a stressful job or very busy lifestyle, you can often have a **weekend or vacation migraine.**

CAN LACK OF SLEEP BE A TRIGGER?
An irregular sleep pattern is a common cause of migraine. Sleeping in on the weekend is often perceived as a good thing, but in reality are as much a trigger for migraine attacks as lack of sleep.

WHAT OTHER FACTORS CAUSE MIGRAINE?
Travel, weather changes, hormonal factors (in women), loud noises, bright or flickering lights, TV, movies, or videos, shopping, and strong smells have all been known to trigger attacks.

WHAT IS THE TREATMENT?
Everyone who suffers has their favorite recipe for a migraine, arrived at by trial and error over the years. For instance, mine was **Stemetil** suppositories (prescription only) and a darkened room; my stepdaughter's is Solpadeine extra strength, two capsules every four hours.

A hard and fast rule is that any headache can develop into a migraine, so never ignore one.

Your pharmacist will advise you about over-the-counter remedies and medicines for children. However, these are largely for the treatment of symptoms – they don't get at the cause.

From your doctor there are many prescription medicines to try, the latest one being a selective serotonin reuptake inhibitor (SSRI), which treats the cause. Some of these medicines are injectable, while others can be inhaled or ingested as wafers. Also, if migraine headaches occur frequently (more than about four times a month) there are medications that you take daily to prevent migraines from coming on.

Your emergency kit: When my migraines were worst I never went anywhere without my migraine remedies. Carry yours with you always so that you can take action fast.

See also:
• **The atopic family of conditions p. 311**

Trigeminal neuralgia

TRIGEMINAL NEURALGIA IS A SEVERE PAIN ON ONE SIDE OF THE FACE DUE TO COMPRESSION, INFLAMMATION, OR DAMAGE TO THE TRIGEMINAL NERVE. THE PAIN IS EXPERIENCED IN BRIEF, RECURRENT EPISODES WHICH, ALTHOUGH SHORT-LIVED, ARE EXCRUCIATINGLY PAINFUL.

The trigeminal nerve carries sensation from parts of the face to the brain and controls some of the muscles that are involved in chewing. Damage or irritation to this nerve causes the repeated **bursts** of sharp, stabbing pain known as trigeminal neuralgia. The pain, felt in the lip, gum, or cheek on one side of the face, may follow the path of the nerve or affect the skin supplied by the nerve. Attacks of trigeminal neuralgia may last from a few seconds to several minutes.

Trigeminal neuralgia is unusual in people under the age of 50, and in young people might be an early sign of multiple sclerosis.

Path of trigeminal nerve

Ophthalmic branch

Maxillary branch

Mandibular branch

Trigeminal nerve

WHAT MIGHT BE DONE?

The pain rarely has a sinister origin but can be triggered by touch, shaving, washing, eating, drinking, even talking.

■ Treatment in the main is symptomatic so you may be given analgesics, such as **acetaminophen**, to relieve the pain.

■ If the pain persists, your doctor may prescribe anticonvulsant drugs, such as **carbamazapine**, which are effective in trigeminal neuralgia.

Unlike analgesics, which should be taken only when the pain is present, both the anticonvulsants and antidepressants must be taken **every day** to **prevent attacks from occurring**.

SURGERY

■ If, rarely, a tumor is found, surgery may be necessary to remove it.

■ Surgery may also be used to separate the trigeminal nerve from a blood vessel if the vessel is compressing the nerve.

■ People who have chronic severe pain that does not respond to drugs may be offered treatment to numb the face. The trigeminal nerve may be cut or alcohol may be injected into the nerve to deaden it. The pain can also be alleviated by using a special heated probe to destroy the nerve.

NB If you have had treatment to numb the

Postherpetic neuralgia

Postherpetic facial pain may be the most serious side effect of having shingles involving the face. The **herpes zoster** virus may damage the facial nerve and about one-third of people can be left with severe pain that lasts a long time. The older the person and the more pronounced the rash the longer the pain lasts. Rarely, steroid hormones may be prescribed because they may help prevent the pain from becoming chronic.

face, trigeminal neuralgia will not recur, but you must avoid hot food or drinks that could burn you.

WHAT IS THE OUTLOOK?

Attacks of neuralgia may stop spontaneously, become more frequent, or persist without change for months or years. However, symptoms usually improve significantly with treatment.

Subarachnoid hemorrhage

BLEEDING INTO THE SPACE BETWEEN THE TWO INNER MEMBRANES COVERING THE BRAIN IS KNOWN AS A SUBARACHNOID HEMORRHAGE. IT TYPICALLY PRODUCES A SEVERE HEADACHE THAT FEELS LIKE A SEVERE BLOW TO THE TOP OF THE HEAD.

Most subarachnoid hemorrhages occur spontaneously rather than as a result of a head injury. They are most common in people between the ages of 35 and 60.

WHAT ARE THE SYMPTOMS?

The onset of symptoms is usually sudden and without warning. However, in a few cases, a headache gradually comes on over a few hours before the hemorrhage occurs. Typical symptoms may include the following:

● sudden, severe headache
● nausea and vomiting
● stiff neck
● dislike of bright light
● irritability.

In a few minutes, these may lead to:

● confusion and drowsiness
● seizures
● loss of consciousness.

The body may react by constricting the arteries in the brain, further reducing its supply of oxygen, and this may cause a stroke, possibly resulting in muscle weakness or paralysis.

WHAT MIGHT BE DONE?

■ If a subarachnoid hemorrhage is suspected, admission to the hospital must be immediate.

■ **Computerized tomography (CT) scanning** is usually carried out to identify the location and extent of bleeding.

■ A **lumbar puncture** may be performed to

look for signs of bleeding into the fluid surrounding the brain and spinal cord.

■ **Magnetic resonance imaging (MRI)** or **cerebral angiography** may also be done to look at the blood vessels of the brain.

■ If a subarachnoid hemorrhage is confirmed, drugs called **calcium channel blockers** are usually given to reduce the risk of a stroke.

■ If cerebral angiography shows that one or more **berry aneurysms** are present, surgery will probably be required to remove them.

WHAT IS THE OUTLOOK?

If another hemorrhage does not occur within the next six months or if surgery is successful, **further bleeding is unlikely**.

Brain tumors

BRAIN TUMORS ARE ABNORMAL GROWTHS THAT MAY DEVELOP IN BRAIN TISSUE
OR IN THE MENINGES, THE MEMBRANES THAT COVER THE BRAIN. THE SERIOUSNESS OF
A BRAIN TUMOR DEPENDS ON ITS LOCATION, SIZE, AND RATE OF GROWTH.

Brain tumors may be cancerous or non-cancerous. However, unlike most tumors elsewhere in the body, cancerous and non-cancerous brain tumors may be equally serious because both types of tumor can compress nearby tissue, causing pressure to build up inside the skull. Brain tumors are more common in men, usually occurring between the ages of 60 and 70.

Tumors that arise from brain tissue or from the meninges that cover the brain are called **primary tumors** and are comparatively rare.

Secondary brain tumors (metastases) are more common than primary tumors. They are always cancerous, having developed from cancer cells that have spread to the brain from tumors in other parts of the body, such as the breast.

Certain types of brain tumor, such as **neuroblastomas**, affect only children.

WHAT ARE THE SYMPTOMS?

Symptoms are usually the result of a primary tumor or a metastasis compressing part of the brain or raising the pressure inside the skull. They include:

- headache that is usually more severe in the morning and is worsened by coughing or bending over
- nausea and vomiting
- blurry vision.

Other symptoms tend to be related to whichever area of the brain is affected by the tumor and may include:

- slurred speech
- difficulty reading and writing
- change of personality
- numbness and weakness of the limbs on one side of the body.

A tumor may also cause **seizures**. Sometimes, a tumor blocks the flow of the cerebrospinal fluid that circulates in and around the brain and spinal cord. As a result, the pressure inside the ventricles (the fluid-filled spaces in the brain) increases and leads to further compression of brain tissue. Left untreated, **drowsiness** can develop, which may eventually progress to **coma** and then **death**.

HOW ARE BRAIN TUMORS DIAGNOSED?

- If a brain tumor is suspected, you will have an immediate assessment by a neurologist.
- You will have computerized tomography (CT) scanning or magnetic resonance imaging (MRI) of the brain to look for a tumor and check its location and size.
- If these tests suggest that the tumor has

spread from a cancer elsewhere, you may need other tests such as **mammography** or **chest X-rays** to check for tumors in the breast or lungs.

- Further **MRI** scans may be done to show the tumor and surrounding tissue in more detail.

- You may also need to have a **brain biopsy**, in which a sample of the tumor is removed and examined under a microscope in order to identify the type of cell from which the tumor has developed.

continued on page 412

TEST

Magnetic resonance imaging (MRI)

The technique of magnetic resonance imaging has been used since the early 1980s to provide highly detailed sectional images of internal organs and structures. These images are created by a computer using information received from a scanner. Unlike X-rays or computerized tomography (CT) scanning, MRI does not involve your being exposed to potentially harmful radiation; instead, it uses magnets and radio waves.

Images from MRI scans are similar to those produced by CT scanning, but MRIs can distinguish abnormal tissue much more clearly. MRI scans can also be taken at a greater range of planes through the body than is possible with CT scanning and therefore can be used to image any part of the body. MRI is radiation-free and is

considered to be one of the safest imaging techniques available.

During an MRI scan, you lie inside a scanner surrounded by a large, powerful magnet. A receiving magnet is then placed around the part of your body that is to be investigated. If large areas, such as the abdomen, are to be imaged, the receiving magnet is fitted inside the MRI scanner; for smaller areas, such as a joint, a magnet may be placed around the part to be scanned. The MRI scanner is operated from an adjacent room because the computer controlling the scanner has to be protected from the powerful magnetic field created during the procedure. MRI scanners can be very noisy and you may be given earplugs or headphones to wear. Each MRI scan lasts only a few minutes, but a full examination may require many scan sequences and may last between 15 minutes and an hour. If you feel anxious about the procedure you may be given a mild sedative; you may also be asked if you would like to bring a relative or a friend for moral support.

MRI scanning is especially useful for looking at the brain and for detecting brain tumors. MRI is also valuable for looking at the spinal cord and may be used to investigate low back pain. Sports injuries, especially in the knee, are increasingly being examined using a MRI. In a small number of cases, a MRI has been used to examine the breasts. MRI scans show the locations of tumors within the breast tissue more accurately than plain two-dimensional X-rays. In addition, since a MRI does not use radiation, MRI scans can be repeated often, allowing doctors to monitor a condition carefully.

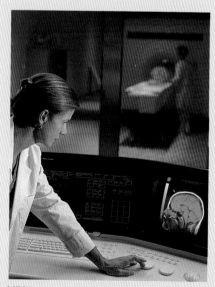

MRI images are viewed by computer in the control room, away from the scanner's magnetic field.

FOCUS *on* chronic fatigue syndrome

The terminology applied to fatigue is confusing for everyone, including doctors. As anyone knows who has gotten chronically tired, there's a range of fatigue which, at one end, may need nothing more than a few early nights to catch up but at the other end of the spectrum may require time off work resting in bed.

So it's important to separate ordinary fatigue from chronic fatigue syndrome (CFS), also known as **myalgic encephalopathy** or ME.

WHAT IS CFS?

Chronic fatigue syndrome is a complex illness with extreme fatigue over a long time. Extreme exhaustion is nearly always a prominent part of CFS, plus muscle pain and a flulike malaise.

Other symptoms can include problems with concentration and memory, loss of balance, digestive problems, sleep disturbances, and mood swings.

CFS affects up to 800,000 people in the US but we know of no exact cause, there's no specific test for it and treatment is purely symptomatic. Many cases arise after a persistent viral infection that has **weakened** the immune system. The association of a viral infection followed by fatigue isn't new of course. We've known for years that the mononucleosis virus, for example, can leave behind it lassitude and depression that can take 9–12 months to get better.

HOW DO WE GET FATIGUED?

Our fight-and-flight system, the release of adrenaline to prepare us to fight an enemy or run from him, was perfect millennia ago, when stress would consist of the occasional sighting of hostile neighboring tribesmen.

But today it's constantly on red alert because of the pressured environment we live in. It simply cannot cope with modern-day stresses.

Our bodies are never given the chance to

How can I help myself?

Along with experts in the field, I'm very concerned that supplements are promoted heavily to a vulnerable group of people whose expectations may be falsely raised. I personally would always recommend good eating combined with exercise to relieve chronic fatigue. Exercise is the only way I know of increasing the amount of energy I have. The cornerstone of fitness, exercise is also the antidote to fatigue and ensures refreshing sleep. Run through the benefits of exercise on p. 21. But here are tables of the **foods that contain carbohydrates** and minerals that can also help boost your energy levels.

Minerals

I personally would always recommend good eating combined with exercise to relieve chronic fatigue. But first – here are foods containing minerals that will help to bump up your energy levels.

Best food source	Nutrient	Quantity	Maximum
Broccoli, canned salmon, cheese, fortified orange juice, milk, soy products, and yogurt	Calcium	1,000mg	1,500mg
Barley, legumes, lobster, nuts, organ meats, and prunes	Copper	1.5 to 3mg	9mg
Beans, fortified breads and cereals, green leafy vegetables, nuts, oysters, and scallops	Magnesium	310mg	700mg
Avocados, beef, dried apricots, fortified breads and cereals, legumes, and shellfish	Iron	15mg	65mg
Chicken, mushrooms, nuts, onions, seafood, seeds, garlic, wheatgerm, and whole grain bread	Selenium	55mcg	200mcg
Beef, fortified cereals, legumes, liver, shellfish, wheatgerm, and yogurt	Zinc	12mg	30mg

Carbohydrates

The best source of energy is carbohydrate, so start loading your diet with it.

Food	Grams of carbohydrates
230g serving cooked pasta	50
60g serving cornflakes	50
150g serving rice	45
2 slices of whole grain bread	30
Toasted bun	30
54g milk chocolate	30
2 scoops of mashed potato	25
1 medium banana, apple, or pear	20
160ml serving orange juice	15

And here's how to eat carbohydrates. Try to eat 5g of carbohydrate per two pounds of body weight each day. For a 155lb man this means having at least 350g of carbohydrates a day and for a 120lb woman, at least 275g. To reach these figures have some carbohydrate foods at each meal. Try bread and bread products, pasta, breakfast cereals, rice, potatoes, beans, root vegetables, fruits, and **crispbreads**. Ideally eat a meal containing carbohydrates 2–4 hours prior to exercise and a small snack such as a banana about an hour before. Try to eat around 50g of carbohydrates within 2 hours of finishing exercise. This helps refuel the muscles and should include some quickly absorbed foods such as fruit bars, bananas, **cornflakes** with skim milk, golden or brown raisins, or a glass of high-energy drink.

recover from an acute (sudden) stress reaction and soon end up in a state of chronic (long-term) stress, which may compromise the immune system.

When the immune system can't fight off infection we're into a vicious downward spiral to exhaustion.

WHAT ARE THE SYMPTOMS OF CFS?

Although the number and severity of symptoms may vary, the major symptoms of chronic fatigue syndrome are:

- **prolonged** severe fatigue lasting at least six months
- **impairment** of short-term memory or concentration
- **sore** throat
- **tender** lymph nodes
- **muscle** and joint pain without swelling or redness
- **unrefreshing** sleep
- **headaches**
- **prolonged** fatigue and feeling ill after even mild exertion.

Many people who have chronic fatigue syndrome also develop symptoms of depression, such as loss of interest in their work and leisure activities, or of anxiety. This in turn can lead to prolonged inactivity, resulting in "deconditioning" of the whole body that affects the muscles particularly. Conditions involving an allergic reaction, such as eczema and asthma, may become worse in people who have chronic fatigue syndrome.

HOW IS CFS DIAGNOSED?

There are specific criteria which must be present before a diagnosis can be made. Just being plain tired doesn't mean you've got CFS. Your doctor may suspect chronic fatigue syndrome if you have had prolonged fatigue for more than six months with no obvious cause, and you also have at least four of the other symptoms listed. Even

if no underlying cause is identified, the diagnosis of chronic fatigue syndrome will only be made if your symptoms meet the diagnostic criteria.

COPING WITH CFS

If you develop chronic fatigue syndrome, you are likely to have fluctuating energy levels. You may find that you need to be flexible and adjust your lifestyle to help you live with the condition. The following actions may be helpful.

- Try to divide the day into sessions of rest and work.
- Graded exercise may be useful. Try to set yourself a progressive increase in activity week by week.
- Set realistic goals for yourself.
- Make dietary changes, in particular by drinking less alcohol and cutting out drinks containing caffeine.
- Try to reduce stress.
- Join a support group so that you do not feel isolated.

WHAT IS THE TREATMENT FOR CFS?

Although there is no specific treatment for chronic fatigue syndrome, there are a number of measures that may help you cope with the condition.

- Your doctor may give you drugs to help relieve some of your symptoms. For example, headaches and joint pain may be relieved by analgesics, such as aspirin, or **nonsteroidal anti-inflammatory drugs**.
- **Antidepressant drugs** may produce an improvement in your condition even if you have not developed the symptoms of depression.
- Your doctor may advise you to have **counseling** to help you cope with your illness and to provide support.
- You may also find **cognitive therapy** and **behavior therapy** beneficial.

WHAT IS THE OUTLOOK?

Chronic fatigue syndrome is a long-term condition. Many people find that symptoms are at their worst in the first 1–2 years. In more than half of all cases, the condition clears up completely after several years. In some people, the symptoms of chronic fatigue syndrome come and go over a number of years.

See also:
- Insomnia p. 296 • Depression p. 298
- Menopause p. 497

TATT syndrome

If you're one of the many in the US population who feels exhausted most of the time and wakes up **unrefreshed**, you're in good company.

You have a **recognized** syndrome – TATT – "tired all the time" syndrome. There's no cure, but you could feel a whole lot better if you eat **well**, get eight hours sleep and set aside time for yourself each day. The simple explanation for present-day long-term fatigue is that we all do too much. We're on overload, even **burned-out**.

A special problem for women Women are often struggling to care for children,

working in the day, doing household chores in the evening, and being a wife at night. And women feel under pressure to perform well in all their roles, so it's hardly surprising that many end up chronically tired.

People with chronic fatigue often work too hard. If, on top of everything, you sleep badly you may never recharge your batteries at the end of the day. The key is to have a balance between work and leisure. It's no bad thing to take an inventory of your lifestyle, the time you go to bed, the quality of sleep you get, and whether you take time off to relax and enjoy yourself.

continued from page 409

WHAT IS THE TREATMENT?

Treatment for brain tumors depends on whether there is one tumor or several, the precise location of the tumor and the type of cell involved.

■ Primary brain tumors are commonly treated **surgically**. The aim of surgery is to remove the entire tumor, or as much of it as possible, with minimal damage to surrounding brain tissue.

■ Surgery will probably not be an option for tumors that are located deep within the brain tissue.

■ **Radiation therapy** may be used in addition to surgical treatment, or as an alternative to it, for both cancerous and noncancerous primary tumors.

■ Since brain metastases are often multiple, surgery is not usually an option. However, in those cases where there is a single metastasis, surgical removal may be successful. Multiple tumors are usually treated with a course of radiation therapy or, less commonly, with **chemotherapy**.

■ Other treatments may be necessary to treat the effects of brain tumors. For example, the drug **dexamethasone** may be given to reduce the pressure inside the skull.

■ **Anticonvulsant drugs** may also be prescribed to prevent or treat seizures.

■ If a tumor blocks the flow of cerebrospinal fluid in the brain so that the fluid builds up inside the ventricles, **a small tube** may be inserted through the skull in order to bypass the blockage.

■ You may also benefit from treatments for the physical effects of the tumor, such as physical therapy to help with mobility problems.

■ Speech therapy is helpful for learning how to deal with speech problems.

WHAT IS THE OUTLOOK?

The future is usually brighter for slow growing, noncancerous tumors, and many will be completely cured. For other tumors, the outlook depends on the type of cell affected and whether the tumor can be surgically removed. About 1 in 4 people is alive two years after the initial diagnosis of a primary cancerous brain tumor, but few people live longer than five years. Most people with brain metastases do not live longer than six months, although in rare cases, a person with a single metastatic tumor may be cured. All types of brain tumor carry a risk of permanently damaging nearby brain tissue.

Multiple sclerosis

MULTIPLE SCLEROSIS (MS) IS INFLAMMATION OF THE BRAIN AND SPINAL CORD, CAUSING WEAKNESS AND PROBLEMS WITH SENSATION AND VISION. IT USUALLY DEVELOPS BETWEEN THE AGES OF 20 AND 40 AND IS MORE COMMON IN WOMEN.

MS is the most common nervous system disorder affecting young adults. Nerves in the brain and spinal cord are progressively damaged, causing a wide range of symptoms that affect sensation, movement, body functions, and balance. Specific symptoms may relate to the particular areas that are damaged and vary in severity between individuals. For example, damage to the optic nerve may cause reduction of vision, especially color vision. If nerve fibers in the spinal cord are affected, it may cause weakness and heaviness in the legs or arms. Damage to nerves in the brain stem, the area of the brain that connects to the spinal cord, may affect balance, causing severe vertigo. Classically, MS symptoms occur intermittently and may be followed by long periods of freedom from symptoms (remission). However, some people have chronic symptoms that gradually get worse. In the US 200 new cases of MS are diagnosed each week. People who have a close relative with MS are more likely to develop the disorder. The condition is much more common in the northern hemisphere, which suggests that environmental factors also play a part.

WHAT ARE THE CAUSES?

MS is an **autoimmune** disorder in which the body's immune system attacks its own tissues, in this case the nervous system. Many nerves in the brain and spinal cord are covered by a protective insulating sheath of material called **myelin**. In MS, small areas of myelin are damaged, leaving holes in the sheath, a process known as **demyelination**. Once the myelin sheath has been damaged, impulses cannot be conducted normally along nerves to and from the brain and spinal cord. At first, damage may be limited to one nerve, but myelin covering other nerves may be damaged over time. Eventually, damaged patches of myelin insulation are replaced by scar tissue.

It is thought that MS may be **triggered** by external factors such as a **viral infection** during childhood in genetically susceptible individuals.

WHAT ARE THE TYPES?

There are **three** types of MS.

■ In the most common form, known as **relapsing–remitting MS**, symptoms last for days or weeks and then clear up for months or even years. However, some symptoms may eventually persist between the attacks.

■ About 3 in 10 people with MS have a type known as **chronic–progressive MS**, in which there is a gradual worsening of symptoms with no remission.

■ The third type is **primary progressive**, in which deterioration is seen from the start.

A person with relapsing–remitting MS may go on to develop chronic–progressive MS.

WHAT ARE THE SYMPTOMS?

Symptoms may occur singly in the initial stages and in combination as the disorder progresses. They may include:

● reduction of vision, especially color vision

● numbness or tingling in any part of the body

● fatigue, which may be persistent

● weakness and a feeling of heaviness in the legs or arms

● problems with coordination and balance, such as an unsteady gait

● slurred speech

● vertigo.

Stress, heat, and fatigue make symptoms worse. About half of the people who have MS find it hard to concentrate, and experience

TEST

MRI images

Magnetic resonance imaging can be used to detect areas of demyelination in the brain that are characteristic of multiple sclerosis.

In these MRI images of brains of people with multiple sclerosis, areas of demyelination appear yellow and orange.

memory lapses. **Depression** is common in advanced multiple sclerosis. Later in the course of the disease, some people with muscle weakness develop **painful muscle spasms**. Nerve damage can also lead to **urinary incontinence**, and men may find it is increasingly difficult to achieve an **erection**. Eventually, damage to myelin covering nerves in the spinal cord may cause **partial paralysis**, and an affected person may need a **wheelchair**.

HOW IS IT DIAGNOSED?

There is no single test to diagnose MS, and, because symptoms are so wide-ranging, a diagnosis is only made once other possible causes of the symptoms have been excluded. Quite often it's possible to make a fairly certain diagnosis from your medical history and a physical examination.

■ If you are having visual problems, such as blurry vision, you may be referred to an ophthalmologist, who will examine the optic nerve, which is commonly affected in the early stages of the disorder.

■ Your doctor may arrange tests to find out how quickly your brain receives messages when certain nerves are stimulated. The most common test uses the visual pathways.

■ You will probably also have an imaging test of the brain, such as MRI, to see if there are areas of demyelination.

■ Your doctor may order a **lumbar puncture**, a procedure in which a small amount of the fluid that surrounds the spinal cord is removed for microscopic analysis. Abnormalities in this fluid may confirm the diagnosis.

WHAT IS THE TREATMENT?

■ There is no cure for MS, but if you have relapsing–remitting MS, **interferon or copaxone** may help lengthen remission periods and shorten the length of attacks.

■ Your doctor may prescribe **corticosteroids** to shorten the duration of a relapse. Mitoxanthrone is used to treat chronic-progressive multiple sclerosis.

■ Your doctor may treat muscle spasms with a muscle relaxant drug.

■ Similarly, incontinence can often be improved by drugs.

■ Problems in getting an erection may be helped by a drug treatment such as **sildenafil**.

■ If you have mobility problems, your doctor may arrange for you to have physical therapy.

■ Occupational therapy may make day-to-day activities easier.

WHAT CAN I DO?

If you are diagnosed with MS, you and your family will need time and possibly counseling to come to terms with the disorder. You should minimize stress in your life and avoid exposure to high temperatures if heat tends to make your symptoms worse. Regular gentle exercise, such as swimming, will help keep your muscles strong without risk of overstraining them.

WHAT IS THE OUTLOOK?

The progression of MS is extremely variable, but people who are older when the disease first develops tend to fare less well. About 7 in 10 people with MS have active lives with long periods of remission between relapses.

Marijuana and MS

Marijuana can be very helpful in MS, relieving muscle spasms and incontinence. Walking and general mobility may become possible after smoking marijuana. Cannabinoids, thought to be the active ingredients in marijuana that help MS, are not as potent as marijuana itself, which contains over 3000 chemically active substances. This use of marijuana makes a strong case for its being available by prescription. A test is currently underway for the use of marijuana in treating MS.

However, some people, particularly those with chronic–progressive MS, become increasingly disabled. Half of all people with MS are still leading active lives 10 years after diagnosis, and the average lifespan from diagnosis is 25–30 years.

See also:
• **Psychological therapies p. 286**

MS and pregnancy

MS does not affect a woman's fertility in any way and has no effect on the course of pregnancy, labor, or delivery. Women with MS have very few complications during pregnancy. In a study of 36 pregnant women with MS, the only complications mentioned were two cases of mild vomiting. There is no increase in spontaneous abortions, complications in pregnancy or delivery, malformations, or stillbirths.

Many research studies suggest that pregnancy is a **protection** for women with MS. This is probably because the natural state of immunosuppression that occurs in pregnancy to prevent a woman from rejecting her baby also suppresses the inflammation that causes nerve and brain damage in MS. On the other hand,

there is a slightly increased risk of a flare-up for 3–6 months after the birth. Between 40 and 60 percent of women have a relapse during this time – 20 percent of these suffer from permanent side effects while 80 percent go back to the state of MS they were in before the pregnancy. The long-term course of MS does not appear to be affected by pregnancy.

MS and the baby

In an area with a high prevalence of MS, 1 person in 1000 out of the normal population would be likely to develop the disease. One study has shown that among children of people with MS, the figure could rise to 1 in 100. Most people feel that the risk of their child having MS is not great enough to stop them from choosing to conceive.

MS medication and the developing baby

Drugs to stop painful muscle spasms would be discontinued before conception, as would long-term anti-inflammatory therapies. Drugs that help to control urinary frequency or incontinence would also be stopped. Very powerful drugs such as steroids, which are only given if the life of either the mother or the baby is in danger, are hardly ever needed during pregnancy.

After the birth

There are no medical reasons for a woman with MS not to breast-feed, except if she is taking medication, and she should insist on doing so. Rest, however, is extremely important, so she should make arrangements to have help and express enough milk for the night feedings so that they can be given by others.

Alzheimer's disease

IN ALZHEIMER'S DISEASE, THERE IS A PROGRESSIVE DETERIORATION IN MENTAL ABILITY DUE TO DEGENERATION OF BRAIN TISSUE.

It is normal to become mildly forgetful with increasing age, but severe impairment of short-term memory may be a sign of Alzheimer's disease, in which brain cells gradually degenerate and deposits of an abnormal protein build up in the brain. As a result the brain tissue shrinks, with progressive loss of mental abilities, known as **dementia**.

Alzheimer's disease is the most common form of dementia and the fourth most common cause of death in the West. In the US, Alzheimer's disease affects about **1 in 10 people over age 65 and nearly half of people over 85**.

WHAT ARE THE CAUSES?

The underlying cause is unknown, although genetic factors are almost certainly involved. Studies have found that 15 in 100 people with Alzheimer's disease have a parent affected by the disorder. In women, lack of estrogen after menopause probably plays a role and hormone replacement therapy (HRT) is advocated to prevent the onset of Alzheimer's.

WHAT ARE THE SYMPTOMS?

The first symptom is usually **forgetfulness**. The normal deterioration of memory that occurs in old age becomes much more severe and begins to affect intellectual ability. Memory loss is eventually accompanied by other symptoms, including:
- impairment of memory, particularly when trying to recall recent events
- gradual loss of intellect, affecting reasoning and understanding
- difficulty engaging in conversation
- reduced vocabulary
- emotional outbursts
- wandering and restlessness
- neglect of personal hygiene
- poor concentration
- difficulty understanding both written and spoken language
- wandering and getting lost, even in familiar surroundings.

In the early stages of the disease people are aware that they have become more forgetful. This may lead to depression and anxiety. Over time, the existing symptoms may get worse and additional symptoms may develop, including:
- slow movements and unsteadiness when walking
- rapid mood swings from happiness to tearfulness
- personality changes, aggression, and feelings of persecution.

Sometimes people find it difficult to sleep and become restless at night. After several years, most people with the disease cannot look after themselves and need full-time care.

HOW IS IT DIAGNOSED?

- New tests can help in the early diagnosis of Alzheimer's disease. However, severe depression may mimic dementia – so-called pseudodementia.
- Tests may be arranged to exclude other possible causes of dementia. For example, blood tests may be carried out to check for vitamin B deficiencies.
- Imaging tests such as CT scanning or a MRI may be done to show shrinkage of the brain and exclude other brain disorders, such as subdural hemorrhage or a brain tumor.
- An assessment of mental ability, including memory and writing tests, may be done to determine the severity of the dementia.

WHAT IS THE TREATMENT?

There is no cure, but drugs such as **donepezil** may slow the loss of mental function in mild to moderate cases. Some of the symptoms that are associated with Alzheimer's disease, such as depression and sleeping problems, can be relieved by antidepressant drugs. A person who is agitated may be given a sedative drug to calm them. HRT may reduce risk for Alzheimer's in women if given at menopause, but there is no evidence that HRT helps Alzheimer's once it begins.

Eventually, **full-time care** will probably be necessary either at home or in a nursing home. Caring for a person who has Alzheimer's disease is often stressful and many caregivers need practical and emotional support, especially if the affected person becomes hostile and aggressive. Support groups can help people cope with caring for an elderly relative with the disease. Most people with Alzheimer's disease survive for 5–10 years from the time of diagnosis.

SELF-HELP

Caring for someone with dementia

If you are taking care of someone with dementia, you need to balance his or her needs with your own. In the early stages, it is important to allow the person to remain as independent and active as possible. As the disorder progresses, there are several measures you can take to help compensate for the person's failing memory, loss of judgement, and unpredictable behavior.
- Put up a bulletin board with a list of things that need to be done during each day.
- If wandering is a problem, persuade the person to wear a badge with your contact details and phone number on it.

- Place notes around the house to help the person remember to turn off appliances.
- Consider installing bath aids to make washing easier.
- Try to be patient – it's common for people with dementia to have frequent mood changes.
- Give yourself a break whenever you can by finding someone who can help for a few hours, so investigate local respite care.
- Join a caregivers' support group and investigate day centers or respite care.

Simple procedures such as leaving notes as reminders can help people with mild dementia.

Parkinson's disease and parkinsonism

PARKINSON'S DISEASE IS A PROGRESSIVE BRAIN DISORDER CAUSING SHAKING AND PROBLEMS WITH MOVEMENT. IT RESULTS FROM A LACK OF DOPAMINE, THE NEUROTRANSMITTER THAT SMOOTHES MUSCLE MOVEMENTS, AND IS MOST COMMON IN MEN OVER THE AGE OF 60.

Parkinson's disease results from degeneration of cells in a particular part of the brain called the **basal ganglia**, which control the smoothness of muscle movements. Cells in the basal ganglia produce a **neurotransmitter** (a chemical that transmits nerve impulses) called **dopamine**, which acts with **acetylcholine**, another neurotransmitter, to fine-tune muscle movements. In Parkinson's disease, the level of dopamine relative to acetylcholine is reduced, and muscle control is lost.

Although the cause of Parkinson's disease is not known, genetic factors are probably involved. About 3 in 10 people with the disorder have an affected family member. About 1 in 100 people over the age of 60 in the West have Parkinson's disease.

Parkinsonism is the term given to the symptoms of Parkinson's disease when they are due to another underlying disorder. Certain drugs, including some **antipsychotic drugs** used to treat severe psychiatric illness as well as antinausea and antivertigo drugs, may cause parkinsonism, as may repeated head injuries.

WHAT ARE THE SYMPTOMS?

The main symptoms of Parkinson's disease begin gradually over a period of months or even years. Symptoms include:
- greasiness of the face and excessive salivation
- expressionless or masklike face
- tremor of one hand, arm, or leg, usually when resting and later occurring on both sides
- muscle stiffness, making it difficult to start moving
- handwriting that gets smaller and smaller
- slowness of movement
- shuffling walk
- stooped posture.

Later, stiffness, immobility, and a constant trembling of both hands can make daily tasks difficult to perform. Speech may become slow and hesitant, and swallowing may be difficult. Many people with Parkinson's disease develop depression. About 3 out of 10 people with the condition eventually develop dementia.

HOW IS IT DIAGNOSED?

Since Parkinson's disease begins gradually, it is often not possible to diagnose immediately.
- Your doctor will arrange for you to see a neurologist. Tests such as CT scanning or magnetic resonance imaging (MRI) may be done to exclude other possible causes.
- Sometimes it is only a positive response to antiparkinsonism drugs that confirms the diagnosis.
- If a specific underlying disorder is found to be causing your symptoms, you will be diagnosed as having parkinsonism rather than Parkinson's disease.

HOW MIGHT THE DOCTOR TREAT IT?

Although there is no specific cure for Parkinson's disease, **drugs, surgery,** and **physical treatments** may relieve symptoms. If you have parkinsonism due to medication your doctor may change your drugs. Symptoms may then disappear in about eight weeks. If symptoms do not resolve, treatment with antiparkinsonism drugs may be needed.

DRUG TREATMENT
- The goal of drug treatment is to restore the balance of dopamine and acetylcholine in the brain. For mild to moderate symptoms, two main types of drugs are prescribed:
1. Drugs such as **amantadine** to increase the activity of dopamine.
2. Anticholinergic drugs, such as **trihexyphenidyl**, to decrease acetylcholine activity.

Together these drugs help reduce shaking and muscle stiffness and improve mobility.
- Amantadine may be effective for only a few months. Side effects include nausea, insomnia, loss of appetite, and occasionally hallucinations.
- Levodopa is usually effective for several years. At first, its side effects are mainly nausea and vomiting, although in some cases involuntary movements and hallucinations may occur.
- Long-term use of levodopa sometimes results in abrupt changes of symptoms known as the **"on–off"** phenomenon. Movements are sluggish and difficult as the drug wears off during the "off" periods. During the "on" periods, mobility is impaired by involuntary movements such as tics, spasms, and writhing.
- Levodopa is often prescribed **in combination with** another drug called **carbidopa**, which reduces the side effects. Carbidopa prevents the breakdown of levodopa, so smaller doses of levodopa provide the same effect.
- Anticholinergic drugs can be effective for several years. However, side effects may include vision problems, difficulty urinating, and a dry mouth.
- If you experience any changes in your symptoms, it is important for you to consult your doctor because your drug regimen may need to be altered.

PHYSICAL TREATMENT
The doctor may arrange **physical therapy** to help with mobility problems, or **speech therapy** for speech and swallowing problems. If you are finding it difficult to manage at home, **occupational therapy** may be useful. The therapist may suggest changes, such as installing grab-rails in your home, to make it easier for you to move around.

SURGICAL TREATMENT
- Younger people may have surgery if the tremor cannot be controlled by drugs and they are otherwise in good health. Surgery for Parkinson's disease involves destroying a part of the brain tissue responsible for the tremor.
- Recent experimental therapies include replacement of damaged brain cells with **transplanted fetal adrenal tissue.**
- Deep brain stimulation with electrical impulses to reduce tremor is proving helpful and holds promise as a future treatment.

WHAT IS THE OUTLOOK?

The course of the disease is variable, but drugs may be effective in treating the symptoms and improving quality of life. People can lead active lives for many years after being diagnosed with Parkinson's disease. However, most people eventually need daily help, and their symptoms may become increasingly hard to control with drugs.

SELF-HELP

Keeping mobile

It is important to continue to exercise and take care of your general health. Try to take a walk each day. Stretching exercises can help you maintain your strength and mobility. However, you should also rest during the day to avoid getting tired. Encouragement and emotional support from family, friends, and support groups is also important.

Creutzfeldt–Jakob disease

CREUTZFELDT–JAKOB DISEASE (CJD) IS AN EXTREMELY RARE CONDITION IN WHICH
BRAIN TISSUE IS PROGRESSIVELY DESTROYED BY AN UNUSUAL INFECTIOUS AGENT.

A general decline in all areas of mental and physical ability leads ultimately to death. CJD affects about one person in a million each year worldwide.

WHAT IS THE CAUSE?

CJD is caused by an infectious agent known as a **prion**, which replicates in the brain and causes brain damage.

■ One type of CJD, accounting for 15 in 100 cases, has been found to run in families. Most people who develop this form of CJD are over age 50. Usually, the source of the infection is unknown. In about 1 in 20 affected people it can be traced to previous treatment with products derived from human tissue. Before the use of artificial growth hormone to treat growth disorders, one source of infection was human growth hormone injections.

■ In the mid-1990s, a new rare variant of CJD that affects younger people was discovered in Great Britain. This form of the disease is believed to be linked with eating contaminated meat from cattle with a disease called **bovine spongiform encephalopathy (BSE)**. It is possible that this form of the disease might be passed from a pregnant mother to her unborn child.

WHAT ARE THE SYMPTOMS?

It is thought that CJD is present for between two and 15 years before symptoms start to appear. Early symptoms develop gradually and may include:
● depression
● poor memory
● unsteadiness and poor coordination.
Other symptoms develop as the condition progresses and include:
● sudden muscle contractions
● seizures
● weakness or paralysis on one side of the body
● progressive dementia
● impaired vision.
Eventually, an affected person may become unable to move and talk. People with late-stage CJD who are confined to bed are also prone to serious lung infections.

WHAT MIGHT BE DONE?

CJD is usually diagnosed from the symptoms. Tests performed on the tonsils and appendix may confirm the presence of the prions associated with the new variant form of CJD. Other tests are:
● magnetic resonance imaging (MRI) to exclude other treatable causes
● brain biopsy, during which a small piece of tissue is surgically removed for microscopic examination.
CJD cannot be cured, but drugs can relieve some of the symptoms.
■ Symptoms of depression may be treated with antidepressant drugs.
■ Muscle contractions may be controlled by muscle relaxants.
The disorder is usually fatal within three years.

Motor neuron disease

IN MOTOR NEURON DISEASE THERE IS PROGRESSIVE DEGENERATION OF THE NERVES IN THE
BRAIN AND SPINAL CORD THAT CONTROL MUSCLE ACTIVITY, LEADING TO WEAKNESS AND WASTING
OF THE MUSCLES. SOME TYPES OF MOTOR NEURON DISEASE ARE INHERITED.

WHAT ARE THE SYMPTOMS?

In the initial stage of the disease, there is weakness and wasting, developing over a few months and usually affecting muscles of the hands, arms, or legs.

Other early symptoms may include:
● twitching movements in the muscles
● stiffness and muscle cramps
● difficulty performing twisting movements, such as unscrewing bottle tops and turning keys.
As the disease progresses, other symptoms may include:
● dragging one foot or a tendency to stumble when walking
● difficulty climbing stairs or getting up from low chairs
● less commonly, slurred speech, hoarseness, and difficulty swallowing if the muscles of the mouth and throat are involved
● mood swings, anxiety, and depression
● recurrent chest infections and possibly pneumonia, if the muscles involved in breathing and swallowing are affected and small particles of food enter the lungs
● the head falling forward because the muscles in the neck are too weak to support it
● eventually, difficulty in breathing due to weakness of the muscles that control respiration.

WHAT IS THE TREATMENT?

Currently, no treatment can significantly slow down the progression of motor neuron disease, although a new drug called riluzole may have a small effect. Treatment for symptoms may include antidepressants to relieve depression and antibiotics to treat chest infections. A gastrostomy may be done to treat difficulty swallowing. This is a surgically created opening through which a permanent feeding tube is inserted directly into the stomach or the small intestine.

Usually, a team of specialists will be available to provide support and care for an affected person and members of his or her family. Counseling may be offered to both, and the affected person may be given physical therapy to help keep joints and muscles supple.

Facial palsy

IN FACIAL PALSY, ALSO CALLED BELL'S PALSY, THERE IS WEAKNESS OR PARALYSIS
OF THE FACIAL MUSCLES ON ONE SIDE OF THE FACE DUE TO DAMAGE TO THE FACIAL
NERVE. THE PROBLEM USUALLY CLEARS UP WITHOUT TREATMENT.

WHAT ARE THE CAUSES?

■ The viral infection **shingles (herpes zoster)** is
a known cause of damage to the facial nerve, and
many other viruses, especially herpes simplex,
also have the potential to cause facial palsy.
■ The bacterial infection **Lyme disease**, carried
by ticks, is also a known cause.
■ Inflammation of the facial nerve is
sometimes due to a middle ear infection.
■ Rarely, the facial nerve may be compressed
by a tumor called an **acoustic neuroma**.

WHAT ARE THE SYMPTOMS?

In some cases, the symptoms of facial palsy
appear suddenly over about 24 hours. In
other cases, including facial palsy caused by
an acoustic neuroma, symptoms may develop
slowly. The symptoms include:
● partial or complete paralysis of the muscles
on one side of the face
● pain behind the ear on the affected side
● drooping of the corner of the mouth,
sometimes associated with drooling
● inability to close the eyelid on the affected
side, and watering of the eye
● impairment of taste.

If facial palsy is very severe, you may have
difficulty speaking and eating. In a few cases,
sounds seem unnaturally loud in the ear on
the affected side. If the eyelid cannot be
closed, the eye may become infected, possibly
leading to ulceration of the cornea, the
transparent front part of the eye. In facial

palsy due to shingles, there is also a rash of
crusting blisters on the face.

WHAT MIGHT BE DONE?

■ If your symptoms have appeared in the last
48 hours, your doctor may prescribe
corticosteroids for up to two weeks to reduce
inflammation of the nerve.
■ Analgesics will relieve pain.
■ To prevent damage to the cornea, you
may be given artificial tears and you will
probably be advised to tape the affected eye
shut when you go to sleep.

WHAT IS THE OUTLOOK?

Bell's palsy usually clears up without further
treatment. If facial palsy has an underlying
cause, it will be treated too. For example, if
facial palsy is due to shingles, antiviral drugs
such as **acyclovir** will be prescribed. To be
effective, treatment with acyclovir should begin
as soon as the rash appears. If there is an
acoustic neuroma, it will be removed surgically
to relieve compression of the facial nerve.

If muscle paralysis persists, **plastic surgery**
may be used to reroute another nerve to the
face. Facial exercises and massage may help
maintain tone and facial symmetry.

With appropriate treatment, facial palsy
usually improves in about two weeks. However,
a full recovery may take up to three months.
Some people are left with weakness in the
affected area, and facial palsy may recur.

Persistent vegetative state

PERSISTENT VEGETATIVE STATE IS A LONG-TERM STATE OF UNCONSCIOUSNESS CAUSED BY DAMAGE
TO THE BRAIN. SUFFERERS ARE PHYSICALLY AND MENTALLY UNRESPONSIVE TO EXTERNAL STIMULI,
BUT REQUIRE NO HELP WITH VITAL FUNCTIONS SUCH AS BREATHING AND HEART RATE.

Coma may result from extensive brain damage
as may occur in head injuries or after a heart
attack when the brain has been starved of
oxygen for too long. The most common cause
is a severe head injury. Persistent vegetative
state can also be caused by infection of the
brain, such as **viral encephalitis**, or by oxygen
deprivation of the brain as a result of **near-
drowning**.

In persistent vegetative state, the parts of the
brain that control the higher mental functions
such as thought are damaged, leaving the areas
that control the vital functions such as
breathing and heart rate intact. So although

someone is physically and mentally unresponsive
to noise, light, and other stimuli, they can
breathe without assistance. They may also move
the head or limbs.

People in a persistent vegetative state appear
to have normal sleep patterns, with their eyes
closing and opening as if sleeping and waking.
However, they do not appear to feel physical
sensations such as pain or experience emotional
distress. Since areas of the brain that control
breathing and other functions are intact, a
person in a persistent vegetative state can
remain alive for months or even years provided
appropriate medical treatment is given.

WHAT MIGHT BE DONE?

The diagnosis of persistent vegetative state is
made if a person who is unconscious fails to
respond to stimulation or to communicate but
vital functions such as breathing are
maintained. It's generally agreed that the mind
of the person is not functioning consciously.

There is no effective treatment for a person
who is in a persistent vegetative state. However,
general supportive measures and nursing care
will ensure that an affected person is kept
as comfortable as possible. A person in a
persistent vegetative state can live for several
years but recovery is unlikely.

Vertigo

VERTIGO IS AN UNPLEASANT SENSATION OF MOVING OR SPINNING, OFTEN COMBINED
WITH NAUSEA AND VOMITING. AN ATTACK OF VERTIGO CAN BE VERY DISTRESSING AND
IN SEVERE CASES MAY MAKE IT IMPOSSIBLE TO WALK OR EVEN TO STAND.

Vertigo is a symptom of many different
disorders, for example:
● a disorder of the organs of balance in the
inner ear (the vestibular apparatus)
● a disorder of the nerve that connects the
inner ear to the brain
● problems in the areas of the brain concerned
with balance
● a condition such as multiple sclerosis (MS)
that requires urgent medical attention.

WHAT ARE THE CAUSES?
There are a number of possible causes.
■ **Infection of the vestibular apparatus**:
labyrinthitis usually begins as a viral infection
of the respiratory tract, such as a common
cold or flu or, less frequently, a bacterial
infection of the middle ear. This type of
vertigo usually **starts suddenly and lasts for
1–2 weeks**.
■ **Ménière's disease**: recurrent vertigo
combined with deafness and **tinnitus** is a
conditional sign of Ménière's disease.
■ **Antibiotics**: vertigo is a side effect of certain
antibiotics.
■ **Acoustic neuroma**: this type of tumor,
affecting the nerve that connects the inner
ear to the brain, is a rare cause of vertigo.
■ **Strokes and head injuries** are other rare
causes of vertigo.

SELF-HELP
You'll relieve vertigo by lying still, closing your
eyes and avoiding sudden movement. If you've
been vomiting, take small sips of water every
10 minutes to avoid dehydration until your
symptoms go. If the vertigo persists for more
than a few minutes, or if it becomes recurrent,
you should consult your doctor.

WHAT TESTS MIGHT BE DONE?
■ Your doctor may examine your ears, eye
movements, and nervous system to look for
a cause.
■ Tests may include a caloric test, in which
water at different temperatures is poured into
the ear to check the function of the vestibular
apparatus of the inner ear.
■ A neck X-ray may be done to look for
cervical spondylitis.
■ If you also have tinnitus, you may have
computerized tomography (CT) scanning or
magnetic resonance imaging (MRI) to rule
out a tumor pressing on the brain.

WHAT IS THE TREATMENT?
Antinausea drugs and antihistamines will
relieve vertigo. If vertigo is a side effect of an
antibiotic, you can be given an alternative.

Bones, joints, & muscles

Image shows a colored scanning electron micrograph of normal spongy bone

Miriam's overview

We take the efficient, comfortable working of the skeleton very much for granted until something goes wrong. It can be a rude awakening when bone, joint, and muscle disorders become extremely painful and disabling.

With arthritis in a knee, going about your everyday activities is curtailed, but with a frozen shoulder, you can't even get out the door since it stops you from putting your clothes on.

Within the body our bony skeleton, our joints, and our muscles work in harmony together to make us uniquely mobile and dexterous. The efficiency of our muscles to move joints and leverage bone is quite astonishing, but all components need servicing.

Muscles can't work efficiently if they're unfit. Joints don't remain frictionless if they're damaged or abused and bones can become thin if not properly nourished and exercised.

So it's our responsibility to keep this whole system in good working order by resisting a sedentary lifestyle and getting regular weight-bearing exercise. If we don't, we, and especially women, pay a heavy price.

Peak bone mass – the intrinsic strength of our bones – reaches a maximum before the age of 35. If we've been a dieter or not had much exercise, or worst of all been anorexic, our peak bone mass is low. This is premature osteoporosis.

When menopause arrives and bones stop gaining mass and begin losing it – the loss can be one-third of their mass in three years due to lack of estrogen – they are at much greater risk of osteoporosis. And brittle bones are painful,

they fracture, they collapse, and can land a woman in the hospital from which she may never come out. 1 in 4 women with a fractured hip bone dies in hospital.

Great strides have been taken with the biotechnology of joint replacement. Nowadays almost any joint can be renewed for sufferers of both osteoarthritis and rheumatoid arthritis. The latter is always the most difficult to treat with its acutely tender and swollen joints, so inflamed that some destruction is inevitable, leaving behind ugly deformities. Newer drugs and newer ways of giving them present much hope that the course of rheumatoid arthritis can be arrested.

"it's our *responsibility* to keep this whole system in *good working order*"

Repetitive strain injury (RSI) is an almost entirely modern phenomenon. Never before have jobs called for repetitive fine movements performed for long periods of time. The main trouble is in the brain, not in the fingers, wrist, or elbows where we feel the pain. The brain apparently gets confused in RSI and calls on our joints and muscles to perform opposing movements at the same time. Retraining your brain therefore is just as essential a part of treatment for RSI as hand rests and careful positioning of keyboards.

INSIDE
your bones, joints, and muscles

The human **skeleton** is made up of 206 **bones** and provides the framework of the body. It protects the internal organs and provides anchor points for the muscles. Bone itself is living tissue, which is constantly being renewed. Inside bone, the soft, fatty substance known as **bone marrow** is responsible for making most of the body's blood cells. A type of connective tissue called **cartilage**, which is not as hard as bone, is also an important component of many parts of the body.

Where two or more bones meet there is a **joint**. Joints that move freely, such as the elbow or the knee, are called **synovial joints** and are lubricated by **synovial fluid** that is secreted by the joint lining. **Semimovable joints**, such as those in the pelvis, do not move freely but are more stable. Certain joints, such as those in the skull, are **fixed** and do not move.

Moving the body is the job of the **muscles**. The skeletal muscles are attached to bones by flexible, fibrous cords of tissue called **tendons**. Muscles normally cross two bones and their joint.

the skeleton

The axial skeleton consists of the skull, spine, and rib cage and protects the brain, spinal cord, heart, and lungs. The remaining bones belong to the appendicular skeleton.

Parietal bone
Frontal bone
Zygomatic arch
Temporal bone
Occipital bone
Mandible
Scapula
Clavicle
Sternum
Humerus
Rib
Radius
Vertebral column
Pelvis
Carpals
Ulna
Metacarpals
Femur
Phalanges
Patella
Tibia
Fibula
Tarsals
Metatarsals
Calcaneus
Phalanges

how the body moves

Muscles can only contract, not expand. For this reason, muscles work in opposing pairs.

To move the forearm down, the triceps contracts while the biceps relaxes.

KEY
Blue arrows show movement of the forearm

Contracted triceps muscle
Relaxed biceps muscle
Humerus
Elbow joint
Radius
Ulna

Contracted biceps muscle

Relaxed triceps muscle

To move the forearm up, the biceps contracts while the triceps relaxes.

the structure of a synovial joint

Bone
Synovial membrane
Articular cartilage
Synovial fluid
Ligament forming capsule

Synovial joints are held together by ligaments and are lubricated by synovial fluid.

the structure of bone

Periosteum
Artery
Compact bone
Nerve
Spongy bone
Bone marrow
Vein

Bone consists of an outer layer of compact bone surrounding an inner layer of spongy bone. An inner core of bone marrow produces blood cells.

BONES

Bone consists of an elastic protein framework stiffened by calcium and phosphate. Bone isn't lifeless and unchanging, it's very much a living tissue that is continually broken down and rebuilt. Bone is also the source of blood; most of our blood cells are made in the marrow. Disorders of bone, therefore, can lead to **anemias**, and abnormal cell growth in the bone marrow to **leukemia**. Bone can be weakened by nutritional deficiencies, especially of calcium and vitamin D. Hormones guarantee the integrity of bone and with the estrogen deficiency that occurs with **menopause** or **eating disorders** and after, bone becomes weak and brittle (**osteoporosis**) unless we take precautions.

Osteoporosis, which affects 1 in 3 women after menopause, is the most common bone disorder. Estrogen normally keeps the natural processes of bone breakdown and replacement in balance. Without estrogen, replacement can't keep pace with breakdown and so bones become fragile and fracture more easily.

Fractures are common and various and so I've explained them in some detail to give you a clear understanding of them. Primary bone cancers are extremely rare, but secondary bone cancers (**metastases**) are relatively common and are mentioned here.

Fractures

A BREAK OR CRACK IN ANY BONE IN THE BODY IS KNOWN AS A FRACTURE.
FRACTURES ARE USUALLY DUE TO INJURY FROM A FALL BUT THEY CAN BE CAUSED BY BOUTS
OF COUGHING OR EVEN A HUG IF THE BONES ARE SERIOUSLY OSTEOPOROTIC.

Types of fracture

Transverse fracture
In a transverse fracture, there is a straight break across a bone. Transverse fractures, often in the arm or leg, are usually due to a powerful blow, such as that sustained in a collision during a traffic accident.

Spiral fracture
Spiral fractures, or oblique fractures, are usually caused by sudden, violent, rotating movements, such as twisting the leg during a fall, especially if there's a ski on the end of it.

Greenstick fracture
If a long bone in the arm or leg bends, it may crack on one side only, producing an incomplete break called a "greenstick" fracture. This type of fracture occurs in children, whose bones are still growing and bendy.

Comminuted fracture
The bone is broken into small fragments, which increases the likelihood of damage to the soft tissues surrounding the broken bone. These fractures are usually caused by severe, direct forces.

Avulsion fracture
A piece of bone is pulled away from the main bone by a tendon that attaches a muscle to a bone. It usually results from a sudden violent contraction of the muscle.

Compression fracture
A compression fracture occurs if spongy bone, like that in the vertebrae of the spine, is crushed; this type of fracture is often due to osteoporosis.

Stress fracture
Fractures are caused by repetitive overload of a bone are called stress fractures. They may occur in the foot bones or shin bones of long-distance runners. In the elderly, fractures may result from minor stress such as a chronic cough, which can break a rib.

Fractures due to a bone being twisted or bent occur in athletic sports such as skiing or football. Susceptibility to fractures increases with the bone disorder **osteoporosis**, which mainly affects women after menopause and results in brittle bones. Fractures that occur in bones affected by tumors are known as **pathological fractures** and may occur after minimal injury or even spontaneously. **Greenstick fractures** occur when a long bone bends and cracks on one side only; these fractures are especially common in children.

WHAT ARE THE TYPES?
There are two main types of fracture: **closed** (simple), in which the broken bone does not break through the overlying skin, and **open** (compound), in which the bone pierces the skin and is exposed. Open fractures are more serious because of the risk of infection and damage to nerves and blood vessels.

WHAT ARE THE SYMPTOMS?
The symptoms of a fracture depend on its type and include:
- deformity in the affected area
- pain and tenderness, which limits movement
- swelling and bruising
- crackling noise caused by grating of the ends of the bones on movement or pressure
- in an open fracture, damage to skin, bleeding, and visible bone.

All fractures cause a certain amount of **internal bleeding** because of damage to blood

continued on page 426

FOCUS *on* osteoporosis

The painful, crippling, and, sometimes, life threatening bone condition known as osteoporosis is the single most important health hazard for women who have reached menopause – it is more common than heart disease, stroke, diabetes, or breast cancer.

The word "osteoporosis" is derived from the Greek and means "bone that has many holes." A special X-ray of affected bones will show they have a "low bone density," which means there may be an increased risk of fracture. Some bones can be so brittle as to fracture with coughing, even a hug. 1 in 4 elderly women who fracture the neck of the thighbone (femur) after a fall die in hospital. So osteoporosis must be taken seriously and prevented if at all possible. Black women, because they have greater bone density, have a lower risk of osteoporosis than white women. Osteoporosis also occurs in elderly men, although much more rarely than in women. Osteoporosis can also occur in female athletes.

WHAT HAPPENS?

As estrogen and progesterone levels fall after menopause, bones begin to lose mass by up to 3 percent a year. By the time a woman is 80, she can easily have lost **half of her bone mass**.

Healthy bone has blood vessels and nerves and a very efficient repair and maintenance system. There are special cells, called osteoblasts, that renew, repair, and lay down new bone, and others, called osteoclasts, that cause bone breakdown. **The activity of osteoblasts is controlled mainly by hormones, including estrogen, which is thought to increase the repair and renewal rate of bone.** If estrogen levels fall, bone is not replaced as efficiently.

AM I AT RISK?

• If you're menopausal, yes. **Menopause** is the main cause of osteoporosis.
• If you have **impaired peak bone density**, yes. Bone density normally peaks at around age 25–27. If your peak bone density is low, less bone loss will be required to develop osteoporosis when you reach menopause. **Anorexia** and **repeated dieting** lower your peak bone density, making you a candidate for osteoporosis later on.
• If your **mother** has osteoporosis your risk is higher than average.

• Osteoporosis occurs in some women with **premenopausal** lack of menstrual periods (**amenorrhea**), because of low estrogen levels.
• Women such as **ballet dancers,** who exercise excessively while on restricted diets, are at risk.
• Women who have an **overactive thyroid gland** are at risk of developing osteoporosis.
• The **earlier the age of menopause**, with its depletion of estrogen, the greater the risk of osteoporosis.

• Menopause may start up to five years early in heavy smokers, so **smoking** is a risk factor for osteoporosis.
• **Hysterectomy** with **removal of the ovaries** leads to loss of bone mass. Most women show early signs of osteoporosis within four years of removal of the ovaries if HRT is not given.
• If you've taken **corticosteroids**, such as **cortisone** or **prednisone**, for longer than six months you're a candidate for osteoporosis so ask for a bone scan when the treatment is over.
• Malignant disease, a chronic liver disorder, or rheumatoid arthritis all increase the risk.

WHAT ARE THE SYMPTOMS?

• There are no symptoms of early osteoporosis. All women should have a bone density test done at menopause.

Bone density tests

Normal bone mass
Normal bone has a T score above -1 SD units.

Below normal bone mass
A T score between -1 and -2.5 SD units is below normal.

Osteoporotic bone
A T score below -2.5 SD units indicates osteoporosis.

This technique uses low-dose X-rays to measure the density of bone. The test is carried out to screen for and diagnose osteoporosis, a condition that is particularly common in postmenopausal women. The varying absorption of X-rays as they pass through the body is interpreted by a computer and displayed as an image. The computer calculates the average density of the bone and compares it with the normal range for the person's age and sex. The procedure takes about 10–20 minutes and is painless. You will be asked to lie still with your legs raised and your back flat. The X-ray generator and detector move along the length of your spine and transmit information to a computer.

● Symptoms that may signal osteoporosis include upper and low back pain, aches and pains in the joints and limbs, swollen joints at the ends of your fingers.
● Fractures are a very common symptom of osteoporosis, often the first sign that a person has the condition.

● If you are over 40 and you fracture your wrist or hip after a minor fall, you are likely to have osteoporosis. (The working rule is if you sustain a fracture after minor trauma, osteoporosis is present.)
● Fractures of the wrist, **Colles' fractures**, in menopausal women are sustained when they

fall and reach out to save themselves.
● **Hip fractures** are one of the most serious types of fracture because they render an elderly person immobile.
● **Compression fractures of the vertebrae** are also common leading to a reduction in height and an outward curvature of the spine, known as **Dowager's Hump**.

DOWAGER'S HUMP
As the bones of the spine gradually lose density, the vertebrae collapse, causing the rib cage to tilt downward toward the hips. A curvature in the upper spine creates a second curve in the lower spinal column, pushing the internal organs forward. Because of the compressed spinal column, up to 8in (20cm) in height can be lost in severe cases. Constipation can be a problem, breathing may become labored, indigestion and acid reflux are common, and pain in the lower back and limbs results from pressure on the nerves by the collapsed vertebrae. Finding clothes that fit isn't easy and day-to-day life can become increasingly difficult.

The structure of bone

Healthy bone
Bone is living tissue that is constantly being broken down and renewed by the body. Bone is made up of a framework of protein fibers with deposits of calcium and phosphate among them.

HOW IS IT DIAGNOSED?
● At the first sign of menopause, usually long, heavy periods, ask your doctor to arrange **bone density tests**.
● If you **suddenly** begin to suffer upper or low back pain, you should ask your doctor to do an X-ray of your spine.
There are several ways of assessing bone density, and a scan is considered the best predictor of fractures.

WHAT IS THE TREATMENT?
The goal of prescription drugs, such as HRT, is to halt bone loss, prevent further fractures, and replace or repair bone whenever possible. **Once fractures occur, at least one-third of bone mass** has already been lost; in some cases as much as 60 percent is gone.

NONHORMONAL TREATMENT
● Ask your doctor about calcium supplements. A general guideline is 1500mg a day after menopause. To **maximize** its benefits, calcium should be taken with other treatments, such as HRT and vitamin D. In parallel you should increase calcium intake through your diet. Eat plenty of calcium-rich foods, including dairy products, canned fish with bones, such as sardines, and vegetables such as broccoli.
● A drug called **etidronate** has been shown to treat effectively established spinal osteoporosis.

Osteoporotic bone
If the mineral content of bone is not adequately maintained, osteoporosis may result, in which the bones become weak and brittle and more prone to fractures.

- A new class of drugs called SERMS for menopausal women treats osteoporosis. It also prevents heart disease but is ineffective against menopausal symptoms such as hot flashes and dry vagina.
- Vitamin D supplements will increase the efficiency of your calcium supplements.

PAIN RELIEF

- Women with vertebral osteoporosis can suffer intense back pain, especially after a new fracture, and may need strong prescription painkillers.
- Curvature of the spine produces ongoing muscular and ligament pain, but this can be treated with nonprescription **painkillers**, such as **acetaminophen**.
- Physical therapists use various forms of **electrotherapy** or **ultrasound** to help relieve pain.
- TENS (**Transcutaneous Electrical Nerve Stimulation**) machines for pain relief are available in most treatment centers and pharmacies.
- **Complementary** techniques such as acupuncture, and the use of heating pads, hot-water bottles, or ice packs at home, are sometimes helpful for pain but they don't correct osteoporosis.
- An occupational therapist can advise you on how to **organize your home and work environment** to **minimize pain**. You should sit in a chair with a high back that gives support to the whole spine, and your bed should be firm, but not so hard that it cannot accommodate the altered shape of your spine.

HOW DO I PREVENT OSTEOPOROSIS?

Since all women are at risk of developing osteoporosis, it is important that we adopt self-help measures early in order to build up our resistance to it.
- **Get regular exercise from the age of 12–13 onward**
Exercise is crucial at menopause. Increased muscle strength, improved spinal power, and posture, maintenance of bone strength, relief of pain, and toning of pelvic floor muscles to cope with stress incontinence are all benefits of exercise. Join an exercise class. Women who get regular weight-bearing exercise – walking will do – twice a week have denser bones than those who exercise once a week, who, in turn, have denser bones than those who never get exercise at all. It is never too late to strengthen your bones.
- **Eat a calcium-rich diet**
From an early age always take the opportunity to eat calcium-rich foods, such as dairy products, fish with bones (such as sardines), and dark green vegetables. Seek them out, keep them in the fridge, choose them from restaurant menus.
- **Consider HRT**
I would suggest that a sensible way of **preventing osteoporosis**, once you are menopausal, is to take enough estrogen to maintain bone mass. HRT in the form of estrogen taken continuously in combination with progestogen for 10–13 days per month seems to **optimize** bone health, and prevent fractures. Ideally, you should have a bone density test to assess your bone health before HRT is prescribed but it isn't mandatory. You should discuss the possibility of taking HRT, orally or through the skin via gel or a skin patch, with your doctor. There are over 50 forms on the market so one should suit you. Be sure to give yourself a four-month trial. You need to take HRT for five years for your bones to benefit and the benefit is lost when you stop.

Natural types of HRT, including progesterone cream, have NEVER been shown to have any effect on osteoporosis.

PREVENTING FRACTURES
As the greatest danger of osteoporosis is a fracture, it is vital that you help yourself prevent it from happening.

- Regular exercise, a balanced diet, and mental alertness can help to maintain overall fitness, which lowers your chance of falling heavily.
- Maintain good vision by having your eyes tested regularly, particularly for a condition known as glaucoma.
- Avoid sedatives and other drugs that might reduce your alertness, such as antihistamines, and try to limit your alcohol intake.
- Reduce the hazards in your home by removing any trailing electrical cords and loose rugs.
- Make sure that there is always a firm handrail on stairs and be particularly on guard when walking on slippery or uneven surfaces.
- Some women avoid going out and, as a result, may suffer from lack of exercise and vitamin D (through lack of exposure to the sun). This may make their osteoporosis worse.
- Counseling, emotional support, and talking to other menopausal women with similar problems can do much to give a woman a more positive attitude to life and help her become more outgoing and confident.
- Have regular health checkups with your doctor.
- Ask your doctor to check your heart and blood pressure annually.

continued from page 422

vessels in the bone. The broken bone ends may cause further bleeding by damaging tissues and blood vessels in the injured area. In some fractures, particularly a break in the thighbone (femur), blood loss may be severe and lead to shock.

Various complications may be associated with a fracture. For example, if you fracture a rib, there is a risk that the broken rib may puncture a lung, causing **pneumothorax**.

Delay in treating a fracture properly may result in failure of the bone to heal, causing permanent deformity or disability. Consult a doctor immediately if you think you have a fracture.

HOW IS IT DIAGNOSED?

Your doctor will arrange for you to have X-rays to reveal the type and extent of the fracture. CT scanning or a MRI may be needed to investigate complex fractures. If a fracture wasn't due to injury, your doctor may check for a possible underlying disorder that may have weakened your bones.

WHAT IS THE TREATMENT?

If the broken ends of the bone have been displaced, they will be brought into line to restore normal shape by manipulation. This process is known as reduction. Each type of fracture has its own manipulation maneuver, which may be performed under local or general anesthetic.

TEST

X-rays

X-ray photography is one of the oldest methods of imaging the body. In this technique high intensity radiation (in the form of X-rays) passes through the body to form an image on film placed on the other side of the body. Hard structures within the body, such as bones, block the radiation and so show up on the X-ray film as white areas. X-rays are therefore useful for imaging hard structures but are not very useful for imaging soft tissues, such as the liver, since they do not block the radiation. However, a special type of X-ray, known as a contrast X-ray, may be used to image certain soft tissues.

During an X-ray, the source of the X-rays is usually positioned directly above the area to be examined. You will be asked to keep completely still during the procedure to ensure that the X-ray picture is clear. You will be exposed to X-ray radiation for less than one second, and the procedure usually takes only a few minutes.

See also:
- **CT scanning p. 401** • **MRI p. 409**
- **Osteoporosis p. 423** • **Pneumothorax 395** • **Shock p. 560**

Bone cancers

THERE ARE TWO TYPES OF CANCEROUS GROWTH THAT OCCUR IN BONE: PRIMARY BONE CANCER, WHICH ORIGINATES IN THE BONE ITSELF AND IS VERY RARE, AND SECONDARY BONE CANCER, WHICH ARISES FROM CANCER ELSEWHERE IN THE BODY AND HAS SPREAD TO THE BONE VIA THE BLOOD.

Secondary cancers, called **metastases**, are much more common than primary bone cancers, especially in older people, who are more likely to have cancer elsewhere.

PRIMARY BONE CANCER

Primary bone cancer is a cancerous tumor that originates in bone. Sarcoma, a form of primary bone cancer, is rare, but myeloma is more common in people 40–60 years old. Primary bone cancers are more common in childhood and adolescence and sometimes run in families.

WHAT MIGHT BE DONE?

In most cases the tumor is removed **surgically**. **Radiation therapy** may help reduce the size of the tumor. Postoperative **chemotherapy** helps destroy any remaining cancerous cells. Removed bone is replaced by metal replacements (prostheses) or by bone taken from elsewhere in the body or from a donor.

Most people treated for primary bone cancer have a very small chance of recurrence in the first five years. Thereafter, recurrence is unlikely.

SECONDARY BONE CANCER (BONE METASTASES)

Secondary bone cancer is a cancerous tumor in bone that has spread from a cancer elsewhere in the body. Cancers that typically metastasize to bone include **breast**, **lung**, and **prostate cancer** and **cancer of the ovary**, and are often called "secondaries."

Metastases most often develop in the ribs, pelvis, skull, or spine. The condition is much more common than primary bone cancer.

WHAT ARE THE SYMPTOMS?

Bone metastases may cause the following symptoms, in addition to those of the main cancer:
- gnawing bone pain that may become worse at night
- swelling of the affected area
- tenderness over the affected area
- proneness of affected bones to fracture easily, often after minor injury.

WHAT MIGHT BE DONE?

If you already have a cancer somewhere else in your body, you may have X-rays or radionuclide scanning to check whether the cancer has spread to the bones. If the site of the primary cancer is unknown, you may need further tests to find out where the metastasis came from. For example, women may be given **mammography** to look for evidence of breast cancer.

Your doctor will probably direct treatment at your original cancer. He or she may also arrange for you to have **chemotherapy**, **radiation therapy**, or **hormonal therapy** to relieve bone pain.

The prognosis for people with bone metastases usually depends on the site of the original cancer and how successfully it can be treated. However, the best that can usually be achieved for bone metastases is a period of remission and relief from pain.

See also:
- **Breast cancer p. 261**
- **Cancer of the ovary p. 260**
- **Chemotherapy p.257** • **Lung cancer p. 394**
- **Mammograms p. 245**
- **Prostate cancer p. 265**
- **Radiation therapy p. 395**

JOINTS

Joints allow our bodies to be flexible. Their perfect engineering is mainly due to an enveloping capsule and a lining, the **synovium**, which produces lubrication in the form of synovial fluid. Within joints, cartilage lines the ends of bones and prevents friction during movement. Fibrous ligaments surround the joints, giving strength, support, and stability. Joints may be damaged by injury, inflammation, and the degeneration of bone, cartilage, and ligaments that comes with aging or disease.

Joint disorders are a major cause of disability and immobility, but the treatment of chronic joint disease has improved enormously in the past 20 years due to the availability of new drugs and safe, reliable artificial joints.

The word **arthritis** means inflammation of one or more joints, although there is little evidence of actual inflammation in the most common form, **osteoarthritis**, which comes to affect most joints as they age and especially if they've been injured. **Spondylosis** is a natural deterioration in the spinal joints affecting the parts of the spine where there's most movement – the neck and lower back – and affects all of us from middle age onward. **Rheumatoid arthritis** is a true inflammatory arthritis and may be the most dramatic feature of a condition in which there is inflammation in many organs of the body other than simply the joints. This kind of disorder is called a **connective tissue disorder** or **autoimmune disease** and rheumatoid arthritis is the most common example. And gout, although comparatively rare, is extremely painful and deserves attention.

Last but not least the common **bunion** gets a mention since it's an inflammation of the tissues around a joint, the bursa of the big toe, affecting many people.

Arthritis

THE TERM ARTHRITIS COVERS A LARGE GROUP OF INFLAMMATORY AND DEGENERATIVE CONDITIONS THAT CAUSE STIFFNESS, SWELLING, AND PAIN IN THE JOINTS.

Arthritis may be linked with skin diseases such as **psoriasis**, intestinal disorders such as **Crohn's disease,** and autoimmune disease such as **lupus**.

WHAT ARE THE TYPES?

There are several different types of arthritis, each having its own characteristics.

■ The most common form is a degenerative type, **osteoarthritis**, usually affecting middle-aged and older people in the weight-bearing joints – the knees and hips – and after menopause, the ends of the fingers. **Spondylosis** is a common form of osteoarthritis that affects the joints in the spine, mainly the neck (cervical) and lower back (lumbar) regions.

■ **Rheumatoid arthritis** results from inflammation in the joints and other body tissues, such as the **heart, lungs,** and **eyes**.

■ Another chronic disorder is **ankylosing spondylitis**, which affects the spine and joints between the base of the spine and the pelvis. As with rheumatoid arthritis, other body tissues, the eyes for example, may be affected. The condition eventually causes the vertebrae (the bones of the spine) to fuse together, making walking extremely difficult.

Living with arthritis

If you have long-term arthritis, you may be able to manage your symptoms so that you can maintain an active lifestyle. Consult your doctor about pain relief and keeping joints mobile. Organizations concerned with arthritis (see Useful addresses, p.567) can also provide valuable information.

Self-help

• If you are overweight, probably the most important single thing you can do is lose weight.

• In addition, exercises to increase muscle power will help stabilize the affected joint and reduce your symptoms.

Mobility

Gentle, regular exercise helps relieve stiffness and improve mobility. Physical activity also helps strengthen the muscles that support the joints. However, if exercise causes swelling or pain, stop the activity and consult your doctor.

Pain relief

Severe joint pain can be improved by applying heat or cold to the area. Heat increases blood flow; cold helps reduce swelling. Both decrease sensitivity to pain.

Specialized equipment

Your doctor or a physical therapist may be able to suggest specially adapted pieces of equipment to help you with household tasks. The equipment may have particular features, such as handles that are easy to grip or extending arms to help you reach objects without bending down.

• If arthritis restricts the movement in your hands, use cutlery with thick handles and glasses with wide stems that will be easier to grip. A plate with a rim may keep the food from spilling, and a nonslip mat will help hold your plate still during a meal.

• Tongs enable you to pick up objects that are out of your reach without bending or stretching. Some types of tongs have a trigger mechanism that operate pincers at the end of the arm.

• A fixed seat in the shower allows you to sit down while you wash. Handrails and a nonslip floor surface reduce the risk of falls.

TREATMENT

Joint replacement

Joints that have been severely damaged by arthritis or injury may be surgically replaced with artificial joints made of metal, ceramic, or plastic. Most joints in the body can be replaced, but the common ones are the hips, knees, and shoulders. During the operation, the ends of damaged bones are removed and the artificial components are fixed in place. The operation usually relieves pain and increases the range of motion in the joint.

Hip replacement

The most commonly replaced joint is the hip. During the operation, both the pelvic socket and the head of the thighbone (femur) are replaced. An epidural anesthetic is used and it involves a short stay in hospital. In the first two weeks following the operation the new joint is unstable and patients must be careful not to dislocate it during this time.

Other joints

Many different types of joints in the body can be replaced, from tiny finger joints to large joints such as the knees.

Knee joint replacement

Most artificial knee joints consist of metal and plastic implants. The remaining cartilage and part of the end of the bone is removed to allow placement of the metal and plastic components. The operation is performed under an epidural anesthesia. The patient can put some weight on the leg beginning on day two.

Finger joint replacement

Artificial finger joints are made of metal, plastic, or silicone rubber and are used to replace damaged joints in the fingers. The operation is done under a local or general anesthetic and stitches are usually removed after about 10 days.

■ **Reactive arthritis** typically develops in susceptible people after they've had an infection, most often of the **genital tract**, such as **nonspecific urethritis**, or of the **intestines**, such as **ulcerative colitis**. This kind of arthritis most commonly causes inflammation in an **ankle** or a **knee**.

■ In **gout**, crystals of **uric acid** are deposited in a joint, leading to swelling and pain. **Treatment** of arthritis depends on the type. **Analgesics** and **nonsteroidal anti-inflammatory drugs (NSAIDs)** may help relieve symptoms. **Physical therapy** helps keep joints mobile. Drugs such as allopurinol or colchicine may help to decrease uric acid levels and prevent gout attacks. Severely damaged joints may need to be surgically replaced with artificial joints.

> See also:
> • Ankylosing spondylitis p. 430
> • Crohn's disease p. 366
> • Gout p. 433
> • Lupus p. 324 • Psoriasis p. 448
> • Rheumatoid arthritis p. 429

Osteoarthritis

THE GRADUAL DEGENERATION OF THE CARTILAGE COVERING THE ENDS OF BONE INSIDE JOINTS, DUE TO WEAR AND TEAR OVER MANY YEARS, CAUSES THE PAIN, SWELLING, AND STIFFNESS OF OSTEOARTHRITIS.

The condition rarely appears before middle age and primarily affects the weight-bearing joints – the hips and knees. Around the age of menopause, the terminal joints of the fingers show osteoarthritic change with the appearance of bony outgrowths on the sides of the joints – **Heberden's nodes**. Any joint that is injured could become osteoarthritic at a later date. The greater the wear and tear in early life the greater the chance of osteoarthritis (OA) setting in.

HOW DOES IT DEVELOP?

OA develops as a result of excessive wear and tear on the joints and it's usually part of the natural aging process. For example, in OA of the knee, where the thigh bone and shin bone meet, the cartilage preventing them from grinding together has worn away and pain is the result.

OA is common in weight-bearing joints that have been subject to injury in youth or that have been used extensively in certain sports or strained due to obesity. Most people over the age of 60 have some degree of OA and three times as many women are affected as men. The areas most commonly affected are the large spinal joints of the lower back, hips, knees, and feet. A thickening of the bone ends causes bony spurs to appear at the edge of joints.

Exactly the same process occurs at the edges of the neck (cervical) vertebrae, often causing a stiff neck that makes movement painful. This condition is known as **cervical spondylosis**.

WHAT ARE THE SYMPTOMS?

■ As well as pain, OA also causes swelling, creaking, and stiffness of the affected joints.
■ Weakness and shrinkage of surrounding muscles may occur if pain prevents the joint being used regularly.
■ Pressure from a bony spur on a nerve in the neck (cervical spondylosis) may cause pain in the shoulder, elbow, and fingers.
■ When bony growths occur in the lower back (lumbar spondylosis), pressure on the sciatic nerve may cause pain in the buttock and the back of the legs down to the sole of the foot, pain known as **sciatica**.

WHAT IS THE TREATMENT?

■ Unfortunately, there is no cure although the symptoms can be relieved by painkillers

Formation of osteophytes on bone

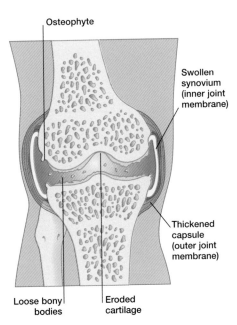

Osteophyte

Swollen synovium (inner joint membrane)

Thickened capsule (outer joint membrane)

Loose bony bodies

Eroded cartilage

Weight-bearing joints may erode and osteophytes (bony outgrowths) may form.

Exercises for people with osteoarthritis

1. Hold your arms straight down but across your body, then lift them upward and outward, uncrossing them as you go. With your arms in this position, clasp your hands behind your head.
2. Push your toes and feet down and then pull them up toward you. Move your toes and ankles around in a large circle.
3. Lie down, preferably on the floor, bend each leg in turn up onto your chest toward the opposite shoulder.
4. Rest your arms on a table or arm of a chair without supporting your hand. Bend your hand down toward the floor and then lift it up. Next, move your hand to the left and then to the right. When you are doing this make sure your hand rests in the mid-position and is in line with your forearm and doesn't fall downward.

5. Bend your fingers and grip tightly, then stretch and spread your fingers. Touch the tip of each finger in turn with your thumb.

If sitting in a cramped seat becomes painful after half an hour or so, stand up and walk around or massage your knees. **Don't** sit with your legs crossed – it isn't good for the knees.

Swimming is an excellent way to strengthen muscles and maintain joint mobility. Because the water supports your body, muscles can be exercised without straining your joints. If you have a heated pool nearby, use it at least once a week since it increases muscle power without putting undue strain on joints.

---

and nonsteroidal anti-inflammatory drugs (NSAIDs).
■ Physical therapy, heat treatment, and exercise are helpful for pain relief and mobility.

■ Corticosteroid injections can sometimes bring instant, if temporary, relief but must be used sparingly.

See also:
• NSAIDS p. 431
• Spondylosis p. 432

Rheumatoid arthritis

THIS FORM OF ARTHRITIS CAUSES CHRONIC INFLAMMATION OF THE CONNECTIVE TISSUES THROUGHOUT THE BODY, BUT PARTICULARLY AROUND THE JOINTS WHERE THE MAIN SIGN IS OFTEN PAINFUL, SWOLLEN, STIFF JOINTS THAT MAY EVENTUALLY BECOME DEFORMED.

Rheumatoid arthritis (RA) affects about 1 in 100 people, is most common between the ages of 40 and 60, and affects three times more women than men. It sometimes runs in families, suggesting a genetic factor is at play. RA almost always affects the same joints on both sides of the body.

WHAT HAPPENS?
In rheumatoid arthritis, the joints become stiff and swollen as a result of inflammation of the synovial membrane, which lines each joint. Gradually, the cartilage covering the ends of the bones is eroded, together with the bone underlying the cartilage. The tendons and ligaments, which give the joints support, become worn and slack, and the joints may become deformed.

HOW DOES RA AFFECT THE BODY AS A WHOLE?
In most cases rheumatoid arthritis affects several joints. It usually starts first in the small joints of the hands and feet but may develop in any joint. RA usually tends to be symmetrical, appearing in similar joints on both sides of the body. It is classified as one of the **autoimmune disorders**, in which the body produces antibodies that attack its own tissues.

Tissues, mainly connective tissue made out of **collagen**, in other parts of the body, such as the **eyes, lungs, heart,** and **blood vessels,** may be affected by inflammation and RA is therefore also described as a **connective tissue disorder**.
RA runs a chronic course and usually recurs in episodes lasting for several weeks or months with relatively symptom-free periods in between. After many years it usually "burns itself out" and becomes quiescent, like an extinct volcano.

WHAT ARE THE SYMPTOMS?
Rheumatoid arthritis usually develops slowly, although very occasionally the onset may be sudden and dramatic. General symptoms include **fatigue, pale skin, shortness of breath** on exertion, and **poor appetite. Specific symptoms** may include:
• stiff, painful, and swollen joints, often of the hands, and classically affecting the middle joint of the fingers so that they become spindle-shaped
• classically, the pain and stiffness is worst when waking and improves as the day goes on.
• painless, small bumps (nodules) on areas of pressure such as the elbows.

ARE THERE COMPLICATIONS?
■ In time, the bones around the affected joint may lose density and strength as a result of reduced mobility, becoming increasingly brittle and more susceptible to fracture.
■ The more **general symptoms** of RA are partly due to **anemia,** caused by a failure of the bone marrow to manufacture enough new red blood cells.
■ **Bursitis** may develop, in which one or more of the fluid-filled sacs around a joint become inflamed.
■ Swelling that compresses the **median nerve in the wrist** may lead to tingling and pain in the fingers. This is called **carpal tunnel syndrome.**
As part of the generalized autoimmune disorder affecting connective tissue throughout the body, complications may include:
• inflammation of the walls of the **arteries** supplying the fingers and toes may result in **Raynaud's phenomenon,** a condition in which the fingers and toes become pale and painful on exposure to cold
• less commonly, the spleen and the lymph nodes may become enlarged
• the membranous sac that surrounds the heart – the pericardium – may also become inflamed (pericarditis)

• some people may also experience inflammation of the eye – iridocyclitis or uveitis.

Symptoms may improve during pregnancy but sometimes flare up again after the birth.

HOW IS IT DIAGNOSED?

■ Joint changes in the hands are so classic as to confirm the diagnosis. However, your doctor may arrange for a blood test to check for the presence of an antibody known as **rheumatoid factor** (RF), which is often associated with RA.

■ Blood tests may also be done to measure the severity of the inflammation.

■ X-rays of the affected joints may be taken to assess the level of bone and joint damage.

WHAT IS THE TREATMENT?

The goal of treatment is twofold: firstly, to relieve your symptoms and, secondly, to reduce further joint damage by arresting inflammation and slowing the progress of the disease. Different drugs are available, and your doctor's recommendation will depend on the severity and progress of your disease, your age, and your general health.

■ **If your symptoms are only mild**, your doctor may simply prescribe a nonsteroidal anti-inflammatory drug (NSAID).

■ **If your symptoms are severe**, drugs that slow the disease process may be suggested, such as **sulphasalazine** or **chloroquine**. Such drugs should limit permanent damage to the joints but may have to be taken over a few months before their full benefits are felt.

■ **If the symptoms persist**, your doctor may prescribe a drug such as **cyclosporin, penicillamine, methotrexate, or gold**. These drugs can have serious side effects so your condition will be monitored closely by your doctor.

Rheumatoid arthritis

Eroded cartilage

Joint swollen by synovial (lubrication) fluid

Thickened capsule (outer joint membrane)

Inflamed synovial membrane

Characteristic changes in rheumatoid arthritis damage the joint.

■ The **anemia** that is commonly associated with RA may be improved by treatment with the hormone **erythropoietin**.

■ Your doctor may recommend that you use a **splint or brace**, particularly at night, to support a particularly painful joint and slow the development of deformities.

■ Gentle, regular **exercise** may help keep your joints mobile and prevent muscle weakness.

■ **Physical therapy** may be given to improve joint mobility and help increase muscle strength.

■ **Hydrotherapy** and **heat or ice treatments** may help relieve pain.

■ If a joint is intensely painful, it may need an **injection** of a corticosteroid.

■ If the joint becomes severely damaged, your doctor may suggest that you have surgery to replace the damaged joint with an **artificial** one.

WHAT IS THE OUTLOOK?

Many people with rheumatoid arthritis are able to lead a normal life, although lifelong drug treatment may be necessary to control the symptoms. About 1 in 10 people have some degree of disability, since repeated attacks gradually destroy the joints.

There are many household items that will help you to lead a normal life so ask your doctor about them.

Regular blood tests will be needed to monitor the progress of the disease and your response to treatment. In some cases, the attacks gradually stop, and the disease is said to **have burned itself out**. After the age of 50, RA quite frequently does so. However, some permanent disability may remain.

See also:
• Autoimmune disorders p. 323
• Carpal tunnel syndrome p. 434
• Joint replacement p. 428
• Living with arthritis p. 427
• NSAIDS p. 431
• Raynaud's phenomenon p. 234

Ankylosing spondylitis

THE CHRONIC, PROGRESSIVE JOINT INFLAMMATION AND STIFFENING (USUALLY OF THE SPINE AND PELVIS) THAT ARE THE MAIN SYMPTOMS OF ANKYLOSING SPONDYLITIS CLASSICALLY AFFECT YOUNG MEN. THE CONDITION TENDS TO RUN IN FAMILIES.

Although the main symptoms are in the joints, ankylosing spondylitis is a connective tissue disorder and also affects other organs in the body. The disorder particularly affects the **sacroiliac joints** that join the back of the pelvis to the bones of the spine (vertebrae). If the spine is severely diseased, new bone starts to grow between the vertebrae and eventually fuses them together so that the spine becomes fixed and immobile.

A variant of ankylosing spondylitis is preceded by the skin disorder **psoriasis** and by inflammatory bowel disease such as **Crohn's disease**.

WHAT ARE THE CAUSES?

The cause of ankylosing spondylitis is unknown, but about 9 out of 10 people with the condition have a particular substance that is capable of stimulating an immune response in the body (**antigen**), called HLA–B27, on the surface of most cells. This antigen is inherited, which helps explain why ankylosing spondylitis runs in families. Nonetheless, most people with HLA–B27 don't develop ankylosing spondylitis so there must be other factors at work.

It's thought that a bacterial infection could trigger ankylosing spondylitis in those who are predisposed.

WHAT ARE THE SYMPTOMS?

The symptoms of ankylosing spondylitis usually appear in late adolescence or early adulthood and develop gradually over a period of months or even years. The main symptoms include:

• low back pain, which may spread down into the buttocks and thighs

• low back stiffness that may be worse in the morning and improves with exercise

• pain in other joints, such as the hips, knees, and shoulders

• pain and tenderness in the heels

• fatigue, weight loss, and mild fever.

Gentle, regular exercise can help maintain flexibility and relieve the symptoms of ankylosing spondylitis.

WHAT ARE THE COMPLICATIONS?
- If left untreated, ankylosing spondylitis can cause the spine to become distorted, forming a convex curvature called **kyphosis** that results in a stooped posture.
- If the joints between the spine and the ribs are affected, **chest expansion** is restricted.
- In some people, ankylosing spondylitis causes inflammation or damage to the tissues in areas other than the joints, such as the **eyes**.

HOW IS IT DIAGNOSED?
- Your doctor may suspect ankylosing spondylitis from the pattern of your symptoms.
- An X-ray will show up evidence of fusion in the joints of the pelvis and the spine.
- Blood tests will be done to measure the level of inflammation and look for the HLA–B27 antigen.

WHAT IS THE TREATMENT?
The treatment of ankylosing spondylitis is directed at relieving the symptoms and preventing the development of deformity.
- Your doctor may prescribe a **nonsteroidal anti-inflammatory drug** (NSAID) to control pain and inflammation.
- You will have physical therapy, probably including breathing **exercises** and daily exercises to improve posture, strengthen the back muscles, and prevent deformities of the spine.

- You may also benefit from gentle regular physical activity, such as **swimming**, which helps relieve pain and stiffness.
- If a joint such as the hip is affected, you may eventually need to have it **replaced** surgically.
- If your mobility becomes severely reduced, you may need **occupational therapy**.
- Your therapist may suggest that you use **specially designed equipment** and furniture to help make your life easier.

WHAT IS THE OUTLOOK?
Most people with ankylosing spondylitis are only mildly affected, causing minimum disruption to their everyday lives. Even in those people with more severe symptoms, the condition tends to become less severe with age. In many cases, early treatment and regular exercise help relieve pain and stiffness of the back and prevent deformity of the spine. However, about 1 in 20 people with ankylosing spondylitis eventually becomes disabled.

See also:
- **Crohn's disease p. 366**
- **Joint replacement p. 428** • **Psoriasis p. 448**

NSAIDs

Nonsteroidal anti-inflammatory drugs (NSAIDs) are a group of nonaddictive drugs used to relieve pain and inflammation, particularly in muscles, ligaments, and joints. They work by limiting the release of prostaglandins, chemicals produced by the body that cause pain and trigger inflammation. One of the best-known NSAIDS is ibuprofen, which is available over the counter.

NSAIDs can cause side effects. One of the most common is irritation of the stomach lining, which may lead to peptic ulcers if NSAIDs are taken for a long period of time. If you are prescribed NSAIDs for a chronic condition, you will probably be prescribed an antiulcer drug in addition to counter this effect. Another side effect of NSAIDs is allergic reaction, which may appear as a rash or swelling. People with asthma or kidney problems should not take NSAIDs because they can make these conditions worse.

Spondylosis

THE BONES AND CARTILAGE IN THE NECK AND LOWER BACK GRADUALLY DEGENERATE
WITH AGE, LEADING TO THE PAIN AND STIFFNESS OF SPONDYLOSIS.

There are two types of spondylosis: if the symptoms are in the neck it is called **cervical** spondylosis, and if they are in the lower back, it is **lumbar** spondylosis. Since everyone over the age of 45 has some degree of cervical and/or lumbar spondylosis, it is considered part of the normal aging process.

Spondylosis is **osteoarthritis** affecting the spine where the vertebrae and the discs of cartilage between them begin to degenerate. Where movement is greatest, that is in the neck and the lower back, the bones become thickened, and bony spurs called **osteophytes** develop on the edges of the vertebrae. Osteophytes may press on spinal nerves, giving

rise to **root pain** radiating down the arms and legs.

WHAT ARE THE SYMPTOMS?
Many people don't have symptoms. When they become apparent, they include:
● restricted movement of the neck and lower back that may be painful
● pain at the back of the head and in the lower back
● aching or shooting pain that travels from the shoulders to the hands and from the lower back to the buttocks, down the back of the legs to the soles of the feet
● numbness, tingling, and muscle weakness in the hands, arms and legs.

Sometimes, if the head is moved too quickly, the bony spurs may temporarily compress blood vessels that supply the brain, resulting in dizziness, unsteadiness and double vision.

HOW IS IT DIAGNOSED?
Since spondylosis may be symptomless, the condition is often only diagnosed when an X-ray is taken for another reason.
■ If you experience neck pain or dizziness, you should consult your doctor, who may order X-rays to look for signs of cervical spondylosis.
■ If your doctor doubts that your symptoms are due solely to cervical spondylosis, he or she may arrange for further tests to look for other causes, such as a prolapsed or herniated (slipped) disk.
■ You may also have **nerve conduction studies**

and electromyography (EMG) to assess the function of nerves in your arms and hands.
■ CT (computerized tomography) scanning or MRI (magnetic resonance imaging) may also be carried out to see whether there have been any changes in the bones of the spine, the disks or cartilage between them, or the tissues around them.

WHAT IS THE TREATMENT?
Degeneration of the spine cannot be halted, but its effects can be reduced with treatment.
■ To relieve pain in mild cases of cervical spondylosis, your doctor may recommend **painkillers**, such as acetaminophen, or prescribe nonsteroidal anti-inflammatory drugs (NSAIDs).
■ Once the initial pain has been relieved, he or she may suggest **neck exercises** to help maintain mobility and increase muscle strength in your neck.
■ If cervical spondylosis has damaged a nerve, **surgery** may be recommended to prevent the symptoms from getting worse. This involves widening the natural opening between the vertebrae through which the nerve passes when it branches off the spinal cord. In some cases, surgery may also be peformed to stabilize the spine by **fusing together** the affected vertebrae.

See also:
● **Osteoarthritis p. 428** ● **Slipped disk p. 437**

Complications

Spondylitis
Occasionally spondylosis goes on to become **inflamed** when the condition is called spondylitis. This may require treatment with anti-inflammatory drugs.

Spondylolisthesis
One spinal bone may slide out of position forward onto another bone, causing pain because the adjacent muscles and ligaments are kept under stretch. This occurs in the lower lumbar region and may be symptomless.

Bunion

A BUNION IS A THICKENED SWELLING AT THE BASE OF THE BIG TOE. IT IS USUALLY CAUSED BY A
MINOR BONE DEFORMITY (HALLUX VALGUS) WHEN THE JOINT AT THE BASE OF THE BIG TOE
PROJECTS OUTWARD, FORCING THE TIP OF THE TOE TO TURN INWARD TOWARD THE OTHER TOES.

This causes a thickening of the soft tissue (bursitis) and a bony overgrowth at the base of the big toe, which often becomes inflamed and painful, making walking difficult. The cause of hallux valgus is multifactorial, that is, due to a number of causes. As a result of pressure on the deformity, the surrounding tissues thicken. The lump caused by a combination of the bony deformity and the thickened soft tissue is called a bunion.

WHAT CAUSES IT?
■ The condition is common in young women as a result of wearing shoes that are too tight or pointed, especially those with high heels. When the big toe joint is compressed it produces a

cushion of fluid that is held in a sac (a bursa) that surrounds the joint of the big toe.
■ In rare cases, the constant rubbing of tight shoes on the skin over a bunion may cause an abrasion and lead to a bacterial infection.
■ People who have **diabetes mellitus** are particularly susceptible to problems involving bunions because of impaired sensation in their feet and skin that tends to heal more slowly.

WHAT IS THE TREATMENT?
Without attention, a bunion may gradually worsen. Pain may be alleviated by wearing comfortable shoes with good cushioning and a special toe pad or corrective sock that straightens the big toe. However, if a bunion

is causing severe discomfort, your doctor may suggest surgery to correct the underlying deformity by realigning the bone.

If the bunion becomes infected with bacteria, your doctor will prescribe antibiotics.

SELF-HELP
Rest the feet whenever possible. Do not wear high-heeled shoes or ill-fitting shoes; go for wide shoes with low heels.

SURGERY
If the bunion is extremely severe and the feet become very deformed, it is possible to have surgical treatment from an orthopedic surgeon. The treatment involves completely

excising the inflamed bursa and the joint. In doing so, the orthopaedic surgeon fixes the joint, so while it will be entirely painless it will be stiff and immovable. This does not mean that you cannot walk properly, you will, but you will not be able to stand on your toes.

HOW CAN IT BE PREVENTED?

A bunion only forms when the joint of the big toe is overstrained. Prevention is therefore not to overstrain the big toe by not wearing high-heeled shoes for long periods of time and by not wearing ill-fitting shoes.

> See also:
> • Diabetes mellitus p. 504
> • Osteoarthritis p. 428

> See also:
> • Diabetes mellitus p. 504
> • Osteoarthritis p. 428

TREATMENT

Bunion surgery

Surgery to treat a bunion is designed to correct the underlying deformity of the bone, known as hallux valgus. One common type of surgical procedure used to treat a bunion involves reshaping and realigning the deformed bone (the first metatarsal bone) at the base of the big toe.

During the operation the protruding part of the bone is cut away and a V-shaped cut is made in the lower part of the bone. This allows the bone to slide sideways and become realigned. In some cases a temporary wire or a permanent screw may be inserted into the bone. To support the toe, the foot is put in a bandage or cast that must remain in place for about six weeks.

The operation is performed under an epidural anesthetic and may require a brief stay in the hospital. Crutches or a cane are required for the period during which the foot is bandaged, but normal walking can usually be resumed about six weeks after surgery.

Gout

A TYPE OF ARTHRITIS, IN WHICH CRYSTALLINE DEPOSITS OF URIC ACID FORM WITHIN JOINTS, GOUT IS 20 TIMES MORE COMMON IN MEN, ESPECIALLY THOSE WHO ARE OVERWEIGHT AND INDULGE IN RICH FOODS AND FORTIFIED WINES, CLASSICALLY PORT.

The base of the big toe is the most common site of gout, but any joint may be affected. Gout causes sudden pain and inflammation, usually in a single joint. In women, it rarely appears before menopause.

WHAT ARE THE CAUSES?

Gout is usually caused by high levels of the waste product uric acid in the blood. Excess uric acid is caused by the over-production and decreased excretion of uric acid and may lead to uric acid **crystals** being deposited in a joint. Why this happens no one knows, but the condition is often inherited. A few people with gout also develop **kidney stones** formed from excess uric acid crystals.

Gout may occur spontaneously or be brought on by surgery, being overweight, drinking alcohol, or excessive cell destruction associated with **chemotherapy**.

WHAT ARE THE SYMPTOMS?

The symptoms of gout usually flare up suddenly. They may include:
• fiery redness, tenderness, warmth, and swelling around the affected area, as in infection
• pain, which may be excruciating, in the affected joint or joints
• mild fever.

In long-standing gout, deposits of uric acid crystals may collect in the earlobes and the soft tissues of the hands, forming small, creamy lumps called **tophi**.

WHAT MIGHT BE DONE?

■ Your doctor will order blood tests to measure your uric acid levels. Severely high uric acid levels are diagnostic of gout.
■ To confirm the diagnosis, a joint aspiration, in which fluid is withdrawn from the affected joint, is examined for uric acid crystals.

WHAT IS THE TREATMENT?

Gout may subside by itself after a few days without treatment. If it persists the following treatments may be offered.
■ To reduce severe pain and inflammation, you may be treated with a nonsteroidal anti-inflammatory drug (NSAID), the antigout drug **colchicine** or with **oral corticosteroids**.
■ If you have recurring gout, you may need **lifelong treatment** with preventative drugs such as **allopurinol** to reduce the production of uric acid, or **probenecid** to increase the excretion of uric acid.
■ Your doctor may recommend that you make lifestyle changes and reduce the amount of alcohol you drink and the richness of your diet; in particular you should try to avoid liver, other offal, poultry, and legumes.
■ Losing excess weight may help reduce the frequency and severity of attacks of gout.

WHAT IS THE OUTLOOK?

Gout can be very painful and disrupt normal physical activities, but attacks tend to become less frequent and less severe with age. Repeated attacks may cause permanent damage to the affected joint and occasionally to the kidneys.

> See also:
> • Chemotherapy p. 257
> • Kidney stones p. 377

MUSCULOSKELETAL DISORDERS

The musculoskeletal system consists of the bones and joints of the skeleton and the hundreds of muscles, tendons, and ligaments attached to them. When one of the components of the system is damaged or strained, the whole system is thrown out of kilter, resulting in pain. For example, most cases of low back pain involve a degree of spondylosis – osteoarthritis – of the spine with some painful **muscle spasm** around the spondylotic vertebra. Similarly there is nearly always **muscle weakness** adjacent to a prolapsed disk.

Carpal tunnel syndrome

COMMONLY AFFLICTING PEOPLE BETWEEN THE AGES OF 40 AND 60, PARTICULARLY WOMEN, CARPAL TUNNEL SYNDROME CAUSES TINGLING AND PAIN IN THE HAND AND FOREARM DUE TO SOFT TISSUE SWELLING AND COMPRESSION OF A NERVE AT THE WRIST.

The carpal tunnel is the narrow space formed by the bones of the wrist (carpal bones) and the strong ligament that lies over them. Nerves and tendons run through this tunnel. In carpal tunnel syndrome, **the median nerve**, which controls some hand muscles and sensation in the thumb, index, and middle fingers, is compressed where it passes through the tunnel. This causes painful tingling in the hand, wrist, and forearm and often affects both hands. In women menopause undoubtedly plays a part. Work involving repetitive hand movements is a risk factor.

WHAT ARE THE CAUSES?

Carpal tunnel syndrome occurs because the soft tissues within the carpal tunnel swell and press on the median nerve at the wrist. Such swelling may occur during **pregnancy**, as part of **rheumatoid arthritis,** and after a **wrist fracture**. It may be a feature of **RSI**. In most cases there is no clear-cut cause.

WHAT ARE THE SYMPTOMS?

Symptoms mainly affect the areas of the hand supplied by the median nerve, that is the thumb, the index, and middle fingers, the inner side of the ring finger, and the palm of the hand. Symptoms initially include:
- burning and tingling in the hand
- pain in the wrist and up the forearm.

As the condition worsens, other symptoms may gradually appear including:
- numbness of the hand
- weakened grip
- wasting of some hand muscles, particularly at the base of the thumb.

Symptoms are usually more severe at night, and pain may interrupt sleep. Shaking the affected arm may temporarily relieve symptoms, but the numbness may become persistent if left untreated.

WHAT MIGHT BE DONE?

The symptoms of carpal tunnel syndrome may be relieved temporarily by **nonsteroidal anti-inflammatory drugs** (NSAIDs), or by wearing a **wrist splint**. Resting the hand and arm on a **pillow** often brings relief. In some cases a **corticosteroid injection** under the ligament may reduce swelling. If symptoms persist or recur, **surgery** may be recommended to cut

the ligament under local anesthetic and release pressure on the nerve. After surgery, most people have no further symptoms.

> See also:
> - Diabetes mellitus p. 504
> - NSAIDs p. 431 • RSI p. 439

Low back pain

MORE WORK DAYS ARE LOST DUE TO LOW BACK PAIN THAN TO ANY OTHER MEDICAL CONDITION – IT AFFECTS ABOUT 3 IN 5 ADULTS.

Low back pain occurs in the back below the waist and it may be sudden and sharp or persistent and dull; it may radiate down to the buttock and then down the back of the leg to the sole of the foot.

In most cases low back pain lasts for only a week or so, but many people find that the problem recurs unless they alter their lifestyle and the way in which they perform daily activities. In a minority of people, persistent low back pain causes chronic disability.

Low back pain is usually caused by minor damage to the ligaments and muscles in the back secondary to minor injury (e.g. a twist), overexertion (e.g. digging in the garden), or lumbar spondylosis (the natural aging process of the spine). The lower back is vulnerable to these problems because it supports much of the body's weight and is under continual stress from movement such as bending and twisting. Less commonly, low back pain may be due to an underlying disorder such as a prolapsed or herniated (slipped) disk in the spine.

WHAT ARE THE CAUSES?

Low back pain may come on suddenly (acute) or develop gradually over a period of weeks. If the pain persists it's described as chronic.

ACUTE

Sudden back pain is often caused by **lifting** or **moving** heavy objects, such as furniture, and is due to a strained muscle or tendon. It may also be secondary to an acute disk herniation. The injury may be aggravated by subsequent activity. In most cases, symptoms subside within 2–14 days.

CHRONIC

■ Back pain that tends to be more persistent is often caused by **poor posture**, such as while sitting at a desk or driving a car, or by excessive muscle tension due to emotional stress.

■ In back pain in **pregnancy** there are two factors at work – changes in posture because of the extra weight of the baby and softening of the ligaments supporting the spine due to high levels of pregnancy hormones.

■ In people over age 45, persistent low back pain is caused by **osteoarthritis** of the spine, while in younger people the joints of the spine may be affected by **ankylosing spondylitis**.

■ **Pain** from compression of the nerve root is due to a prolapsed disk or spondylosis exerting pressure on a spinal nerve. Back pain of this type may have a gradual or sudden onset and is often accompanied by **sciatica**, a disorder where severe pain shoots down the back of one or, rarely, both legs.

■ Back pain may rarely come from the **bone** itself, for instance, where cancer has spread to bone from a tumor elsewhere in the body.

■ Conditions affecting the **pelvic organs** can cause pain in the lower back. Examples are **pelvic inflammatory disease** and **kidney infection**. **Peptic ulcers** and gallbladder disease can cause "referred" pain that is felt in the back.

WHAT ARE THE SYMPTOMS?

Low back pain can take various forms. You may experience:

● a sharp pain localized to a small area of the back

● a more general aching pain in the back and buttocks, made worse by sitting and relieved by standing

● back stiffness and pain when bending

● pain in the back that radiates to the buttock, leg, and foot, sometimes accompanied by numbness or tingling.

WHAT CAN I DO?

In most cases, you should be able to treat low back pain yourself.

■ An over-the-counter **nonsteroidal anti-inflammatory drug** (NSAID) should reduce the pain, and a heating pad or wrapped hot water bottle or sometimes ice placed against your back may provide additional relief.

■ If the pain is severe, you may be more comfortable resting in bed, but you should not stay in bed for more than two days. Start moving around as soon as possible and gradually return to normal activities.

■ If the pain worsens or is still too severe to allow you to move around after a few days, you

Back-strengthening exercises

The key is to strengthen your **abdominal** muscles so they will "splint" and support your back from the front. You can help prevent back pain by gently exercising the muscles in your back and abdomen. Consult a doctor or ask for a referral to a physical therapist before starting an exercise program. You should not continue any exercise that causes you pain. The movements shown below should make your back muscles stronger and your spine more flexible. Repeat each one 10 times if you can, and try to exercise daily. Do the exercises on a comfortable but firm, flat surface, such as a mat laid on the floor.

Lower back stretch

This stretch may relieve aching joints and muscles in the lower back. Lie on your back with your feet flat on the floor and your knees bent. Lift your knees toward your body. With your hands, pull your knees into your chest. Hold for seven seconds and breathe deeply. Keeping your knees bent, lower your feet to the floor one at a time.

Hump and sag

The movements in this exercise should increase suppleness in the joints and muscles of the back. Support yourself on your hands and knees, your knees slightly apart.

Tuck your chin into your chest, then gently arch your back. Hold for about five seconds. Look up, allowing your back to sag, and hold again for about another five seconds.

Pelvic tilt

This movement helps to stretch the muscles and ligaments of the lower back. Lie on your back with your knees bent and your feet flat on the floor. Press the small of your back into the floor.

Tighten your buttock and abdominal muscles so that your buttocks rise slightly off the floor and your pelvis tilts upward. Hold for six seconds, then relax. Once you've learned this exercise you can do it standing at any time.

should consult your doctor.

■ Once the pain has subsided, you can help prevent any recurrences by paying attention to your posture, learning to lift correctly and doing **regular exercises** to strengthen the muscles of your back and lower abdomen and make your spine more flexible (see box, above).

WHAT MIGHT THE DOCTOR DO?

■ Your doctor will do a full physical examination to assess your posture, the range of movement in your spine, and any areas of local tenderness.

■ Your reflexes, the strength of different leg

TREATMENT

Self-help: Preventing back pain

Driving position: Angle your seat backward a little so it supports your spine, and position the seat so that you can reach the hand and foot controls easily.

Sitting position: Sit with your back straight and both feet on the floor. Use a chair that supports the small of your back. When using a computer, position the monitor so you can look straight at it.

Lifting position: Keep your back straight and hold the object to be lifted as close to your body as possible. Use the muscles of your legs, not your back, to lift the object.

Most people have experienced back pain at some time in their lives, but in many cases the problem could have been avoided. Back pain is often due to poor posture, weak abdominal or back muscles, or sudden muscle strain. You can improve your posture by wearing comfortable shoes, by standing or sitting with your spine properly aligned, and by choosing a supportive mattress for your bed. Gentle, regular exercises may strengthen abdominal and back muscles, and losing excess weight may relieve stress on joints and muscles. Learning how to perform physical tasks safely, such as lifting and carrying objects, can prevent back strain. Ask your doctor or physical therapist for advice on posture, exercises, and diet.

Correct body posture

To break bad postural habits, you should be constantly aware of the way in which you stand, sit, move, and even sleep. The pictures on the left show how to carry out everyday activities comfortably, with minimal strain on your spine and back muscles.

Lifting an object

When lifting, pushing, or pulling a heavy object, keep the object close to you so you can use your full strength to move it. To lift an object, hold the bottom edge so that you support the full weight of the object, and keep your body balanced as you lift to avoid straining your spine.
1. Squat close to the object with your weight evenly on both feet and the object between your legs. Grasp the base of the object.
2. Keep your back straight and lean forward slightly. Stand up in a single, smooth movement, pushing yourself up with your leg muscles and keeping the object close to you.
3. Once you are upright, keep the weight close to your body. Keep your back straight and head up, so that your body is balanced over its center of gravity.

muscles, and the sensation in your legs will be tested to look for evidence of pressure on spinal nerves or the spinal cord.
■ A **pelvic or rectal examination** may also be performed to rule out disorders of the internal organs.
■ You may have various **blood tests and X-rays** to look for underlying causes of the pain, such as joint inflammation or bone cancer.
■ If there is evidence of pressure on the spinal cord or spinal nerves, MRI (magnetic resonance imaging) or CT (computerized tomography) scanning may be done to detect abnormalities requiring special treatment, such as a prolapsed or herniated disk.

WHAT IS THE TREATMENT?
■ Unless the physical examination and other tests indicate that there is a serious underlying cause for your back pain, your doctor will probably advise you to continue taking a non-steroidal anti-inflammatory drug (NSAID).
■ You may be given **physical therapy** to mobilize stiff and painful joints between the vertebrae.
■ A local anesthetic combined with a corticosteroid may be injected into the tender areas.
■ **Osteopathy** may be effective for treating low back pain and an osteopath is worth consulting.

WHAT IS THE OUTLOOK?
You may think your low back pain will never get better but even the worst episodes do, given time. Most clear up without any specific treatment, but the problem recurs in many people unless factors such as poor posture or ways of lifting are improved.

In a small number of people, low back pain may be a long-standing condition, severely disrupting their work and social life and sometimes leading to depression. Effective pain control is essential in these situations, and many people find that taking the newer **antidepressants**, SSRIs, helps them cope and allows tense muscles to relax.

Once you have "a back" you'll always have a back. As we get older, episodes of pain may get more severe and take longer to resolve but with heat, back-strengthening exercises, painkiller, and physical therapy most resolve after several months. Being careful with posture, sitting, and moving or lifting heavy weights should be part of our lives.

See also:
• Ankylosing spondylitis p. 430
• Back-strengthening exercises p. 435
• CT scanning p. 401
• Infection of the kidneys p. 376
• MRI p. 409 • Osteoarthritis p. 428
• Peptic ulcer p. 353 • Slipped disk p. 437
• X-rays p. 426

Slipped disk

WHEN ONE OF THE SHOCK-ABSORBING PADS THAT LIE BETWEEN THE VERTEBRAE OF
THE SPINE BECOMES DISPLACED AND PROTRUDES, IT IS KNOWN AS A SLIPPED DISC.
DOCTORS REFER TO THE CONDITION AS A PROLAPSED OR HERNIATED DISC.

A slipped disk is most common between the ages of 25 and 45 and is slightly more common in men. Being overweight and lifting objects incorrectly are risk factors.

The shock-absorbing discs between the vertebrae consist of a strong, fibrous outer coat and a soft, gelatinous core. A prolapsed disk occurs when the core pushes outward, distorting the shape of the disc. If the outer coat ruptures, the condition is termed a **herniated disc**. When a disk prolapses or herniates, the surrounding tissues become inflamed and swollen. Together with the disc, the tissues may press on a spinal nerve, causing pain down the length of that nerve, the most common being the **sciatic nerve**, giving rise to **sciatica**.

WHAT ARE THE CAUSES?
After about the age of 25, the discs begin to **dry out**, being driest on waking, so strenuous activity involving the back shouldn't be undertaken without a good warm-up routine. Discs also become more vulnerable to prolapse or herniation as a result of the normal stress of daily life and minor injury. Sometimes damage to a disk is caused by a sharp bending or twisting movement or by lifting a heavy object incorrectly. From about the age of 45, fibrous tissue forms around the discs, eventually stabilizing them and making them less likely to be damaged.

WHAT ARE THE SYMPTOMS?
Symptoms of a prolapsed or herniated disk may develop progressively over a period of weeks or may appear suddenly. They include:
● dull pain in the affected area
● muscle spasm and stiffness around the affected area that makes movement difficult and pain much worse.

If the disk presses on a spinal nerve, you may also have the following symptoms:
● severe pain, tingling, or numbness in your leg or, if the neck is affected, in your arm
● weakness or restricted movement in your leg or arm.

The pain is usually relieved by rest but can be made worse by walking upstairs, sitting, coughing, sneezing, or bending. Bowel movements can also aggravate the pain. Impaired bladder or bowel function may indicate pressure on the spinal cord, and you should consult a doctor immediately.

WHAT MIGHT BE DONE?
■ X-rays will rule out other causes of back pain, such as spondylosis.
■ MRI (magnetic resonance imaging) or CT (computerized tomography) scanning will locate the position of the prolapsed or herniated disk accurately.
■ Even if the disk is permanently damaged, the pain usually improves over 6–8 weeks as the swelling subsides. Your doctor will suggest bed rest and pain medication. If you are free of pain, physical therapy and exercises may help reduce muscle spasms and hasten recovery. For persistent pain, you will require referral to a hospital.
■ Rarely, pain may be relieved with **traction**,

TREATMENT

Microdiscectomy

Microdiscectomy is a surgical procedure used to treat a prolapsed or herniated disk pressing on a spinal nerve or the spinal cord. The protruding part of the disk is removed through an incision in the fibrous outer coat of the disk using an operating microscope. The operation is performed under general anesthetic and requires a brief stay in the hospital.

in which the spine is gently stretched with weights to create more space around the nerves, reducing pressure on and around them.
■ Some people may benefit from a selective **nerve root block**, in which a local anesthetic, sometimes combined with a corticosteroid drug, is injected around the compressed nerve to decrease swelling. Occasionally surgery is needed to decompress the affected nerve root.

See also:
● CT scanning p. 401 ● Low back pain p. 434
● MRI p. 409
● Spondylosis p. 432

Restless legs syndrome

RESTLESS LEGS SYNDROM CAUSES A BURNING SENSATION IN THE LEGS AND FEET THAT
MAY BE RELIEVED BY MOVING THEM, SOMETIMES CONTINUOUSLY.

We still have a lot to learn about this distressing condition but around 5 percent of the population can expect to experience some or all of the symptoms during their lives.

WHAT CAUSES IT?
Mainly associated with elderly women, restless legs can also affect men and children and there is evidence to suggest that it runs in families. The first symptoms may occur mildly or infrequently in the teenage years, occur again in pregnancy to fade away after the birth, only to reappear later in life.

Some studies have suggested an association with **anxiety, depression,** and **stress**. It is known that about one-third of all patients with **rheumatoid arthritis** also suffer from this condition.

WHAT ARE THE SYMPTOMS?
Unpleasant creeping, prickling, or burning sensations in one or both calves that can sometimes be felt in the feet, thighs, trunk, and arms. The sensations can begin soon after sitting or lying down but usually come on in the evening and at night, causing severe

disruption of sleep.
Although symptoms can vary widely, the one consistent factor is that short-lived relief can be achieved by movement.

If you, or someone you know, suffers frequently from this kind of distressing discomfort, it is important to consult your doctor so a diagnosis can be made. Other disorders – for example, iron deficiency anemia, circulatory, or disk problems – can give rise to similar symptoms.

A similar painful condition, common in the elderly, is **meralgia paraesthetica**, or pain in the outer leg. Unlike restless legs, it can be easily treated by conservative treatment so you can see the importance of an accurate diagnosis.

WHAT CAN I DO?
As yet there is no cure for restless legs, but some sufferers have found regular gentle exercise, swimming, cool showers, yoga, and relaxation exercises and vitamin B_{12} helpful.

It is wise to avoid standing or sitting for long periods, catnaps during the day, heavy meals before bedtime, coffee, restrictive clothing, and clothing made from synthetic materials. Treatment with certain drugs has proved effective, in particular **ropinirole**. No clinical trials have been carried out on ropinirole as a therapy for restless legs (although trials are about to start soon) but there is considerable anecdotal evidence indicating that it has brought relief to many sufferers. It was developed to control leg tremors in people with Parkinson's disease and it has been discovered to have a wider application. Since it is not licensed as a therapy for restless legs, a doctor may need to prescribe it privately on a "named patient" basis. This is where a doctor notifies the health authorities that he is administering an unlicensed drug to his patient and that you both accept responsibility for the decision.

The support group for sufferers (see Useful addresses p. 567) can provide a wealth of information and practical advice on remedies that other people have found effective. Through newsletters it shares information about current medical research and investigations.

MUSCLES AND TENDONS

When skeletal muscles contract and relax they move the body by making joints bend and straighten. Muscles are connected to bones by fibrous tissue known as tendons. Both muscles and tendons can be temporarily or permanently damaged by injury and overuse, leading to pain, weakness, restricted movement, and fatigue.

Although our muscles account for half the weight of the body they are only rarely affected by disease. Overexertion of a muscle or tendon, through very strenuous exercise, unusual activity, or as a result of repetitive movements or immobilization, will cause many of the disorders described in this section, including **muscle cramps**, **frozen shoulder**, **repetitive strain injury**, and **tennis elbow**. Inflammation of a tendon (tendinitis) or tendon sheath (tenosynovitis) is really quite common and quite painful so I've included some personal observations. Probably the most common cause of muscle pain is **fibromyalgia**, a condition whose precise origin remains a mystery but there is nearly always a psychological component.

Some disorders that affect the muscles are covered in other parts of the book. So you'll find **immune system** disorders such as **polymyositis and dermatomyositis** on page 326 and the inherited disease **muscular dystrophy** on page 523. Musculoskeletal conditions are on page 434.

Muscle cramps

PAINFUL SPASMS IN A MUSCLE OR GROUP OF MUSCLES, USUALLY IN THE LOWER LEG, ARE COMMONLY KNOWN AS CRAMPS; THIS UNPLEASANT BUT TEMPORARY CONDITION AFFECTS ALMOST EVERYONE FROM TIME TO TIME.

WHAT CAUSES IT?
Painful spasms of cramping, often lasting only a few minutes, make the muscle become hard and tender; this is usually due to overuse. Protracted pain from muscle spasm is normally because a muscle is protecting an injured part underneath it, as in spondylosis and spondylitis, and won't go until the injured part improves. Muscle cramps may occur in any muscle in the body but they are most common in the large groups of leg muscles, such as the quadriceps on the front of the thighs, the hamstrings at the back of the thighs, and the calf muscles. When abdominal muscles are affected, the condition is also known as a "stitch."
■ Muscle cramps often develop during **exercise**, because the working muscle outstrips its oxygen supply or builds up lactic acid during anaerobic exercise.
■ Another possible cause is the loss of salt and water due to heavy sweating during hot weather or strenuous exercise.
■ Muscle cramps may also develop if you have been sitting or lying in an awkward position for a long time.
■ Cramping is not the only cause of attacks of muscle pain. If you develop recurrent muscle pain in the calves when you are walking, you should consult your doctor; the cause may be poor blood flow when the arteries that supply blood to the leg muscles become clogged by atherosclerosis.

WHAT MIGHT HELP?
■ The immediate self-help treatment for muscle cramps is to stretch and rub the affected area and to apply a heating pad.
■ You should drink plenty of fluids and eat something salty.
■ If you regularly have muscle cramps at night, your doctor may prescribe a low dose of **quinine**, an antimalarial drug that effectively relieves the symptoms.
■ Muscle relaxing drugs are sometimes helpful.
■ Flunitrazepam, a sedative with muscle-relaxing effects, may give you a pain-free night's sleep.

See also:
• **The heart and atherosclerosis p. 222**
• **Spondylosis p. 432**

FOCUS *on* RSI

Any person whose work or hobby involves repeated physical movements, particularly of the hands and arms, is at risk of causing damage to tendons, nerves, muscles, and other soft body tissues. This type of injury is commonly known as repetitive strain injury (RSI).

Workers ranging from packers to musicians can develop RSI as a result of the tasks they perform. The computer, with the flat, light-touch keyboard that permits high-speed typing has produced an epidemic of injuries to the hands, arms, and shoulders.

WHAT ARE THE SYMPTOMS?
- **Tightness**, discomfort, stiffness, soreness, and burning in the hands, wrists, fingers, and forearms or elbows.
- **Tingling**, coldness, or numbness in the hands.
- **Clumsiness** or loss of strength and **coordination** in the hands.
- **Pain** that wakes you up at night.
- **Need to massage** your hands, wrists, and arms.

RSI CONDITIONS
Specific conditions include **nerve compression, tendonitis,** or inflammation of the tendons, **carpal tunnel syndrome** – which causes numbness and pain in the hand – and involuntary movements and spasms of the hand and fingers.

All have different symptoms, from pain and stiffness to jerky movements and cramping.

WHAT IS THE CAUSE?
Researchers around the world have been searching for explanations for RSI. Some doctors aren't so sure that RSI has a single cause and believe that a variety of factors, including genes and personality, could play a part.

One theory says it's psychological and another says it's physical. A third theory says it's an interaction between physical and mental. There isn't just one cause – some people get RSI, others don't while performing an identical task. It may even stem from the brain becoming confused by the repetitive task.

SELF-HELP
Wrist splints, arm rests, split keyboards, and spinal adjustment won't get you back to work quickly. Your RSI will relapse unless you make long-term changes in technique and work habits.

If, as some experts think, RSI turns out to be a problem of the brain rather than the hands and arms, reeducating the brain could be more useful. So exercises such as using **Braille** cards or **playing dominoes with the eyes closed** – what the experts call **sensory retraining** – may be the answer for some people (see box, below).

WHAT IS THE TREATMENT?
Treatments range from anti-inflammatory drugs to surgery, but for some people the only cure is a change of job. And compensation can be hard to come by.

HOW DO I AVOID RSI?
- Eliminate unnecessary computer usage. No **amount of ergonomic changes, fancy keyboards, or exercises** are going to help if you are simply typing too much.
- **Don't** use computer/video games that often involve long, unbroken sessions of very intense keyboard usage.
- Increase your font sizes. Small fonts encourage you to hunch forward into the monitor to read, putting pressure on nerves and blood vessels in the neck and shoulders.
- Don't pound on the keys. Use a light touch.
- Use two hands to perform double-key operations instead of twisting one hand to do it. Move your whole hand to hit function keys instead of stretching.
- Take a lot of breaks to stretch and relax. This means both momentary breaks every few minutes and longer breaks every hour or so.
- Hold the mouse lightly, don't grip it hard or squeeze it. Place the pointing device close to the keyboard. Pace and plan your computer work.
- **Don't** tuck the telephone between your shoulder and ear so you can type and talk on the phone at the same time, because it's a great strain on your neck, shoulders, and arms.
- Keep your arms and hands warm. Cold muscles and tendons are at much greater risk from overuse injuries.
- Take care of your eyes.
- Look at other things you're doing. Problems may be caused or aggravated by other things you do frequently. Sports, carrying children, hobbies requiring intense small work like knitting, and excess effort/tension in other daily things may have enormous impact too.
- Pay attention to your body. Pain is a symptom that your body is in trouble, but learning what's comfortable or awkward for your body before you're in pain may prevent injury.
- Kids are at risk, too, with increasing hours in front of the computer at home and school, using equipment that rarely is set up correctly for people of their size.

Handy hints

- Exercise to teach your fingers how to discriminate again.
- Play dominoes with your eyes shut.
- Match a shape to an opening with eyes closed.
- Put together puzzles that have a raised surface with eyes closed.
- Play cards using a Braille deck.
- Ask someone to draw letters and numbers on your fingers and, with eyes closed, try to guess what they are writing.
- Get someone to rub different objects on your hand and try to identify them.
- Carry pairs of different shaped objects in your pocket and try to match them.
- Make a grab bag of different shaped items and try to identify them.
- Play games requiring orientation, such as pinning the tail on the donkey, blindfolded.

Fibromyalgia

THIS IS A MUSCLE DISORDER THAT CAUSES WIDESPREAD MUSCLE PAIN, ACHING, STIFFNESS, AND
FATIGUE ASSOCIATED WITH MUSCLE TENDERNESS.

Although the condition has no obvious cause, and no visible abnormality has ever been identified in the muscle itself, fibromyalgia is more common in females, and often develops during periods of stress.

WHAT ARE THE SYMPTOMS?
The symptoms of fibromyalgia develop slowly over weeks and occur in a distinct pattern around the body. They may include the following:
● muscle pain in the upper back, head, thighs, abdomen, and hips
● particularly tender areas of muscle, typically at the base of the skull, the neck, and near the shoulder blades.
  Fibromyalgia is commonly associated with headaches, fatigue, depression, anxiety disorders, and disturbed sleep patterns. Some people have irregular bowel movements (irritable bowel syndrome). All of these symptoms usually become worse when levels of stress increase.

WHAT MIGHT BE DONE?
■ The diagnosis of fibromyalgia is often based on the symptoms and a physical examination, but your doctor may arrange for blood tests to rule out other disorders, such as rheumatoid arthritis.
■ Although there is no specific treatment, the pain may be relieved by deep tissue massage and locally applied moist heat, ultrasound treatment,

or an injection with a local anesthetic.
■ Your doctor may also prescribe a low dose of amitriptyline, which is effective in relieving pain in this condition.
■ Regular exercise is also important to maintain muscle tone and flexibility.
  Most people make a full recovery, but in some cases the symptoms recur.

Deep tissue massage can help relieve the pain of fibromyalgia.

> **See also:**
> ● **Irritable bowel syndrome p. 362**
> ● **Rheumatoid arthritis p. 429**

Polymyalgia rheumatica

THE PROMINENT COMPLAINT IN POLYMYALGIA RHEUMATICA IS PAIN AND STIFFNESS
IN THE SHOULDERS AND HIPS, ASSOCIATED WITH A LOSS OF ENERGY
AND A GENERAL SENSE OF NOT FEELING WELL.

The condition, which may run in families, is rare under the age of 60 and is twice as common in females. Polymyalgia rheumatica is an **autoimmune disorder** in which antibodies attack the body's own tissues, in this case the muscles. It may occur in association with another autoimmune disorder, **temporal arteritis**.

WHAT ARE THE SYMPTOMS?
The symptoms usually appear over a few weeks but sometimes develop suddenly. They include:
● painful, stiff muscles, often causing difficulty getting out of bed and moving around and usually affecting the neck and shoulders

● profound fatigue
● persistent or intermittent fever; night sweats
● weight loss
● depression.
  If temporal arteritis is also present, there could be severe headaches on one or both sides of the head and tenderness of the scalp.

WHAT MIGHT BE DONE?
It is important to get advice because treatment is simple and effective.
■ Your doctor will probably be able to make a diagnosis simply on a physical examination and the results of blood tests to look for inflammation.

■ Additional blood tests will be performed to exclude other disorders, such as rheumatoid arthritis.
■ **Oral corticosteroids** reduce the inflammation and pain dramatically. If you also have temporal arteritis, the initial doses may be high. In either case, the dose will be reduced to a maintenance level once the symptoms subside.
  Take heart! Symptoms are usually relieved soon after starting corticosteroid treatment. However, polymyalgia rheumatica may persist, in which case you will need to continue taking low doses of a coricosteroid, such as prednisone.

Tennis elbow and golfer's elbow

THIS IS INJURY OF A TENDON AT ITS ATTACHMENT TO THE BONE
AT THE ELBOW DUE TO UNACCUSTOMED REPETITIVE MOVEMENT.

The disorder is rare among professionals but common among recreational tennis players, golfers, keyboard users, gardeners, anyone who uses their arms repetitively, and among people doing repetitive unaccustomed activities like cleaning windows and hanging wallpaper. Music conductors get tennis elbow too!

Tennis elbow and golfer's elbow both occur when the tendon attachment of the muscle to the bone at the elbow becomes damaged. In tennis elbow, the tendon on the outer side of the elbow is injured; in golfer's elbow, the tendon on the inner side of the elbow is affected. It depends if the movement is mainly **backhanded** using the extensor tendon (tennis elbow) or **forehanded** using the flexor tendon (golfer's elbow).

Both conditions are caused by vigorous and repeated use of the forearm against resistance, which can occur when playing certain sports, such as tennis, using a screwdriver, or using pruning shears. The tendon is repeatedly pulled at the point at which it is attached to the bone, which may cause small tears to develop. The resulting damage leads to tenderness and pain in the affected arm.

WHAT IS THE TREATMENT?

■ You should rest the affected painful arm as much as possible.
■ Physical therapy, ice packs, and simple exercises to stretch and strengthen the muscles may help.
■ Ultrasound treatment may help relieve symptoms.

■ You may also find that a non-steroidal anti-inflammatory drug (NSAID) helps.
■ If the condition does not improve within 2–6 weeks, your doctor may inject a corticosteroid drug into the tender area.

■ Once the symptoms have subsided, you should seek advice from a physiotherapist on ways to change your technique before resuming the sport or activity that gave rise to the condition.

Frozen shoulder

PAIN AND RESTRICTION OF MOVEMENT IN THE SHOULDER JOINT, COMMONLY FOLLOWING
A MINOR INJURY, IS CALLED FROZEN SHOULDER. THE CONDITION IS MORE COMMON IN WOMEN
THAN MEN. ANY INJURY TO THE SHOULDER CAN END UP AS FROZEN SHOULDER.

WHAT CAUSES IT?

Frozen shoulder may be caused by inflammation as a result of an injury to the shoulder region. The condition may also occur if the shoulder is kept immobilized for a period of time, for example after a minor injury or stroke. However, frozen shoulder may also develop for no apparent reason. People with **diabetes mellitus** and **thyroid disease** are more susceptible to the condition. The pain is due to inflammation inside the shoulder joint made worse by muscle spasm to protect an injured part underneath them.

WHAT ARE THE SYMPTOMS?

The symptoms of frozen shoulder often begin gradually over a period of weeks or months. They include:
● pain in the shoulder, which can be very severe in the early stage of the condition and often worse at night
● with time, decreasing pain but increasing stiffness and restricted joint movement
● in severe cases, pain traveling down the arm to the elbow and up into the neck.

If you have pain in the shoulder that lasts for more than a few days, consult your doctor

without delay. The longer a frozen shoulder is left, the harder it is to treat. It's quite common for a frozen shoulder to last a year or longer, but it does always get better. Most specialists prescribe hydrocortisone injected into the joint.

WHAT MIGHT BE DONE?

■ A painkiller or a nonsteroidal anti-inflammatory drug (NSAID) will relieve pain and reduce inflammation.
■ If the pain persists or is severe, you may be given a corticosteroid drug by a **direct**

injection into the shoulder joint to treat the inflammation.

■ You may also be referred for physical therapy, hydrotherapy, massage and heat treatment. If night pain is severe, codeine may be prescribed for short-term use.

■ Despite these measures, your shoulder may remain stiff for up to a year or longer.

■ In very severe, persistent cases you may have to have your shoulder stretched to its limits under a general anesthetic.

Whatever the severity of the condition, recovery is usually slow and may take up to another six months after the disappearance of stiffness to be back to normal.

See also:
• **Diabetes mellitus p. 504** • **NSAIDS p. 431**

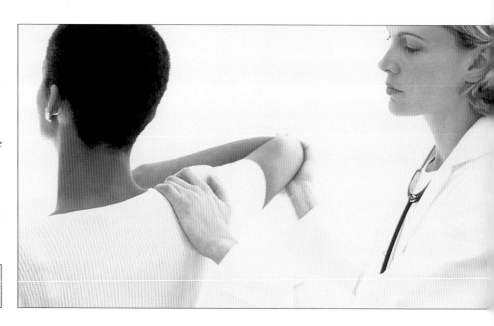

Dupuytren's contracture

IN DUPUYTREN'S CONTRACTURE, THE FIBROUS TISSUE IN THE PALM OF THE HAND
BECOMES THICKENED AND SHORTENED, RESULTING IN DEFORMITY.

One or more of the fingers, often the ring and little fingers, are pulled towards the palm into a bent position and, sometimes, painful lumps develop on the palm and the overlying skin becomes puckered. In about half of all cases, both hands are involved. Rarely, the disorder affects the soles of the feet. Dupuytren's contracture is much more common in men over age 50; alcohol abuse is a risk factor. The disorder may run in families.

The tissue changes in Dupuytren's contracture develop slowly over months or years. The cause is unknown, but it occurs more commonly in people with **diabetes mellitus** or **epilepsy**, and in people who **drink to excess**. About 1 in 10 people with Dupuytren's contracture has a relative with the disorder, so there may be a **gene** at work.

WHAT MIGHT BE DONE?

■ In mild cases no treatment may be needed.

■ If your fingers are slightly bent you may benefit from stretching exercises or short-term splinting.

■ For lumps in your palm, a corticosteroid drug may be injected into the affected area.

■ In severe cases, surgery is the most effective treatment, especially if performed early. Under regional or local anesthetic, the thickened tissue in the palm is removed to allow the fingers to straighten.

■ Further treatment may be needed if the disorder recurs.

See also:
• **Diabetes mellitus p. 504**
• **Epilepsy p. 538**

Skin, Hair, and Nails

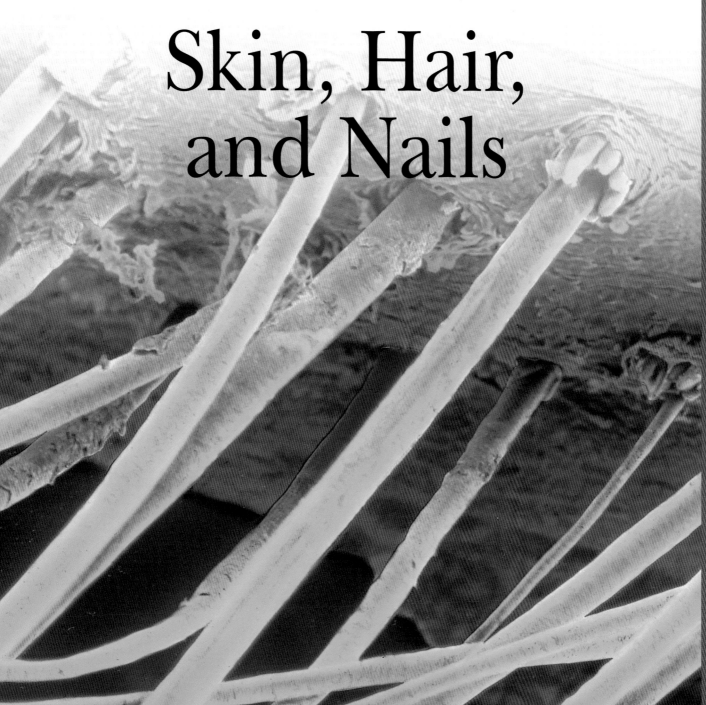

Image shows a colored scanning electron micrograph of eyelashes

Miriam's overview

The skin is the largest organ in the body. When it gets hot and pink it siphons off half our blood, which is why we can feel faint when we get hot and bothered – there's not enough blood left over to nourish the brain.

The skin is the body's first defense, it's a protective layer that stops harmful things from getting in and useful things from getting out.

Among other vital jobs it keeps our core temperature constant by conserving heat when we cool down and throwing off calories when we get too hot.

These two main functions of the skin may go awry with dire consequences.

● When more than half the skin is damaged as in severe burns the body loses its ability to keep the temperature steady and we may become dangerously superheated.
● With most of its covering gone the body can't hang on to vital components, they seep away. An example of this is protein which may be lost from burned skin so quickly that life is threatened.

The main message of this millennium about the skin is to stay out of the sun. Wear sunscreen on exposed parts every day, yes, every day. Exposure to sunlight causes skin cancers and the sunshine on a bleak winter's day still counts as part of your TOTAL LIFE DOSE.

It's this cumulative dose that causes cancer. You will get your total life dose quickly if you live in Australia or slowly if you live in England. That means in Australia you'll still be quite young when your skin has soaked up its total life dose of sunshine. Once that's happened you're vulnerable to skin cancer. As the ozone layer gets thinner you get the total life dose earlier and earlier. So the watchword is sun protection at all times, starting as a baby.

"*wear sunscreen* on exposed parts every day, yes, *every day*"

That's crucially important because we've learned that severe sunburn as a child can cause damage so that you have an increased tendency to develop skin cancer later in life. I've never understood the obsession with getting a tan. Every day in the sun means a wrinkle later. The sun ages the skin like nothing else. And it can't be undone.

The skin has accessories in the form of hair and nails, both of which are dead. It follows that you can only affect their basic quality while they're growing in the hair follicle and nailbed respectively. That's about two months before their condition becomes visible to the naked eye so it's a retrospective judgement. Put another way, if you want healthy hair and nails for your summer vacation you make your plans and take action (mainly what you eat) at Christmas.

Inflammation of the skin, such as eczema (dermatitis), is generally part of genetically programmed reaction to stress and other factors called atopy, found on p. 312.

INSIDE
your skin, hair, and nails

The skin is the largest organ of the body and provides our first line of defense against injury and infection. Hair and nails, which grow from the skin, provide the body with further protection.

Skin consists of two layers of tissue: the outer **epidermis**, which is quite thin, and the thicker **inner dermis**. The upper layer of the epidermis consists mostly of dead cells, while the dermis is made of strong, elastic tissue and contains **blood vessels**, **glands**, and **nerve endings**. Hair, which is composed mainly of a protein called **keratin**, grows from **follicles** in the skin. Nails are also composed mainly of keratin and grow from an area beneath the nail's **cuticle** called the **matrix**.

the parts of a nail

external view

free edge

nail plate

lunular

cuticle

nail matrix

cross section

free edge

nail plate

cuticle

nail matrix

nail bed

skin

bone

The nail itself is dead tissue made up of keratin, the same protein as hair. Nails provide the sensitive ends of the fingers with a protective covering.

the structure of the skin and hair

The skin is the body's largest organ. Skin has two layers, the outer epidermis, and the thicker dermis that lies beneath it.

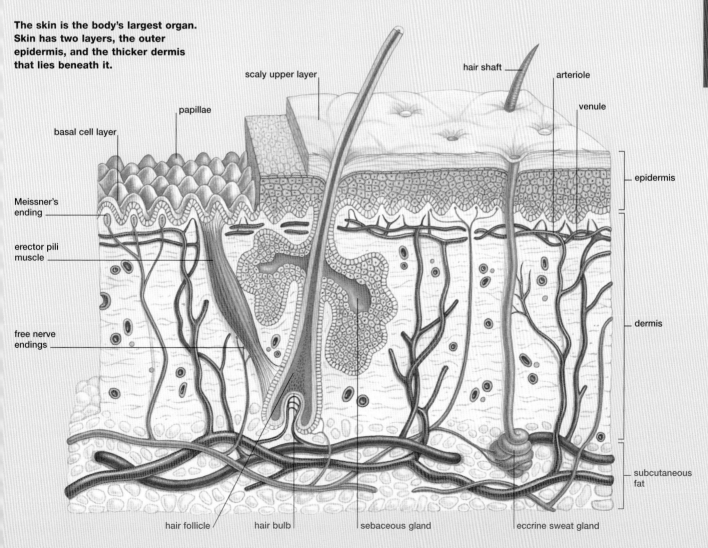

scaly upper layer

hair shaft

arteriole

venule

papillae

basal cell layer

epidermis

Meissner's ending

erector pili muscle

dermis

free nerve endings

subcutaneous fat

hair follicle

hair bulb

sebaceous gland

eccrine sweat gland

Teenage acne

THE GREASY SKIN WITH BLACKHEADS, PUS-FILLED PIMPLES, PURPLISH-RED LUMPS, AND
POSSIBLY SCARRING THAT CHARACTERIZES ACNE IS MOST COMMON IN ADOLESCENTS,
MORE COMMON IN BOYS, AND MAY RUN IN FAMILIES.

Acne mainly affects the face, chest, and back and is caused by blockage and inflammation of the grease glands in the skin. There is a persistent adult form of acne.

Our skin contains grease (sebaceous) glands that secrete an oily substance (sebum) to keep the skin supple and moist. If the exits from these glands become blocked, sebum bursts into the deeper layers of skin. Here it's highly irritating and causes inflammation, which can become infected. The result is pus-filled pimples and the classic tender, purplish lumps of acne. When the lumps heal, scars and pitting may be left behind.

WHAT ARE THE CAUSES?
■ **Male hormones** are the cause of acne, and this goes for adolescent girls as well as boys. Under the influence of these male hormones (androgens), the best known of which is **testosterone**, cells at the exit from the sebaceous gland overgrow and block the outlet. At puberty, androgens pour into the blood and reach their highest levels in both sexes. In girls, they're even higher than estrogens. So at **adolescence**, with all those androgens rushing about, sebaceous glands get blocked very easily. To make matters worse, androgens cause overproduction of sebum so sebaceous glands are stretched to bursting and some do.
■ Many women have acne in a mild form just prior to **menstruation,** when estrogen levels are low.
■ People who take **steroids** may get acne.
■ Skin **bacteria** are important too in the formation of the red and yellow pimples. After puberty, the skin of the face and upper trunk, with or without acne, contains many bacteria. The most important bacteria in acne are called *Propionibacterium acnes*. They get into the ducts

of the grease glands where they make chemicals that eventually escape into the deeper parts of the skin and cause more inflammation. This does not mean that acne is infective: it isn't. It's not a question of hygiene either. Washing, or the lack of it, does not cause acne.

Sometimes acne persists into the late teens and 20s and, rarely, into the 30s. It's no joke because **adult acne** is more difficult to treat.

FACTORS THAT AFFECT ACNE
■ No matter what you're told or have read, acne **isn't** caused by eating rich or fatty foods, not washing thoroughly, or by drinking too much alcohol.
■ There seems to be a tendency for acne to run in families.
■ In girls, a flare-up of acne is common just before the **monthly period**.
■ Pregnancy does not usually influence acne.
■ **Sunshine** may help acne, but tanning booths give little benefit.
■ **Diet** probably has no role in acne.
■ **Poor personal hygiene** does not worsen it.
■ **Squeezing pimples** usually aggravates the problem.
■ **Stress** may make acne worse.
■ Overcleansing, too much rubbing or using products that contain abrasives worsen acne because they liberate bacteria from the grease glands onto the skin and promote more pimples.

If acne starts after adolescence, for example in women over the age of 25, the factors above also apply.

SHOULD I SEE A DOCTOR AND WHAT HE CAN DO?
Yes, do, acne can be totally cured these days. But effective treatments are only available by prescription, **not over the counter**. The basis of treatment is four-fold:
1. To reduce the number of bacteria on the skin
2. To stop the multiplication of cells in the sebaceous glands, which results in blockage
3. To unblock pores
4. To lower sebum production.

GENERAL PRINCIPLES OF TREATMENT
With prescription treatment – not over-the-counter remedies – pimples can usually be kept under excellent control and scarring prevented. **90 percent of patients show a 50 percent improvement in three months**

and an 80 percent improvement within six months, but **continuous treatment** is necessary **for many years**.

There are three types of oral therapy: **antibiotics**, **hormones**, and **retinoids**. All are available only by prescription and, with the exception of retinoids, should be combined with topical therapy. People who respond to oral antibiotics may need repeat courses, each lasting at least six months.
■ Gels and creams containing **benzoyl peroxide** are often recommended to help unblock pores.
■ Long-term therapy with **oral antibiotics** often helps. The antibiotics are prescribed regularly for up to six months at a time. They have an effect not only on the bacteria in the skin but may also have a direct effect on inflammatory cells in acne pimples, as well as on sebum production. A daily dose of the antibiotic **tetracycline** (750mg once a day) has been shown to help acne sufferers a great deal. There are usually no side effects and the dose is reduced according to the progress of the treatment.
■ Creams based on **vitamin A** reduce sebum production but may have side effects such as reddening of the skin, and should only be used under medical supervision.
■ The treatment of severe acne has greatly improved with the use of oral **retinoid drugs**, such as **isotretinoin** (related to vitamin A), which are prescribed only when antibiotics and other measures haven't helped. Oral

Stages of acne

Acne is graded in stages of severity:

Stage 1: An oily skin with blackheads

Stage 2: Stage 1 with pus-filled pimples

Stage 3: Stage 2 with deep, tender, hard purplish lumps

Stage 4: Stage 3 with pitted and scarred skin.

WARNING:
SIDE EFFECTS OF ISOTRETINOIN
All patients develop considerable drying of the lips and skin (especially of the face); some have mild aches and pains in their joints, and headaches. However, all these side effects can be easily and well controlled, for example by using a moisturizing cream or a simple painkiller, such as acetaminophen. It is very rare to have to stop treatment. BUT the **drug will harm an unborn baby and contraception must be used** for two months before, during, and three months after treatment. Oral isotretinoin can also cause liver damage and your doctor will monitor you for this.

isotretinoin is very effective but it can only be prescribed by a dermatologist, whose instructions must be strictly followed. A five-month course is usually needed, **after which most acne will be virtually clear**. These drugs must be used cautiously because they may cause liver damage and will cause malformations in an unborn baby. Depression has also been reported as a possible side effect.

■ Acne cysts can often be treated by **intralesional therapy** (direct injection of a drug into the acne pimples), which also helps to reduce scarring.

■ In some cases of severe and extensive scarring, **dermabrasion** (that's the removal of the top layer of skin under a general anesthetic) may help get rid of pits and scars.

■ A special form of the **oral contraceptive pill** may be prescribed for women because it's often successful in settling acne down. Ordinary contraceptive pills have little or no effect on acne. However, your doctor can prescribe one particular oral contraceptive that is often helpful. The rationale is that the estrogen in the pill reduces the production of sebum. It also opposes the effect of male hormones in blocking sebaceous glands and frees them up. It is usually taken for 12–36 months. The side effects of this medication are the same as those of an ordinary contraceptive pill; ask your doctor to explain these to you if you want further information. A doctor is unlikely to prescribe the pill before the age of

17, unless it's for contraception, because the hormones may interfere with growth.

ESCAPE ROUTE

If you're unhappy with the results of treatment, ask your doctor if you can see a **dermatologist** who'll tell you about the very latest advances in acne treatment and special procedures that are available only in hospitals.

Acne is a condition that can be virtually cured in expert hands and if it's really bothering you, insist that you see a dermatologist.

TREATMENT OF SCARS

Carefully selected patients with bad scarring may be considered for dermabrasion. This operation is usually performed by plastic surgeons or dermatologists, under a local or general anesthetic. The success rate is between 25 and 70 percent. Only patients who are strongly motivated to have the operation should be recommended for it. If in doubt, surgery should be avoided.

HOW SUCCESSFUL IS TREATMENT FOR ACNE?

Acne is usually one of the easiest of the persistent skin conditions to treat, but it must be treated sooner rather than later. Early treatment minimizes the risk of scarring.

Don't give up your treatment. Doctors can now offer therapies that can guarantee a satisfactory result in virtually everyone.

Rosacea

Rosacea is a long-term, possibly permanent skin condition and is most common in women between the ages of 30 and 55 and after menopause. The features of rosacea include redness and pimples on the cheeks and forehead. The condition often runs in families. Alcohol, coffee, and spicy foods may trigger attacks so it's best to avoid them, as well as temperature extremes in winter.

Special treatment will be prescribed by a dermatologist (a skin specialist).

WHAT ABOUT ALTERNATIVE METHODS?

Herbalists will almost certainly recommend special diets and special creams and possibly certain natural or herbal medicines to take by mouth, none of which are proven to work. Sage, plantain, verbascum, and ground ivy are said to have useful astringent properties. Shepherd's purse has cleansing properties. Aromatherapists advocate the use of bergamot, camphor, cedarwood, juniper, and lavender.

SELF-HELP

Coping with acne

■ **Cleanse** your skin meticulously. Use an **antiseptic soap** or soap solution, brought up to a lather in the palm of your hand, and gently massage it into your skin for at least two minutes, then rinse off. The aim is to de-grease the skin. Wash this way at least three times a day.

■ **Don't** use commercial acne cleansers since they scrape the skin, break down the pustules, and spread germs all over the skin, thereby encouraging acne lesions elsewhere.

■ You can treat blackheads by **steaming** your face. Hold your face about 12in (30cm) above a bowl of hot water from the tap and cover your head with a towel. The steam will cause the pores to open. You can then very gently nudge out the blackhead with a clean fingertip.

■ You should never squeeze anything but a blackhead. Try to keep your fingers away from the acne pimples – touching and rubbing simply spreads germs into the

surrounding skin. Much worse, squeezing forces sebum out of the gland and into the skin, causing those hard, tender, purple lumps.

■ Don't put anything greasy on your skin. It'll make your acne worse.

■ If you're female, wear heavy-textured oil-free makeup to cover the pimples. Many people mistakenly believe that makeup blocks the pores. That's completely wrong. Nothing put on the skin (except paint) can block pores. Makeup won't make acne worse and it does improve morale, which in turn makes acne better.

■ Moderate exposure to sunlight is helpful since it dries out the skin. Doctors advocate a **mild peel** from mild sunburn to unblock the pores.

■ Don't let acne affect your diet. Research has shown that foods such as chocolate don't have the slightest effect on acne. So eat a balanced diet to improve your general health.

Mild acne can often be successfully controlled using simple self-help measures.

Psoriasis

ABOUT 1 IN 50 PEOPLE SUFFERS FROM PSORIASIS. THE RED, THICKENED, SCALY RASH THAT CHARACTERIZES THIS CONDITION TENDS TO FLARE UP AT DIFFERENT TIMES THROUGHOUT LIFE.

If psoriasis affects many parts of the body, commonly the fronts of the knees, the backs of the elbows, trunk, scalp, and back, it may cause physical discomfort as well as embarrassment in public due to shedding skin scales. The nails can be involved as can the joints. Psoriasis often runs in families and infections and stress can trigger an attack.

In a psoriasis plaque, new skin cells are produced about ten times faster than normal and at a much faster rate than dead cells are shed. The skin cells pile up to form thick, creamy colored scales. The cause is not known, but psoriasis often has a genetic component. A flare-up of psoriasis may be triggered by infection, injury or stress. Certain drugs, such as **antidepressants**, especially lithium, **antihypertensives**, **beta blockers,** and **antimalarial drugs**, can trigger psoriasis in some people. Drinking alcohol can worsen existing psoriasis.

WHAT ARE THE TYPES?

There are **four** main types of psoriasis, each of which has a distinctive appearance. Some people may be affected by more than one type. Here are the characteristics of each type.

1. PLAQUE PSORIASIS

■ Areas called plaques, consisting of thickened, red skin with cream-colored scaly surfaces, usually occur on the knees, elbows, lower back, and scalp, behind the ears and at the hairline.
■ There is intermittent itching.
■ Nails become discolored and covered with small pits. In severe cases, the nails thicken and lift away from the nail beds.
■ Plaques tend to last for weeks or months and may recur intermittently.

2. GUTTATE PSORIASIS

This form most commonly affects **children** and **adolescents**, often occurring after a bacterial **throat infection**.
■ Numerous coin-shaped, pink patches of scaly skin, each about ⅜in (1cm) across, appear mainly on the back and chest.
■ There is usually intermittent itching.

These symptoms usually disappear in 4–6 months and do not recur, but more than half of those affected later develop another form of psoriasis.

3. PUSTULAR PSORIASIS

■ Small blisters filled with pus may appear abruptly on the palms of the hands and the soles of the feet.
■ There may be widespread areas of red, inflamed, and acutely tender skin.
■ There may be some thickening and scaling of the inflamed areas.

4. INVERSE PSORIASIS

Elderly people are commonly affected by this type of psoriasis in which large, moist, red areas develop in **skin folds**, rather than widespread body areas. The rash often affects the groin, the skin under the breasts, and sometimes the armpits. Inverse psoriasis usually clears up with treatment but may recur.

ARE THERE COMPLICATIONS?

About 1 in 10 people with psoriasis of any type develops a form of **arthritis** that usually affects the **fingers** or **knee joints**. In **pustular** and **exfoliative** psoriasis, a massive loss of cells from the surface of the skin may lead to loss of protein, infections, and high fever; if it is left untreated, the condition can be life threatening.

WHAT MIGHT BE DONE?
TOPICAL TREATMENT

■ Psoriasis is commonly treated with **emollients** to soften the skin. Other common treatments are preparations containing **coal tar** or a substance called **anthralin.** These reduce inflammation and scaling. Coal tar and anthralin are effective but have an unpleasant smell and can stain clothing and bed linen. Anthralin should be applied to affected areas only because it can irritate healthy skin.
■ Alternatively, your doctor may prescribe a topical preparation containing the vitamin D derivative **calcipotriol** to be applied twice a day. It has no smell, does not stain skin or clothes, and is normally effective within about four weeks. You should follow the advice of your doctor or dermatologist because this treatment should not be used on the face or in the creases of the skin.

A diet high in whole grain cereals and low in saturated fats and sugar may help in the treatment of psoriasis.

- Topical corticosteroids may also be used, sparingly.

SPECIAL TREATMENTS

- For widespread psoriasis that does not respond to topical treatments, therapeutic exposure to **ultraviolet (UV) light** is often effective. PUVA therapy involves using UV therapy together with **psoralen**, an oral drug that is taken before the ultraviolet light treatment and helps make the skin more sensitive to the effects of light.
- Regular, short doses of **sunlight** often help clear up psoriasis. Moderate exposure of affected areas to sunlight can be beneficial during the summer months.
- In very severe cases of **pustular psoriasis**, for which topical preparations may not be effective, treatment with oral or intravenous drugs may be recommended. The drugs used for this treatment include **retinoids**, the cancer fighting drug **methotrexate,** and the immunosuppressant drug **cyclosporin**. However, both retinoids and methotrexate can cause abnormalities in a developing fetus. For this reason, you should not take either of these drugs if you are pregnant or you are planning to have a child.
- Chinese herbs in pill, infusion, and cream form can be very successful and are always worth trying.
- The Dead Sea treatment claims a three-year remission. No one knows how it works but it's not solely due to immersion in the Dead Sea. Fellow patients lend support akin to group therapy. But then you have to travel to the Dead Sea for the treatment.

WHAT IS THE OUTLOOK?

Although there is no cure for psoriasis, treatment normally relieves the symptoms and helps many people with the condition lead a normal life. If psoriasis is a long-term problem, you may want to join a support group or the Psoriasis Association (see Useful addresses, p. 567).

SELF-HELP

It may help to reduce your intake of meat, animal fats, sugar, and alcohol and increase intake of fiber – that is, whole grain cereals, fruit, vegetables, cooked dried beans and peas, and nuts and seeds. Eat more oily fish, particularly mackerel, sardines, herring, and salmon. An oatmeal bath can help to soothe irritated skin. Put 2lb (1kg) of oatmeal in cheesecloth bags in a hot bath and soak for 15 minutes. Apply your treatment afterward.

Photosensitivity

ABNORMAL SENSITIVITY OF THE SKIN TO ULTRAVIOLET LIGHT, RESULTING IN REDNESS AND DISCOMFORT, IS CALLED PHOTOSENSITIVITY.

Various substances may cause photosensitivity, including **drugs** such as **tetracyclines, diuretics,** and **oral contraceptives**, as well as **chemicals** used in the manufacture of cosmetics. The rare metabolic disorder porphyria can also cause photosensitivity.

WHAT ARE THE SYMPTOMS?

The reaction occurs in areas of skin frequently exposed to sunlight, such as the face and hands. Not much exposure is needed. The effects usually develop shortly after exposure, but may be delayed for 24–48 hours. The symptoms include:
- red, often painful, rash
- small, itchy blisters
- scaly skin.

WHAT IS THE TREATMENT?

- To relieve symptoms, the doctor may prescribe topical corticosteroids.
- Oral **antihistamines** may be prescribed.
- Severe cases are treated with controlled exposure to ultraviolet light, sometimes combined with drugs, to desensitize the skin.
- If a particular drug is causing photosensitivity, your doctor may be able to prescribe a different drug.

SELF-HELP

You can help control the reaction by avoiding sunlight as much as possible. When outdoors, cover your skin, wear a hat and use a high SPF sunscreen.

Purpura

THE CHARACTERISTIC RASH OF PURPURA CAUSES REDDISH-PURPLE SPOTS THAT DON'T DISAPPEAR WHEN PRESSED BY A GLASS.

The spots are small areas of bleeding under the skin, and may be caused by damaged blood vessels or by an abnormality in the blood, such as **thrombocytopenia**, that affects clotting. They can range from the size of a pinhead to about 1in (2.5cm) in diameter. Purpura is a classic sign of one kind of bacterial meningitis. The most common of all types of purpura – senile purpura – mainly affects middle-aged and elderly women.

Purpura is sometimes a sign of a potentially serious disorder so you should always consult your doctor as a matter of urgency if you note a purpuric rash.

See also:
- **Meningitis p. 404**
- **Thrombocytopenia p. 239**

Chilblains

WHEN THE SKIN OF A COLD-SENSITIVE PERSON IS EXPOSED TO COLD AND DAMP, THE BLOOD VESSELS CLOSE UP TO CONSERVE HEAT, CAUSING THE SKIN TO BECOME NUMB AND PALE OR PIMPLY.

When the blood vessels dilate again with warmth, the skin becomes red and itchy. The resulting chilblains, due to hypersensitivity to cold, are irritating, but they are not serious. They usually appear on the extremities and other parts of the body where circulation is poor, such as the ankles, hands, and feet, and on the back of the legs.

Consult your doctor if chilblains cause a great deal of discomfort. He may prescribe a vasodilator cream to improve circulation.

SELF-HELP

- Keep all the susceptible parts of your body covered up and warm in damp and cold weather.
- Put thermal insoles in your shoes if you suffer from chilblains on your feet.
- If you have been out in the cold without warm clothing and develop chilblains, dust the skin with talcum powder or corn starch to ease the irritation.

SKIN INFECTIONS

Although the skin's surface provides protection from the environment, infectious organisms can enter the skin in various ways. Natural openings, such as a hair follicle or sweat gland, or broken skin at the site of an insect bite or a cut may provide a gateway for bacteria. Warm and moist areas, such as the skin between the toes, are susceptible to fungal infection. Some viral skin infections can easily be spread from the skin on one part of the body to another or passed between people.

Boil

ONE OF THE MOST COMMON TYPES OF SKIN INFECTION IS A BOIL. THIS IS A TENDER LUMP SURROUNDING A HAIR FOLLICLE THAT HAS BECOME INFECTED WITH BACTERIA, USUALLY STAPHYLOCOCCI. BOILS MAY BE LARGE OR SMALL.

The pus-filled lump gradually comes to a head and bursts after about two or three days. It may also heal on its own without bursting and slowly disappear. Because the hair follicles are so close together, the bacteria can infect a wide area, causing more boils to occur. This is most likely to happen on the face, especially the shaving area and the back of the neck near the hairline where the hairs may grow back into the skin. Boils usually appear on areas where there are pressure points, such as where a collar rubs or on the buttocks.

Although unsightly, a boil is not serious. However, it can be extremely painful, especially if it develops over a bony area such as the jaw or forehead where the skin is stretched tight. Consult your doctor as soon as possible if a boil does not come to a head within five days, if the boil is causing a lot of pain or if you notice red streaks spreading out from the center of the boil, which may mean that the infection is spreading.

WHAT IS THE TREATMENT?

■ Your doctor will examine the boil and the surrounding area. If he can feel pus under the skin, your doctor will probably lance the boil with a small scalpel and drain the pus, thus reducing the pain immediately.

■ If there is a spreading infection, or if you have had a number of boils over the previous months, your doctor may prescribe an **anti-infective cream** to treat the skin's surface, or **oral antibiotics** to prevent the internal spread of the infection lower down into the skin.

■ If there are crops of boils, your doctor may prescribe a special **antiseptic** to put in the bath water.

■ If the boils are recurrent, you will be referred to a **dermatologist** to find out if there is an underlying cause, such as diabetes mellitus.

SELF-HELP

■ Don't scratch or touch the area around the boil. Wash the skin with rubbing alcohol or a solution of one teaspoonful of salt in a glass of warm water to prevent infection from spreading.

■ **Do not squeeze** the boil, even when it comes to a head. Squeezing will spread the infection to the surrounding area and make the problem much worse.

■ Once the boil has burst, keep the area clean

and covered with a dressing for a few days.

■ Keep your towel and face cloth **separate** from those of the family.

■ If the boil is in a place where clothing might rub it, put a **thick pad** over the dressing to prevent any friction.

Candidiasis

CANDIDIASIS IS A YEAST INFECTION THAT USUALLY AFFECTS ONLY ONE PART OF THE BODY BUT CAN BE SERIOUS IF IT SPREADS AROUND THE BODY.

In healthy people, the yeast *Candida albicans* normally exists on the surface of certain areas of the body, including the mouth, throat, and vagina. Sometimes, the yeast overgrows in localized areas, causing minor forms of candidiasis such as oral thrush. In people with reduced immunity, such as those with acquired immune deficiency syndrome (AIDS) or diabetes mellitus, the yeast may spread into the blood and other tissues. Infection that spreads throughout the body may also affect people who have long-term urinary catheters or intravenous catheters, or people who have had prolonged courses of antibiotics or use intravenous drugs.

Widespread candidiasis may be diagnosed by culturing the yeast from a sample of blood or other body fluids or tissue specimens. A chest X-ray may also be done to look for signs of infection in the lungs. Antifungal drugs may be given either orally or intravenously, depending on the severity of the infection.

Untreated, the infection can spread through the body and may eventually be fatal. The prognosis depends on the extent of infection and on the person's general health.

See also:
• **Diabetes mellitus p. 504**
• **HIV infection and AIDS p. 338**
• **Vaginal yeast p. 279**

Impetigo

IMPETIGO IS A BACTERIAL SKIN INFECTION THAT IS MOST OFTEN
SEEN AROUND THE LIPS, NOSE, AND EARS.

Impetigo is caused by common bacterial organisms (staphylococcus and streptococcus), which are carried in the nose. The rash starts as small blisters, which break and crust over to become yellow-brown scabs. Impetigo is most often seen in school children and is highly contagious. It should be treated immediately for this reason, although the condition rarely has serious effects.

WHAT IS THE TREATMENT?

■ Your doctor will prescribe an **antibiotic cream** that should clear up the impetigo within five days.
■ Your doctor might also prescribe a course of **antibiotics** to be taken by mouth to eradicate the infection from your body, or a nasal cream to prevent the infection from being spread from the nose.

SELF-HELP

■ Before applying the ointment, **wash away** any yellow crusts and pat dry with a paper towel.
■ Be meticulous about hygiene. **Wash your hands** before and after treatment.
■ When the infection has cleared up, keep the area soft with emollient cream.

Athlete's foot

A CONTAGIOUS FUNGAL INFECTION, ATHLETE'S FOOT IS USUALLY PICKED UP BY WALKING BAREFOOT
IN COMMUNAL AREAS, SUCH AS SHOWER ROOMS, GYMS, AND SWIMMING POOLS.

Athlete's foot affects the soft area between and underneath the toes and seems to have a preference for sweaty feet. The infection is aggravated by **sweaty feet** because the fungus, **tinea**, which also causes ringworm elsewhere in the body, thrives in warm, moist conditions. Athlete's foot may also affect the toenails. Not everyone exposed to the fungus gets the infection.

WHAT ARE THE SYMPTOMS?

■ White, blistered skin between and underneath the toes. The area is itchy and, when scratched, splits and leaves raw, red skin underneath.
■ Dry, peeling skin.

■ Thick, yellow toenails.
Athlete's foot is a common condition requiring simple treatment and good hygiene to cure it. However, since it is contagious, you should act quickly so that the infection is not spread. Consult your doctor as soon as possible if the underside of the foot is already affected, or if the nails are distorted or yellowing. Consult your doctor if self-help measures (see box, below) fail to improve the condition within two or three weeks.

WHAT MIGHT BE DONE?

If the fungus has affected the toenails, they turn whitish, thicken and sometimes detach from the nail bed. Usually, debris from the

infected nail collects under its free edge. The diagnosis is confirmed by examining a sample of the nail debris under a microscope, where the fungus can be seen growing, and culturing it to determine which fungus is causing the infection.
■ If you have consulted your doctor because self-help measures failed, your doctor will prescribe another **antifungal powder** or cream and will advise you on the correct procedure for good foot hygiene.
■ If your toenails are affected, your doctor will prescribe an antifungal medication that may need to be taken for **three months**. The infected nails will eventually grow out in about 70 percent of cases.

Treating athlete's foot

■ Check the area between and underneath the toes for blisters, redness, and cracking.
■ Check the condition of the toenails.
■ Buy an **antifungal powder** or cream from your pharmacist, and, after washing and drying the feet thoroughly, apply it, following the manufacturer's instructions.
■ Keep your towel and bathmat **separate** from those of the rest of the family and wash them every day.
■ **Don't go barefoot** until the condition has cleared up.
■ Make sure you wear **clean socks every day**, preferably made from natural fibers such as cotton or wool.
■ Rotate your shoes, especially sneakers, so they dry out between wearings.

Keeping your feet clean and dry, particularly the area between the toes, helps prevent athlete's foot.

Warts and plantar warts

WARTS ARE SMALL BENIGN LUMPS CAUSED BY THE WART VIRUS.
A PLANTAR WART IS A PAINFUL WART ON THE SOLE OF THE FOOT THAT HAS BEEN
PUSHED DEEP INTO THE FOOT BY THE PRESSURE OF WALKING.

Warts are made up of an excess of dead cells that protrude above the surface of the skin. They can appear singly or in alarming numbers over all parts of the body, including the face and genitals.

It usually takes about two years for the body to build up a resistance to the wart virus, and after that time warts usually disappear spontaneously. Warts are spread by direct contact with an infected person.

WHAT ARE THE SYMPTOMS?

■ Hard lumps of dried skin that appear spontaneously and grow singly or in clusters anywhere on the body. Warts are usually round and have a raised surface; planar warts are flat with a thickened surface.

■ Both warts and plantar warts may have small black dots within the lumps (these are blood vessels not dirt).

Warts in the skin are neither serious nor painful, but consult your doctor if the warts continue to multiply or appear on the face and you want them removed. Plantar warts can cause pain and discomfort, depending on where they appear on the sole of the foot.

WHAT IS THE TREATMENT?

■ Your doctor may advise you to ignore the warts, or refer you to a dermatologist.
■ Methods of removal include freezing, cauterization, and surgical removal.

See also:
• Genital warts p. 282

• Genital warts p. 282

SELF-HELP

Wart cures

You can try commercial wart cures from the pharmacy. These work by the application of a weak acid solution to the wart and the daily removal of the resulting burnt skin. You should follow the manufacturer's instructions carefully and avoid applying the solution to healthy skin. Don't use patent wart cures on warts that appear on the face or genitals; you may cause scarring.

SKIN INFESTATIONS

Like other parts of the body, skin can become infested with minute creatures that feed off human blood. The creatures lay eggs and multiply and, when sufficient numbers are reached, irritating symptoms arise, most notably rash and itching.

The most common skin infestations are scabies and lice (head, body, and pubic). While none of these causes harmful effects, they are all highly contagious and the itching and scratching they lead to may be embarrassing and a nuisance.

Scabies

SCABIES IS AN IRRITATING, ITCHY RASH CAUSED BY A TINY MITE. THE BURROWING AND EGG-LAYING
OF THESE MITES PRODUCE A RASH THAT NEARLY ALWAYS AFFECTS THE HANDS AND FINGERS,
PARTICULARLY THE CLEFTS BETWEEN THE FINGERS.

Scabies is visible as a fine gray line where the mite has burrowed into the skin, ending in a black dot – the mite. Scabies may also affect the ankles, feet, toes, elbows, and the area around the genitals. When the eggs hatch, they are easily passed to another person by direct contact. They can also be picked up from bedding or linen that is infested with the mites.

WHAT ARE THE SYMPTOMS?

■ Intense itching.
■ Burrows – fine, short lines on the backs of the hands and the sides of the fingers that end in a black spot the size of a pinhead.
■ Scabs on the itchy areas.

Scabies is not serious but it is contagious and could run through a family if not treated promptly. Consult your doctor as soon as possible if you suspect scabies or if you are scratching a lot.

WHAT IS THE TREATMENT?

Your doctor will prescribe an **antiparasitic lotion** in sufficient quantity for the whole family to be treated. All the skin must be treated for the lotion to be effective.

SELF-HELP

■ Try **not to scratch** affected areas. This may hinder the doctor's diagnosis and cause sores to form that could become infected.

■ After thorough washing, you should apply the lotion to the **whole body** below the neck and let dry. Do not wash it off for 24 hours. To ensure disinfestation, repeat the procedure for another 24 hours in a day or two.
■ Carry out the treatment for **other members of the family** simultaneously.
■ **Launder or air all bedding and clothing** to eradicate the mite. The mite does not live for longer than five or six days after it is removed from human skin.

Lice

LICE ARE WINGLESS INSECTS THAT FEED ON HUMAN BLOOD. THERE ARE THREE KINDS OF HUMAN LICE – PUBIC LICE (ALSO CALLED CRABS), BODY LICE, AND HEAD LICE.

PUBIC LICE

Pubic lice need the bodily heat of a person to keep them alive – hence they don't live very long on a toilet seat, although they may survive on warm bed clothes or garments for a short time.

Medical textbooks state that crabs are nearly always passed from one person to another during **sexual contact** because they actually live on pubic hair, and sometimes body hair, where they feed on blood and lay eggs called nits. Rarely, infestation can be spread through contact with bed linens, towels, or clothers.

With crabs, the most common symptom is itching in the pubic area and around the anus, especially at night. Some people have no symptoms and only realize that they are infested when they see the nits (eggs) or the tiny insects. Normal washing does not remove the nits since they are firmly stuck to the pubic hair.

If you think that you or your partner has pubic lice, you should consult your doctor or go to a clinic specializing in sexually transmitted diseases (STDs).

BODY LICE

Body lice, on the other hand, live on clothing and bed linen and are easily picked up by someone sharing a bed or garments. Body lice do, of course, occasionally stray to the pubic area. Many people confuse the two.

WHAT IS THE TREATMENT?

Your doctor will probably prescribe a preparation containing **lindane** or **permethrin** to apply to affected areas. A second application is needed about **10 days after** the first to destroy freshly hatched lice.

To prevent the spread of lice, **sexual partners** should be checked and treated if necessary. **The clothing and sheets** used by an infested person should be machine washed in hot water.

HEAD LICE

Head lice affect all social classes and have absolutely nothing to do with personal hygiene. They like clean heads as much as they do dirty ones and there is nothing shameful about being infected. If you have a child there is a good chance you will come into contact with head lice at some stage.

Head lice live and suck blood from the scalp, leaving tiny red spots that cause intense itching. Adult lice can live for several weeks and the females lay a daily batch of tiny pale eggs (nits) close to the scalp. These hatch out after several days. Lice are spread through direct contact, but it doesn't necessarily have to be head-to-head.

WHAT IS THE TREATMENT?

The traditional treatment for an outbreak of head lice is the application of powerful lotions containing pesticides. The main advantage is that such lotions can penetrate the hard casing of the lice eggs and kill the nits inside.

However, scientists and parents are beginning to think again, for the following reasons.

■ It seems that with repeated use these pesticides are losing their effectiveness. There are reports from some areas that live nits are not being destroyed and it is suggested that some adult lice may also be resistant.

■ There is concern about using powerful chemicals on young children.

■ They are expensive and unpleasant to use.
However, there are effective alternatives.

ALTERNATIVE TREATMENTS

■ The first and most important weapon against head lice is the **small fine-toothed comb** (often called a nit comb because the teeth are so close together it can remove the lice eggs). Plastic combs are recommended rather than metal because they are more flexible and therefore can get nearer to the scalp. They are also easier to clean and less likely to pull or snag hair.

Use the nit comb every time you wash your own and your children's hair. But do use plenty of **conditioner** after shampooing. Using conditioner makes the procedure simple and painless (no tangles) and makes it possible to dislodge lice from the slippery strands. Pay special attention to anyone with curly hair since it's harder to see the lice or get a comb through and so they may be more vulnerable.

■ The use of Quassia chips is an alternative remedy that is becoming popular with parents. Quassia chips look like pieces of dried wood. They are cheap, natural and don't smell or leave a greasy residue. To use Quassia chips:

1. Place 1oz (25g) of Quassia chips in a saucepan and pour 1 pint (560ml) of boiling water over them. This loosens the oil in the chips. Leave overnight and the next day bring to a boil and simmer for 10–15 minutes. Let it cool and transfer to a spray bottle.

2. Shampoo hair, rinse, and apply conditioner. Comb through with the nit comb. Rinse off the conditioner and towel dry. Spray the Quassia solution all over the hair. Let dry naturally. Spray again when dry.

3. Spray again the following morning after brushing and repeat over the next couple of days. You can also use the Quassia solution as a preventive because it creates a bitter, hostile environment that lice do not like.

■ There are natural remedies that blend essential oils such as citronella, geranium, eucalyptus, lavender, and rosemary. They claim to get rid of lice and act as a repellent.

ABNORMALITIES OF PIGMENTATION

The pigmentation of the skin is due to a substance known as melanin. Melanin filters out ultraviolet rays and so helps to protect the skin from damage by the sun (a suntan is caused by the extra melanin the body produces in response to exposure to sunlight). Some conditions, such as vitiligo and chloasma, are caused by changes in the amount of melanin in the skin in localized areas.

Vitiligo

THE CONDITION KNOWN AS VITILIGO IS CHARACTERIZED BY PATCHES OF WHITE SKIN DUE TO LOSS OF NORMAL PIGMENT (MELANIN) FROM PATCHES OF SKIN, MOST COMMONLY OCCURRING ON THE FACE AND HANDS. VITILIGO IS MORE OBVIOUS IN PEOPLE WITH DARK SKIN.

WHAT IS THE CAUSE?

Vitiligo is thought to be an **autoimmune disorder**, in which the body produces antibodies that react against its own tissues. The antibodies destroy the cells in the skin that produce melanin. About 1 in 3 people with vitiligo has a **family history** of the condition. About the same proportion also have **another type** of autoimmune disorder, such as **pernicious anemia.**

SELF-HELP

■ In mild vitiligo, the discolored areas can be hidden with concealing cosmetics. No other treatment is needed.
■ The affected areas cannot tan. To prevent sunburn, you should avoid exposure to the sun and use sunscreen in direct sunlight.
■ Phototherapy using ultraviolet (UV) light can help but it takes several months to work.
■ Before UV treatment, you may be given a drug called **psoralen** to increase the sensitivity of the skin to light. This treatment, usually used for psoriasis, is called PUVA (psoralen and ultraviolet light).

WHAT IS THE OUTLOOK?

There is no cure for vitiligo and often the depigmented patches continue to enlarge slowly. However, about 3 in 10 affected people regain their natural skin color spontaneously.

Chloasma

ALSO CALLED THE MASK OF PREGNANCY, CHLOASMA IS A SPECIAL FORM OF PIGMENTATION THAT CAUSES BROWN PATCHES TO APPEAR ON THE BRIDGE OF THE NOSE, CHEEKS, AND NECK.

The only way to handle chloasma is to camouflage it with a cover stick or the cover-up cosmetics that are used for birthmarks. Never try to bleach out the pigment; the patches will begin to fade within three months of childbirth. In black women, patches of paler skin develop on their faces and necks. These will probably disappear after delivery and can be camouflaged during pregnancy.

SKIN CANCERS

There are several types of skin cancer, most of which are associated with prolonged exposure to sunlight. Fair-skinned people are most at risk. Exposure to the sun is a risk factor and should be avoided from babyhood; the use of tanning booths is also a risk factor and should likewise be avoided.

Skin cancer is now the **most common** form of cancer in the world. In recent years, the incidence around the world has escalated, and the condition now affects millions of people worldwide. The good news is that skin cancer can usually be cured if it is diagnosed early, though preventive measures are always preferable.

WHAT ARE THE RISKS?

The usual cause of skin cancer is prolonged exposure to the harmful ultraviolet radiation in sunlight. The risk is higher if you are fair-skinned and if you live or take vacations in areas with intense sun; the closer you are to the equator, the greater the risk. It's the **cumulative** hours of sunshine that count so if you live in a very sunny place you'll reach your "**cancer-inducing dose**" earlier than somewhere like Seattle where there isn't so much sun. The recent depletion of the ozone layer is thought to have played a part in increasing the incidence of skin cancer because the ozone layer acts as a shield against harmful ultraviolet (UV) light. Tanning booths, which emit ultraviolet light, may also cause skin cancer. You should also keep in mind that the more times you have been sunburned, the greater your chance of developing malignant melanoma, the most dangerous form of skin cancer.

If you work outside or have been sunburned (particularly in childhood), you could be vulnerable to skin cancer. People who have fair skin are especially susceptible because they have low levels of melanin, the pigment that give the skin its color and helps protect it from the sun's harmful ultraviolet rays.

To reduce the risk of developing skin cancer, try to avoid exposure to the sun and protect your skin when outside. Examine your skin regularly, and ask someone else to check your back and scalp. Wear UV-resistant clothing in areas of intense sunshine and where there's a lot of reflection, for example on snow or water.

WHAT ARE THE TYPES?

There are three main types of skin cancer all linked to overexposure to the sun.
1. The most common type is **basal cell carcinoma**, which can be easily treated. It rarely spreads.
2. **Squamous cell carcinoma** is a form of skin cancer that may spread and is occasionally fatal, but can be cured completely if detected early.
3. **Malignant melanoma** is still rare but getting more common all the time. It can spread

rapidly to other parts of the body and causes more deaths than other skin cancers.

An uncommon skin cancer, known as Kaposi's sarcoma, usually occurs only in people with acquired immune deficiency syndrome (AIDS).

WHAT MIGHT BE DONE?

Skin cancer can usually be cured if it is diagnosed early. You should consult your doctor promptly if you notice any changes in your skin, such as enlarging lumps or sores that do not heal. You may need to have a skin biopsy. During this procedure, a small area of

skin is removed and examined under a microscope for abnormal cells.

The type of skin cancer and spread of the disease determines the treatment and prognosis. Sometimes, only the affected area of skin needs to be treated.

It is possible to remove most types of skin cancers **surgically**. However, **skin grafting** may be necessary if a cancer has invaded large areas of surrounding skin tissue. If the cancer has spread to other parts of the body, **radiation therapy** or **chemotherapy** may also be needed.

Malignant melanoma

OF ALL THE TYPES OF SKIN CANCER, MALIGNANT MELANOMA IS THE MOST SERIOUS. MALIGNANT MELANOMA HAS BECOME MORE COMMON WITH OUR OBSESSION WITH GETTING AND KEEPING A TAN.

A melanoma may begin as a new growth on normal skin or may develop from an existing mole. Left untreated, the cancer can spread rapidly to other parts of the body and may be fatal. As with most other skin cancers, exposure to the sun and the use of tanning booths are risk factors, and fair-skinned people are most at risk. Malignant melanoma is most common between the ages of 40 and 60, increasingly common in young adults, and more common in women.

Worldwide, the number of cases of malignant melanoma, particularly in young adults, has increased dramatically over the past 10 years. This rise is probably due to the growing popularity of outdoor activities. However, the condition is still most common in people aged 40–60. There will be about 88,000 new cases of melanoma diagnosed in the US. One person each hour dies from melanoma.

WHAT IS THE CAUSE?

Malignant melanoma is thought to result from damage to **melanocytes** (the skin cells that produce the pigment melanin) by sunlight. The cancer occurs more frequently in people with **fair skin** than in those with dark skin.

People who continually expose themselves to intense sunlight or who live in sunny climates are at greater risk of developing the cancer.

Severe sunburn in childhood has been shown to double the chance of developing malignant melanoma in later life. Reducing exposure to the sun can help decrease the risk of developing any type of skin cancer.

WHAT ARE THE RISKS?

If caught early, most cases of skin cancer can

be treated successfully through surgery, although some can prove fatal.

Skin cancers have increased by 7 percent in fair-skinned people worldwide over the last 10 years. A person's risk of developing skin cancer is increased by several factors, including:
- having fair skin
- having skin that has a tendency to freckle
- having many moles
- a family history of malignant melanoma
- having had one or more episodes of severe sunburn during childhood
- being aged over 30 years
- many years of exposure to strong sunlight.

WHAT ARE THE SYMPTOMS?

Malignant melanomas can develop on any part of the body but appear most commonly on sun-exposed areas. Some melanomas spread across the skin in irregular flat patches, others appear as fast-growing lumps. In older people, they may occur on the face as frecklelike spots, known as **lentigo maligna**, that grow slowly over many years. If they are not removed, all of these types of melanoma will grow down into the underlying layers of the skin.

continued on page 458

Wearing a high sun protection factor sunscreen and a hat helps reduce sun damage to the skin.

FOCUS *on* sun protection

More than one million people in the US are diagnosed with skin cancer every year, and around 9,600 people die of it. It's the second most common cancer in the country. Unlike many cancers, skin cancer is a disease that's mostly avoidable. The main cause, exposure to sunlight, is widely recognized.

By taking simple precautions in the sun we can ensure that the rise in the number of skin cancers is brought to a halt, if not reversed.

As you soak up the sun at home or abroad this summer, remember you're damaging your skin. You don't have to sunbathe to get sunburned. Simply walking around in the sunshine can be enough. A tan may make you feel healthy, but it's a sign that your skin is being damaged and it is trying to protect itself, regardless of how gradually you acquire it.

A burned face and hot, painful sunburn on your body isn't attractive, it's painful and unsightly and can cause permanent damage to collagen in your skin, leading to wrinkles.

WHAT SUN DOES TO SKIN

- Exposure to UV rays causes the outer layer of the skin to thicken as more cells are produced, causing wrinkles.
- The elastic tissue of the skin also breaks down, resulting in sags and bags.
- On top of this, the sun tends to dry out the skin, making it coarse and leathery.

- Dark patches or liver spots can appear, due to an overproduction of melanin (a pigment produced by skin cells). These patches are normally seen in older people, but can also be found in young people who sunbathe frequently.

PROTECTING YOURSELF

Staying safe is easy – follow these simple tips and you'll greatly reduce your risk of getting skin cancer.

- Clothing is the ideal barrier from the sun – it's cheaper than sunscreens and it doesn't rub off. Cover up with loose-fitting, cool garments and a hat. Take special care of your ears and neck since these are the most common places for skin cancers. You can buy clothes in UV-resistant materials at sports shops.
- On parts of your body you can't cover up, always use sunscreen, with an SPF of 15 or

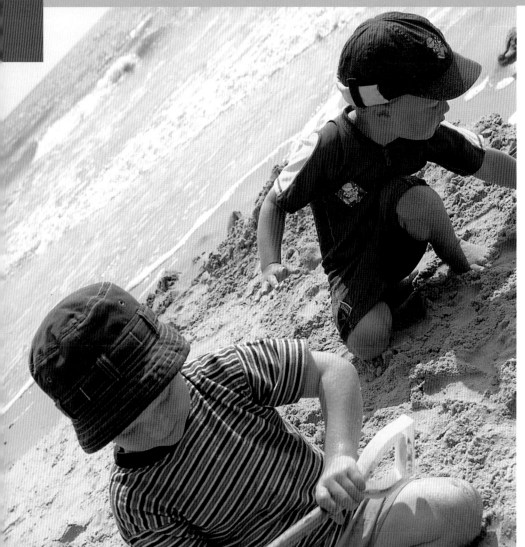

Ultraviolet rays

Sunlight contains visible rays, infrared rays, and ultraviolet rays. The latter are mainly responsible for tanning and skin damage.

There are three types of ultraviolet rays in sunlight – UVA, UVB, and UVC. UVA are longer, tanning rays and UVB are shorter, burning rays. Both easily injure the DNA of cells and the pigment-forming **melanocytes** causing skin damage and cancer.

Very little UVC radiation, which is potentially very dangerous, reaches Earth as it is filtered out by the ozone layer; the development of holes in this layer is of increasing concern.

UV rays can also damage the **Langerhans** cells in the skin's epidermis that scavenge for invading bacteria or cancer cells.

above. Apply it an hour before you go out, and reapply it frequently and generously.

- Find some shade during the hottest part of the day, usually between 11am and 3pm.
- **Never** fall asleep in the sun unprotected – even after a late night. Keep an eye on how much time you spend in the sun and reapply sunscreen often.
- **Don't** be fooled by an overcast day – the sun can penetrate through cloud, so you can still get burned.
- If you're a **watersport** fanatic, remember that the reflection of the sun's rays on the water can make it even stronger. Protect your skin with a wet suit and use a waterproof sunscreen.
- **Always** wear good-quality sunglasses in bright sunlight. Look for those that block 99 percent of UV light.

WHAT DOES SPF MEAN?

SPF stands for Sun Protection Factor and is a measure of how much a sunscreen protects your skin from burning in the sun. The higher the SPF, the greater the protection. The rating may range from 2 to 30 or even higher. You can get many brands of sunscreen that have an SPF of 45.

HOW MUCH SUNSCREEN?

Most people apply sunscreen too thinly and generally end up with less protection than the SPF on the bottle suggests.

WHEN USING A SUNSCREEN

- **apply it thickly and evenly** over all exposed areas
- **remember,** those parts of the body that aren't usually exposed to the sun will tend to burn more easily. Pay particular attention to ears, neck, bald patches, hands, and feet.
- reapply regularly, especially after swimming.

AFTER-SUN CREAM

After-sun creams and lotions may help to soothe sunburned or dry skin caused by the sun, but they can't help repair serious skin damage.

PROTECTING CHILDREN

Babies and young children need special care because they can't protect themselves and aren't aware of how the sun can damage their skin. So it's important that you take precautions for them.

Getting sunburned as a child leads to greater risk of skin cancer in later life. It's important

that children, especially babies and toddlers, are given the protection they deserve.

Babies: Keep babies less than 12 months old out of the sun and in the shade. Loose-fitting clothing will help keep babies cool. Remember that babies cannot move around by themselves and may get hot and uncomfortable if they become overheated. Be sure to give your baby frequent drinks to help prevent dehydration.

Toddlers and young children: Dress young children in loose-fitting, UV-resistant clothing and a wide-brimmed hat when they're in the sun. Generously apply sunscreen – before they go out in the sun – to the parts of the body that remain exposed. Select a sunscreen with an SPF of at least 15 and make sure it's water-resistant if they will be going into the water.

Encourage children to play in the shade when the sun is at its strongest. You can create

your own shade with a beach umbrella or canopy, or take advantage of natural shade under trees.

Choose sunglasses for children that block 99 percent of UV light. If taking children in the car, make sure they have adequate ventilation and never leave them in the car unattended.

TREATING SUNBURN

Calamine lotion or sunburn cream can **soothe burned skin**, which should be protected from further exposure to the sun until healing takes place. A **nonsteroidal anti-inflammatory painkiller** such as ibuprofen may be needed to relieve tenderness. A person with severe sunburn should consult a doctor, who may prescribe a cream containing a **corticosteroid drug** to relieve the symptoms.

continued from page 455

SELF-HELP

■ You should inspect your skin regularly and note the location and size of any moles. Get help from another person to examine your back and scalp. Changes in existing moles or the appearance of a new and enlarging spot should be reported to your doctor as soon as possible. A mole that is more than ¼in (6mm) across or shows variation in shade or color needs to be checked by your doctor immediately.

■ If you have a **mole or freckle** in a spot where there's **friction**, for example under a bra strap, around the waist, or on the side of the foot, have it excised immediately.

■ Always wear **sunscreen** on the face and backs of hands, a floppy hat, and ultraviolet (UV) resistant clothing in very bright sun or where there's a lot of reflection, as on snow or water.

WHAT MIGHT BE DONE?

If your doctor suspects that you have a malignant melanoma, he or she will arrange for a sample to be removed for microscopic examination (a biopsy). If the sample is found to be cancerous, a wider area of skin may then be removed to decrease the risk of malignant cells remaining. If a large portion of skin has to be removed, you may need skin grafting.

Samples may also be removed from the lymph nodes near the melanoma and examined for cancerous cells, the presence of which would indicate that the cancer has spread. If the cancer has spread and other areas of the body are affected, you may have **chemotherapy** or **radiation therapy**.

WHAT IS THE OUTLOOK?

The outlook depends on where the melanoma is situated, how far the lesion has grown down into the skin and whether the cancer has spread to other areas. People with superficial melanomas who receive early treatment are usually cured. If melanomas are particularly aggressive or penetrate deep into the skin, the outlook is less optimistic. Melanomas that have spread to other parts of the body are often fatal.

WARNING:

You may have a malignant melanoma if a quickly growing, irregular, dark-colored spot develops on your skin. If you notice any of the following changes in an existing mole, seek immediate medical advice:

- increasing size
- irregular and asymmetrical edges
- itching, inflammation, or redness
- thickening of the surface
- bleeding or crusting
- variation in shade or color.

See also:
• Tissue tests p. 259
• Sun protection p. 456

TAKING CARE OF YOUR HAIR

As hair is such a prominent part of a person's appearance, many people, particularly women, spend a lot of time and money looking after it. This is not necessary and a simple regime of gently washing and conditioning your hair every other day combined with a healthy well-balanced diet should ensure a healthy head of hair. Hair problems can usually be avoided by following a few simple rules about hairstyles and hair-coloring products. Tension on the hair caused by styles such as tight braiding, or by wearing curlers for prolonged periods, may produce bald patches, and both perming and bleaching may damage hair.

SHAMPOOING

Most people should wash their hair every other day.

1. Use the mildest shampoo you can find and only shampoo your hair once – shampoos are so efficient that shampooing twice is unnecessary.

2. Mix two teaspoonfuls of shampoo in a glass of warm water and pour it over your wet hair.

3. Then massage the shampoo very gently into your hair.

4. Don't scrub hard to work up a lather, just leave the shampoo on for about a minute and then rinse until the hair is free of soap.

5. Always use a conditioner after hair washing to prevent tangling.

6. After you have washed your hair, dab it dry with a towel rather than rubbing it vigorously.

Hair-care tips

Don't scrub the scalp with your fingertips when you wash your hair since you will loosen hairs from the soft wet hair follicles.

Don't tug or pull at wet hair when you comb it since this will remove or tear it. Use a wide-toothed brush or comb.

Don't brush or comb your hair too frequently since this may irritate the scalp and stimulate oil glands to produce more oil, making your hair look lank and dull.

Don't use a medicated shampoo for dandruff unless your doctor advises it.

Don't use antidandruff shampoos more than once every two weeks since they may contain ingredients, such as selenium, that can irritate the scalp and make dandruff worse.

Alopecia

HAIR LOSS, OR ALOPECIA, CAN OCCUR IN ANY BODY AREA BUT IS PARTICULARLY
NOTICEABLE WHEN IT AFFECTS THE SCALP, CAUSING BALDNESS.

Alopecia may be localized (in which hair is lost in patches) or generalized (in which there is thinning or total hair loss over the whole scalp). Hair loss can be temporary or permanent. Alopecia is not always associated with ill health but it may cause embarrassment.

WHAT ARE THE CAUSES?

■ The most common cause of alopecia in men is oversensitivity to the hormone **testosterone**, producing a characteristic pattern of hair loss (**male-pattern baldness**). Male-pattern baldness is an **inherited** condition and the most common form of alopecia. The process starts when normal hair at the temples and crown is replaced by fine, downy hair. The hairline then gradually recedes. Only a trained dermatologist can determine if the hair follicle (the pit in the skin from which the hair grows) is so badly damaged that hair loss is permanent.

■ Patchy hair loss is usually due to **alopecia areata**, an **autoimmune** disorder that causes bald patches to appear on the scalp, surrounded by short, broken hairs. The hair will usually regrow within six months, but in rare cases alopecia areata can cause permanent loss of all body hair – **alopecia universalis**.

■ Hairstyles that pull on the scalp are a common cause of patchy hair loss. If the pulling is continuous hair loss may be permanent.

■ Patchy hair loss may be the result of a rare psychological disorder in which the hair is compulsively pulled – trichotillomania.

■ Burns or skin disorders, such as ringworm, that scar the scalp may cause permanent patchy hair loss.

■ Generalized thinning of the hair is noticeable after **menopause**, and hair loss is normal in elderly people.

■ Hair loss may occur temporarily after pregnancy for up to a period of 18 months and is a common side effect of **chemotherapy** and **hypothyroidism**.

■ Other causes of thinning hair include **acute illness**, **stress**, and **malnutrition**.

WHAT IS THE TREATMENT?

The hair usually regrows once the underlying cause has been treated. Your doctor will probably be able to diagnose alopecia areata by the appearance of your scalp.

1. This condition does not usually require treatment, but corticosteroids injected into the hairless patches may be effective in promoting regrowth. In most cases of hair loss, the hair usually regrows once the underlying cause has been treated.

2. If your scalp has **patchy scarring** you may need a skin biopsy to diagnose the underlying cause. Scarred areas may be treated with topical corticosteroids or antifungal drugs, but if the damage is severe and has affected the hair follicles it is unlikely that new hair will grow.

POSSIBILITIES FOR PERMANENT HAIR LOSS

Over the years, a number of different strategies have been used with varying degrees of success. Here is a brief summary of those currently available.

HAIRPIECES

This is the safest and least painful way (in terms of health and money) to camouflage hair loss. Some can be permanently attached to the head, either by being tied to existing hairs or by being sewn onto the scalp. The latter can cause infection and are not recommended for that reason. The only other possible side effect is that occasionally people are sensitive to the adhesive that is sometimes used.

HAIRWEAVING

This is a nonsurgical procedure that adds replacement hair to existing hair in order to cover bald patches. The new hair is braided strand by strand onto the edges of the hair in place. Hairweaving requires maintenance and careful cleansing.

HAIR IMPLANT

This is a quasi-surgical procedure where strips of hair are attached to the scalp in the form of surgical threads implanted in the balding area. The implants are usually synthetic so a hairdryer mustn't be used.

HAIR TRANSPLANT

This is a surgical procedure that generally results in permanent replacement of hair – although even when well established, it is not as luxurious as the hair you've lost. Plugs of hair are cut from the remaining healthy hair on the sides and back of the head and implanted in bald spots. This hair normally falls out after transplant but is replaced by new hair. Quite a few follicles must be transplanted in the same session and the process needs to be repeated if the total bald area is to be covered.

SCALP COLORANTS

A spray available from the pharmacy covers the head in an organic dust to disguise any bald patches. Colored creams can darken the scalp to camouflage pale, hairless skin.

SELF-HELP

If possible, try not to worry about your hair loss because anxiety makes the problem worse. Very often it is worth considering wearing a wig so that the psychological effect of the hair loss doesn't take too great a toll.

MEDICATION

During research on a drug to control high blood pressure, it was discovered that **minoxidil** promoted hair growth. It has to be applied to the scalp twice daily for a minimum of four months for any effect to be noticeable. Treatment has to be continued or hair loss will reoccur.

The one thing that all these treatments have in common is the expense involved over a long period of time. It is sensible to seek advice before committing yourself to any particular form of treatment (see the organizations listed under Useful Addresses on p. 567).

HAIR LOSS AND WOMEN

■ **Estrogen** receptors in hair follicles maintain the health of each hair, which is why problems can occur at the time of menopause if estrogen levels are low. So it's possible that if you have a problem with hair loss it may be due to a hormone imbalance and hormone replacement therapy might help. Consult your doctor for advice about this.

■ It's also possible you have an **underactive thyroid** since hair loss is one of the symptoms. A simple blood test can diagnose this.

■ **Iron-deficiency anemia** can also cause hair loss. Women who suffer with heavy periods are often deficient in iron.

■ **Rapid weight loss and stress** is also thought to affect the hair follicles by constricting the blood vessels that supply them and so limiting their supply of oxygen.

■ General thinning of the hair is common after **pregnancy**. The pregnancy hormones drive most of the scalp hair into a growing phase. Under normal circumstances, hairs are at different stages of resting and growing phases and therefore hair loss is gradual and imperceptible. The dramatic hair loss associated with pregnancy is because great numbers of hairs come out of the resting phase at the same time and are lost simultaneously. This may go on for anything up to 18 months or two years. Although very disturbing, it is no cause for alarm because it is self-limiting and reversible – although hair may take a long time to grow back, and straight hair may become curly and vice versa.

■ **Chronic scratching of the scalp**, particularly at the back near the nape of the neck, is quite a

common symptom of anxiety and can give rise to hair loss. However, this is rarely complete and always recovers when scratching stops.

■ **Hair pulling**, or **trichotillomania**, can occasionally cause bald patches but it can always be diagnosed because hair loss is never complete and there are often broken hairs of

different lengths present in the bald patches. Like chronic scratching, trichotillomania nearly always has a **psychological** cause.

See also:
• **Hypothyroidism p. 507**

Excessive hair

HAIR GROWTH THAT OCCURS IN AREAS THAT WOULD NOT NORMALLY HAVE HAIR, OR EXCESSIVE HAIR GROWTH, IS MORE COMMON IN WOMEN AND OCCURS ONLY AFTER PUBERTY. IT IS MORE FREQUENT WITH INCREASING AGE AND SOMETIMES RUNS IN FAMILIES.

There are two types of excessive hair growth: **hirsutism** and **hypertrichosis**. **Hirsutism** affects women only. In this condition, excessive hair develops particularly on the face, trunk, and limbs. This type of excessive growth is more common in women over the age of 60, due to estrogen deficiency, especially those who are of Mediterranean, Asian, Hispanic, or Arab descent. **Hypertrichosis** can affect both males and females. In this condition, the hair grows all over the body, even in areas that do not normally have hair.

WHAT ARE THE CAUSES?

■ Mild hirsutism in women is often considered normal, especially following menopause when there is a relative excess of male hormones (androgens) as estrogen levels fall.

■ Hirsutism may be the result of an increase in normally occurring androgens in women with disorders such as **polycystic ovarian syndrome** (PCOS).

Hypertrichosis may occur with **anorexia nervosa** or may occur as a side effect of **immunosuppressant** or **antihypertensive drugs**.

WHAT MIGHT BE DONE?

■ If you are a young woman with hirsutism, you doctor may arrange for a blood test to measure your male hormone levels and exclude PCOS.

■ If androgens are high, you may be given a drug to block the hormone's effects and be treated for an underlying disorder such as polycystic ovarian syndrome.

■ If hypertrichosis occurs as a side effect of a drug, a change of treatment usually reverses the condition.

TREATMENT

Hair removal

You can deal with excessive hair yourself by bleaching it or by shaving, plucking, waxing, or using depilatory creams. The only way to remove hair permanently is by electrolysis and laser treatment but they are slow and can be uncomfortable.

Unlike other body hair, facial hair can actually be made worse by some methods of removal, so it is always wise for a doctor to identify the cause of facial hirsutism before any attempt at treatment is made.

Sugaring and waxing

Sugaring involves painting the skin with a mixture of lemon, sugar, water, and herbs, waiting for it to dry and then pulling it off, with the hairs attached. It works on the same principle as waxing, in which warm melted wax is applied to the skin and allowed to dry before removing along with excess hair, but because the mixture is cold it is less likely to cause a reaction on sensitive skin. It doesn't usually cost as much as waxing and lasts for 4–5 weeks.

There are home kits available for both sugaring and waxing but play safe and have it done at a reputable beauty salon. Sugaring

and waxing, as well as depilatory cream, can be used to remove hair in the bikini line area.

Bleaching

This won't remove the hair but it will disguise it. It is most suitable for women with light-colored hair. Coarse hair is likely to show after bleaching but is not likely to be quite as noticeable because it will be a lighter shade.

Depilatory creams

Hair removal creams specifically designed for the face should be the only ones used on this sensitive part of the body. Normal creams are likely to be too strong and will cause irritation. Regrowth usually occurs between two and three weeks. Hair lighteners and removal creams vary in price and are available from most pharmacies.

Lasers

Extensive research has recently been carried out into the use of a laser system that can safely slow down or stop hair growth without damaging the surrounding skin. A ruby laser is used that produces a red light. This is highly absorbed by hair and only minimally absorbed by skin. The light is applied for less than a thousandth of a second – enough

time to destroy the hair but not to heat the skin. Any part of the body can be treated and it has proved particularly popular with women who have a problem with facial hair.

Electrolysis

This is a very effective and relatively cheap method for removing facial hair. It involves passing an electrical current through the hair, cutting it off at the root. It can take some time to remove all the hair and must be carried out by a qualified operator.

Epilight

The latest concept in permanent hair removal works on the principle of intense pulsed light (IPL) technology. Using camera flash bursts of multiple light wavelengths pulsed through a quartz crystal, the result is superfast, long-term removal of all types of hair anywhere on the body. A slight reddening of the skin may be apparent after treatment, but this usually subsides within 24 hours.

Hormone replacement therapy (HRT)

Excessive hair can be counteracted by estrogen in the form of HRT. A woman who takes female hormones should have few problems with unwanted hair.

NAILS

The nails, like the hair, are dead, except for the growing root, and are made up of compacted **keratin**, the same protein as in hair. It takes a nail nine months to grow out so the nail plate is, in fact, a week-by-week photograph of what's going on inside the body. Consequently, internal events can be "read" in the nails. The chart on the right describes some of them.

Internal disorders that show up in the nails

Nail feature	Significance
Horizontal ridge	Illness, psychological trauma, surgery
Pits like the surface of a thimble	Psoriasis
Pale nail beds	Liver disease
Spoon-shaped nails	Iron deficiency
Brown longitudinal marks (splinter hemorrhages)	Bleeding disorder, septicemia
Highly curved nails ("clubbing")	Lung, heart, or liver disease

Ingrown toenail

MOST COMMON IN MEN, AN INGROWN TOENAIL IS PAINFUL GROWTH OF THE INNER EDGES OF A TOENAIL INTO THE SURROUNDING SKIN. TIGHT OR BADLY FITTING SHOES INCREASE THE RISK.

WHAT CAUSES IT?

An ingrown toenail curves under on one or both sides and cuts into the surrounding skin, causing pain, inflammation, and sometimes infection. A small toenail with a very fleshy toe predisposes to it. The big toe is particularly vulnerable to badly fitting shoes pressing on an incorrectly cut nail. In some cases, injury can cause the skin around the nail to overgrow and engulf part of the nail. Poor foot hygiene can also increase the risk of infection, leading to inflammation.

WHAT ARE THE SYMPTOMS?

The symptoms of an ingrowing toenail may include the following:
● pain, redness, and swelling around the toenail
● broken skin at the nail edge, which oozes clear fluid, pus, or blood.

You should consult your doctor as soon as you notice a toenail has become ingrown because it is possible that your toe will get infected.

WHAT IS THE TREATMENT?

■ You can relieve the pain of an ingrown toenail by **bathing** your foot **in warm salt water daily** and by taking **painkillers**.
■ You should protect the affected toe by keeping it covered with **clean, dry gauze**.
■ If your toenail is infected, **oral antibiotics** or **topical antibiotics** will be prescribed.

A couple of simple measures can help prevent an ingrown toenail from recurring.
■ Keep your feet clean and wear **correctly fitting shoes.**

■ **Cut straight across** your toenails, rather than along a curve, to prevent them growing into the skin.

If the problem recurs, a section or all of the toenail will be removed to prevent the toenail from growing into the flesh of the toe again.

SELF-HELP

■ Examine the skin around the nail to see if the nail has penetrated the skin.
■ Cut a tiny V-shape in the top edge of the nail to relieve pressure on the sides of the nail.
■ Apply an antiseptic cream to the sides of the nail to prevent infection.
■ If there is any sign of redness or pus, lie down with your foot propped up. Apply a sterile dressing to the toe.
■ Cut your toenails straight across and not too short. Cut them regularly; don't let them get too long.
■ Make sure that your shoes and socks are not too tight – you should have enough space to wriggle your toes.
■ If your toenail has become infected, don't wear socks; cut the toe out of an old shoe or wear sandals while the infection clears up.

TREATMENT
CHIROPODY

A podiatrist will cut your toenail to prevent further problems. It's important not to leave splinters of nails at the side but they're best removed by an expert.

Good foot hygiene keeps the feet healthy and reduces the chance of developing ingrown toenails.

REMOVAL OF THE INGROWN EDGES

Under a local anaesthetic your doctor or podiatrist can lift up the ingrown edges at the sides of the nail and cut them away so that none is left growing into the skin. This allows the infection to subside and the nail bed to heal. If you adhere to self-help measures the nail should not grow inward again.

REMOVAL OF AN INGROWN TOENAIL

Minor surgery may be needed for an ingrown toenail. Your toe will be anesthetized and cleaned with antiseptic. The nail, or part of it, will be removed, and phenol will be applied to the exposed nail bed to seal the blood vessels. You should be comfortable enough to walk within 24 hours of surgery, and the wound should heal completely within a week.

Eyes and Vision

Image shows a macrophotograph of a human iris and pupil

Miriam's overview

The eyes are equipped with one of the most potent antiseptics known to science – the tears. Not only do tears bathe the eyeball continually so that blinking is comfortable, they help keep the eye free of infections. The powerful natural antiseptic in tears is called lysozyme – if only we could bottle it.

We think of diminishing sight as a sign of getting old but it isn't. It's a sign that the eyeball is changing shape. The images of objects then fall in front of or behind the retina at the back of the eye and appear blurry.

If the eyeball elongates in the horizontal plane, the image falls in front of the retina and when the eyeball elongates vertically, the reverse happens.

Glasses and contact lenses pull the image back into the right place and laser surgery can alter the shape of the eyeball by shaving off thin slivers of the cornea.

The treatment of cataracts has leapt forward recently so that modern cataract surgery is quick and highly effective. Very few people these days should have compromised vision because of cataracts.

"modern *cataract surgery* is quick and *highly effective*"

Glaucoma is a treatable condition caught early enough so it's important to have regular tonometry tests and optic nerve evaluations done by your eye doctor to measure the pressure inside your eyes. Any "red eye" should take you to your doctor immediately because it could be a sign of acute glaucoma.

INSIDE your eyesight

The sensory cells of the eye are an extension of the brain, budding out from the brain during fetal development. The eye shows less growth than any other organ between birth and adulthood.

The eye is sensitive to light, which is focused through the **cornea** and the **lens** onto the **retina** at the back of the eye. The retina contains 137 million **cells**, of which 130 million are **rod-shaped** and used for black and white vision, sensing movement and seeing in poor light, while seven million are **cone-shaped** and used to sense color and pattern in bright light. Cones are concentrated in the parts of the retina called the **fovea centralis** (central depression) and the **macula**. A network of nerve cells on the surface of the retina changes the light signals into electrical nerve impulses and then relays them to the brain via the **optic nerve**. The eye contains 70 percent of the body's sensors and can deal with one and a half million simultaneous messages. The **pupils** automatically dilate or contract to control the amount of light that falls on the retina.

the parts of the eye

Choroid
Retina
Macula
Retinal blood vessel
Cornea
Pupil
Lens
Aqueous humor
Iris
Conjunctiva
Optic nerve
Focea centralis
Eye muscle
Vitreous humour
Sclera

Light rays enter the eye through the pupil and are focused by the cornea. The image that falls on the retina is transmitted to the brain via the optic nerve.

Focusing and sight

The human eye is more efficient at accommodation (ability to resolve fine detail) than the eyes of most mammals. Light enters the eye through the pupil, which dilates or constricts according to lighting conditions, lens adjustment, and emotions. The lens then focuses the light on the retina by changing shape. When focusing over long distances (over 20ft/7m), the lens is at its flattest and thinnest. When focusing on near objects, the lens becomes rounder and thicker.

The closest point at which the eye can focus varies with age – from about 3in (7cm) in infancy to about 16in (40cm) in early adulthood. The lens focuses an image upside down on the retina; the conscious mind interprets the image and "sees" it in its true position.

The eye's strength of accommodation is determined by the lens' ability to change shape. We have 200,000 receptors/mm^2, giving excellent resolution as long as vision during infancy has not been impeded in any way. Some creatures have an even higher resolution – the buzzard's retina, for example, contains one million receptors/mm^2.

how we see

Light rays reflected from an object are partly focused by cornea before entering the eye through the pupil. The im is focused further by the lens onto the retina, where it appears upside down. Electrical signals from the retina transmit the image to the brain, which interprets it as up

Field of vision

Since our eyes are placed on the front of the head we have binocular (three dimensional, or 3D) vision. Binocular vision means that we can see through 180° without moving the head, with an overlap of about 90° between the right and left visual fields. This enables us to judge distances and pick out detail, and improves the sensitivity of vision when light is poor.

90° overlap between right and left visual fields

Color vision

Detail of the retina

Connecting nerve cells

Connecting nerve cells

Light entering the eye

Pigment cells

Cones   Rods

In response to light, the rods and cones in the retina produce electrical signals that trigger impulses in the nerve cells to which they connect. These impulses travel along the optic nerve to the brain. Pigment cells behind the rods and the cones prevent reflection of light within the eye.

In common with other primates, we see only part of the color spectrum since some wavelengths, such as infrared and ultraviolet, are invisible to us. The color pigments we perceive are blue, green, and red. Color is registered by the **cones** in the retina; the cones are concentrated in the **fovea centralis** and the **macula**, which surrounds it. Each cone has a particular sensitivity for blue, green, or red, and intermediate sensitivity to the rest of the color spectrum. These sensitivities overlap so that wavelengths other than blue, green, or red also trigger color perceptions; for example, where light hits an overlapping curve of red and blue, the color purple is "seen." We can only see color in bright light. **Rods** in the retina cannot distinguish colors and are responsible mainly for night vision.

DISORDERS OF THE EYE ITSELF

The eye is a complex organ made up of several highly specialized components. Many eye disorders do not threaten sight, but a few serious conditions such as glaucoma may damage the eye and lead to loss of vision. A few eye disorders, such as conjunctivitis, are very common and early diagnosis usually leads to successful treatment.

I've chosen to start with the condition that is most common, **floaters**, because virtually all of us will get them and they are nothing to worry about. Other common problems, such as **styes** and **crossed eyes**, mainly affect children and you will find them in the childhood section. Several conditions, including acute glaucoma, can cause "**red eye,**" the most common being **conjunctivitis** due to an infection, which is easily remedied with local antibiotics. **Glaucoma**, both acute and chronic, is an often treatable condition but left undiagnosed and untreated can cause serious loss of vision, so I give both forms prominence in this section.

Floaters

IT'S QUITE COMMON TO SEE SMALL SPECKS THAT APPEAR TO FLOAT IN THE FIELD OF VISION. ALTHOUGH FLOATERS SEEM TO LIE IN FRONT OF THE EYES, THEY ARE IN FACT FRAGMENTS OR CONDENSATION OF THE JELLYLIKE FLUID THAT FILLS THE BACK OF THE EYE.

Floaters move rapidly with any eye movement but when the eyes are still, they drift slowly. No treatment is usually necessary.

The reason for most floaters isn't known. They rarely affect vision, but you should consult your doctor immediately if floaters suddenly appear.

In an older person or in someone with preexisting eye problems a sudden increase in the number of floaters, which may be combined with the sensation of flashing lights, could indicate a serious eye disorder that requires urgent treatment, such as the separation of the retina from the back of the eye (retinal detachment).

See also:
• **Retinal detachment p. 467**

Conjunctivitis

ALSO CALLED PINK OR RED EYE, CONJUNCTIVITIS IS A COMMON CONDITION. THE CONJUNCTIVA, THE MEMBRANE COVERING THE WHITE OF THE EYE AND THE INSIDE OF THE EYELIDS, BECOMES INFLAMED CAUSING THE EYE TO BECOME RED AND SORE.

Conjunctivitis may look alarming but it is rarely serious. One or both eyes may be affected, and in some cases it begins in one eye and then spreads to the other. Wearing contact lenses and using cosmetics are risk factors.

WHAT ARE THE CAUSES?
• Conjunctivitis may be caused by a **bacterial** or **viral** infection. **Bacterial conjunctivitis**, which is common, may be caused by any of several types of bacteria. **Viral conjunctivitis** can occur in epidemics and may be caused by one of the viruses responsible for the common cold. It may also be due to the **herpes simplex virus** that causes cold sores. Conjunctivitis due to a viral infection can be spread by hand-to-eye contact and is usually highly contagious.
• Conjunctivitis may result from an allergic reaction or irritation of the conjunctiva, for example by smoke, pollution, or ultraviolet light. **Allergic conjunctivitis** is a common feature of hay fever and of allergy to dust, pollen and other airborne substances. The condition may also be triggered by chemicals found in eye drops, cosmetics, or contact lens solutions. Allergic conjunctivitis often runs in families.
• Newborn babies sometimes develop conjunctivitis. This occasionally happens if an infection is transmitted to the baby's eyes from the mother's vagina during birth.

WHAT ARE THE SYMPTOMS?
The symptoms of conjunctivitis usually develop over a few hours and are often first experienced when waking. The symptoms generally include:
• redness of the white of the eye
• gritty and uncomfortable sensation in the eye
• swelling and itching of the eyelids
• discharge that may be yellowish and thick or clear and watery
• crusts on the eyelashes and eyelid margins due to discharge that has dried out during sleep. As a result, the eyelids sometimes stick together on waking.

WARNING:
If an eye becomes painful and red, you should consult your doctor as soon as possible to rule out the possibility of a more serious condition.

WHAT CAN I DO?
The symptoms of conjunctivitis can often be relieved by bathing the eye with artificial tears, "comfort" drops, from the pharmacy. To avoid spreading infection, wash your hands after touching the eye and do not share towels or washcloths. Once the conjunctivitis has cleared up, vision is rarely affected.

If you are susceptible to allergic conjunctivitis, avoid exposure to triggering substances. Antiallergy eye drops can be used to ease the symptoms.

Conjunctivitis caused by a bacterial infection can be easily treated using antibiotic eyedrops, which your doctor may prescribe. Symptoms usually clear up within 48 hours of starting treatment.

WHAT MIGHT THE DOCTOR DO?

■ If infection is suspected, a sample of the discharge may be taken to identify the cause.

■ Bacterial conjunctivitis is treated by applying antibiotic drops or ointment. In such cases, the symptoms usually clear up within 48 hours. However, the treatment should be continued for 7–10 days, even if the symptoms improve, to ensure the infection is eradicated.

■ Viral conjunctivitis that occurs because of a herpes infection may be treated with eye drops containing an antiviral drug. Although the treatment of other types of viral conjunctivitis is mostly palliative, their symptoms usually clear up within 2–3 weeks.

■ Your doctor may prescribe eye drops or oral antiallergy drugs for allergic conjunctivitis.

See also:
- Allergies p. 315
- Hay fever p. 319
- Herpes simplex infection p. 336

Acute glaucoma

NORMALLY, THE FLUID THAT IS SECRETED INTO THE FRONT OF THE EYE TO MAINTAIN THE EYE'S SHAPE AND NOURISH THE TISSUES DRAINS AWAY CONTINUOUSLY.

However, in acute glaucoma, the drainage system suddenly develops a blockage, and the fluid pressure inside the eye rises rapidly, causing pain and a "red eye." Acute glaucoma is a medical emergency. Without prompt treatment, the eye can swiftly become damaged and a permanent reduction in vision can result. Acute glaucoma is rare under the age of 40 and most common over the age of 60. The tendency to develop it sometimes runs in families.

WHAT ARE THE CAUSES?

The fluid in the front part of the eye is produced continuously by a ring of tissue called the **ciliary body**, behind the eye's colored iris. Normally the fluid flows out through the pupil and drains away through the sievelike meshwork behind the drainage angle at the outer rim of the iris. In acute glaucoma, the iris bulges forward and closes the drainage angle, so that fluid is trapped within the eye. The pressure inside the eye rises as more fluid is secreted and as the pressure rises damage may occur to the optic nerve.

WHAT ARE THE RISKS?

■ Having an eyeball that is smaller than normal is a common cause of farsightedness and increases the risk of developing acute glaucoma.

■ The disorder is more common in older

people because the lens of the eye thickens throughout life and may eventually press against the iris. Fluid then builds up behind the iris, which bulges forward and blocks the drainage angle.

■ Occasionally, acute glaucoma may be triggered when dim light causes the pupil to widen. The iris then thickens and the drainage angle can close.

■ Acute glaucoma sometimes runs in families.

WHAT ARE THE SYMPTOMS?

Mild episodes of acute glaucoma tend to occur in the evening. Symptoms include pain in the eyes and haloes appearing around lights; seek medical attention. Full-blown attacks usually develop suddenly and include these symptoms:

- rapid deterioration of vision
- intense pain in the eye
- redness and watering of the eye
- sensitivity to bright light
- haloes appearing around lights
- nausea and vomiting.

WHAT IS THE TREATMENT?

Applanation tonometry, which measures the pressure inside the eye, is used to detect acute glaucoma. Laser iridotomy (see box, right) is usually performed to correct the condition.

See also:
- Eye tests p. 468 - Nearsightedness and farsightedness p. 469

Chronic glaucoma

CHRONIC GLAUCOMA IS A GRADUAL, PAINLESS INCREASE IN THE FLUID PRESSURE INSIDE
THE EYE, USUALLY STARTING AFTER THE AGE OF 40 AND SOMETIMES RUNNING IN FAMILIES.
IT IS MORE COMMON IN PEOPLE OF AFRICAN DESCENT.

Chronic glaucoma is also known as **open-angle glaucoma**. The condition causes a gradual deterioration of sight due to a progressive buildup of fluid pressure inside the eye over a period of several years. There are often no symptoms until late in the disease, when loss of vision may be permanent. Although the condition can lead to total blindness, early treatment often prevents severe damage. In most cases, both eyes are affected, although symptoms may only occur in one eye initially.

WHAT ARE THE SYMPTOMS?
By the time symptoms appear, it is probable that your vision has been permanently affected. At this late stage, symptoms may include:

● bumping into objects because of loss of the outer edges of vision (peripheral vision)
● blurring of objects that are straight ahead of you.

WHAT MIGHT BE DONE?
Your eye doctor will probably perform a test called applanation tonometry to measure the pressure inside your eye. Various other tests may be done, including a visual field test to check for loss of peripheral vision.

WHAT IS THE TREATMENT?
■ If chronic glaucoma is diagnosed early, eye drops to reduce the pressure in the eye will probably be prescribed. You will probably have to continue using these eye drops for the rest of your life.
■ If the condition is advanced, or if eye drops do not lower the pressure sufficiently, surgery may be needed to make a drainage channel in the white of the eye.
■ In another surgical technique, called **laser trabeculoplasty**, a laser beam is used to increase the flow through the trabecular meshwork, allowing fluid to drain away.

See also:
• Eye tests p. 468

Retinal detachment

THE LIGHT-SENSITIVE RETINA OF THE EYE IS NORMALLY ATTACHED TO THE UNDERLYING TISSUE,
BUT IN RETINAL DETACHMENT PART OF THE RETINA PEELS AWAY FROM THIS TISSUE.

Retinal detachment usually affects one eye only but, without rapid treatment, can cause partial or total blindness in the affected eye. Retinal detachment is more common in people over the age of 50 and sometimes runs in families. Participating in sports that may lead to a blow to the eye, such as boxing, is a risk factor. Severe nearsightedness is also a risk factor.

Retinal detachment usually begins with a small tear in the retina. Fluid is then able to pass through the hole and separates the retina from the supporting tissues underneath.

WHAT ARE THE SYMPTOMS?
■ Flashing lights in the corner of the eye.
■ Sudden appearance of a large number of dark spots (floaters) in the field of vision.
■ Shadow affecting vision.

WHAT MIGHT BE DONE?
Your doctor can diagnose retinal detachment using an ophthalmoscope, an instrument used to examine the back of the eye. If only a small area of retina has detached, the tear may be sealed by laser surgery, which may require local anesthetic. However, if a large area has become detached, microsurgery (see box, right) under a local anesthetic will be necessary. If treated early, normal vision may be restored, but if treatment is delayed, recovery is less certain.

TREATMENT

Microsurgery

Microsurgery is a technique that enables surgeons to operate on extremely small and delicate tissues in the body. In microsurgery a binocular microscope is used to view the operating site and surgeons operate with specially adapted operating instruments.

Microsurgery is often used to operate on tissue such as nerves and blood vessels and on small structures in the eye, middle ear, and reproductive system. For example, microsurgery is regularly used in the repair of detached retinas. It is also used routinely to remove a cataract (a diseased eye lens) and replace it with an artificially made lens. In an operation to reattach a severed limb or digit, microsurgery is used to repair severed nerves and blood vessels. Microsurgery may also be used to try to reverse sterilization operations such as tubal ligation in females and vasectomy in males.

Microsurgery is usually performed under general anesthesia, but for some procedures, such as cataract operations, regional local or topical anesthesia may be used instead. Since some microsurgical operations take longer than other similar surgical procedures, the time under anesthesia is longer and this may extend the recovery time from anesthesia.

Microsurgery is usually highly successful for procedures such as cataract removal and repairing a detached retina. In other procedures, the success of microsurgery often depends on the extent to which tissues were damaged initially.

IMPERFECT VISION

Most people have a visual problem at some time in their lives so it's important to have regular eye checkups with your eye doctor throughout your life. The most common disorders of vision are **nearsightedness** (myopia) and **farsightedness** (hypermetropia), which are **focusing** (refractive) errors. If you have a refractive error it means that the image of an object cannot be focused clearly on the retina at the back of the eye and so the object appears fuzzy. Either the eye can't bend the light accurately enough or the eye is the wrong shape and refracted light misses the retina. Another refractive error, **presbyopia**, may develop as you get older for a different reason – the rigidity of the lens increases as it ages so that the lens can no longer focus near images on the retina. Most refractive errors can be corrected by glasses or contact lenses, or cured by surgical techniques.

In this section, I include **color blindness**, which affects more men than women, and serious visual problems including double vision.

TESTS

Eye tests

Regular eye exams are important, not just to check on your sight but also because a routine checkup will include tonometry to check your eye pressure (a test for glaucoma) and an examination of the optic nerve at the back of the eye to make sure the retina is healthy.

Vision tests

You should have your vision tested once every two years, especially if you are over 40 years old. The most common vision tests assess the sharpness (acuity) of your distance vision and how well your eyes focus on near objects. The tests also show which corrective lenses you may need. An additional test for glaucoma (see Applanation tonometry, below) should be performed, depending on your age and medical history.
Phoroptor This device holds different lenses in front of each eye, allowing the optometrist to test each eye separately.
Snellen chart The sharpness of your distance vision is tested separately for each eye. The test involves reading letters of decreasing sizes on a Snellen chart.
Near-vision test Wearing your glasses or contact lenses, if you use them, you will be asked to read very small print on a chart held at normal reading distance. This tests how well you can focus on near objects.
Having a vision test Lenses in the phoroptor are changed until you can read letters near the bottom of the Snellen chart, enabling the eye doctor to make the appropriate prescription for your corrective lenses.
Applanation tonometry The condition glaucoma, in which the pressure inside the eye is often raised, can be detected using an instrument called an applanation tonometer. Anesthetic drops are put into your eye and

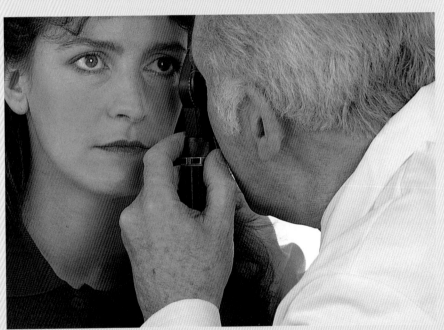

A phoroptor, which can hold lenses of different strengths in front of the eyes, is used with a Snellen chart to test distance vision. Each eye can be tested separately.

the tonometer is then gently pressed against the cornea (the transparent front part of the eye) to measure the force needed to flatten the cornea. The test lasts only a few seconds and is painless.

Vision tests for children

Vision tests in children are designed according to their age and ability and are performed on a regular basis to look for defects that may delay normal development and learning. Vision can be assessed in infants using special tests, while older children can match shapes or letters. Once a child can read, adult vision tests can be used (see Snellen chart, above).
Retinoscopy This test may be performed on infants. About 30 minutes before the test,

eye drops are given to dilate the pupils and prevent focusing, and a beam of light is shone into each eye in turn from an instrument called a retinoscope. The effect of different lenses on the beam of light tells whether the child needs glasses. The test is performed in a darkened room.
Letter-matching test This test is usually used for children from about the age of three who are able to recognize letters. A child is given a card with letters printed on it. The optometrist then holds up cards with letters of decreasing size at a distance of 10ft (3m) and asks the child to identify the same letters on the card he is holding. Each of the eyes should be tested separately using an eyepatch.

Nearsightedness and farsightedness

NEARSIGHTEDNESS (MYOPIA) IS THE INABILITY TO SEE DISTANT OBJECTS CLEARLY DUE TO A MISMATCH BETWEEN THE SIZE OR SHAPE OF THE EYEBALL AND THE FOCUSING POWER OF THE EYE.

In nearightedness, the eyeball is too long and the image forms in front of the retina. Nearsightedness can be corrected with glasses using **concave** lenses or contact lenses (see box, below).

Farsightedness (hypermetropia) is the inability to see close objects clearly because the image cannot be focused precisely on the retina. In farsightedness, the eyeball is too short and the image falls behind the retina. Farsightedness can be corrected with glasses using **convex** lenses or contact lenses (see box, below). Farsightedness in children may interfere with reading and early learning and must be corrected when very young.

WHAT MIGHT BE DONE?
NEARSIGHTEDNESS
■ Your optometrist will check your visual acuity and the level of detail you can see and then assess the severity of any visual defect.
■ Nearsightedness can be corrected by wearing contact lenses or glasses that have concave lenses. The focusing power of your own lenses decreases gradually with age, and your prescription may need to be updated regularly.

It's very important to treat nearsightedness in children, particularly once they are in school. Nearsightedness can prevent a child from following lessons written on the blackboard or from participating fully in sports that involve catching a ball.

FARSIGHTEDNESS
■ Your optometrist will check your visual acuity and the level of detail you can see, and then assess the severity of any visual defect.
■ Farsightedness can be corrected by wearing contact lenses or glasses that have convex lenses. The focusing power of your own lenses decreases gradually with age, and your prescription may need to be updated regularly.
■ Some people who have farsightedness may be helped by laser treatment, which reshapes the surface of the cornea with a laser beam to increase its focusing power.
■ Farsightedness doesn't cause complications, but people who have it are more prone to **acute glaucoma**, a serious condition that must be treated promptly. You should, therefore, see an eye doctor regularly, so that any problems can be spotted early and dealt with.

It's crucial to treat farsightedness in children. Although it may be detected during routine vision tests at school, children with a family history of farsightedness should have a vision test before the age of 3 because early treatment is important for early learning.

Presbyopia

Many of us find that the normal reading distance becomes longer and longer as we get older; this is known as **presbyopia**. As our eyes age they lose the power to focus; deterioration starts around the age of 40 years and by the age of 65 little focusing power remains. Presbyopia can be corrected by simple reading glasses with convex lenses or by contact lenses (see Glasses and contact lenses, below). Lenses may need to be changed four or five times over 20 or 30 years until eventually all focusing is done by glasses or contact lenses.

Focusing errors

Nearsightedness

In nearsightedness, the eyeball is too long relative to the focusing power of the cornea and lens. Light from distant objects is focused in front of the retina and the image is blurry.

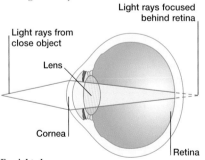

Farsightedness

In a person with farsightedness, the eye is too short relative to the focusing power of the cornea and lens. Light rays are focused behind the retina and the image is blurry.

See also:
• **Acute glaucoma p. 466** • **Chronic glaucoma p. 467** • **Surgery for refractive errors p. 470**

TREATMENT

Glasses and contact lenses

Most focusing (refractive) errors can be corrected by glasses or, for older children and adults, contact lenses. Glasses can correct most refractive errors and do not cause complications. Contact lenses are most effective for nearsightedness and farsightedness. They require careful cleaning to reduce the chance of an infection of the cornea, over which they are placed.

How corrective lenses work
Glasses and contact lenses correct refractive errors by altering the angle of light rays before the rays reach the surface of the cornea, the transparent front layer of the eye, allowing the lens to focus the rays correctly on the retina.
■ Nearsightedness is corrected by concave lenses, which make light rays diverge, so that they are focused on the retina and not in front of it.
■ Farsightedness requires a convex lens to make light rays converge, focusing them on the retina and not behind it.

Contact lenses
Three types of contact lenses are available: rigid (hard), gas-permeable, and soft. Soft lenses are the most widely used type of contact lens. Disposable soft lenses are worn only once or for a few days, then thrown away. Nondisposable lenses should be disinfected and cleaned daily, unless worn for an extended period of time (not usually recommended). If an eye becomes red or painful, stop wearing your lenses and consult your eye doctor immediately.

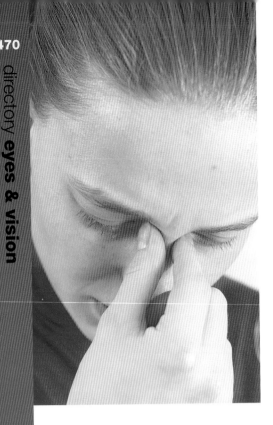

Eyestrain

MOST PEOPLE SUFFER FROM TEMPORARY DISCOMFORT OR ACHING IN OR AROUND THE EYES EVERY SO OFTEN.

Eyestrain is neither a medical term nor a diagnosis. In contrast to widespread belief, you cannot damage or strain your eyes by using them under difficult conditions, such as reading small print in poor light or wearing glasses of the wrong strength. Although aching and discomfort are commonly attributed to eyestrain, more often the cause is a headache due to tension or fatigue of the muscles around the eye as a result of frowning or squinting.

The symptoms normally attributed to eyestrain don't require treatment and normally disappear on their own, but if the problem worsens or persists, you should consult your doctor.

Tips for tired eyes

■ When you're doing close work, rest your eyes by glancing up now and then.
■ If your eyes become sore and dry after close work (as a consequence of forgetting to blink often enough), simply blink a few times to sluice out the eyeball with tears and cure the dryness.
■ "Palming" – the practice of cupping the hands over the eyes to rest them – will do no harm, but shutting the eyes to rest them every so often is just as effective a method of refreshing and relieving them.
■ After a long bout of crying, cold water compresses on the eyelids should help to relieve the discomfort of swollen eyes.
■ It does no harm to rub the eyes, as long as there is no foreign body in either of them and that rubbing them does not cause any pain.

Ophthalmic migraines

THE CLASSICAL SYMPTOMS OF MIGRAINES INCLUDE VISUAL DISTURBANCES, HEADACHE AND, POSSIBLY, NAUSEA WITH VOMITING.

Ophthalmic symptoms may include **blurred vision**, **flashing lights**, **haloes** around light sources, and **sensitivity** to light lasting 20–30 minutes. Neither the headache or nausea develop. When the visual symptoms disappear, the migraine attack resolves too.

Astigmatism

AN UNEVEN CURVATURE OF THE TRANSPARENT CORNEA AT THE FRONT OF THE EYE CAUSES ASTIGMATISM, WHICH IS DISTORTED VISION THAT CAN RESULT IN BLURRING OF SMALL PRINT.

You may notice difficulty with both near and distant vision and should seek an eye test from your optometrist. Most astigmatism is present from birth.

WHAT IS THE TREATMENT?
■ Vision can usually be corrected by glasses that have specially curved lenses to compensate for the unevenly shaped cornea.
■ Rigid contact lenses are also effective for astigmatism because in effect, they smooth out the surface of the cornea.
■ Conventional soft contact lenses mold to the shape of the cornea and can normally only correct for mild astigmatism. However, soft contact lenses that are specially designed to correct the condition (known as **toric lenses**) are also available.
■ Astigmatism may be corrected by surgical treatment that reshapes the cornea (see box, right). One of the most widely used surgical treatments for this condition is laser surgery.

See also:
• **Glasses and contact lenses p. 469**

TREATMENT

Surgery for refractive errors

Surgery can be used to correct some refractive errors. The three main surgical techniques are:
● laser-assisted in-situ keratomileusis (LASIK), in which the cornea is reshaped by a laser
● radial keratotomy (RK), in which the cornea is flattened by multiple cuts
● photorefractive keratectomy (PRK), in which areas of the cornea are shaved away by laser.

Warning:
Radial keratotomy (RK) can **weaken** the cornea. Photorefractive keratectomy may cause mild corneal scarring. LASIK causes the least scarring and is the most widely used method.

Double vision

IF YOU HAVE DOUBLE VISION, THAT IS, SEEING TWO IMAGES OF ONE OBJECT, YOU MAY
FIND THE DEFECT DISAPPEARS WHEN YOU CLOSE ONE OF YOUR EYES.

However, you should consult your doctor immediately if you suddenly start to experience double vision because it may indicate that you have a serious underlying disorder.

WHAT ARE THE CAUSES?
■ The most common cause of prolonged double vision is weakness or paralysis of one or more of the muscles that control the movements of one eye.
■ Many serious conditions that affect the brain and nervous system may cause impaired eye movements leading to double vision. Potential causes include **multiple sclerosis**, **head injuries**, **brain tumors,** and bulging of an artery inside the head due to a weakness in the vessel wall (**aneurysm**).

■ In older people, impaired eye movement resulting in double vision may be linked to **diabetes mellitus** and to **atherosclerosis** and **high blood pressure**.
■ Double vision can also occur as a result of a **tumor** or **blood clot** behind one of the eyes, causing the movement of that eye to be affected.

HOW IS IT DIAGNOSED?
■ Your doctor may ask you to shut one eye at a time to see whether the double vision disappears.
■ Your doctor will probably observe the movements of your eyes closely in order to establish whether any of the eye muscles are weak or paralyzed and do special vision tests to identify weak eye movement.

■ If double vision has come on suddenly, or if no obvious cause can be found, urgent computerized tomography (CT) scanning or magnetic resonance imaging (MRI) may be done to check for any abnormality in the eye sockets or brain that might be affecting the alignment of the eyes. You may also have a neurological examination.

See also:
• **CT scanning p. 401**
• **MRI p. 409**

YOUR EYELIDS AND TEARS

Eyelids and tears work together to protect the eye against damage. The eyelids act as shutters, closing to prevent foreign material from entering the eyes. Tears contain one of the most potent antiseptic substances known, called **lysozyme**. It keeps the surface of the eyes moist and helps prevent infection. Disorders of the eyelids or tear system can damage the eyes, but most are easily treated if detected early.

The upper and lower eyelids provide essential protection for the eyes. If anything approaches the eye or face rapidly, the eyelids close together as a reflex action. Furthermore, each eyelid has two or three rows of

eyelashes, which help prevent small particles from entering the eye.
Tears are another important part of the eye's defenses. They are made up of salty fluid produced by the lacrimal (tear) glands, which are located above the upper eyelids. Tears lubricate the exposed surface of the eye and wash away potentially harmful materials, such as dust and chemicals. The production of tears tends to decrease with age, which is why wearing contact lenses can become increasingly uncomfortable as we age. However, dry eyes per se can be part of a serious syndrome called Sjögren's syndrome.

Blepharitis

BLEPHARITIS IS INFLAMMATION, REDNESS, AND SCALING OF THE MARGIN OF THE UPPER OR LOWER
EYELID OR BOTH, OFTEN ASSOCIATED WITH THE SEBACEOUS GLANDS OF THE EYELASHES AND
WITH THE COMMON SKIN DISORDER SEBORRHEIC DERMATITIS.

Blepharitis is generally caused by bacterial infection or may be due to an allergy to cosmetics.
If you have blepharitis, your eyelids will be swollen, red, and itchy. The margins of the eyelids may be covered with soft, greasy scales that dry into crusts, sticking the eyelashes together. In some cases, the roots of the eyelashes become infected, causing styes to form.

WHAT IS THE TREATMENT?
■ You can relieve the symptoms by holding a clean, warm, damp cloth against the eyelid.
■ The healing process may be helped by cleaning the eyelids twice a day with baby shampoo diluted half and half with water, or you could use an over-the-counter eyelid wash.
■ If you have seborrheic dermatitis, treating it should also help the blepharitis.
■ If the blepharitis recurs repeatedly, see your

doctor, who may prescribe topical antibiotics. The condition often clears up after 2 weeks of treatment but it may recur.
■ Allergic blepharitis usually improves on its own, but you should try to avoid contact with the substance that triggered the condition.

See also:
• **Seborrheic dermatitis p. 315** • **Stye p. 543**

FOCUS *on* cataracts

As we get older, cataracts (loss of transparency of the lenses in the eyes) are the most common cause of impaired vision. Cataracts form due to changes in the delicate protein fibers within the lens, in the way that an egg white becomes solid when we cook it.

With increasing loss of transparency, the clarity and detail of what we see gets progressively less. Cataracts usually occur in both eyes, but one eye is nearly always more severely affected than the other.

Almost everyone over the age of 65 has cataracts to some degree, but they're usually minor and often confined to the edge of the lens where they don't interfere with sight. Most people over the age of 75 experience some visual impairment due to cataracts.

WHAT ARE THE CAUSES?

You shouldn't be fearful of getting cataracts – they are so common that they could almost be considered part of the normal aging process.
- Exposure to the **ultraviolet radiation in strong sunshine** increases the risk, and cataracts are more common in tropical countries than in Europe or North America. They occur more often in those who spend most of their lives outdoors, especially if the eyes are unprotected.
- Exposure to other types of radiation,

including **infrared** radiation and **X-rays**, may cause cataracts to form.
- Cataracts may be caused by **direct injury** to the eye, and are almost inevitable if a foreign particle, such as a shard of metal or glass, gets into the lens.
- Cataracts are common in people with **diabetes** and may develop early if the diabetes isn't well controlled and blood-sugar levels get very high.
- The formation of cataracts is promoted by long-term treatment with **corticosteroid drugs**, poisoning by substances such as **naphthalene** (found in mothballs) or **ergot** (formed in stored grain contaminated by a certain type of fungus).
- Mixing **sunshine** and the herbal antidepressant **St.-John's-wort** may lead to cataracts. **Hypericin**, the active ingredient in St.-John's-wort, reacts with visible and ultraviolet light to produce free radicals that damage the lens. Once proteins are damaged they produce cloudiness in the lens, forming a cataract. Hypericin does not cause any protein damage when kept in the dark, so at the very least, those taking St.-John's-wort should wear hats and wraparound sunglasses.

WHAT ARE THE SYMPTOMS?
- Cataracts are entirely painless.
- The onset of visual symptoms is almost imperceptible, and progress is nearly always very slow.
- The main symptom is blurring of vision and **nearsightedness,** which gradually becomes worse. So a person who was previously farsighted may be able to read without using their reading glasses.
- Colors become distorted, with dulling of blues and accentuation of reds, yellow, and oranges; the full perception of color is dramatically restored after surgery.
- Beware! Night driving can be impaired. Often the lens opacity causes scattering of light rays and, even at a fairly early stage, may seriously affect night driving.

WHAT IS THE TREATMENT?
Once a cataract has developed, changes to the lens are irreversible. Nowadays, the need to have thick glasses can be avoided by replacing the removed lens with a tiny plastic implant that is fixed permanently in the eye during surgery. Cataract surgery gives excellent results in most cases.

Cataract surgery

A cataract is an opaque region in the lens of the eye causing loss of vision. During cataract surgery, the affected lens is removed and replaced with an artificial lens using microsurgical techniques. The operation is usually performed under topical or local anesthetic, and you will probably be able to go home the same day. **The lens is first softened by an ultrasound probe** and then the softened tissue is extracted. The back of the natural lens capsule is left in place, and an artificial lens is placed inside it. The incision in the cornea is either closed with surgical **stitches** or will gradually heal on its own.

Dry eye (keratoconjunctivitis sicca)

PERSISTENT DRYNESS OF THE EYE DUE TO INSUFFICIENT PRODUCTION OF TEARS
IS KNOWN MEDICALLY AS KERATOCONJUNCTIVITIS SICCA; THE CONDITION BECOMES
INCREASINGLY COMMON IN WOMEN OVER AGE 35.

WHAT ARE THE CAUSES?

Dry eye can be a feature of certain autoimmune disorders in which the tear glands can be damaged, such as:
- rheumatoid arthritis
- Sjögren's syndrome (see below)
- lupus.

If you notice that your eyes are becoming dry frequently, you should consult your doctor so that he can exclude any possible related condition.

WHAT ARE THE SYMPTOMS?

Symptoms of dry eye include:
- blurred vision
- burning and itching
- grittiness.

If left untreated, corneal ulcers and eventually scarring of the cornea may occur.

WHAT IS THE TREATMENT?

■ Your doctor will prescribe artificial tears to restore moisture to the eye.

■ Investigations should be done to find any underlying cause of the dry eyes and appropriate treatment given.
■ In some cases, surgery may be performed to plug the channel through which the tears normally drain away from the eyes.

> **See also:**
> - **Lupus p. 324**
> - **Rheumatoid arthritis p. 429**

Sjögren's syndrome

DRY EYES ARE A MAJOR SYMPTOM OF THE AUTOIMMUNE CONDITION
SJÖGREN'S SYNDROME.

Other normally moist parts of the body – the nose, mouth, throat, and vagina – also tend to be dry, causing a range of problems. Arthritis, resembling rheumatoid arthritis, occurs as the autoimmune process begins to destroy glands that produce protective lubricating fluids. 9 out of 10 sufferers are postmenopausal women.

WHAT IS THE TREATMENT?

■ Artificial tears are essential to treat dry eyes.
■ Frequent dental checkups will avoid tooth decay due to lack of saliva.
■ Dry vagina responds to vaginal moisturizers, HRT, and ostrogen cream or suppositories used vaginally.

■ Arthritis should be treated in the same way as rheumatoid arthritis.

Color blindness

Some people have a defect in the cones, the specialized cells in the retina at the back of the eye, that reduces their ability to tell certain colors apart. An inability to distinguish between red and green is the most common type of color blindness, and this is a gender-linked genetic disorder. It is much rarer in women than it is in men.

Noninherited causes of colour blindness include certain eye conditions, such as macular degeneration. It may also be a side effect of certain drugs, for example some antimalarial drugs.

Color blindness rarely causes serious problems but it can exclude people from certain jobs where being able to distinguish between colors is essential, such as flying an airplane.

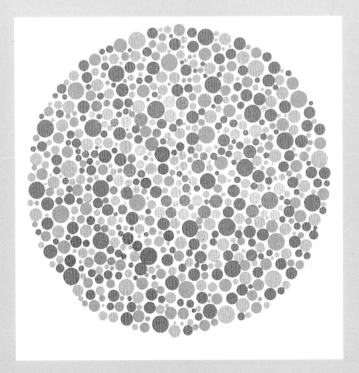

People who are color blind cannot discern the number in the circle.

Ears, Nose, and Throat

Image shows a CT (computerized tomography) section through a human head showing the brain and ear canal

Miriam's overview

When I was a child Ears, Nose, and Throat (ENT) or otolaryngology was a major speciality, even though it spans a comparatively small anatomical area.

The popularity of ENT as a medical speciality was mainly due to tonsillectomy – taking out the tonsils – a procedure that enjoyed a great vogue until about 30 years go.

It was felt that infected tonsils were a "bad thing" and every child would be better off without them. That approach seemed logical at the time. But then we realized that the tonsils were, so to speak, the guardians of the throat and chest and by becoming infected they were only doing their job preventing the infection from going any further.

I remember when this approach was first adopted, one ENT surgeon regretting the "tons of tonsils" he had removed unnecessarily.

More medical knowledge means practices change. In the 1990s the ENT operation in vogue was the insertion of tubes. This followed on the realization that much middle ear disease, otitis media, was referable to glue ear, a new description coined to describe the thick gluey mucus that filled the middle ear in small children, causing deafness and difficulty at school later on.

A new operation was devised to drain away this mucus allowing the ear to work normally and hearing to be restored. This was the insertion of tiny tubes in the eardrum that ventilate the middle ear.

But this fashion too, it would seem, has had its day. Tubes aren't that easy to maintain and they drop out but they're still widely used.

Snoring is the butt of jokes and the cause of sleepless

> *"we realized that the tonsils* were, so to speak, the guardians of the *throat and chest"*

nights for wakeful partners. But recently we've realized that some snorers could be in danger of heart attacks. These are people, mainly men, who have periods of "sleep apnea," spells when they stop breathing. The amount of oxygen in their blood drops, putting heart health in jeopardy.

Snoring needs urgent attention from your doctor, not teasing or jokes.

INSIDE
your ears, nose, and throat

The ears are responsible for two different senses: hearing and balance. The ear consists of the outer, middle, and inner ear. The visible outer part of the ear is called the **pinna**, and the opening into the middle ear is called the **ear canal**. At the end of the ear canal is the **eardrum**, which vibrates in response to sound waves. Beyond the eardrum is the **middle ear**, which contains the **ossicles**, three tiny bones that transmit vibration from the eardrum to a membrane known as the **oval window**. Beyond this membrane lies the **inner ear**. This contains the **cochlea**, which transforms vibration into electrical impulses that are then relayed along nerves to the brain. The inner ear also contains structures responsible for detecting movement and balance.

The **eustachian tube** connects the middle ear to the back of the nose and throat and allows equal air pressure to be maintained on both sides of the eardrum. The nose consists of the visible outer structure, the **nostrils** and the **inner nasal cavity**, which warms and moistens air that is breathed in. Within the skull bones around the nose and eyes are the **sinuses**, cavities that have little use in humans. The back of the nasal cavity connects to the **throat**, or pharynx. At the top of the throat are the **tonsils**, which help protect the body against infection. At the bottom of the throat is the **voice box** (larynx), the structure that contains the **vocal cords** and allows speech to be produced.

how the ear works

KEY

Sound

Electrial signals

Sound waves are transmitted along the path of the blue arrows and are transmitted to the brain as electrical signals.

the nose and throat

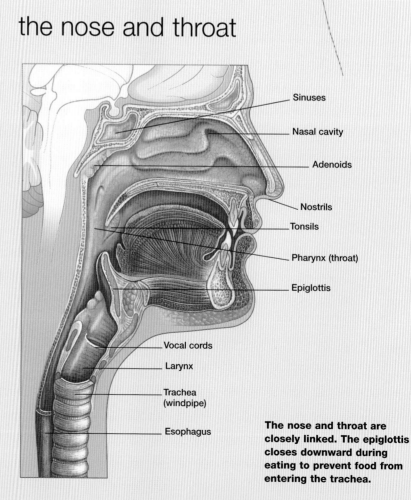

The nose and throat are closely linked. The epiglottis closes downward during eating to prevent food from entering the trachea.

connecting passageways

The ears, nose, and throat are interconnected. The eustachian tube maintains equal air pressure on both sides of the eardrum.

Wax blockage

EARWAX IS PRODUCED BY GLANDS IN THE EAR CANAL AND ITS JOB IS TO CLEAN, MOISTEN, AND PROTECT THE CANAL. IF WAX IS PRODUCED IN LARGER THAN NORMAL QUANTITIES, IT MAY CAUSE A BLOCKAGE AND INTERFERE WITH HEARING.

Usually, earwax is produced in small quantities and emerges naturally from the ear. If the canal becomes blocked with wax, it causes a feeling of blockage, itchiness, and sometimes hearing loss.

WARNING:
Under normal circumstances the ear canal is a self-cleansing organ and needs no special attention. Never use a cotton swab, hair clip or finger to remove wax from your ears – that simply compacts the wax, making it hard.

WHAT IS THE TREATMENT?
■ Wax blockage can be treated with over-the-counter eardrops, and following the maker's instructions will usually dissolve the earwax in about 4–10 days.
■ If the ear remains blocked, you should consult your doctor.
■ Your doctor will probably use a viewing instrument (an otoscope) to inspect the ear canal.
■ You may have the wax removed with a probe or suction device.
■ The ear may be gently flushed out with warm water from a syringe.
■ Wax blockage sometimes recurs after treatment because some ear canals just produce more wax than others.

Ménière's disease

IN MÉNIÈRE'S DISEASE, THE FLUID IN THE INNER EAR INCREASES FROM TIME TO TIME. THE RAISED PRESSURE IN THE INNER EAR DISTURBS THE ORGANS OF HEARING AND BALANCE, CAUSING SUDDEN ATTACKS OF RINGING IN THE EARS AND SEVERE DIZZINESS.

Attacks of Ménière's disease occur suddenly and may last from a few minutes to several days before gradually subsiding.

WHAT ARE THE SYMPTOMS?
The symptoms may include:
● sudden, severe dizziness and loss of balance (vertigo)
● nausea and vomiting
● abnormal, jerky eye movements
● ringing or buzzing noises in the affected ear (tinnitus)
● loss of hearing, particularly of low-pitched sounds
● feeling of pressure in the affected ear.
The time between attacks of Ménière's disease ranges from a few days to years. Tinnitus may be constant or occur only during an attack. Between attacks, vertigo and nausea cease and hearing may improve. With repeated episodes, hearing can deteriorate progressively.

HOW IS IT DIAGNOSED?
■ Your doctor may arrange for hearing tests to assess your hearing loss.

■ Tests such as CT (computerized tomography) scanning or MRI (magnetic resonance imaging) may also be done.

WHAT IS THE TREATMENT?
■ You may be prescribed drugs to relieve nausea (antiemetic drugs).
■ An antihistamine may give further relief from nausea and vertigo and reduce the frequency of the episodes.
■ Sedative drugs such as diazepam may be prescribed to relieve vertigo, and diuretic drugs may be used to help prevent further attacks.

SELF-HELP
■ During an attack, lie still with your eyes closed and avoid noise, perhaps by wearing ear plugs.
■ Between attacks, try to avoid stress.
■ Relaxation techniques may be helpful.
■ A low-salt diet may help – don't add salt to cooking or use with food, and avoid very salty foods such as smoked fish and sausage.

For people with disabling vertigo, an operation to sever the nerve between part of the inner ear and the brain is the last resort. The operation cures the vertigo.

WHAT IS THE OUTLOOK?
■ The symptoms of Ménière's disease are usually improved with medication.
■ The frequency and severity of the episodes tend to decrease over a period of years.
■ However, hearing usually worsens progressively with each successive attack, and permanent hearing loss may be the end result.
■ By the time hearing loss becomes severe, the other symptoms have usually disappeared.

See also:
● **CT scanning p. 401** ● **MRI p. 409**
● **Relaxation p. 292**
● **Tinnitus p. 478** ● **Vertigo p. 418**

Otosclerosis

IN OTOSCLEROSIS, BONE OVERGROWS AROUND ONE OF THE THREE TINY BONES (OSSICLES) IN THE MIDDLE EAR, PREVENTING TRANSMISSION OF SOUND VIBRATIONS TO THE INNER EAR AND CAUSING DEAFNESS. USUALLY BOTH EARS ARE AFFECTED, THOUGH NOT ALWAYS EQUALLY.

Abnormal growth of bone in the middle ear, or otosclerosis, affects about 1 in 12 Caucasian people. It is less common in African Americans. It sometimes leads to hearing loss, but is often symptomless. When symptoms develop it's usually between the ages of 20 and 30. We do not understand why otosclerosis develops but the condition is twice as common in females, and in 3 out of 5 cases someone in the family also has it.

WHAT ARE THE SYMPTOMS?

The symptoms of otosclerosis develop gradually and may include:

● hearing loss in which sounds are muffled but are sometimes clearer if there's background noise
● ringing or buzzing noises in the ears (tinnitus, see below)
● in severe cases, dizziness and imbalance (vertigo).

WHAT MIGHT BE DONE?

Your doctor will probably be able to diagnose otosclerosis from the results of hearing tests and from your family history. The disease can't be halted but a hearing aid may be helpful. If not, consult your doctor about possible surgery to free up the ossicles. There is some evidence that fluoride and calcium pills may slow the progression of otosclerosis.

See also:
● Vertigo p. 418

Tinnitus

PEOPLE WITH TINNITUS HEAR SOUNDS THAT ORIGINATE IN THE EAR ITSELF. THESE SOUNDS MAY INCLUDE RINGING, BUZZING, WHISTLING, ROARING, OR HISSING NOISES. THEY MAY PULSE IN TIME WITH THE HEARTBEAT OR, MORE COMMONLY, OCCUR CONTINUOUSLY AND PERMANENTLY.

WHAT ARE THE CAUSES?

Tinnitus may have no apparent cause, but it's commonly part of **Ménière's disease**. People with anemia, an overactive thyroid gland, or head injuries may have tinnitus, and treatment with various drugs, such as aspirin and antibiotics, can also cause it.

If you develop tinnitus, particularly if it affects one ear only, you should consult your doctor right away. When tinnitus is continuous and permanent it may lead to depression and anxiety disorders.

WHAT MIGHT BE DONE?
TESTS
After looking at your eardrum with an otoscope, your doctor may arrange for hearing tests and a blood test for anemia as well as CT (computerized tomography) scanning or an MRI (magnetic resonance imaging).

TREATMENT
■ If an underlying cause, such as thyroid disease, is found and successfully treated, the tinnitus may improve.
■ If tinnitus persists, your doctor may recommend a device called a **masker**. This device, worn in or behind the ear like a hearing aid, produces sounds that distract you from the tinnitus.
■ If tinnitus accompanies hearing loss, a hearing aid may provide relief by increasing your awareness of background noise while masking the internal sounds.

■ Many people with tinnitus find that background noise, such as playing music, reduces their awareness of the sounds in their ears.
■ If tinnitus is very distressing or leads to depression or anxiety, counseling, support groups, or relaxation exercises may help.

See also:
● CT scanning p. 401
● Ménière's disease p. 477
● MRI p. 409

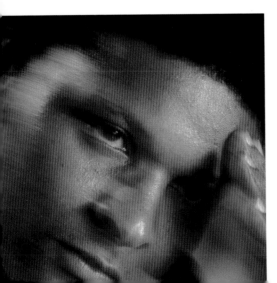

Labyrinthitis

IN LABYRINTHITIS, THE PART OF THE INNER EAR KNOWN AS THE LABYRINTH IS INFLAMED.

Because the labyrinth contains the organs of balance and hearing, inflammation in this part of the ear leads to dizziness, nausea, vomiting, and tinnitus.

WHAT IS THE TREATMENT?
Labyrinthitis can often be diagnosed from your symptoms. Your doctor may suggest:
● antibiotics for bacterial labyrinthitis, though most cases are viral
● you lie in a darkened room
● an antiemetic drug to ease the nausea.
It may take several weeks to recover completely from labyrinthitis, so go slowly.

Motion sickness

MOTION SICKNESS OCCURS WHEN THE BALANCE ORGANS IN THE EAR ARE UPSET BY MOVEMENT, CAUSING SYMPTOMS RANGING FROM SLIGHT QUEASINESS TO VOMITING AND FAINTING.

Motion sickness is very common in some families. When the sensation of movement doesn't correspond with what the eyes see, it causes confusion in the brain and may lead to motion sickness. The problem may occur, for example, if you ride a roller coaster or travel in a car, boat, or plane. Children tend to suffer from motion sickness more than adults, though why is not known; most outgrow it by adolescence.

IS IT SERIOUS?

Motion sickness is not serious, but it is inconvenient. With a young child there is a risk that prolonged vomiting could cause dehydration.

WHAT SHOULD I DO FIRST?

1. Lie down flat.
2. Close your eyes to minimize the confusing signals being received by the brain.

POSSIBLE SYMPTOMS

- Nausea.
- Vomiting.
- Pale, clammy forehead.
- Weakness or dizziness.
- Fainting.

SHOULD I CONSULT THE DOCTOR?

Consult your doctor if you suffer from motion sickness even on short trips, or if commericial brands of motion-sickness medicine do not help.

WHAT MIGHT THE DOCTOR DO?

After questioning you about the symptoms and their frequency, your doctor may prescribe a drug such as an **antihistamine**, though some antihistamines can have side effects such as drowsiness.

SELF-HELP

- Prevent motion sickness by taking a motion sickness medicine before you start the trip. There are several good over-the-counter medications available from the pharmacy.
- Have a small snack before setting out. Don't travel on a full stomach.
- Take plenty of drinks with you, or check that they will be available en route, to prevent the possibility of dehydration through vomiting. Fresh drinks can also reduce the feeling of nausea.
- Carry suitable "sick bags" (strong paper bags are best) in case of vomiting.
- Some people find copper bands worn on the wrist can help.

Nosebleed

BLEEDING FROM THE NOSE MAY OCCUR FOR VARIOUS REASONS, INCLUDING INJURY, NOSE-PICKING, FORCEFUL NOSE-BLOWING, A FOREIGN BODY AND AS A SYMPTOM OF SOME ILLNESSES. NOSEBLEEDS OCCUR MOST COMMONLY IN CHILDREN AND IN PEOPLE OVER 50.

Bleeding from the nose, usually from one nostril only, is most common in children, but the bleeding usually stops by itself and is minor. It comes from a patch of blood vessels just inside the nostril and just under the nasal lining. Nosebleeds are also common, and sometimes very serious, in people over age 50, when bleeding may come from the back of the nose and be hard to stop, especially when accompanied by high blood pressure.

WHAT ARE THE CAUSES?

Nosebleeds may occur from injury to the nose or from nose-picking or forceful nose-blowing. In children, nosebleeds often occur as a result of rough play. A foreign body in the nose or an infection in the upper respiratory tract may also result in a nosebleed.

continued on page 481

Nasal polyps

Benign fleshy growths of the mucus-secreting lining of the nose, known as nasal polyps, have no known cause. They can block the nose and produce a nasal voice, runny nose, and diminished sense of smell.

What might be done?

- A small sample of a single polyp may be removed and examined under a microscope in order to exclude anything sinister.
- Small nasal polyps may be treated by using a corticosteroid spray, which shrinks the polyps over a few weeks.
- Larger polyps may be removed during an endoscopic procedure. A corticosteroid spray may also be necessary for several months after surgery to prevent the polyps from recurring.
- In more severe cases, a course of oral corticosteroids may also be prescribed.

FOCUS *on* snoring

Snoring is a noise caused when floppy tissue at the back of the throat, such as the uvula, blocks the upper air passages during sleep. It may be a symptom of the more serious disorder sleep apnoea, more common in men.

Turbulent airflow creates quite violent vibrations of the soft palate or other structures in the **mouth**, **nose** and **throat**. Depending on how flappable these structures are, vibrations can produce snoring sounds of such resonance that the decibels can be heard throughout the house and curtail the sleep of anyone who's in it.

Most causes of snoring are easily remedied, and there's a good chance that simple treatment or a change in lifestyle will significantly improve things. But other causes are more complex and need specialist investigation and treatment.

WHAT ARE THE CAUSES?
Some factors make us more likely to snore. Smoking, being overweight, consumption of alcohol, use of sleeping pills, poor sleeping position and reaction to house dust and dust mites are all implicated. Avoiding these factors may reduce the likelihood of snoring.

Several things make us more likely to snore:
- obstruction by the tongue if it drops back
- small or collapsing nostrils
- deviated nasal septum, say from a sports injury
- overnight catarrhal congestion
- large, floppy soft palate or uvula
- enlarged nasal bones in the nostrils
- nasal polyps
- in children, enlarged adenoids and mouth breathing.

IS SNORING DANGEROUS?
Snoring in itself isn't serious but it can be a symptom of a more serious disorder, sleep apnoea, in which the snorer stops breathing several times an hour during sleep. The point is that people with sleep apnoea are prone to irregular heartbeats, even possibly heart attacks.

The most vulnerable person is a man over the age of 45 or a woman who's gone through the menopause and isn't taking hormone replacement therapy. So if you're a middle-aged **snorer**, ask your doctor to check you over.

WHAT IS SLEEP APNOEA?
Apnoea literally means a temporary inability to breathe. Sleep apnoea is when a sufferer stops breathing during sleep. The cessation of breathing causes a drop in the blood oxygen level, which arouses the body to start breathing again.

The sleep/arousal cycle is repeated during the night and sufferers get up feeling **unrefreshed** and continually tired. More often than not, they're unaware of their condition.

WHAT ARE THE SYMPTOMS OF SLEEP APNOEA?
Common symptoms are:
- loud snoring
- feelings of choking and shortness of breath at night
- restless, unrefreshing sleep
- excessive daytime sleepiness
- personality changes
- morning headaches.

WHAT CAN BE DONE TO HELP?
Several hospitals have **sleep apnoea and snoring clinics** that can investigate the cause of snoring and diagnose sleep apnoea. Your GP can refer you for special tests to diagnose the cause of your snoring and recommend treatment.

LIFESTYLE CHANGES
Some overweight patients are described as **"weight-sensitive" snorers**. You'll be given a weight-loss programme, and weight reduction alone may provide a complete cure.

HOW DOES LOSING WEIGHT HELP?
Snoring problems are often made worse if you're slightly overweight. Significant relief can often be obtained by some degree of weight reduction, so a sensible eating plan may be of help.

Treating snoring

Surgery
There are a number of new surgical operations for snorers who are found to have obstructions or deformities of the mouth, nose and throat. Such operations are not always guaranteed to work, however.

If snoring is accompanied by sleep apnoea, which is detrimental to your health, treatment may be available on the NHS from an ear, nose and throat surgeon or a respiratory physician. Ask your GP about the possibility.

Somnoplasty
A revolutionary new treatment using low-power, low-temperature, radio-frequency energy will reduce the size of the soft palate.

Laser-assisted uvuloplasty – LAUP
Carbon dioxide laser treatment that will reduce the length and floppiness of the palate and uvula. The technique reshapes your soft palate and is an effective treatment for palatal snorers.

Corrective nasal airway surgery – septoplasty/nasal polypectomy
Minor surgery that opens up the nasal passage by removing a polyp or correcting a deformity that is responsible for reducing the size of the nasal passage.

Tonsillectomy
Where the tonsils and the walls of the pharynx (throat) are causing an obstruction, this operation will be of benefit in a small number of snorers and mild sleep apnoea sufferers.

continued from page 479

WHAT CAN I DO?

■ Put direct pressure on the soft part of your nose by pressing both sides together for at least 15 minutes while breathing through your mouth.

■ Avoid sniffing and/or blowing your nose afterward because you may dislodge the blood clot that has formed and cause another nosebleed.

■ If bleeding persists for half an hour or more, you should seek medical attention.

■ If membranes in the nose are dry and cracked, rubbing water-based ointment in your nose a few times a day or using a saline spray may help prevent recurrent nosebleeds.

WHAT MIGHT THE DOCTOR DO?

A persistent nosebleed will probably require medical treatment.

■ The doctor may pack your nose with nasal sponges, which are left in place for about two days.

■ Alternatively, a flexible tube with a small balloon at the tip may be inserted into the back of your nose and inflated to stop the bleeding by applying pressure to leaking vessels.

■ Bleeding vessels may also be cauterized (sealed using heat or a chemical) under local anesthesia.

■ Blood tests may be done to check how well your blood clots.

Sinusitis

SINUSITIS MEANS INFLAMMATION OF THE SINUSES – THE AIR-FILLED CAVITIES IN THE SKULL SITUATED BEHIND THE NOSE AND EYES AND IN THE CHEEKS AND FOREHEAD. THE PROBLEM USUALLY RESULTS FROM A SECONDARY BACTERIAL INFECTION IN BLOCKED SINUSES.

The sinuses are lined with a mucus-secreting membrane and are connected to the nasal cavity by a number of narrow channels. They have little function in humans.

WHAT ARE THE CAUSES?

The most common primary cause of sinusitis is a viral infection, such as the common cold. If the channels connecting the nose to the sinuses become blocked due to the viral infection,

mucus collects in the sinuses. When mucus can't drain away it can become infected with bacteria.

Blockage of the channels is more likely in people with an abnormality in the nose, such as nasal polyps or a deviated nasal septum (twisting of the cartilage that divides the nose internally into two). People with hay fever or cystic fibrosis are also more likely to develop sinusitis.

WHAT ARE THE SYMPTOMS?

In adults, symptoms depend on which sinuses are affected and may include:

● headache
● pain and tenderness in the face that tends to worsen when bending down
● toothache, if the sinuses behind the cheeks are affected
● thick, yellow nasal discharge
● nasal congestion or obstruction.

SELF-HELP

Steam inhalation

Inhaling steam from a bowl of hot water can help relieve the symptoms of colds, sore throats, sinusitis, and laryngitis. The moisture in the steam loosens secretions in congested upper airways, making them easier to clear. You can also run hot water while you are in the bathroom and inhale the steam. Children shouldn't do steam inhalation unless they are under adult supervision.

Preparation

Fill a bowl about one-third full with hot water. Lean forward, pull a towel over your head as well as the bowl, and inhale steam for several minutes.

My mom used to put Friar's Balsam into the water and you can use mentholated over-the-counter products to suit your taste. Some people prefer herbal aromatic oils dissolved in the hot water.

Inhaling steam is a good way to clear a blocked nose or sinuses and soothe a sore throat.

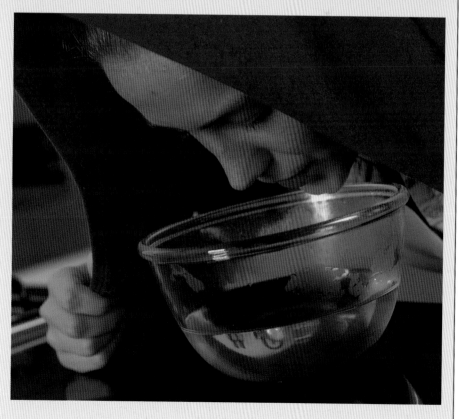

In a few cases, the infection spreads and may cause redness and swelling of the skin around an eye.

SELF-HELP

In many cases, sinusitis clears up without treatment.
- Painkillers and a decongestant, both available over the counter, may alleviate symptoms.
- Steam inhalation, which usually helps clear the nose, may also relieve symptoms.
- If symptoms become worse or do not improve within three days, you should consult a doctor.

WHAT MIGHT THE DOCTOR DO?

Treatments and tests might include:
- antibiotics prescribed to clear up a secondary bacterial infection
- if sinusitis recurs or doesn't clear up completely, X-rays to look for thickening of the lining of the sinuses and excess mucus
- endoscopy of the nose
- CT (computerized tomography) scanning to look for a specific cause, such as nasal polyps
- surgery may be necessary to enlarge drainage channels from the sinuses to the nose or create new ones.

Acute sinusitis usually clears up in a few weeks, but the symptoms of chronic sinusitis may last for a couple of months and need a prolonged course of antibiotics.

See also:
- Hay fever p. 319
- CT scanning p. 401
- Cystic fibrosis p. 521

Laryngitis

INFLAMMATION OF THE LARYNX (VOICE BOX) IS KNOWN
AS LARYNGITIS OR A "SORE THROAT."

Laryngitis is usually caused by infection, often a viral infection, and results in hoarseness. It's more common in smokers and drinkers.

WHAT ARE THE SYMPTOMS?

The symptoms of laryngitis usually develop over 12–24 hours and vary depending on the underlying cause. Symptoms may include:
- hoarseness
- gradual loss of the voice
- pain in the throat, especially when using the voice.

Sometimes laryngitis is associated with vocal cord nodules due to overuse or misuse.

WHAT CAN I DO?

When vocal cords are inflamed they need rest. For both forms of laryngitis, resting your voice can help relieve pain and avoid further damage to the vocal cords. Acute laryngitis that's caused by a viral infection usually clears up without treatment. There's no specific treatment for chronic laryngitis.

Sudden hoarseness in middle or older age must always be investigated by your doctor since it may indicate cancer or an underlying lung disease.

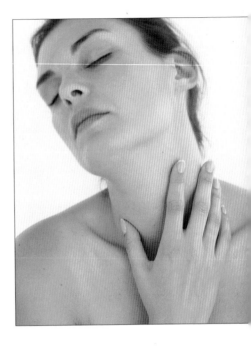

Cancer of the larynx

CANCER OF THE LARYNX (VOICE BOX) OFTEN CAUSES PERSISTENT HOARSENESS.
IT'S MOST COMMON BETWEEN THE AGES OF 55 AND 65, AND IS FIVE TIMES MORE COMMON
IN MEN, ESPECIALLY IF THEY SMOKE AND DRINK.

In about 3 out of 5 cases, the cancer develops on the vocal cords.

WHAT IS THE TREATMENT?

- You may be offered surgery to remove part or all of the larynx and/or radiation therapy.
- If the larynx has to be removed, I'm afraid ordinary speech will no longer be possible.

However, several techniques have been developed to allow you to speak without a larynx. Speech therapy may enable you to

speak using your esophagus, or you may be able to learn to speak with the help of a handheld electromechanical device that generates sounds. Alternatively, a small device known as a tracheoesophageal implant may be fitted to help you speak.

GOOD NEWS!

In more than 9 of out 10 cases, treatment is successful if the tumor develops on the vocal cords and is detected and treated early.

WARNING:
Any hoarseness starting for no reason in middle age or older must be checked out by your doctor.

Teeth and Gums

Image shows a polarized light micrograph of molar teeth in the lower jaw

Miriam's overview

The old joke goes, "Dentist looking into patient's mouth, 'Your teeth are all right but your gums will have to come out.'" And there's more than a grain of truth in that.

Without healthy gums the teeth cannot stay healthy. Infections in pockets around the gum margin, caused by the bacteria in plaque, eventually loosen the sealing of the tooth in the jawbone, leading to infections, "sensitive" teeth, pain, difficulty chewing, and eventually loss of teeth – they simply fall out.

"without *healthy gums* the teeth cannot stay healthy"

There are two main ways to maintain gum health – preventing the accumulation of plaque around our children's teeth by cutting down on sugary foods and making sure all youngsters grow up with good dental hygiene habits and continue them through life.

As we get older this requires more than brushing. Spaces open up between the teeth where fermenting food can lodge, creating the conditions where gum-destroying bacteria can thrive. Each meal therefore requires the ritual of tooth brushing and flossing (or the use of dental sticks or micro-brushes) to get rid of all food fragments.

Cosmetic dentistry caught on 20 years ago and is now the prerogative of everyone. It goes a lot further than teenage braces to straighten uneven front teeth. Discolored teeth can be bleached or whitened with a veneer, teeth can be filed down, built up, replaced, capped, crowned, implanted both to conserve and enhance.

Teeth are seen as accessories whose appearance is important not just for personal morale but also for professional reasons. An attractive smile is just as important to someone whose looks are their fortune as any other part of their body.

"*each meal* requires the ritual of *tooth brushing* and *flossing*"

INSIDE
your teeth and gums

A child's first set of 20 teeth, called **primary, deciduous,** or **milk teeth**, erupt from the gums between the ages of about six months and three years. These start to be replaced by 32 **secondary teeth** at about the age of 6, with most secondary teeth in place by the age of 21.

All teeth have the same structure. Each tooth has a hard shell, made of enamel and dentin, that surrounds an inner structure filled with soft tissue, known as **pulp**. The exposed part of the tooth, or the **crown**, is covered by a layer of tough **enamel**, which is similar to ivory, and underneath the enamel is a substance called **dentin**. Long, pointed **roots** extend from the dentin and pulp into the jaw and are sealed by a layer of firm, fleshy tissue called the **gums**.

the structure of a tooth

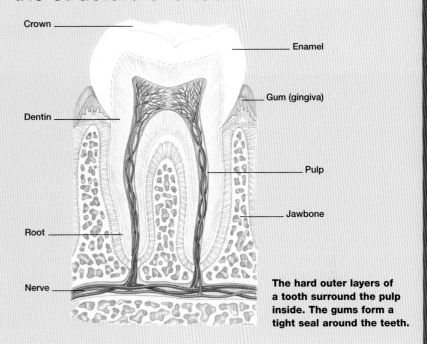

Crown

Enamel

Gum (gingiva)

Dentin

Pulp

Jawbone

Root

Nerve

The hard outer layers of a tooth surround the pulp inside. The gums form a tight seal around the teeth.

Caring for your teeth and gums

THE HEALTH OF THE TEETH IS AT LEAST 50 PERCENT DEPENDENT ON THE HEALTH OF THE GUMS; IN THE WESTERN WORLD, MORE TEETH ARE LOST THROUGH GUM DISEASE THAN THROUGH TOOTH DECAY.

Brushing the teeth regularly and frequently (at least twice a day) is the best possible way to maintain and protect the health of the teeth and gums.

Most dentists would agree that the single most important thing is to use a method that is right for you and that is efficient. At one time, a rolling action was propagated, with a downward motion for the upper teeth and an upward motion for the lower teeth. This, however, was shown to be only about 50 percent as effective as the technique that is now generally recommended – a gentle, rapid, short, elliptical action using the **side and edge** of the brush. Don't press too hard or seesaw the toothbrush backward and forward – this may damage the delicate gum margin. If you cannot brush between meals, chewing sugar-free gum may help. Avoid sugary foods and drinks. If your water does not contain fluoride, ask your dentist about using a fluoride rinse or drops.

DENTAL FLOSS
Using dental floss is an excellent adjunct to tooth brushing. It has to be used carefully so as not to damage the delicate margins of the gum. Use it as follows:
1. Wind a 4–6in (10–15cm) length of floss around the first two fingers of each hand.
2. Slide it gently down between two teeth, pressing it against the side of the tooth (but do not seesaw it against the gum). Then swing it upward, pressing against the side of the other tooth and removing any debris with it.

DENTAL CARE
■ Your hygienist will scale the teeth and remove any deposits of tartar from the gum margins. Visits should preferably be at six-monthly intervals.
■ Children, whose teeth and bones are still forming, need to have an adequate intake of calcium and vitamin D in their diets.

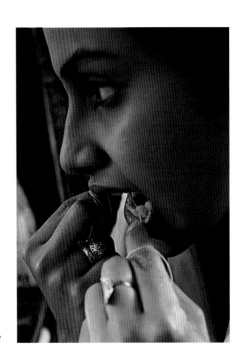

continued on page 488

FOCUS *on* fear of dentists

One of the most common phobias is fear of dentists. At the thought of walking into a dentist's waiting room many of us break out into a cold sweat. It's very important to keep our teeth and gums in good shape and that requires regular dental checkups. But overcoming our fear of dentists can be an uphill struggle.

These days dentistry is a pretty painless exercise. Indeed some dentists go to extraordinary lengths to make sure the procedure is as comfortable as possible. I've come across one dentist, for example, who provides his patients with a headphone so they cannot hear the sound of the drill – so-called white noise – and another who sits and chats until the anesthetic works.

● Another possibility is to ask the dentist to smear a **local anaesthetic gel** on your gums before he injects them. Ask for just half the injection of anesthetic to begin with, wait for five minutes, then have the rest and you shouldn't feel a thing.

● There is also the **needleless syrijet** or **electrical dental analgesia**, which delivers a mild electrical pulse that the patient controls and that stops their senses sending pain messages to the brain.

● Some dentists now use a technique called **inhalation sedation** when taking out teeth. The patient remains conscious throughout but is calmed by breathing in a mixture of nitrous oxide and oxygen.

● In extreme cases a **general anesthetic** may be available, but can only be administered in a hospital setting.

● One solution chosen by many people is to have a **valium** injection in the arm to relax

them. So although they are awake they are so relaxed they don't feel a thing. The only problem is you have to be accompanied since it can take several hours for the effects to wear off. This type of injection isn't addictive.

SELF-HELP
Practice the drill for instant relief from a panic attack (see p. 287).

Visualization

1. Imagine you are going to the dentist and visualize the trip from the moment you are leaving your house until you get to the dentist's door. Note your reactions. Use relaxation (see right) to reduce anxiety. As you familiarize yourself with what you see, venture closer, observing and coping as before.

2. Visualize being in the reception area, waiting room, or office. Imagine that your dentist says you need to have some tests. Stay with this and observe your reactions even though you may want to escape. Observe what you are thinking – perhaps you are imagining

some complicated treatment. If your mind is racing along these lines, again don't stop. Stay with the thoughts until they no longer have any effect.

● One of the best ways to find **a dentist sympathetic to nervous patients** is through a friend's recommendation. Doctors can sometimes provide useful guidance on where to find sympathetic dentists. Or contact several local dental practices and explain you are nervous and ask what treatment is available for someone like you.

● To start with, just book a consultation appointment so you can discuss your fears before making any commitment to treatment. Try to take someone with you for moral support.

The American Dental Association can provide more information on what's available to relieve any pain and discomfort and has a variety of **free brochures**, including some that deal with fear, treatment options, and caring for your teeth.

● Try and get ahold of a **relaxation tape**. Play it at home and take it to the dentist with you.

● **Hypnotherapy** can work wonders for some people. You may require several sessions so it can be expensive. If you would like to explore this avenue, I suggest you do some investigation first because it is crucial to find a qualified hypnotist.

Relaxation exercises

Head: Sit in a chair with arms, shoulders, and head supported. Clench fists, hold tension, and relax. Repeat until hands feel relaxed. With mouth open, take a deep breath, hold it for five seconds and let the air out. Repeat six times. You will feel more calm and relaxed.

Legs: Stretch both legs out, holding them in the air. Point toes away from yourself, holding the tension. Pull toes to point toward yourself and tense leg muscles. Relax, letting legs flop onto the floor. Repeat until legs feel loose and relaxed.

Stomach: Contract stomach muscles and take a deep breath and hold the tension. Relax, letting breath out. Repeat five times

Arms: Clench fists, hold tension, and relax. Stretch arms up (as if to touch the ceiling) and tense muscles, reaching as high into the air as possible. Relax, letting arms drop to sides. Repeat until your arms feel very loose and relaxed.

Shoulders: Shrug shoulders so that they touch your ears. Then let them drop and relax. Repeat five times. Push shoulders forward and inward to meet each other, making a "hump" in your back (pushing arms forward). Push shoulders backward and inward, arching your back. Hold the tension and then relax, falling back into the chair. Repeat five times.

Neck: Move head to left, hold tension. Turn head to right and hold tension. Press head forward with your chin on your chest and tense back of neck. Relax, allowing head to fall back onto chair. Repeat five times.

Head and face: Raise eyebrows, tense, and then frown and tense. Repeat until scalp and forehead are relaxed. Close eyes very tightly. Clench up eyes and hold tension. Relax, letting eyelids drop and close eyes. Clench teeth, feel the tension and then relax, letting the jaw drop slightly. Tighten mouth into a whistling shape or "O," then tense lips as if to make an "E" sound. Relax mouth.

● Concentrate on breathing deeply and regularly, letting breath out when breathing out.
● Let yourself sink, relaxed, into the chair. Remain like this for about 10 minutes – and let yourself enjoy it.
● Pick your favorite relaxing scene and fill your mind with it.

Remember
● When you have finished relaxing, slowly open your eyes.
● Never jump up and rush around immediately.
● Use relaxation on any part of your body that feels tense during the day.
● Deep breathing is useful anywhere to help you feel calm.
● Begin by relaxing when you are on your own. Soon you will find you can do it quite easily with other people around you.
● Begin by doing each exercise in turn. Later you will find that you can just sit down and relax in a moment, doing a few exercises.

ARMS
Stretch arms up and tense muscles

SHOULDERS
1. Push shoulders forward and inward

2. Push shoulders backward and inward

continued from page 485

■ While it is a myth that your teeth suffer during pregnancy, your gums certainly do – one of the effects of the high level of circulating estrogen and progesterone that occurs during pregnancy is softening of the gum margins. For this reason alone, you should visit your dentist two or three times during pregnancy to make sure all is well.

■ There is unequivocal evidence to show the kind of diet we eat affects the health of our gums and teeth, and that dental decay is caused in mainly by sugary foods containing sucrose. Such foods include most refined foods and sweet drinks, candy, chocolate, sticky foods, such as gummies or fruit roll-ups, and ice cream. If you want healthy teeth do not have sweet, sugary foods or drinks between meals – within 20 minutes of eating such foods, damage to your gums and teeth has already begun.

■ Dentists agree that "**safe snacks**" would include any fresh, raw fruits and vegetables, corn chips, nuts, or cheese. Cheese is a particularly useful and healthy food for the mouth, gums, and teeth, since it stimulates the production of saliva and it is a very good way to end a meal. Saliva helps prevent the production of plaque acid, which is caused by bacterial fermentation of sugar in the diet (the initial process that starts tooth decay).

■ There is clear evidence that fluoride, in all its forms, protects the teeth against decay and it is most effective if the fluoride is actually incorporated in the teeth during their development. By far the best way of taking fluoride, of course, is in drinking water. Also make sure that you always use fluoride toothpaste and consult your dentist about giving fluoride tablets, drops, or rinse to your children to protect their developing teeth.

■ The arch villain of tooth decay is **plaque** which corrodes the outer protective enamel of the teeth and eventually works its way through to the inner living part of the tooth, the pulp cavity (causing pulpitis).

■ Smoking upsets the natural bacterial flora of the mouth; it causes unpleasant mouth odor and stains the teeth, mouth, and even the skin surrounding the lips, an unpleasant yellowish color. It also increases the risk of gum disease and mouth cancer.

■ Certain drugs can affect the health of the gums and teeth. For example, antiepileptic drugs, such as hydantoins, can make the gum margins red, soft and swollen. Some drugs used to treat heart conditions can also cause the gums to swell. Tetracyclines, if taken by a pregnant mother, may be deposited in her baby's developing teeth and may stain the teeth a yellowish color.

Dental cavities

GRADUAL, PROGRESSIVE DECAY OF A TOOTH IS KNOWN AS DENTAL CAVITIES.

Dental cavities usually starts as a small cavity, or hole, in the enamel (the hard, protective outer covering of a tooth).

If left untreated, the decay eventually penetrates the outer layer of enamel and attacks the dentine (the softer material that makes up the bulk of a tooth). As the tooth decay progresses, the pulp (the living core of the tooth that contains the nerves and the blood vessels) may be affected. If the pulp is exposed to decay and becomes infected, it may die.

WHAT ARE THE CAUSES?

■ Tooth decay is usually caused by a buildup of **plaque** (a deposit of food particles, mucus, and bacteria) on the surface of the teeth. The bacteria in plaque break down the sugar in food to produce an acid that erodes the tooth enamel. If sugary foods and drinks are consumed regularly and the teeth are not cleaned thoroughly soon afterward, eventually a cavity is likely to form.

■ The condition is especially common in children, adolescents, and young adults since they are more likely to have a diet high in sugar and fail to clean their teeth regularly.

■ Babies who frequently fall asleep with a bottle of juice, milk, or formula in the mouth may also develop severe cavities, especially in the front teeth, called "bottle mouth."

WHAT MIGHT BE DONE?

■ Your dentist will examine your teeth with a probe and a mirror to look for areas of decay. An X-ray may also be taken to reveal decay

that may be developing beneath the surfaces of the teeth.

■ If you have superficial dental cavities that is restricted to the surfaces of the enamel, your dentist may only apply fluoride to the area and advise you to be more careful about oral hygiene.

■ If tooth decay has penetrated further into the enamel, or if it has affected the dentine, your dentist will probably need to fill the affected tooth. An injection of local anesthetic may be used to numb the tooth and nearby gum to prevent you from feeling pain. When the area is numb, the decayed parts of the tooth are drilled out, and the cavity is cleaned and filled to stop further decay.

■ If you have pulpitis (inflammation of the pulp) and it is found that the pulp cannot be saved you may need root canal treatment.

CAN IT BE PREVENTED?

Your teeth and gums should be brushed and flossed regularly to keep them clean and free from plaque. You can also help prevent dental cavities from developing by resisting the temptation of sugary foods and drinks and eating safe snacks.

See also:
- **Root canal p. 489**
- **X-rays p. 426**

Toothbrushes

The dental profession is fairly well united on the type of toothbrush you should use and the frequency with which you should use it. Here are some guidelines.

■ The toothbrush should have a short handle so that it is easy to control, so that you know exactly where the head of the brush is and so that it doesn't waggle around in your mouth.

■ The handle of the brush should be straight, without any bends in it, so that again you can direct the head accurately.

■ The head of the brush should be fairly small and the bristles ideally should be fairly short.

■ Choose nylon bristle, not pure bristle, because it resists splitting and bending better than natural material.

■ Make sure that the heads of the bristles are round-ended. On no account choose a toothbrush with a serrated edge.

■ The bristles should not be too hard; choose one labeled "soft."

■ Brush your teeth twice a day. Buy a new toothbrush at least every six weeks, or as soon as the bristles become misshapen.

■ Use a fluoride toothpaste.

Dental abscess

AN ACCUMULATION OF PUS IN OR AROUND THE ROOT OF A TOOTH IS KNOWN AS A DENTAL ABSCESS. A DENTAL ABSCESS CAN BE EXTREMELY PAINFUL AND MAY CAUSE THE AFFECTED TOOTH TO LOOSEN IN ITS SOCKET.

WHAT ARE THE CAUSES?

An abscess usually develops as a complication of dental cavities, which gradually destroys the layer of enamel on the outside of the tooth and the inner dentine, allowing bacteria to invade the soft central core or pulp of the tooth. Eventually, a dental abscess may form, which is agonizingly painful and may cause the gum adjacent to the tooth to swell and become very tender (a gum boil).

An abscess may also form as a result of certain forms of gum disease (periodontitis). Periodontitis is usually caused by a buildup of dental plaque (a deposit including food particles, mucus, and bacteria) in a pocket that forms between a tooth and gum.

WHAT ARE THE SYMPTOMS?

The main symptoms of a dental abscess develop gradually and may include:
- throbbing pain in the affected tooth
- severe pain on touching the affected tooth and on biting or chewing
- loosening of the affected tooth
- red, tender swelling of the gum over the root of the tooth
- release of pus into the mouth.

If the abscess is not treated, the infection may make a channel from the tooth to the surface of the gum, and a painful swelling, known as a gum boil, forms. Should the gum boil burst, foul-tasting pus is released and the pain decreases. In some cases the channel may persist, which leads to a chronic abscess that discharges pus periodically. If the infection spreads to surrounding tissues, your face may become swollen and you may develop a fever. If you suspect you have an abscess, you should consult your dentist as soon as possible.

WHAT CAN I DO?

If there is a delay before you are able to see your dentist, you can try taking painkillers such as acetaminophen, which may relieve pain. Rinsing your mouth with warm salt water may also help decrease the pain and possibly encourage a gum boil to burst. If a gum boil does burst, wash away the pus thoroughly with more warm salt water.

WHAT MIGHT THE DENTIST DO?

- Your dentist will ask you about your teeth and gums. He or she may take an X-ray of your mouth to confirm the diagnosis.
- If the abscess has been caused by tooth decay, your dentist will always try to save the tooth. Under local anesthesia, a hole is drilled through the top of the tooth to release the pus, which will have the effect of relieving the pain. If there is a gum boil, a small cut may be made in the boil to drain the pus. The cavity is then cleaned with an antiseptic solution.
- To treat an abscess caused by gum disease, your dentist may use a probe to scrape out the plaque from the pocket between the affected tooth and gum. Afterward, the pocket is washed out with an antiseptic solution.
- Pockets are treated with several weeks of intensive oral hygiene, including frequent brushing, flossing, and the use of antiseptic gel on the floss. Most can be eradicated.

TREATMENT

Root canal

Sometimes, decay invades and destroys the pulp, containing nerves and blood vessels, at the center of the tooth, and root canal treatment may be performed. The pulp is removed and an antiseptic solution is used to sterilize the cavity. If infection within the tooth is severe, a temporary filling may be inserted for a few days before the cavity is sterilized again. The root canals and the remaining tooth structure are then filled.

- Whatever the cause of the abscess, you will probably be prescribed a course of antibiotics.
- Once the infection has cleared up, you may need root canal treatment (see box, above).
- If it is not possible to save the tooth, an extraction is the only remaining option.
- An extracted tooth can be replaced with a removable partial denture, bridge, or an implant.

WHAT IS THE OUTLOOK?

Most treatment is successful, but a small area of infection may persist and further treatment may be required.

> **See also:**
> • **Dental cavities p. 488** • **Gingivitis p. 493**

Malocclusion (poor bite)

IDEALLY, THE UPPER FRONT TEETH SHOULD SLIGHTLY OVERLAP THE LOWER FRONT TEETH AND THE MOLARS SHOULD SLIGHTLY OVERLAP THE LOWERS AS WELL. HOWEVER, PERFECT TEETH ARE RARE AND MOST PEOPLE HAVE SOME TEETH THAT ARE OUT OF POSITION.

Imperfections are not usually a pressing problem unless appearance is adversely affected or biting and chewing are impaired.

A poor bite may occur if teeth are crowded and overlap each other, making them crooked. Another cause is misalignment of the jaws, so that the upper front teeth protrude excessively in front of the lower teeth, or the lower jaw juts out in front of the upper jaw. The back teeth may prevent the front teeth from meeting, a condition known as an open bite.

WHAT ARE THE CAUSES?

Malocclusion often runs in families and usually develops in childhood when the teeth and jaws are growing. The condition is usually caused by a discrepancy between the number and size of the teeth and the growth of the jaws. Protrusion of the front teeth may also be caused by children who persistently suck their thumbs beyond about age 6. If the primary teeth are lost early (before age 9 or 10) because of decay or trauma, the secondary molars that are already in position may move forward to take up some of the space meant for the new front teeth. The new teeth then become crowded and misaligned.

WHAT ARE THE SYMPTOMS?

The symptoms develop gradually from about age 6 onward. They may include:
- out-of-line, crowded, or abnormally spaced teeth

continued on page 492

FOCUS *on* cosmetic dentistry

If you want to have a perfect white smile when you are 20, you (and your parents) will need to start working on it when you are a baby. It is no good thinking that primary or milk teeth are unimportant simply because children start to lose them around the age of 6.

Strong, well-positioned primary teeth guide the secondary or permanent teeth as they erupt and grow to take their lifelong positions in the jawbones. If the primary teeth are crowded, the permanent ones may grow in crookedly. If a gap has been left by the removal of a decayed primary tooth, the permanent teeth on either side of the gap will not be encouraged to grow upright.

It is therefore worthwhile taking good care of primary teeth from the moment that they appear. Never offer a child a bottle filled with fruit juice or milk as a pacifier – the sugar or lactic acid content rapidly decays the teeth and encourages a "sweet tooth" in later life. It is helpful to give a baby hard foods to chew on as soon as he or she develops the liking for **chomping,** since chewing movements exercise the jaw muscles and help to make the teeth grow in straight.

The chances of serious tooth decay can be **minimized by attention to diet** (avoiding a lot of sweet and starchy foods), careful tooth-brushing with the right kind of toothbrush, (see p. 488) and regular visits to the dentist. The use of fluoride either in the form of tablets or drops or as toothpaste also helps stop decay.

WHITENING THE TEETH

According to the best dental opinion, no good "cosmetics" for the teeth can be bought over the counter. **Toothpastes** that claim to whiten teeth usually do so by two methods.

The first is really an optical illusion: the toothpaste contains a red pigment that turns the gums deep pink, so that the teeth look whiter in comparison.

Toothpastes that use the second method, and claim to give a polished, gleaming smile, make the teeth shine by use of abrasives (including one known as "**jeweler's rouge**"). These substances are much too harsh to use on our teeth – they work by scratching the surface enamel, which may be damaged or worn away through prolonged use of such toothpastes. Since there has been a move away

from using abrasives on stainless steel kitchen sinks and ceramic baths and basins, it seems astonishing that we should continue to consider using them on our teeth.

The best and safest way to give your teeth a new look is to visit a **dentist** or **dental hygienist**. To keep your gums and teeth healthy you should go at least every six months – every three months is even better. The hygienist will remove from between the teeth **calculus** (hardened plaque), which irritates the gums and makes them bleed. The hygienist does this by **descaling** your teeth and giving them a good polish. This treatment makes everyone's teeth look several shades whiter, particularly smokers'.

Repositioning teeth

In cosmetic dentistry much can be achieved by the use of simple methods and materials. It is quite possible to move the roots of teeth within the jawbone by perhaps a fraction of a **millimeter**, if they are pushed or pulled in one direction for any length of time. Even such a tiny adjustment makes a great difference to the overall effect. Very often, sufficient force can be applied to a **misaligned** tooth simply by the expert use of elastic bands. For more severe deformities, wires and braces can be fitted to manipulate the teeth over a period of months into the desired position.

WHAT THE COSMETIC DENTIST CAN DO

It is possible for a good, skilled cosmetic dentist to alter completely not just the look of your teeth or your smile, but also the set of your mouth and therefore, to some degree, your facial expression. If, for instance, your teeth have been ground away over the years either because you are a "night grinder" or simply because you have especially strong masticating muscles, your jawbones will tend to come closer together. This accentuates the folds on either side of your mouth and may have an **aging** appearance. A cosmetic dentist can open up the distance between the jawbones by repositioning or crowning the teeth, thereby stretching out the skin in your laughter lines. This procedure can also relieve pain and tenderness in the joints of the jaw, which become over-stressed when the teeth are ground away.

Cosmetic dentistry can also change the shape, color, and arrangement of your teeth to give a more pleasing appearance.

CAPS AND CROWNS

A broken, ugly or severely **malpositioned** tooth can be given a new appearance and a new lease of life by capping or crowning (the two terms are synonymous). This is usually done by filing the tooth away to form a "core" onto which the cap is cemented. Even a tooth that has snapped off or has had to be removed at the line of the gum margin can be capped. In such cases one or more "posts" onto which the cap can be fixed are drilled into the remnants of the tooth.

Caps and crowns are made of a variety of materials. The most modern ones are composed of extremely strong porcelains or metals covered in porcelain, which come in a number of **colors** so that the finished cap will exactly match the rest of the teeth. The cap can be made in any shape to conform to the size and contour of the original tooth – indeed its shape may even be slightly imperfect in order to maintain a natural appearance.

REPLACEMENT TEETH

If one or more teeth have to be extracted, or if they are lost, they can be replaced by one of three different types of artificial teeth: a bridge, dentures, or a dental implant.

A bridge consists of one or more artificial teeth that are fixed permanently in the mouth, usually by being attached to adjacent natural teeth. This may require the adjacent teeth to be crowned.

A denture can be removed and may replace any number of teeth. Dentures have a metal and/or plastic **baseplate** and stay in place by resting on the gum ridges or are held in place by clasps that fit onto the natural teeth. They can be removed for cleaning, either with a sterilizing solution or with a brush.

An implant is a permanent and effective method of replacing a single tooth. A hole is drilled in the jaw at the site of the missing tooth, and a screw is firmly fixed into the hole. A few weeks to several months later when the site has healed, an artificial tooth is fitted to the top of the screw.

"SHORTENING" OR "LENGTHENING" TEETH

In some people with periodontal disease the gums recede, exposing the root surfaces of the teeth. This can make the teeth very sensitive to hot and cold foods and make the crown of the tooth look very long. If excellent oral hygiene can be achieved it is possible to reposition the gum surgically to cover the exposed root surfaces and improve the appearance. Alternatively it may be possible to crown or reshape the teeth to hide the appearance.

Some people have the reverse problem – the gums grow too far up the teeth so that they are, or appear to be, too short, or heavy grinding or clenching of the teeth may wear the teeth away. Again it may be possible to improve the appearance by crowning teeth.

BUCK TEETH

Ideally, buck teeth should be treated before the age of 14 by an **orthodontist** who will use braces and wires to pull the teeth into line with the rest. If you reach adulthood with buck teeth, orthodontics and/or cosmetic dentistry can sometimes correct the deformity by the use of caps or crowns. The **malpositioned teeth** are filed away and the caps fitted to follow the normal line.

Cosmetic dentistry at its best is highly creative and good practitioners will rise to almost any challenge to find an inventive way of correcting tooth deformity. One of the most beautiful and effective examples I have seen was the correction of malpositioned teeth in a person with a cleft palate. Because of the cleft, there were fewer teeth than is normal; in addition, the teeth had moved round the jaw so that the front teeth were off-center. The dentist transformed the appearance by using each of the existing teeth as the basis for a cap, but moving the position of every cap on its tooth a **millimeter** or so along in the direction that brought them all back to center.

See also:
• **Malocclusion p. 489**

Cosmetic teeth whitening

Cosmetic teeth whitening is a noninvasive procedure that uses a bleaching agent to lighten the color of the teeth. Your dentist begins by making a mold of your teeth, from which a plastic tray that fits over your teeth is made. Your dentist then shows you how to fill this tray with a bleaching gel. You will be instructed to wear the tray at home for a few hours each day or possibly overnight. The length of treatment depends on the gel that is used and the degree of lightening to be achieved, but it usually lasts from a week to 10 days. A similar technique may be used to lighten teeth in the dentist's office in one visit.

Before teeth whitening

After teeth whitening

continued from page 489

- excessive protrusion of the upper teeth in front of the lower teeth
- a protruding lower jaw
- front teeth that do not meet.

Some children have some mild symptoms, but these are often temporary and tend to result from a growth spurt.

In severe cases of malocclusion, speech and chewing may be affected. An abnormal bite may be painful or cause discomfort in or around the jaw joint. A severe malocclusion may also affect the facial appearance.

WHAT MIGHT BE DONE?
■ The dentist will look for malocclusion as part of a dental checkup.

■ If malocclusion is found, a specialist dentist called an **orthodontist** may take casts of the teeth to study the bite in detail. The orthodontist may also take X-rays of the teeth, especially if some of the teeth have not erupted.

■ Treatment is usually only necessary if malocclusion is severe and causing difficulties when eating and speaking or affecting appearance.

■ If the teeth are overcrowded, some of them may be extracted.

■ Rough or irregular teeth are often reshaped or capped.

■ If required, the teeth may then be aligned and straightened using an orthodontic appliance such as a brace.

■ Surgery is very rarely necessary but may be an option.

It is best to treat malocclusion during childhood, when the teeth and jaw bones are still developing. However, if malocclusion is caused by a severe mismatch in the size of the jaws and teeth, surgery may be needed and treatment may be delayed until adulthood.

See also:
• **Temporomandibular joint disorder p. 494**

TREATMENT

Orthodontic treatment

Orthodontics is the correction of crowded or unevenly spaced teeth. Orthodontic treatment is usually performed on older children and adolescents while the teeth are still developing, adults can also benefit.

Casts of the teeth are taken before an orthodontic appliance, also called a brace,

is applied to move or straighten the teeth gradually. In some cases, it is necessary to extract one or more teeth to make space for others. The treatment is usually long-term and may take several months or years to complete, with regular visits to the orthodontist for checkups.

Close-up of a child's mouth fitted with a fixed dental brace.

Close-up of a child's mouth fitted with a removable dental brace.

TYPES OF MALOCCLUSION
There is a wide range of malocclusions, which can be divided into a small number of groups depending on the position of the first molars. Some common types of malocclusion are shown below.

Misalignment of the molars, causing a slight overbite

Overbite (also known as overjet), with the molars misaligned

Incisors retroclined (no overlap with lower teeth); lateral incisors proclined (leaning forwards)

Underbite (also known as underjet), with the molars misaligned

GUM DISORDERS

Healthy gum forms a tight seal around the base of the crown of a tooth and protects the sensitive root area below from bacterial infection and corrosion. If the gums are damaged or form pockets, the teeth are more likely to decay. Most gum disorders are caused by plaque (a deposit of food particles, mucus, and bacteria on the surfaces of the teeth) and can be prevented by good oral hygiene.

Most adults have some degree of gum disease which, if left untreated, may eventually lead to loss of teeth. Good oral hygiene is essential to help prevent gum disorders. During regular dental checkups, most dentists and dental hygienists provide information on the correct way to brush and floss teeth and on general mouth care.

Gingivitis and **periodontitis**, both of which can lead to loosening and loss of teeth, are mainly caused by poor oral hygiene. Inadequate teeth cleaning leads to a buildup of **plaque** on the teeth. If the plaque is not removed, it causes the gums to become inflamed (gingivitis). In more serious cases, pockets form in which bacteria can erode tooth enamel and cause tooth decay and inflammation of the bony membrane around the tooth (periodontitis). The teeth may be affected and loosen or come out, either because the periodontal tissues are inflamed and detach from the teeth or because the gums recede, exposing the roots and leading to tooth decay.

Gingivitis (gum disease)

MILD INFLAMMATION OF THE GUM MARGINS (GINGIVITIS) IS VERY COMMON AND OCCURS IN ABOUT 9 OUT OF 10 ADULTS. HEALTHY GUMS ARE PINK AND FIRM. IN GINGIVITIS, THE GUMS BECOME PURPLE-RED, SOFT, AND SHINY AND BLEED EASILY, ESPECIALLY WHEN BRUSHED.

The condition is usually caused by a buildup of plaque (a deposit of food particles, mucus, and bacteria) where the gum meets the base of the tooth.

Gingivitis can be made worse by taking some drugs, such as phenytoin for epilepsy and antihypertensives. These drugs may cause overgrowth of the gums, making the removal of dental plaque difficult. Some contraceptive drugs can also make the symptoms worse. Pregnant women are particularly susceptible to gingivitis because of dramatic changes in their hormone levels.

If gingivitis develops suddenly in acute form, it is known as "**trench mouth,**" usually occurring in teenagers and young adults. The condition sometimes develops from chronic gingivitis and is caused by an abnormal growth of the bacteria that normally exist harmlessly within the mouth. Trench mouth is more common in people who are stressed or run down and in people with AIDS.

WHAT ARE THE SYMPTOMS?
The symptoms of gingivitis develop gradually and usually include:
- purple-red, soft, shiny, swollen gums
- gums that bleed when brushed.
- foul odor
- mobility
- pain

If gingivitis is not treated, a pocket develops between the tooth and the gum in which more dental plaque can form. Bacteria in the plaque may cause the inflammation to spread. Eventually, chronic periodontitis or receding gums may develop. In severe cases, one or more teeth may be lost.

Symptoms of trench mouth usually develop over 1–2 days and may include:
- bright red gums that are covered with a grayish deposit
- craterlike ulcers on the gums

- gums that bleed easily
- bad breath and a metallic taste in the mouth
- pain in the gums.

As trench mouth, or ANUG (acute necrotizing ulcerative gingivitis), progresses, the lymph glands in the neck may become enlarged and you may develop a fever.

WHAT IS THE TREATMENT?
■ Gingivitis is treated and prevented by effective brushing and oral hygiene to remove plaque from around the gum margin.
■ If you have gingivitis, your dentist will probably scale your teeth to remove the plaque and **calculus** (hardened plaque). The procedure involves using an **ultrasonic scaler** to remove the calculus and scraping away at resistant areas with a hand tool. After scaling, the teeth are polished. Regular follow-up visits to the dentist may be necessary to monitor the condition of your gums. Your dentist may also recommend using an antiseptic mouthwash.
■ If you have trench mouth, your dentist will clean carefully around all the teeth. He or she will also prescribe antibiotics and an antiseptic mouthwash. Analgesics may be prescribed to relieve pain. Once your teeth have been scaled and cleaned, your gums will gradually return to normal.

See also:
- **Caring for your teeth and gums p. 485**

Receding gums

HEALTHY GUMS FORM A TIGHT SEAL AROUND THE TOOTH WHERE THE CROWN OF THE TOOTH MEETS THE ROOT. IF THE GUMS RECEDE, THE ROOT OF THE TOOTH BECOMES EXPOSED, CAUSING THE ATTACHMENT BETWEEN THE TOOTH AND THE SOCKET TO WEAKEN.

When the gum recedes, the tooth may eventually become loose and, in severe cases, may have to be extracted by the dentist.

If the roots are exposed, the teeth may be sensitive to hot, cold, or sweet substances. Since the roots are softer than the enamel on the crown of the tooth, they are also more susceptible to decay.

Periodontitis affects many people over 55 and is a major cause of tooth loss. In this condition, the periodontal tissues that secure teeth in their sockets become inflamed, and the teeth loosen. Eventually, teeth may fall out. The damage from periodontitis is irreversible, but further inflammation can be prevented with treatment and by improving oral hygiene.

WHAT ARE THE CAUSES?
■ Severely receding gums are usually a symptom of chronic gingivitis or periodontitis.
■ These disorders are usually a result of **poor oral hygiene** and a **buildup of plaque** (a deposit of food particles, mucus, and bacteria) and calculus (hardened plaque) between the base of the teeth and gums. The gums will eventually become inflamed and recede, exposing the roots of the teeth.
■ Vigorous, abrasive tooth brushing along the margins of the gums, particularly in a horizontal direction with a hard toothbrush, may also cause the gums to recede.
■ Toothpastes containing abrasives contribute.

WHAT MIGHT BE DONE?
■ Improving your oral hygiene is important in order to stop the gums from receding further.
■ Your dentist or dental hygienist will probably use a procedure known as scaling to remove plaque and calculus from your teeth. Scaling should help prevent your gums from receding any further.
■ She will also advise you on your tooth brushing and flossing techniques to avoid further damage to the exposed roots.
■ Your dentist or dental hygienist may also suggest that you use a desensitizing toothpaste or fluoride mouthwash, which will also reduce the risk of decay.
■ If your teeth are very sensitive, the dentist may treat them with a desensitizing varnish and/or an adhesive filling material.
■ Gum-grafting procedures may be used to help cover exposed root surfaces and prevent further recession of the gums.
■ If severely receding gums cause your teeth to loosen, they can sometimes be fixed to teeth that are more firmly anchored in the jawbone.

> **See also:**
> • **Caring for your teeth and gums p. 485**
> • **Gingivitis p. 493**

Temporomandibular joint disorder

THE TEMPOROMANDIBULAR JOINT CONNECTS THE MANDIBLE (LOWER JAWBONE) TO THE PART OF THE SKULL KNOWN AS THE TEMPORAL BONE. THE JOINT ALLOWS THE LOWER JAW TO MOVE IN ALL DIRECTIONS SO THAT THE TEETH CAN BE USED TO BITE OFF AND CHEW FOOD EFFICIENTLY.

In temporomandibular joint disorder, the joint, the muscles and the ligaments that control the joint do not work together properly, causing pain. The condition is three times more likely to occur in women.

Temporomandibular joint disorder is most commonly caused by **spasm** of the chewing muscles, often as a result of **clenching the jaw** or **grinding the teeth**. Clenching the jaw and grinding the teeth may be increased by stress. A poor bite (malocclusion) places stress on the muscles and may also be the cause of temporomandibular joint disorder, as may an injury to the head, jaw or neck that causes displacement of the joint. In some cases, arthritis is a cause.

WHAT ARE THE SYMPTOMS?
You may notice one or more of the following symptoms:
● headaches
● tenderness in the jaw muscles
● aching pain in the face
● severe pain near the ears.

In some cases, pain is caused by chewing or by opening the mouth too widely when yawning. There may be difficulty in opening the mouth, locking of the jaw, and clicking noises from the joint as the mouth is opened or closed.

WHAT MIGHT BE DONE?
■ Your dentist may take X-rays of your mouth and jaws.
■ He may also arrange for you to see a specialist for treatment and investigations such as a CT scan or a MRI.
■ Treatment is aimed at eliminating muscle spasm and tension and relieving pain.
■ There are several self-help measures that you can adopt, including applying a warm, wet towel to the face, massaging the facial muscles, eating only soft foods and using a device that fits over the teeth at night to prevent you from clenching or grinding your teeth.
■ Taking analgesics, such as aspirin, acetaminophen, and anti-inflammatories may also help relieve pain.
■ Your doctor may prescribe muscle relaxant drugs if tension of the muscles used for chewing is severe.
■ If stress is a major factor, relaxation techniques may help.
■ If your bite needs to be adjusted, your dentist may recommend wearing a fixed or removable orthodontic appliance for a period of time.

WHAT IS THE OUTLOOK?
In approximately 3 out of 4 people with temporomandibular joint disorder, symptoms improve within three months of treatment. However, if symptoms do not improve, further treatment may be required. In a few cases surgery to the joint may be necessary.

> **See also:**
> • **Malocclusion p. 489** • **MRI p. 409**
> • **Rheumatoid arthritis p. 429**

Hormones

Image shows a polarized light micrograph of crystals of the hormone progesterone

Miriam's overview

When I was a medical student hormones were a difficult concept for me to get my head around. They're defined as:

"Chemical messengers which are formed in one part of the body, usually a hormone gland, passed into the bloodstream to be carried to a part of the body where they exert an effect." But that definition fails to describe their intricacy.

They control most of the vital functions of the body. They certainly regulate every aspect of metabolism. And they keep all our organs in working order.

What's more, each hormone is bespoke. It's like a laser beam, focusing on one small area of our overall health. Together hormones are like an orchestra and by a myriad ingenious checks and balances they play in tune most of the time. Naturally they require a conductor and we have one, the pituitary gland in the brain, a tiny organ that has the power to switch hormones on and off.

If a rogue hormone gland gets out of control we soon know about it. An overactive thyroid gland or adrenal gland makes us ill. An underactive pancreas gives us symptoms of diabetes; and failing ovaries, menopause. We label this kind of hormonal failure a hormone deficiency state and correct it with hormone supplements as different as insulin for diabetes and HRT for menopause.

So hormones are very potent body regulators, some so

"together *hormones* are like *an orchestra*"

powerful that they are life-giving and curative. We've harnessed steroid hormones from the adrenal glands to arrest inflammation in conditions as different as arthritis and psoriasis.

The sex hormones we've synthesized into potent forms to control basic mechanisms such as ovulation to give us virtually 100 percent effective contraception.

INSIDE your metabolism

Hormones are chemicals that influence or change the activity of particular cells in the body. They are produced by a number of different **glands** besides the pituitary gland and hypothalamus and are carried in the bloodstream to reach their target cells. The production of hormones is regulated by feedback mechanisms, which help to ensure that the correct levels of hormones and other substances are maintained in the blood. The **pituitary gland**, a pea-sized organ located at the base of the brain and regulated by the **hypothalamus**, orchestrates most of the body's hormone secretion.

Major hormone-secreting glands and organs include the **thyroid, parathyroid,** and **adrenal glands,** the **pancreas** and the **testes** in men, and **ovaries** in women. Other organs that secrete hormones include the **kidneys,** the **heart,** the intestines, and the **stomach**.

hormone-secreting glands and cells

Hypothalamus
Pituitary gland
Pineal gland
Parathyroid gland
Thyroid gland
Thymus
Duodenum
Pancreas
Intestines
Ovary
Heart
Stomach
Adrenal gland
Kidney

Pituitary gland

Nerve fibers
Blood vessels
Skull
Pituitary stalk

The pituitary gland is linked to the hypothalamus by a stalk of nerve cells and blood vessels.

The endocrine (hormonal) system is coordinated largely by the pituitary gland, located beneath the hypothalamus at the base of the brain.

MENOPAUSE

Most women reach menopause between the ages of 40 and 55 in the US. The average age is 51. The production of sex hormones slows down; the ovaries stop producing eggs; and monthly periods become less frequent and eventually stop entirely, so after menopause a woman can no longer get pregnant. Menopause is an estrogen-deficiency state and the symptoms that arise are due to lack of estrogen. Most of them are cured by taking estrogen in the form of hormone replacement therapy (HRT). The symptoms most commonly associated with the "change" include hot flashes and night sweats; dryness and soreness of the vagina and consequently some pain on intercourse; anxiety, depression, irritability, and fatigue; an inability to sleep at night; a fall in sexual interest; dry skin and thinning hair; and urinary and bladder problems due to the thinning of the bladder lining.

Women going through menopause have a tendency to put on weight – particularly around the waist, "middle-age spread." This change in shape with loss of the waistline is a sign that carries an increased risk of heart disease, a side effect of menopause along with stroke, osteoporosis, and Alzheimer's disease. All of these long-term health hazards of menopause are ameliorated by HRT.

I believe in women managing their menopause and taking steps to have the menopause they want. There are many tools all women can use in taking responsibility for their own menopausal health. The single most effective tool available is HRT.

SELF-HELP

As well as vitamins and herbal remedies available for menopausal women, there are a number of useful things that you can do to help yourself.

To cope with hot flashes, for example, try to keep the room temperature fairly low and wear loose rather than tight clothing (cottons are good). At night it may be useful to have blankets that you can peel off easily if you get very hot. And keep spare night clothing by the bedside in case you have a night sweat. Avoid strong coffee, alcohol and salt. A glass of cold water may help.

If you feel that you are getting hot and red, then you may also be able to help yourself by "thinking cold". Imagine that you are standing in several inches of snow, or wandering around at a ski resort or taking part in an Arctic expedition. Your skin temperature will fall in response to your imagination and the amount of flushing that takes place will be kept to a minimum.

Finally, even though you feel bright red during a flush, do remember that the flush will probably be hardly noticeable to people around you.

To cope with a dry vagina and make intercourse more comfortable, try using an oil or jelly. You can buy special products from your local pharmacy or you can use an unscented body oil or baby oil. (Avoid anything too thick or greasy or lubricants containing alcohol or medicaments.) Remember that saliva makes a useful and effective lubricant.

Annoying or persistent menopausal symptoms merit a visit to the doctor since HRT is considered by many doctors to be safe and effective for most women who have problems. HRT can ease the symptoms women find most troublesome and, despite some controversy in the past, the majority of doctors now agree that replacing missing hormones is sensible, natural, and acceptable. Where necessary the treatment can be continued for several years. Indeed I personally see no reason to stop.

Finally, remember that although most women do get one or two symptoms, many women go through menopause with no unpleasant symptoms at all.

Coping with menopause the nonhormonal way

SOME WOMEN SAIL THROUGH MENOPAUSE WITHOUT ANY PROBLEMS BUT MOST EXPERIENCE SYMPTOMS RANGING FROM MILD TO VERY SEVERE.

Hormone replacement therapy can make all the difference – but what are the options if HRT is unsuitable for you or your personal preference is not to interfere with nature? The good news is there is a lot you can do to help yourself, and homeopathic and herbal treatments can go a long way in relieving symptoms.

HOMEOPATHY

This is a form of natural healing based on the principle that a substance that produces the same symptoms as an illness will, in a very dilute form, help to cure that illness.

Homeopathic remedies are derived from mineral, animal, or vegetable matter. The homeopathic view of menopausal problems is that they are a manifestation of existing imbalances that can only be treated with regard to the mental and physical makeup of an individual. Women are encouraged to prepare for menopause by looking at their overall health and developing a positive attitude before its onset.

If you would like to treat your symptoms homeopathically, it is a good idea to consult a homeopathic practitioner. If you decide to treat yourself, keep in mind the following things.

■ You should stop taking a remedy as soon as your symptoms start to improve.

■ If your symptoms are not relieved after six doses, seek medical advice.

■ Homeopathic remedies should be kept in a cool, dark place away from smells.

■ Some substances, such as coffee, peppermint, menthol, and camphor, counteract the effects of homeopathic remedies and should be avoided.

■ Some homeopathic pills are coated in milk sugar and you should avoid them if you are allergic to milk.

■ If your symptoms are very acute, you can take a remedy hourly. For longer-term problems, remedies can be taken in the morning and at night.

HERBALISM

Some of the oldest methods of healing the sick are based on herbalism. Herbal lore was handed down through families who had their own recipe books of tonics and teas.

Like homeopathy, the goals behind herbal treatment are to remove the cause of the symptoms rather than merely the symptoms themselves and to improve the patient's general standard of health. A disadvantage of herbalism is that agreement over which remedies should be used for particular disorders is still surprisingly limited.

However, herbalism does offer an attractive alternative to other forms of treatment in that it allows for experimentation with a variety of herbs without the complication of serious side effects. It is also recognized that herbal remedies can work as a complement to conventional medicine. However, it is important to mention that few remedies have been subjected to tightly controlled clinical trials.

AT-A-GLANCE HOMEOPATHIC REMEDIES

Symptom	Remedy
Hot flashes	Lachesis
Insomnia, PMS, joint pain	Pulsatilla
Dry vagina, prolapse, flashes, thinning hair	Sepia
Dry, itchy vulva and skin	Sulphur
PMS, breast pain (mastalgia)	Bryonia
Hot flashes and night sweats	Belladonna

AT-A-GLANCE CHINESE HERBAL REMEDIES

Symptom	Remedy
Night sweats	Nuo dao gen
Night sweats	Wu wei zi
Hot flashes	Quing huo
Hot flashes	Mu dan pi
Thinning hair	Bao shao yao
Thinning hair	Sang shen zi
Dry, itchy skin	Di fu zi
Dry, itchy skin	Chi shao yao
Sore, dry vagina	Tu fu ling
Sore, dry vagina	Chaung zi

If you plan to treat your symptoms with herbs you would be wise to follow these guidelines.
■ Always use herbs in moderation.
■ Discontinue use if you start to experience side effects.
■ Give each herb a week or two to assess its effect.
■ Start by taking a herb in tea form. Increase the amount from half a cup a day to several cups a day, over a period of a week.
■ Don't take herbs for longer than a few months without a break.
■ If you are taking medication, you should check with your doctor before you take a herbal remedy.
■ Don't defer seeking medical advice because you are taking a herbal remedy.

CHINESE HERBS

Chinese medicine views illness as a result of an imbalance or disturbance in the body's two energy forces, yin and yang. Chinese medicine tailors its remedies and dosages to the individual woman and her symptoms. You should consult a Chinese doctor for an individual diagnosis.

VITAMINS AND MINERALS

We all know how important it is to eat a balanced diet to stay healthy but it is especially important during the menopausal years to have a sufficient daily intake of vitamins and minerals.

AT-A-GLANCE HERBAL REMEDIES

Symptoms and effects	Remedy
Swelling, hot flashes	Sage; drink as tea for hot flashes
Menstrual irregularities, PMS	Alfalfa
Heavy or irregular periods	Beth root
Depression, lethargy, insomnia, poor memory, hypertension	St.-John's-wort
Prolapse, weak ligaments, dragging pains	False unicorn root
Nervousness, irritability, anxiety	Scullcap. Combine with balm for anxiety.
Anxiety, emotional symptoms	Vervain. Take as a tea or tincture
Skin inflammation	Elderflower. Use as elderflower water on skin.
Menstrual irregularities, PMS, cyclical skin complaints	Black cohosh
Ovarian and uterine pains, increased production of female hormones	Wild yam
Hot flashes, night sweats	Vitex agnus-castus
Urinary symptoms	Wintergreen, blackberry root, coleus

WHAT ARE THE SYMPTOMS?
NIGHT SWEATS

The nighttime equivalent of the hot flash is the night sweat, in which you wake up hot and drenched in perspiration. Most women who experience night sweats also have hot flashes during the daytime, but the reverse isn't always so. Night sweats can very occasionally be a symptom of stress, or of a disease that is unrelated to menopause – if you consult your doctor he will be able to make a diagnosis.

Sleeplessness in menopausal women is nearly always linked to night sweats.

Self-help

■ Keep your bedroom temperature fairly cool. Leave a window open; try to create a draft.
■ Avoid night clothes and bed linens that are made of nylon or polyester – they can act like sheets of plastic, holding the sweat next to your body. Cotton fabrics will be more comfortable.
■ Keep a battery-operated fan, a bowl of lukewarm water, and a sponge on your bedside table so that you can cool yourself down quickly and easily. Never use cold water since it can cause you to overheat after you have applied it. Allow the lukewarm water to evaporate from your skin – as it evaporates it will take the heat from your skin, which will make you feel cooler and bring the feeling of fever to a more rapid end.

continued on page 500

MINERALS THAT WILL BENEFIT MENOPAUSAL COMPLAINTS

Always take minerals as foods, not as synthetic supplements.

Complaint	Mineral	Source
Osteoporosis, high concentration of blood fat, hypertension	Calcium	Milk and milk products, dark green leafy vegetables, citrus fruits, dried peas and beans
Osteoporosis, fatigue, diabetes mellitus, coronary heart disease, anxiety, depression,	Magnesium	Green leafy vegetables, nuts, soy beans, whole grain cereals
Fatigue, heart disease, hypertension, anxiety, depression	Potassium	Orange juice, bananas, dried fruits, peanut butter, meat
Osteoporosis	Zinc	Meat, liver, eggs, poultry, seafood
Excessive menstrual bleeding	Iron	Nuts, liver, red meats, egg yolk, green leafy vegetables, dried fruits
Hypothyroidism, fibrocystic disease of the breast	Iodine	Seafood, fish, seaweed
Low blood glucose	Chromium	Meat, cheese, whole grains, breads
Fibrocystic disease of the breast and breast cancer	Selenium	Seafood, meat, whole grain cereals
Atherosclerosis	Manganese	Nuts, fruit, and vegetables, whole grain cereals
Hot flashes, excessive menstrual bleeding, vaginal problems, anxiety, irritability, and other emotional problems	Bioflavonoids	All citrus fruits, especially the pulp and pith

VITAMINS THAT WILL BENEFIT MENOPAUSAL COMPLAINTS

Vitamins should be taken in the form of foods, not as pills or capsules.

Complaint	Vitamin	Source
Excessive menstrual bleeding, cervical abnormalities, fibrocystic disease and cancer of the breast	Vitamin A	Carrots, spinach, turnips, apricots, fresh liver, cantaloupes, sweet potatoes
Cervical abnormalities and cancer, osteoporosis, diabetes mellitus	Folic acid	Green leafy vegetables, nuts, peas, beans, liver, and kidney
High concentration of blood fat	Vitamin B_3	Meat and poultry, fish, legumes, whole wheat bran
Cervical abnormalities and cancer, diabetes mellitus	Vitamin B_6	Meat and poultry, fish, bananas, whole grain cereals, dairy products
Anxiety , depression, mood swings, fatigue	Vitamin B_{12}	Fish, poultry, eggs, milk, B_{12}-enriched soy products
Excessive menstrual bleeding, cervical abnormalities and cancer, chloasma	Vitamin C	Citrus fruits, strawberries, broccoli, green peppers
Poor calcium absorption, leading to an increase in the risk of osteoporosis	Vitamin D	Sunlight, oily fish, fortified cereals and bread, fortified margarine
Hot flushes, anxiety, vaginal problems, hypothyroidism, chloasma and other skin conditions, atherosclerosis, osteoarthritis, fibrocystic disease of the breast	Vitamin E	Vegetable oils, green leafy vegetables, cereals, dried beans, whole grains, bread

continued from page 498

■ Relaxation is particularly therapeutic – it calms the mind and body, which in turn normalizes body chemistry and makes the skin sweat less.

MUSCLE AND JOINT SYMPTOMS

Collagen is a protein that provides the scaffolding for every tissue in the body and when it begins to disintegrate at menopause, muscles lose their bulk, strength and co-ordination and joints become stiff.

Self-help

■ If you keep your muscles strong with exercise you will stave off osteoporosis and bone fractures, you'll be more agile and, if you do trip up, muscle strength and coordination will help you to fall with less impact.

■ If you are suffering from rheumatoid arthritis or osteoarthritis, your doctor will advise you about self-help aids for use in the home.

■ If you are suffering from stiff and swollen joints, a poultice made with cayenne pepper may be helpful.

PREMENSTRUAL SYMPTOMS

If you have suffered from premenstrual syndrome all your life, you are more likely to experience intensified symptoms as you become menopausal. The symptoms of PMS usually include fatigue, anxiety, irritability, tearfulness, breast soreness, water retention, skin problems, sugar cravings, and insomnia. If you suspect your mood swings are PMS-related, you can confirm this by charting your menstrual cycle for three months and recording your symptoms on a day-to-day basis.

Self-help

■ Avoid sugar cravings by eating several small meals a day – you will find that your cravings lessen if your blood sugar level is stable.

■ Eat less salt since it increases water retention and bloating.

■ Avoid alcohol and caffeine; they aggravate many of the emotional symptoms of PMS.

■ Make sure you are getting enough calcium, magnesium, vitamin B_6, and vitamin E, since these may reduce emotional symptoms.

■ Get plenty of exercise.

■ Aromatherapists recommend the oils of ylang-ylang, lavender, and lemon grass, which you can use in a warm bath.

SKIN, HAIR, EYE, MOUTH, AND NAIL SYMPTOMS

The lowered estrogen levels that occur at menopause cause changes in the skin, hair, nails, eyes, mouth, and gums.

Self-help

■ Moisturizing is important as you grow older. Avoid soap, which strips skin of its natural oils, and use special cleansing creams and lotions.

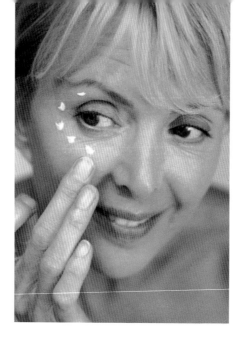

■ Toenails and fingernails need special care, so give yourself a manicure and a pedicure at least every six to eight weeks.

■ Ulcers in the mouth and on the tongue should be treated immediately. Rinse your mouth with salty water or use a commerical ointment. If rough edges on your teeth are causing ulcers, have them filed down.

■ Guard your skin from the sun. As the years pass, you will be less protected from exposure to sunlight. Avoid direct sun at all times and when you go out in sunny weather, wear sunscreen. If possible, limit your exposure to the sun to the early and late parts of the day.

■ The health of the skin, nails and hair, and eyes is largely dependent on a diet rich in vitamins, minerals, and trace elements. It is essential you have a sufficient intake of the vitamins A, B, C, and E as well as potassium, zinc, magnesium, bioflavonoids, iron, calcium, and essential fatty acids. Particular attention should be paid to the B vitamins, especially B_1, B_2, B_3, B_6, B_{12} and folic acid.

INSOMNIA

If you are feeling depressed or anxious or you are suffering from night sweats it can become difficult to get to sleep and common to wake early in the morning.

Self-help

■ If you take a long walk or some other form of aerobic exercise an hour before bedtime the quality of your sleep should noticeably improve.

■ Warm milk at bedtime works for many insomniacs. This may be due to the action of calcium on the nerves.

STOMACH AND BOWEL SYMPTOMS

Bloating with abdominal distension may be a problem during the menopausal years. It is usually due to gas in the large intestine produced by fermentation in the bowel. Constipation is another frequent symptom at

menopause because intestinal motility (movement) is affected by the sex hormones.

Self-help

■ A high-fiber diet, plenty of fluids and frequent exercise will keep the bowels normal. Cutting down on sugar, dairy products, and alcohol will also help.

■ Eat foods that cause fermentation, such as foods containing yeast and sugar, only in the early part of the day.

■ A fast, effective remedy for constipation is to eat lots of prunes and figs, fruits that are both high in fiber.

EMOTIONAL SYMPTOMS

Feelings such as tension, anxiety, depression, listlessness, irritability, tearfulness, and mood swings can occur at any age, but they rarely occur together or as frequently as they do during menopause.

Self-help

■ Severe mood swings and irritability can distance you from your partner and, occasionally, can jeopardize a relationship. However, if you share your feelings you may find your partner is very supportive. Several studies have shown that partners are eager to understand menopausal symptoms and would prefer to have insight into potential problems before the onset of menopause.

■ Women who go to support groups may be better able to deal with depression. Think about joining such a group, or starting one up yourself.

■ 20–30 minutes of strenuous exercise results in the release of endorphins, producing an "exercise high" that lasts for up to eight hours.

■ Yoga, relaxation techniques, and meditation all promote tranquility and combat anxiety.

INTELLECTUAL SYMPTOMS

Forgetfulness is one of the most common symptoms that menopausal women complain about and they may experience it long before they actually stop menstruating. The ability to concentrate can also become impaired.

Self-help

Any sort of work or studying will go a long way to preserve your intellectual ability. It's never too late to get a job, although many women in their menopausal years express fear about how to go about finding one. Many universities, colleges, and evening classes offer courses in a range of subjects, including employment retraining.

BREAST SYMPTOMS

A majority of American women suffer from breast pain at some time in their lives but particularly in the premenopausal and perimenopausal years.

■ Ask your doctor to examine you to exclude a lump.

■ Wear a good supportive bra and if necessary go to a special bra fitter. Wearing a bra in bed may relieve pain during the night.

■ Cut down on the amount of saturated fat you eat.

■ One of the essential fatty acids, gamolenic acid, which is found in evening primrose oil, significantly reduces breast pain in up to 70 percent of women and has not been found to have any side effects.

■ If the breast pain is very severe it may be treated by drugs such as danazol and bromocriptine, which alter hormone balance. However, these drugs can have side effects, including nausea, weight gain, and sometimes hirsutism (excess body hair) and lowering of the voice.

WEIGHT GAIN

The weight we may gain at menopause is due to a slower metabolism – something that affects both men and women as they grow older – and a decline in estrogen levels, which affects the way that fat is distributed. It is important to have a realistic outlook and be aware that changes in body shape happen to all postmenopausal women. Excessive or fad dieting is unhealthy.

Self-help

If your weight is over the recommended weight for your height and age, the following tips may help you to lose weight.

■ Drink two cups of water before you start to eat. This will make you feel more satiated at the end of the meal.

■ Put your food on a small plate. This controls the amount you can reasonably eat at one sitting.

■ The more time you take eating food, the more satisfied you're likely to feel. People who overeat usually eat quickly; they don't taste the food and have to eat more in order to feel satisfied.

■ Getting exercise an hour or so before a meal is a potent appetite suppressant. Eat your largest meal early in the day when you have the most time to burn up the calories you've eaten. Avoid eating large meals late in the evening – sleeping during the night does not burn off many calories.

SEXUAL SYMPTOMS

A common myth about menopause is that it marks the beginning of a woman's sexual decline. Nothing could be further from the truth. The majority of women can continue to experience sexual pleasure well into old age.

Self-help

■ Before sex put some sterile, water-soluble jelly on your vaginal entrance. Water-based jellies are better than oil-based ones because they are less likely to promote bacterial growth and infections and they will not cause the rubber of a condom to disintigrate.

■ Avoid douches, talcum powder, perfumed toilet paper, and any fragranced bath oils and foams, which can irritate the vagina.

■ Avoid washing the inside of your labia with soap since it will dry the skin.

■ Avoid remedies for genital itchiness containing an antihistamine or perfume.

■ Spend longer on foreplay to give your body more time to produce its own lubrication.

■ Women who have low histamine levels may find it difficult to reach orgasm. Women who take antihistamines regularly need to be aware of the possibility of decreased sexual desire and delayed orgasm.

■ Zinc is a mineral associated with histamine production and deficiency can be common in women who suffer from heavy bleeding or women who diet a lot. You can increase your zinc intake by including more zinc-rich foods, such as sardines and wheatgerm, in your diet.

FOCUS *on* HRT

Hormone replacement therapy (HRT) is the main method of treating the troublesome symptoms that arise during menopause. It is also an important preventive medicine since it effectively reduces the risk of certain life-threatening or painful conditions such as bowel cancer and osteoporosis.

HRT is not right for everyone but understanding the advantages and disadvantages and gathering as much information as possible will help you make an informed choice about managing your menopause.

There is hardly an organ in a woman's body whose health is not maintained by **estrogen**. So most organs in a woman's body can benefit from estrogen supplements when her ovaries fail at the end of her fertile life.

WHAT IS THE TREATMENT?

HRT is a combination of the female hormones estrogen and synthetic progesterone (**progestogen**). Estrogen is given to maintain the health of vital organs such as the brain, bones, and also the female sex organs. It also keeps the lining of the vagina and other body tissues elastic, the brain active, relieves anxiety, and promotes sleep. It's helpful in preventing osteoporosis and possibly Alzheimer's disease.

Progestogen causes the uterine lining to shed, which means with some types of HRT you will still have a monthly period, but there are other no-bleed forms for you to choose from. When hormonal medication was first prescribed in the 1960s and 1970s only estrogen was used. It was then discovered that women on this treatment had a slightly higher risk of uterine cancer than nonusers. Since then, progestogen has also been prescribed since it eliminates the risk of uterine cancer and can even protect against it.

HOW DO I TAKE IT?

Types of HRT

Pills – Most HRT is prescribed in pill form, is highly effective in combating physical and emotional symptoms, and can be stopped immediately if it isn't right for you. It may not be appropriate if you have a history of high blood pressure, blood clotting, liver trouble, breast lumps or breast cancer, and diabetes. Some women experience breast tenderness and nausea and you may get breakthrough bleeding if you forget to take a pill.

Creams – An applicator delivers measured doses

of estrogen-impregnated cream directly into the vagina. It reduces genital itching, thinning, discomfort, and urinary problems.

Vaginal approaches – Pellets deliver low doses of estrogen directly into the vagina, reducing vaginal dryness and pain when urinating. Both creams and pellets are easy to use but doses are too low to deal with general menopausal symptoms or to act as a preventive medicine.

Transdermal (skin) patches – A low dose of hormone enters the body through the skin. Patches need to be changed every three to four days. A very few women develop red, itchy skin underneath the patch and this may get worse in a hot climate.

Skin gel – The lowest and most physiological form of HRT is delivered from a gel rubbed into the skin of the thighs and upper legs. It has the fewest side effects and you can alter the dose yourself. It's the form I favor.

Implants – In Europe, pellets containing a **six-month supply** of estrogen are inserted under the skin of the abdomen or buttocks. Pills of **progestogen** are usually taken as well. Implants give excellent relief from physical symptoms and a high level of protection against osteoporosis, but insertion requires a minor surgical procedure. You can have a testosterone implant at the same time to increase your sex drive.

WAYS OF TAKING IT

Continuous therapy – The most common method. Estrogen is absorbed daily either by taking a pill or by wearing a skin patch twice a week. Progestogen is taken in pill form or in a combination skin patch for 12–14 days. Over 90 percent of women will have a monthly bleed but many women find periods dry up after a few months.

Combined continuous therapy (no-bleed HRT) – Continuous daily doses of estrogen with a very low dose of progestogen. Some women bleed at first but this usually stops after a few months. This method is popular with women on long-term treatment and women who start HRT when they're older, say, after

osteoporosis develops.

Cyclical therapy – In Europe, estrogen is sometimes taken from the first to the 21st day of the cycle and progestogen for the last 12 or 13 days; both medications are stopped on the 21st day. Most women will experience a withdrawal bleed between the 22nd and 28th day but it usually disappears over time. Alternatively, progestogen may be taken once every three months. This means that you have four bleeds a year.

SERMs – A nonestrogen form of HRT is called **raloxifene** and is one of a group of drugs called SERMs (Selective Estrogen Reuptake Modulators). It protects the bones and has no risk of breast cancer. But it doesn't treat hot flashes, dry vagina, or bladder symptoms as well as conventional HRT does. Nor does it protect against Alzheimer's disease.

HOW LONG DO I TAKE IT?

Treatment is usually continued for between two and five years as the body gradually adjusts to estrogen deficiency. However, HRT must be taken for at least five years if it is to prevent bone loss. If you stop after a short time, symptoms such as hot flashes may return in a more severe form. Since there is a small increased risk of breast cancer after five years and again after 10 years, many doctors would say 10 years is the longest you should take

HRT. However, the increase in risk is about the same as delaying your first child until after 30 and I, personally, am prepared to live with that risk to enjoy the benefits of HRT.

GALLBLADDER DISEASE
Between ages 50 and 75, 3 women in 100,000 not on HRT are estimated to die from complications of gallbladder disease. This figure doubles to 6 women in 100,000 among women on HRT.

WOMEN AT RISK
Women who fall into one or more of the following categories may be advised by their doctors not to take HRT, though if your menopausal symptoms are very severe you and your doctor can weigh the pros and cons.
- High blood pressure.
- History of thrombosis.
- Diabetes.
- Chronic liver disease.
- History of breast, vaginal, cervical, or endometrial cancer.

THE LATEST PERSPECTIVE ON THE RISKS OF HRT
In July 2002, a US study was published suggesting an increased risk of invasive breast cancer (by 26 percent), heart attacks (by 29 percent) and strokes (by 41 percent) on long-term HRT. Several points need to be made to clarify the report's findings.
- When we assess the risk of breast cancer we do so against a baseline of 1.0 – every woman has a risk of breast cancer of 1.0. That means the risk of getting breast cancer for every woman is 1.0 per 1,000 women over 10 years.
- If, for some reason, that risk goes up to 1.50 per 1,000 women over 10 years that increase is reported as a 50 percent increase.

So, in simple terms, the 26 percent increase in risk of breast cancer in the US study means that the risk went from 1 woman in 1,000 to 1.26 women in 1,000 over a 10-year period, which by any accounting is not a huge jump.

RESULTS
The results are not a surprise, British studies in 1997 and 1998 revealed similar figures and we didn't panic then.

We didn't panic for good reason: the increased risk is no more than the increased risk you impose on yourself if you're overweight, put off your first child until you're over 30, drink too much alcohol, or have no children at all.

Among 10,000 women the new figures represent 8 extra cases of breast cancer, 8 extra strokes, and 7 extra heart problems over the period of a year.

BENEFITS OF HRT
Some benefits are confirmed in this study:
- A 37 percent reduction in bowel cancer.
- A 33 percent reduction in hip fracture.
- A 24 percent reduction in all fractures.
Add to this the emerging evidence that HRT can probably prevent Alzheimer's, and proof that HRT is 98 percent effective in treating menopausal symptoms such as hot flashes, night sweats, and dry vagina.

It keeps women's genital organs healthy, including the bladder, and therefore protects against cystitis. Then there's the sound sleep, strong muscles, increased stamina, and mental tonic effect that many women claim.

ALTERNATIVES TO HRT
If you're worried about HRT, keep in mind there are alternatives with no increase in breast cancer risk.

- Not yet available in the US, tibolone relieves symptoms and doesn't affect the breast.
- Another group of drugs, SERMs, doesn't help symptoms but appears to strengthen bones and protects you from heart disease.

THE LATEST RESEARCH
- In February 2003 a UK study of 13,000 women stated that women wth diabetes should not take HRT, and found no increased risk of heart disease on HRT but no protection either.
- In March 2003 a US study reported no improvement in quality of life on HRT, though the authors admitted there were limitations to the study.

LIVING WITH THE RISK
I personally have decided not to sacrifice the benefits of HRT and to live with any perceived risk. I'm reassured that, despite the frightening headlines, the researchers state that, for each individual woman, the risks of HRT are still very low.. It's only when you lump thousands of women together that they become a concern. I, personally, will live with that, in exchange for vigor, an active brain, a certain fearlessness, and a zest for life.

How HRT can help

- **Hot flashes and night sweats** – Over 90 percent of women find complete relief when they are prescribed estrogen regardless of the form it takes; over 98 percent report that their symptoms have lessened.
- **Vaginal dryness, soreness, and painful intercourse** – Can be relieved.
- **Intellectual problems** (poor concentration/ability to make decisions) – may improve within a month or so.
- **Sleep** – Research indicates that women may dream less when they are estrogen deficient. As this type of sleep is important to your sense of well-being HRT should help make you feel rested after sleep. Take your HRT last thing at night for a really sound sleep.
- **Libido** (sexual drive) – This varies from woman to woman. Testosterone – the male hormone – is also manufactured by the ovaries and is thought to be largely responsible for the female sex drive. Daily low doses of testosterone – or a testosterone implant – can bring about a subtle return of sexual vitality without side effects.

Other benefits
- **Osteoporosis** – This is a bone-thinning process that occurs in postmenopausal women. It can result in fractures, curvature of the spine, and severe back pain. HRT is thought to be an important form of protection against osteoporosis.
- **Reduces risk of developing cancer of the colon by a third and may delay the onset of Alzheimer's disease.**

Diabetes mellitus

DIABETES MELLITUS IS THE INABILITY OF THE BODY TO USE GLUCOSE FOR ENERGY DUE TO
INADEQUATE AMOUNTS OF, OR LOSS OF SENSITIVITY TO, THE HORMONE INSULIN.

In diabetes mellitus the pancreas either produces insufficient amounts of insulin or body cells become resistant to the hormone's effects.

Diabetes mellitus is one of the most common long-term diseases occurring in the Western world, affecting more than 1 in 20 people. It sometimes runs in families.

WHAT ARE THE TYPES?

There are two main forms of diabetes mellitus, designated as **type I diabetes** and **type II diabetes**.

TREATMENT

Insulin

Normally, insulin is produced by the pancreas and enables the body's cells to absorb its main energy source, glucose, from the bloodstream. In diabetes, cells have to use other sources of energy, which may lead to a buildup of toxic by-products in the body. The most dramatic of these is **acetone**, which can be smelled on the breath as **juicyfruit gum** or nail polish remover. Unused glucose accumulates in the blood and urine, leading to high blood sugar levels and **symptoms** such as **passing a lot of urine, thirst, and loss of weight**.

Treatment is designed to keep glucose levels in the blood steady. Among people treated for diabetes mellitus, 1 in 10 depends on self-administered injections of insulin for life. The rest need a carefully managed diet and often oral drugs.

As long as their diabetes is well controlled, most people can then lead normal lives. However, complications may eventually develop, although their onset may be much delayed by careful treatment. Complications may affect the **eyes, kidneys, cardiovascular system** and **nervous system** and include **peripheral nerve disorders**. Poorly controlled diabetes mellitus also weakens the **immune system** and thus increases susceptibility to infections such as **yeast infections, skin infections, and bladder infections**. Diabetes mellitus is usually a permanent condition.

TYPE I DIABETES

This form of diabetes occurs when the pancreas produces too little insulin or none at all. It usually develops suddenly in childhood or adolescence, before age 30. Although dietary measures are also important, it must be treated with insulin injections. Type I diabetes accounts for 5 to 10 percent of diagnosed diabetes in the US.

TYPE II DIABETES

Type II is by far the most common form of diabetes. The pancreas continues to secrete insulin but cells in the body become resistant to its effects. This form of diabetes mainly affects people over the age of 40 and is more common in overweight people. It develops slowly and often goes unnoticed for many years. Sometimes the condition may be treated with dietary measures alone, but oral drugs and sometimes insulin injections may become necessary. Up to 95 percent of people with diabetes have type II.

Diabetes mellitus can sometimes develop during **pregnancy**. This condition is called **gestational diabetes** and is usually treated with insulin to maintain the health of the mother and baby. Gestational diabetes usually disappears after childbirth; however, women who have had it are at increased risk of developing type II diabetes in later life.

WHAT ARE THE CAUSES?

■ **Type I diabetes** is usually caused by an abnormal reaction in which the immune system destroys insulin-secreting cells in the pancreas. This kind of diabetes can be thought of as an **autoimmune disorder**.
■ The trigger of the abnormal reaction is unknown, but it may be a **viral infection**.
■ In some cases, destruction of the insulin-secreting tissues occurs after inflammation of the pancreas during acute pancreatitis.
■ Genetics may also play a role, but the pattern of inheritance is complicated. The child of a person who has type I diabetes is at greater risk of developing it. However, most affected children do not have a parent with diabetes.
■ The causes of **type II diabetes** are less well understood, but genetics and obesity are important factors. About 1 in 3 diabetics has a relative with the same type of diabetes.
■ Type II diabetes is a growing problem in societies that are becoming more affluent. In such societies, food intake increases, leading to a rise in the number of overweight people and the prevalence of this condition.
■ Type II diabetes can also be caused by corticosteroid drugs, or by excess levels of

natural corticosteroid hormones, as occurs in overactivity of the adrenal glands (Cushing's syndrome), which oppose the action of insulin.

WHAT ARE THE SYMPTOMS?

Although some of the symptoms of both forms of diabetes mellitus are similar, type I diabetes tends to develop more quickly and become more severe. The symptoms of type II may not be obvious or may go unnoticed until a routine blood test. The main symptoms of both forms may include:
● excessive urination
● thirst and a dry mouth
● insufficient sleep because of the need to urinate at night
● lack of energy
● blurry vision
● weight loss.

In some people, the first sign of type I diabetes is **ketoacidosis**, a condition in which toxic chemicals called **ketones** build up in the blood. These chemicals are produced when body tissues are unable to take up glucose from the blood due to inadequate production of insulin, and have to use **fats** for energy. Ketoacidosis can also occur in people with type I diabetes who are taking insulin if they miss several doses or develop another illness (because any form of illness increases the body's requirement for insulin). The main symptoms of ketoacidosis include:
● nausea and vomiting, sometimes with abdominal pain
● deep breathing
● acetone smell to the breath (like juicyfruit gum or nail polish remover)
● confusion.

These symptoms constitute a medical emergency because they can lead to severe dehydration and coma if not treated urgently. Emergency treatment for ketoacidosis includes:
● intravenous fluids to correct dehydration and restore the chemical balance in the blood
● Intravenous insulin injections to enable cells to absorb glucose from the blood.

ARE THERE COMPLICATIONS?

Diabetes mellitus may give rise to both **short-term** and **long-term complications**. Short-term problems are usually easy to remedy, but long-term complications are hard to control and can lead to shorter life expectancy.

SHORT-TERM COMPLICATIONS

Poorly controlled or untreated type I diabetes may lead to ketoacidosis, the symptoms of which are described above.

Living with diabetes

People with diabetes mellitus can lead normal lives, and they can continue to exercise and to eat most foods. However, it is very important to eat a healthy diet, maintain fitness, and, if necessary, lose weight. Following a healthy regimen helps minimize the risk of developing complications over time, including heart disease, circulatory problems, and kidney failure.

A healthy diet: For some people with diabetes, a healthy diet and weight loss are enough to keep blood glucose levels normal. Your diet should be high in complex carbohydrates, such as rice, pasta, and legumes, and low in fats, particularly fats of animal origin.

Drinking and smoking: Alcohol in moderation is safe for most people, but in excess it may lower blood glucose levels. In addition, it is high in calories and may cause weight gain. Smoking is very harmful because it greatly increases the risk of long-term complications, such as heart disease and stroke.

Special care for your feet: Diabetes can increase the risk of skin infections and ulcers on the feet. You can reduce the risk by wearing cotton or wool socks, shoes that breathe and fit comfortably, visiting a podiatrist regularly, not walking barefoot, and cutting your toenails straight across. You should inspect and clean and dry your feet daily and consult a doctor promptly if you develop a sore on your foot.

Exercise and sports: Regular exercise makes you feel healthier, reduces the risk of heart disease, stroke, and high blood pressure, and can help if you need to lose weight. If you have type I diabetes, you may need to monitor your blood glucose before, during, and after exercise to check how the activity affects your requirements for both insulin and food.

Strenuous exercise: Blood glucose levels usually drop during strenuous exercise. You may need to adjust your dose of insulin or eat more before strenuous activity.

Moderate exercise: Regular moderate exercise reduces the chance of developing coronary artery disease and may improve the control of your diabetes.

Your medical checkup: You should visit your doctor every few months so that she can detect problems related to diabetes at an early stage and treat them effectively. Management includes a neurological examination, measurement of your pulse and blood pressure, and a full physical examination at least once a year. Your levels of blood sugar and glycosylated hemoglobin will be tested. Your urine will be tested to check for kidney disease.

Eye examination: Inspection of the retina (the light-sensitive membrane at the back of the eye) can detect early retinal damage caused by diabetes.

Blood pressure measurement: People with diabetes mellitus have an increased risk of high blood pressure, and regular monitoring is important.

LONG-TERM COMPLICATIONS

Certain long-standing problems pose the main health threat to people with diabetes and eventually affect even people with well-controlled diabetes. Close control of the blood sugar level reduces the risk of developing these problems, and early recognition of complications helps in their control. For these reasons, all affected people should see their doctor at least four times a year. Type II diabetes is often not diagnosed until years after its onset. As a result, complications may be evident at the time of initial diagnosis.

■ People with diabetes are at increased risk of **cardiovascular disease**. Large blood vessels may be damaged by **atherosclerosis**, which is a major cause of **coronary artery disease** and **stroke**.

■ Elevated levels of **cholesterol** in the blood, which accelerates the development of atherosclerosis, is more common in people with diabetes.

■ Diabetes is also associated with **high blood pressure**, another risk factor for cardiovascular disease.

■ Other long-term complications result from damage to small blood vessels throughout the body. Damage to blood vessels in the light-sensitive retina at the back of the eye may cause **diabetic retinopathy and blindness**.

■ Diabetes also increases the risk of developing **cataracts** in the eyes. People with diabetes mellitus should have their eyes examined yearly by an ophthalmologist.

■ If diabetes affects blood vessels that supply nerves, it may cause **nerve damage**, so there may be a gradual loss of sensation, starting at the hands and feet and sometimes gradually extending up the limbs.

■ Symptoms may also include **dizziness** upon standing.

■ There may be **impotence** in men.

■ Later in life, loss of feeling combined with poor circulation makes the legs more susceptible to **ulcers**, even **gangrene**, so routine checkups with your doctor are vital.

■ Damage to small blood vessels in the kidneys may lead to **chronic kidney failure** and **end-stage kidney failure**, which requires lifelong dialysis or a kidney transplant.

HOW IS IT DIAGNOSED?

High blood glucose is the underlying cause of the symptoms associated with Type I and Type II diabetes. Urine tests alone are not used to diagnose diabetes, although a high level of sugar in the urine may indicate that blood tests such as the random plasma glucose test, the oral glucose tolerance test (OGTT), and the fasting plasma glucose test are in order. If you have one test and the results are positive, it is advisable to have the results confirmed by one of the other tests

WHAT IS THE TREATMENT?

For anyone with diabetes mellitus, the aim of treatment is to maintain the level of glucose in the blood within the normal range without marked fluctuations. This goal may be achieved with dietary measures, a combination of diet and insulin injections, or of diet and pills that lower blood glucose levels. Treatment is usually lifelong and you will have to take responsibility for the daily adjustment of your diet and medication on the basis of daily blood sugar tests, which you perform yourself.

TREATMENT FOR TYPE I DIABETES

■ This form of diabetes mellitus is nearly always treated with **insulin injections**. Oral drugs alone are ineffective.

■ Insulin is available in various forms, including **short-acting, long-acting** and combinations of both forms.

■ Treatment regimens need to be individually tailored and they may include **combinations** of insulin and oral drugs.

■ Your doctor will talk to you about your needs and arrange for you to learn how to **inject yourself**.

■ You will also have to **control your diet** and **monitor your blood glucose** as described below.

■ If the diabetes is difficult to control you may be given an **insulin pump**, which dispenses insulin through a catheter that is inserted into your skin.

POSSIBLE TRANSPLANT

The only way to **cure** type I diabetes is by a pancreas transplant, but this surgery is not routinely offered because the body may reject the new organ and because lifelong treatment with immunosuppressant drugs is needed afterward. Some people are given a pancreas transplant at the same time as a kidney transplant. A method is currently being devised to transplant insulin-secreting cells isolated from a normal pancreas, but this technique is still at an experimental stage.

Injecting insulin

If you need regular injections of insulin, you will be shown how to inject yourself. You can use a syringe and needle, but many people prefer insulin pens, which are easier to use and more discreet. Insulin can be injected into any fatty area, such as the upper arms, abdomen, or thighs. Insert the needle quickly into a pinch of skin and then inject the insulin slowly. You should try not to use exactly the same site each time for the injection. After about age 10, children with diabetes can be taught how to inject themselves.

Insulin pen: This device for carrying and delivering insulin holds an insulin cartridge and has a dial that lets you set the required dose. Disposable needles attach to one end.

TREATMENT FOR TYPE II DIABETES

Many people with this form of diabetes can control their blood glucose levels by **exercising** regularly and following a **healthy diet** to maintain ideal weight.

■ You should follow general guidelines for a healthy diet and seek the guidance of a dietitian if necessary. Try to keep fat intake low, and obtain energy from complex carbohydrates (such as bread and rice) to minimize fluctuations in the blood glucose level. The diet should have a fixed calorie content. The proportions of protein, carbohydrate, and fat must be consistent to keep a balance between food intake and medicine.

■ You must also check your blood glucose regularly. If the glucose level is higher or lower than recommended, you may need to alter your diet or adjust your insulin or drug dose with the help of your doctor. Effective monitoring is especially important if you develop another illness, such as influenza, and in other situations, such as exercising or planning to eat a larger meal than usual.

■ When diet is not sufficient to control your blood sugar, one or more drugs may be

prescribed. You may begin with oral drugs, such as **sulphonylureas**, which stimulate the pancreas to release insulin, or **metformin**, which helps body tissues absorb glucose. You may also be given **acarbose**, which slows absorption of glucose from the intestine and prevents fluctuations in the blood level. If oral drugs are ineffective, you may need insulin injections.

WHAT IS THE OUTLOOK?

If cardiovascular complications develop, diabetes mellitus can cause heart disease, stroke, peripheral vascular disease. High blood pressure can result from kidney disease. However, advances in monitoring blood glucose levels, combined with a healthy lifestyle, have made diabetes easier to control, allowing people to lead a more normal life. Support groups exist for affected people.

See also:
• **The heart and atherosclerosis p. 222**
• **Cataracts p. 472** • **Cystitis p. 378**
• **High blood pressure p. 226**
• **Acute, chronic, and end-stage kidney failure p. 380**

TEST

Monitoring your blood glucose

You can monitor your blood glucose level using a **digital meter**. The method of use varies, depending on the type of meter, but usually involves applying a drop of blood to a test strip impregnated with a chemical that reacts with glucose. Checking your blood glucose **at least once a day,** or as often as your doctor recommends, allows you to monitor your treatment to confirm that it is effective and to alter it as necessary.
1. Before starting, wash your hands thoroughly and dry them. Once your hands

are clean, obtain a drop of blood by using a spring-loaded pricking device on a fingertip.
2. Cover the chemically impregnated target area of the test strip with the drop of blood.
3. Finally, insert the strip into the digital glucose meter. The meter analyzes the blood and gives an instant reading of the glucose level. Some meters allow you to use alternative sites for testing.

Hyperthyroidism and Graves' disease

WHEN THE THYROID GLAND PRODUCES AN EXCESS OF HORMONES, MANY OF THE BODY'S FUNCTIONS ARE STIMULATED AND METABOLISM SPEEDS UP.

An excess of thyroid hormones, known as hyperthyroidism, is one of the most common hormonal disorders. It's most common in women between ages 20 and 50 and can run in families.

About 3 out of 4 cases of the condition are due to Graves' disease, an **autoimmune**

disorder in which the immune system produces antibodies that attack the thyroid gland, resulting in overproduction of thyroid hormones. Graves' disease tends to run in families and is thought to have a genetic basis. In rare cases, hyperthyroidism

may be associated with other autoimmune disorders, in particular the skin disorder **vitiligo, prematurely gray hair,** and **pernicious anemia**, a disorder of blood formation. In some cases thyroid nodules, often called "hot" nodules, secrete excess thyroid hormones, leading to hyperthyroidism. Inflammation of the thyroid gland in thyroiditis may also temporarily produce the symptoms of hyperthyroidism.

WHAT ARE THE SYMPTOMS?

In most cases, symptoms of hyperthyroidism develop gradually over several weeks and may include:

- weight loss despite increased appetite and food consumption
- rapid heartbeat, which is sometimes also irregular, felt as palpitations especially in thigh muscle
- tremor (persistent trembling) affecting the hands
- warm, moist skin as a result of excessive sweating
- intolerance to heat
- anxiety and insomnia
- frequent bowel movements
- swelling in the neck caused by an enlarged thyroid gland (goiter)
- muscle weakness
- in women, irregular menstruation.

People with hyperthyroidism caused by Graves' disease may also have bulging eyes, a condition called exophthalmos. In the elderly, these symptoms are not as obvious.

HOW IS IT DIAGNOSED?

If your doctor suspects you have hyperthyroidism, a blood test to check for abnormally high levels of thyroid hormones and for antibodies that can attack the thyroid gland will be ordered. Your doctor will also feel around your neck for enlargement of the gland. If swelling is detected, you may have radionuclide scanning to check for a hot nodule.

WHAT IS THE TREATMENT?

- Symptoms of hyperthyroidism can initially be relieved by **beta blocker drugs**,(propranolol) which reduce tremor and anxiety but do not affect thyroid hormone levels.
- There are three main treatments aimed at reducing the production of thyroid hormones.
- The most common is **antithyroid drugs**, such as **carbimazole**, which are used when hyperthyroidism is due to Graves' disease and work by suppressing production of thyroid hormones. These drugs need to be taken daily for 12–18 months, after which the thyroid gland often functions normally.
- **Radioactive iodine** may be the most effective treatment for thyroid **nodules** that secrete hormone, and is also commonly used to treat Graves' disease. Treatment involves drinking a dose of radioactive iodine in solution or swallowing a radioactive iodine

capsule. The iodine is absorbed and accumulates in the thyroid gland, destroying part of it.
- Rarely, if drug treatments cause side effects, surgical removal of part of the thyroid gland may be necessary.

WHAT IS THE OUTLOOK?

Many people recover fully following treatment. However, hyperthyroidism may recur, particularly in people who have Graves' disease. If the treatment involves surgery or radioactive iodine, the remaining part of the thyroid may not be able to produce sufficient hormones, leading to hypothyroidism (see below). It is therefore important for thyroid hormone levels to be monitored regularly after treatment so that hormone supplements can be given if needed. The autoimmune form of hyper-thyroidism may "burn out," leaving behind a hypothyroid state.

See also:
- Anemias p. 236
- Arrhythmias p. 231
- Autoimmune disorders p. 323
- Radionuclide scanning p. 508
- Vitiligo p. 454

Hypothyroidism

IN HYPOTHYROIDISM, ALSO KNOWN AS MYXEDEMA, THE THYROID GLAND DOES NOT PRODUCE ENOUGH THYROID HORMONES. THESE HORMONES ARE IMPORTANT IN REGULATING THE BODY'S METABOLISM. A DEFICIENCY CAUSES A SLOWING DOWN OF MANY OF THE BODY'S FUNCTIONS.

Hypothyroidism is more common in women, particularly over age 40, and runs in families.

WHAT ARE THE CAUSES?

- A common cause of hypothyroidism is **thyroiditis**. The most common type of thyroiditis leading to hypothyroidism is an **autoimmune disorder** known as **Hashimoto's thyroiditis**, in which cells damage the thyroid gland. Antibodies are produced to the damaged and dying tissue. Other forms of thyroiditis may lead to temporary or permanent hypothyroidism in about 10 percent of cases. Thyroiditis occurs in women after the birth of a baby but is usually a temporary condition.
- **Treatments for an overactive thyroid gland** that involve **radioactive iodine** or **surgery** can also lead to permanent hypothyroidism. These treatments destroy part of the gland, and the tissue that remains may not produce sufficient hormones.
- **Insufficient dietary iodine**, which is essential for the production of thyroid hormones, can cause hypothyroidism but is rare in developed countries.

- In rare cases, hypothyroidism is due to the pituitary gland releasing insufficient amounts of **thyroid-stimulating hormone** (TSH), which stimulates the thyroid gland to secrete hormones. The underproduction of TSH is often due to a pituitary tumor.

WHAT ARE THE SYMPTOMS?

The symptoms of hypothyroidism vary in severity, usually develop slowly over months or years and may initially go unnoticed. Symptoms include:

- fatigue, which may make even minimal physical activity difficult
- weight gain
- constipation
- hoarseness of the voice
- intolerance to cold
- swelling of the face and puffy eyes
- generalized hair thinning
- in women, heavy menstrual periods.

Some people with hypothyroidism develop a swelling in the neck (a goiter) due to an enlarged thyroid.

WHAT MIGHT BE DONE?

Your doctor may arrange for you to have blood tests to measure the levels of thyroid hormones and TSH and to check for antibodies that act against the thyroid gland.

WHAT IS THE TREATMENT?

Treatment is aimed at the underlying cause. Permanent hypothyroidism may be treated with **replacement synthetic thyroid hormones**, which you will need to take for life. The symptoms should begin to improve about three weeks after drug treatment starts. Hormone treatment must be monitored regularly to ensure that the correct dosage is maintained. If a pituitary tumor is the cause, further tests will be done.

Temporary hypothyroidism does not usually need to be treated, but short-term hormone replacement may be given in some cases, for instance if thyroiditis occurs after giving birth. A deficiency in dietary iodine can be treated with supplements.

Radionuclide scanning

The technique of radionuclide scanning produces images using radiation emitted from a substance within the body. The radioactive substance, called radionuclide, is introduced into the body (orally) and taken up by the organ or tissue to be imaged. A counter positioned outside the body detects the radiation that is emitted by the radionuclide and transmits this information to a computer. The computer then converts the information into images. Radionuclide scanning is used both to image the structure of many internal organs and to provide a measure of their function. SPECT scanning and PET scanning are two specialized forms of radionuclide scanning.

Radionuclide scans show parts of the body as areas of color of varying intensity. Areas of intense color are called hot spots; these are areas where there is a high uptake of radionuclide. Areas of less intense color,

called cold spots, are areas where the radionuclide uptake is low. The greater the amount of tissue activity, the greater the uptake of radionuclide.

How it is done
During a radionuclide scan you will be asked to lie on a motorized bed that will move you past a special camera that can detect the radiation emitted by the radionuclide. The camera relays the information to a computer that builds up an image. Most radionuclide scans take about 45 minutes to an hour to perform.

Radionuclide scanning may be used to detect abnormal levels of activity in organs such as the thyroid gland, where it is used to look for thyroid nodules, and the kidneys. Changes in the function of a tissue or organ often develop before structural changes occur, and radionuclide scanning can detect

some diseases at a significantly earlier stage than most other imaging techniques. For example, a radionuclide scan of bone can detect infection of bone tissue weeks before it would become apparent on an ordinary X-ray. Radionuclide scans are particularly useful for assessing how well a treatment has worked. Scans may be done before and after a particular treatment to compare the function of an organ.

Two particular types of radionuclide scanning may be used to look at the function of the heart. **Thallium scanning** reveals areas of the heart muscle with a poor blood supply and is used to look at the activity of the heart muscle during exercise. **MUGA** (multiple-gated acquisition scanning) is a technique in which the blood flow into and out of the heart is measured to assess how efficiently the heart pumps blood around the body.

ADRENAL GLANDS

The body has two adrenal glands, one sitting above each kidney. Hormones produced by the adrenal glands are vital in controlling body chemistry. If adrenal hormone levels become imbalanced, the effects can be serious, widespread throughout the body and even life-threatening. However, these disorders are fortunately rare.

Adrenal gland disorders may involve either the **overproduction** or **underproduction** of adrenal

hormones, leading to **Cushing's syndrome** and **Addison's disease**. The overproduction of adrenal hormones is most commonly due to the presence of an adrenal tumor, simply removed by surgery.

Adrenal disorders are sometimes due to a pituitary tumor that affects the pituitary gland's production of hormones called adrenal-stimulating hormones, which control the outflow of hormones from the adrenals.

Addison's disease

ADDISON'S DISEASE IS A DISORDER IN WHICH THE ADRENAL GLANDS UNDERPRODUCE HORMONES. THE LACK OF ADRENAL HORMONES (CORTICOSTEROIDS AND FLORINEF) IS FREQUENTLY CAUSED BY AN AUTOIMMUNE DISORDER THAT DAMAGES THE GLAND.

WHAT ARE THE SYMPTOMS?
The symptoms of Addison's disease appear gradually but become increasingly obvious over several weeks or months. You may develop:
● vague feelings of ill health
● fatigue and weakness
● gradual loss of appetite, nausea, even vomiting
● weight loss
● skin pigmentation similar to suntan, especially in the creases of the palms and on

the folds of the knuckles, elbows, and knees.
● salt craving

WHAT IS THE OUTLOOK?
People with Addison's disease usually develop low blood pressure (hypotension) especially when getting up rapidly.

If the levels of corticosteroids become very low, a crisis may occur, particularly during an illness or after an injury. The crisis is caused by

an excessive loss of salt and water and results in dehydration, extreme weakness, abdominal pain, nausea, vomiting, and confusion. Left untreated, a crisis may lead to coma and death. Addison's disease is often treated successfully with synthetic hormones.

See also:
● **Low blood pressure p. 234**

Cushing's syndrome

CUSHING'S SYNDROME IS THE NAME FOR A CHARACTERISTIC COMBINATION OF SYMPTOMS
CAUSED BY EXCESSIVE PRODUCTION OF ADRENAL HORMONES.

WHAT ARE THE SYMPTOMS?

The symptoms appear gradually and become increasingly obvious over a period of weeks or months. Any of the following symptoms may develop:
- changes in the face, which may become red and rounded
- weight gain concentrated around the chest and abdomen
- excessive growth of facial or body hair (more noticeable in women)
- in women, irregular menstruation; eventually, menstruation may stop
- reddish-purple stretch marks on the abdomen, thighs, and arms
- pads of fat between the shoulder blades at the base of the neck
- difficulty climbing stairs associated with muscle wasting and weakness of the legs; the arms may also be affected
- tendency to bruise easily, especially on the limbs
- acne
- lack of sexual drive; men may become impotent
- depression and mood swings.

WHAT IS THE OUTLOOK?

If the disorder is left untreated, it may lead to complications such as **high blood pressure** (hypertension), **thinning of the bones** (osteoporosis), **diabetes mellitus,** and **chronic heart failure.**

See also:
- **Chronic heart failure p. 233**
- **Diabetes mellitus p. 504**
- **High blood pressure p. 226**
- **Osteoporosis p. 423**

Pituitary gland disorders

The pituitary gland is a tiny gland at the base of the brain that produces a large number of the hormones controlling growth, sexual development, and water balance. The gland also produces hormones that control many other hormone-secreting glands, such as the thyroid gland. Most pituitary disorders are caused by tumors that alter the output of particular pituitary hormones.

Some pituitary disorders
PITUITARY TUMORS
Pituitary tumors are generally benign growths in the pituitary gland that may cause hormonal disturbances in many other hormone glands in the body including the ovaries, thyroid, and adrenals.

A prolactinoma is a pituitary tumor that causes excessive secretion of prolactin, a hormone that influences fertility and breast milk production. It is more common in women, where it is usually associated with disturbances to the menstrual cycle.

ACROMEGALY
This is excessive growth of parts of the face and body due to overproduction of growth hormone by the pituitary gland.

HYPOPITUITARISM
Hypopituitarism is insufficient production initially of pituitary hormones. It rarely occurs before puberty, when it may lead to dwarfism or short stature from lack of growth hormone.

DIABETES INSIPIDUS
Diabetes insipidus is inadequate production of, or resistance to, the effects of the pituitary hormone involved in controlling water balance, antidiuretic hormone (ADH or vasopressin), so that large volumes of urine are lost from the body.

Children's conditions

Image shows a colored scanning electron micrograph of the measles virus

Miriam's overview

I have three guiding principles when approaching illness in children.

● Children are not little adults. It follows that illness in children has to be looked at in a different way from illness in adults – children's illness isn't adult illness in miniature. So childhood asthma, childhood diabetes, childhood migraines are different from their adult equivalents and must be managed appropriately.

Then again, there are childhood diseases for which there is no exact adult equivalent. Cystic fibrosis, hydrocephalus, undescended testes are a few examples. These conditions are outside the orbit of any discussion of adult diseases.

● As a junior doctor I very quickly learned there was one person whom I could not ignore when faced with a sick child. That person is you, mom. No one in the world (not even dad) knows your child as you do. You are sensitive to small, subtle signs of being off color when no one else notices and even when drawn to their attention, no one else can spot. Armed with this knowledge you should understand that your child's well-being depends more on you than anyone else. Even though doctors and nurses may be skeptical of what you're saying you must insist if you're convinced your child is ill or doesn't seem right. Never be put off. Don't take no for an answer. Hang on until you get the attention and treatment you want for your child. If you don't look after your child's interests no one else will.

"if you *don't look after* your child's interests *no one else will*"

● Ill children can go downhill very quickly so prompt medical attention is mandatory – delay could always be costly so never hesitate to seek urgent medical advice if you're worried. Better safe than sorry. No doctor will mind if all they're called upon to do is reassure you that all is well.

A child's condition can deteriorate rapidly for several reasons.

● One of the most important is that children are built on a much smaller scale than adults so organs that are far enough apart to resist spread of infection in us are so close together in children that any infection of one part often has to be treated as an infection of the whole. The ear, nose, throat, sinuses, and the chest are such a system: any infection of one, in a small child, threatens involvement of all.

● The immune response in children lags behind that of adults so a baby may develop a very high temperature quite suddenly, made worse by the fact that children can't regulate their temperature as efficiently as can adults.

The corollary of this is that children recover very fast too, faster than adults, because their bodies are resilient and heal quickly. A cause for celebration is that a sick, pale, limp child can be up, running around and asking for a grilled cheese sandwich in half an hour.

Genetic tests

The nucleus of each cell in your body normally contains 23 pairs of chromosomes – 22 pairs of autosomes and one pair of sex chromosomes (XX in women, XY in men). Each chromosome is made up of a number of genes, which are chemical codes that control the way every cell in the body functions. A faulty gene or chromosome may result in a disease or disorder. A wide range of genetic abnormalities can now be identified, and more sophisticated genetic tests are being developed all the time. Some of the best known genetic tests are the screening tests used to detect Down syndrome and other chromosomal disorders during pregnancy. In these tests, the number of chromosomes and their structure are analyzed to determine whether

the correct number of chromosomes is present and whether any of the chromosomes is abnormal.

Other genetic tests look specifically at the genes that make up each chromosome. For certain genetic conditions, such as cystic fibrosis and sickle-cell anemia, the exact genetic abnormality and the way in which it is inherited are known.

Genetic tests are usually performed on white blood cells taken from a blood sample or on cells from tissue taken by gently scraping the inside of the cheek. In prenatal tests, the cells are taken from the amniotic fluid (by amniocentesis) or from the placenta (by chorionic villus sampling).

Genetic tests can identify many genetic conditions including Down syndrome, in which 47 chromosomes are present instead of the usual 46.

CARING FOR A SICK CHILD

Most parents seem to know instinctively when their child isn't well. For example, your child may not be as lively as she usually is, she may refuse her food, she may be clingy.

The problem is that moms and dads can't always diagnose exactly what's wrong with their child, nor can they necessarily recognize whether the symptoms are serious.

Calling the doctor

AN ILL CHILD IS ALWAYS A DISTRESSING SIGHT AND THE SITUATION CAN BE EVEN MORE TENSE IF YOU CANNOT DECIDE WHETHER TO CALL THE DOCTOR.

There are some circumstances, for example after a serious injury, when medical help obviously should be sought immediately. There are, however, many more situations where the seriousness isn't quite as clear-cut. This is where the worry starts: "Are my child's symptoms nothing to worry about or are they potentially serious?"

You must remember that most doctors won't mind if you seek their advice. Always follow your instincts and if you're ever in doubt contact your doctor. If your child's already undergoing treatment from the doctor and you're worried about his progress, call your doctor again. Only take your child to the emergency room if you become very worried about their symptoms or if they show any signs of meningitis (see p. 405).

WHAT TO TELL YOUR DOCTOR
■ Your child's age.
■ Whether your child has a temperature.

Emergencies

Always get your child to the nearest hospital by ambulance or car if you notice any of the following:
■ Your child has stopped breathing.
■ Your child is breathing with difficulty and his lips are becomming blue.
■ Your child is unconscious.
■ Your child has a deep wound that is bleeding badly.
■ Your child has a serious burn.
■ Your child has a suspected broken bone.
■ Your child has a chemical in his eyes.
■ Your child's ear or eye has been pierced.
■ Your child has been bitten.
■ Your child has eaten a poisonous substance.

If so, what it is; how long he has had it; have there been any fluctuations and, if so, what they were. If your child has a fever, did it come on quickly?
■ Are your child's neck glands swollen?
■ Has your child vomited or had diarrhea?
■ Does your child have a rash?
■ Has your child complained of any kind of pain? If so, where is it?
■ Has your child suffered from dizziness or blurred vision (particularly if he's recently had a bump on the head)?
■ Has your child had a convulsion? If so, how long did it last?
■ Has your child lost consciousness?
■ Did your child eat the last meal offered and has he eaten within the past three hours?

WHAT TO EXPECT FROM YOUR DOCTOR
Once the doctor has arrived he should examine your child thoroughly and give you an honest opinion of what's wrong. If your doctor doesn't know what's wrong, he should tell you what further tests are necessary to get a clear diagnosis. He should also advise you on the implications of the illness or condition. If, for example, your child has an acute attack of sinusitis or a middle ear infection, your doctor should tell you that your child may need antibiotics to eradicate it completely. On the other hand, your doctor should not give you medicine if he's sure there's nothing wrong. He would be wrong to give you something simply because you have gone to his office expecting to be treated. Respect him for not being pressured into giving you a prescription.

That said, he should answer all your questions – so persist until you are completely satisfied. If medicine is required, the doctor should give you as much information as possible about what he has prescribed. He should also tell you whether to give it before or after a meal, whether there may be side effects, whether there are any special precautions to take, and he should warn you about possible complications and danger signs to look out for.

THINGS TO ASK YOUR DOCTOR
If your child has a recurrent condition, such as cold sores or boils, ask your doctor what you can do yourself if you notice any symptoms occurring. You can also ask your doctor for any home nursing tips.

If your child has a chronic condition, find out if there's anything you can do at home to help it. For example, with infantile eczema there's quite a lot you can do, such as adding oil to the bathwater, using special soap, gently rubbing in moisturizing ointments and creams, even when the skin is clear. If your child has an infectious disease, ask about the incubation period – could friends be infected too? – the length of time your child will be infectious and how long he will have to stay out of school.

PICK UP THE PHONE NOW
These are the circumstances under which you should **always** call the doctor.

TEMPERATURE
■ Temperature over 102.2°F (39°C).
■ Temperature with drowsiness and a purplish rash.
■ Temperature with a convulsion, or if your child has had convulsions in the past.
■ Temperature with a stiff neck and headache.
■ Temperature below 95°F (35°C) with cold skin, drowsiness, quietness and listlessness.
■ Temperature that drops, rising again suddenly.
■ Temperature of more than 100.4°F (38°C) for more than 24 hours.

DIARRHEA
■ Diarrhea that lasts longer than six hours.
■ Diarrhea accompanied by pain in the abdomen, a temperature, or other obvious signs of illness.

NAUSEA AND VOMITING
■ Vomiting that lasts longer than six hours.
■ Prolonged, violent vomiting.
■ Nausea plus dizziness and headaches.
■ Nausea and vomiting accompanied by right-sided pain in the abdomen.

LOSS OF APPETITE

■ If your baby doesn't want food suddenly, or is under six months and doesn't seem to be thriving.
■ If your child usually has a hearty appetite, but refuses all food for a day and seems listless.

■ Loss of appetite with pain and discomfort.
■ Headaches, along with feeling sick and dizzy.
■ If your child complains of blurred vision, especially after a head bang.
■ Severe griping pains at regular intervals.
■ Pain in the right side of the abdomen and feeling sick.

BREATHING

■ If your child's breathing is labored and his ribs draw in sharply with each breath.
■ If your child is wheezing.

Taking your child's temperature and pulse

IN CHILDREN, NORMAL BODY TEMPERATURE RANGES FROM 96.8°F (36°C) TO 98.6°F (37°C). ANY TEMPERATURE OVER 100°F (37.7°C) IS CLASSED AS A FEVER. HYPOTHERMIA DEVELOPS IF THE TEMPERATURE FALLS BELOW 95°F (35°C).

Body temperature will vary according to how active your child has been and the time of day: it is lowest in the morning because there is little muscle activity during sleep, and highest in the late afternoon after a day's activity.

An abnormally hot forehead could be the first indication you have that your child has a temperature. To be accurate, however, you must take your child's temperature with a thermometer. Because the temperature control center in the brain is primitive in young children, the temperature can shoot up more rapidly than in adults. When a fever is present, you should take your child's temperature again after 20 minutes, just in case it was only a transitory leap. Never regard a high temperature as the only accurate reflection of whether your child is ill or not; a child can be very ill without a high temperature or quite healthy with one.

THERMOMETERS

There are two main types of thermometer that are used for children: **digital** and **liquid crystal**. The old-fashioned mercury thermometer is rarely used for children these days.
Digital thermometers are easy to use with children of all ages and are safer than mercury thermometers to use orally since they are unbreakable. Digital thermometers are battery-operated, so be sure to keep spare batteries on hand. Some digital thermometers, known as ear sensors or aural thermometers, are designed to read the temperature from the inside of the ear and can obtain a temperature reading in a few seconds. However a digital rectal thermometer is the most accurate way to take a baby's temperature. If you use an ear sensor, be sure to use the same ear each time.

Liquid crystal thermometers have a heat-sensitive panel on one side and panels with numbers on the other side. When the sensitive side is placed on the forehead, the numbers (your child's temperature) light up. Liquid crystal thermometers are not as accurate as mercury or digital thermometers but are safe and easy to use.

Mercury thermometers are the most accurate means of assessing temperature but are not ususally recommended anymore. Made of glass, they register the temperature when the mercury expands up the tube to a point on the scale. There are two different ways to take a child's temperature with a mercury thermometer, under his armpit or under his tongue, as long as you can trust your child not to bite the thermometer. To read a mercury thermometer, hold it between your finger and thumb and turn it until you can see the point on the scale.

TAKING YOUR CHILD'S PULSE

The pulse is the wave of pressure that passes along each artery every time the heart beats. You can feel the pulse wherever an artery lies close to the skin. The most common site for taking the pulse is at the wrist (radial pulse). The pulse can also be taken in the neck (carotid pulse), although this is normally only done if you suspect the heart has stopped beating altogether, and on the inside of the upper arm (brachial pulse).

The pulse rate will vary with age. It is normally faster after exercise and slower after resting. A young baby's heart will beat about 160 times a minute; by the time he is one year old it will beat about 100–120 times per minute and by the time he is about seven or eight years old, it will have slowed down to the

Taking your child's temperature

Using an ear sensor (aural thermometer)

Using a liquid crystal thermometer

Tips

■ Never take your child's temperature if he has just been running around.
■ Never leave your child alone with a thermometer in his mouth.
■ If using a mercury thermometer, make sure there is no break in the mercury – it will affect the reading.
■ If your thermometer is cracked, throw it away immediately.

Taking a radial, brachial and carotid pulse

Radial pulse
The radial pulse is found on the inside of the wrist below the thumb. Use your index and middle fingers to find it and not your thrumb, which has a pulse of its own.

Brachial pulse
The brachial pulse is found on the inside of the upper arm in the groove between the biceps and triceps muscles (on the front and back of the arm). Use your index and middle fingers to find the pulse.

Carotid pulse
The carotid pulse is found at the top of the neck just to the right or left of the windpipe. Use your index and middle fingers to find it and not your thumb, which has its own pulse.

adult rate of 80–90 beats per minute. A normal pulse is regular and strong; any abnormality, such as a fast, weak pulse or a slow pulse, may indicate that your child is ill.

When taking your child's pulse, use the first two fingers, not your thumb, which contains a pulse of its own. Count the beats over a 15-second period and multiply this figure by four

to get the rate per minute. If your child is under one, it is generally easier to find the brachial pulse, located on the inside of the upper arm.

Giving your child medicine

WHEN YOU TAKE YOUR CHILD TO THE DOCTOR HE MAY PRESCRIBE SOME FORM OF MEDICINE FOR HER.

Ask for as much information as possible about the medicines: ask if there are likely to be any side effects, whether there are foods that should be avoided or special precautions that should be observed while your child is taking the medication, and clarify whether to give the medicine before or after a meal.

Most medicines for young children are made

up in a sweetened syrup to make them more palatable and can be given with a spoon, tube, or dropper. Droppers and tubes are often more suitable for babies who haven't learned to swallow from a spoon. Some medicines for older children are supplied as pills or capsules.

On most occasions your child will be co-operative but there may be an occasion when

she simply refuses to take her medicine. It is very important that your child takes the medicine prescribed when she is ill. In fact, I think that this is one occasion when bribery is justified. So don't hesitate to give the medicine with ice cream or another favorite food. Very occasionally a child will resist physically; there really is no alternative but for you to be forceful.

Giving medicine

Using a spoon
Hold your baby in a semi-reclining position, gently pull his chin down with your finger, and place the spoon on his lower lip. Raise the angle of the spoon and trickle the medicine into his mouth. Don't let the medicine run directly into his throat or he may choke.

Using a dropper
Hold your baby in the crook of your arm and put the filled dropper into the corner of his mouth. Squeeze the bulb slowly and gently to release the medicine. Don't let the medicine run directly down your baby's throat or he may choke.

Using a medicine tube
Hold your baby in the crook of your arm and put the filled tube into the corner of his mouth. Raise the angle of the tube slowly and gently to release the medicine. Don't let the medicine run directly down your baby's throat or he may choke.

Tips for giving medicines

Giving medicines to babies
■ Enlist the help of another adult or older brother or sister.
■ If you are alone, wrap a blanket around your baby's arms so that you can stop him from struggling and hold him steady.
■ Only put a little of the medicine in his mouth at a time.
■ If your baby spits the medicine out, get the other person to hold his mouth open while you carefully trickle the medicine into the back of his mouth. Then, gently but firmly, close his mouth.

Giving medicines to older children
■ Suggest that your child holds her nose while taking the medicine, so lessening the effect of the taste.
■ Don't forcibly hold your child's nose, since she may inhale some of the medicine.
■ Mix liquid medicine with another syrup such as honey.
■ Don't add liquid medicine to a drink, since it will sink to the bottom of the glass or stick to the sides and you won't be sure that your child has had the whole dose.

■ Show your child that you have her favorite drink ready to wash the taste of the medicine away; do this even if you do not normally allow her to have this drink.
■ Help your child to clean her teeth after taking any liquid medicine to prevent syrup from sticking to her teeth.
■ Crush pills (never capsules, however) between two spoons and mix the powder with something sweet, such as honey, jam, or ice cream.

Giving drops

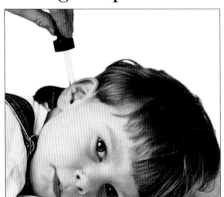

Ear drops
Ask your child to lie on his side. Using a dropper and ear drops that have been warmed to body temperature, squeeze the bulb and let the drops fall into the center of his ear.

Nose drops
Ask your child to lie on his back with his head tilted backward. Using a dropper and nose drops that have been warmed to body temperature, squeeze the bulb and let two or three drops fall into each nostril.

Eye drops
Ask your child to lie on her back. Gently pull down the lower lid of the affected eye and squeeze the dropper's bulb, letting one or two drops fall inside the eyelid.

On the whole, older children do not generally mind medicine too much and often want to pour it out for themselves rather than let you give it to them. I have listed a few tips (see box, above) that may help if your child is difficult. For example, pills can be crushed and mixed with jam or ice cream. Capsules, however, should not be broken.

GIVING DROPS
Ear, nose, or eye infections are generally treated with external drops. It is always easier to administer drops to a baby or young child if you lay her on a flat surface before you begin and enlist some help to keep her still and hold her head steady. An older child will probably be more cooperative and you will only need to ask her to tilt her head back or to the side, while you put the drops in.

Tips for giving drops

Giving drops
■ Warm nose drops and ear drops by standing the container in a bowl of warm, not hot, water for a few minutes, so that your child doesn't get too much of a shock when the liquid drops into his nose or ear.
■ Be careful not to let the dropper touch your child's nose, ear, or eye, or you will transfer the germs back to the bottle. If the dropper does touch your child, make sure you wash it thoroughly before putting it back into the bottle.
■ Commericial drops should not be used for longer than three days without consulting a doctor – if they are used for too long, they can cause irritation and inflammation that is worse than the condition you were treating.

Your medicine chest

You should always keep some medicines in the house in case of an emergency in the middle of the night when you may not be able to get to a pharmacy easily. Keep them somewhere obvious so that you can find them quickly when you need them. Never mix different pills up in the same container and never keep any leftover prescription medicines. Keep all medicines well out of reach of children, in a high, locked cupboard, if necessary. You should also have a first aid kit (see p. 565). Keep all the equipment in a clean, dry, airtight box and put it somewhere it can be found in an emergency.

The items listed below would all be useful to have in emergencies and are therefore well worth keeping in the house.

Medicine cabinet
■ Digital or liquid crystal thermometer – keep two for safety.
■ Junior acetaminophen.

■ Acetaminophen – depending on age and weight of the child, use infant drops or liquid form.
■ Calamine lotion.
■ Mild antiseptic wipes.
■ Cotton balls.
■ Mild antiseptic cream.
■ Gauze dressings – keep dry and paraffin-coated ones.
■ Surgical tape.
■ Crepe bandages for sprains and strains.
■ Open-weave bandages.
■ Triangular bandage.
■ Safety pins, scissors, and blunt-edged tweezers.

Useful household items
■ Package of frozen peas, or ice cubes in plastic bags for cold compresses.
■ Newspaper (folded it can make a splint).
■ Elastic belt to support a strain/sprain.
■ Rehydration fluid to replace fluid lost after vomiting or diarrhea.

■ Bicarbonate of soda to add to a bath to relieve itching.
■ Salt to add to a bath to clean wounds and deter infection.
■ Vinegar to mix with water to soothe jellyfish stings.

Medicines to avoid
The following items, commonly given as useful, should be avoided:
■ Any commerical product containing a local anesthetic, such as lidocaine, because they can cause allergies. They are most generally found in creams for mouth ulcers or insect stings.
■ Any skin creams containing antihistamines (unless prescribed by your doctor); they can cause skin allergies.
■ Any commerical product that contains aspirin.
■ Mouth washes, gargles, eye drops, nose drops, and ear drops, unless recommended by your doctor.

Nursing a sick child

YOU DON'T NEED ANY SPECIAL SKILLS OR MEDICAL KNOWLEDGE TO CARE FOR YOUR SICK CHILD. IT HELPS IF YOU RELAX THE RULES AND TRY TO HIDE YOUR ANXIETY FROM HER. DON'T INSIST THAT SHE EATS WHILE SHE IS ILL, BUT DO ENCOURAGE HER TO DRINK A LOT OF FLUIDS.

In addition to as whatever treatment the doctor recommends, the following routines will help your child to feel more comfortable while she is ill.
■ Air your child's room and bed at least once a day.
■ Leave a bowl by your child's bed if she is vomiting or has whooping cough.
■ Leave a box of tissues by your child's bed.
■ Give small meals frequently; your child may find large portions off-putting.
■ Give liquid acetaminophen for pain relief.

SHOULD YOUR CHILD BE IN BED?
At the beginning of an illness when your child is feeling quite poorly she will probably want to stay in bed and she may sleep a lot. As she starts to feel better she will still need bed rest, but she will want to be around you and she may want intervals of playing. The best way to accommodate this is to make up a bed on the sofa in a room near where you are working so that she can lie down when she wants to. Don't insist that your child goes to bed just because she is ill – children with a fever, for example, don't recover faster if they stay in bed. When your child is tired, however, it is

time to put her to bed. But don't just leave her alone. Make sure that you visit her at regular intervals (every half an hour), and find time to stay and play a game, read a book, or do a puzzle.

When she's on the road to recovery make sure that enough happens in her day to make the distinction between night and day. If she hasn't been watching television, let her watch it before bedtime.

GIVING DRINKS
It is essential that your child drinks a lot when she's ill – when she has a fever, diarrhea or is vomiting – because she will be dehydrated and will need to replace lost fluids. The recommended fluid intake for a child with a fever is 1–2 fluid ounces per pound (100–150 milliliters per kilogram) of body weight per day, which is the equivalent of 20 ounces (1 liter) per day for a child who weighs 20 pounds (9 kilograms).

Encourage your child to drink by leaving her favorite drink at her bedside (preferably not sugary, carbonated drinks such as cola), by putting drinks in glasses that are especially appealing, and by giving her bendable straws to drink with.

OCCUPYING YOUR CHILD
Illness is an occasion when you can completely indulge your child. When she is not resting, spend time playing games and talking to her. Relax all the rules and let her play whatever games she wants to, even if you've previously disallowed them in bed. If your child wants to do something messy like painting, just spread an old sheet or a sheet of plastic over the bed. If you can, move a television into her room temporarily – this will keep her entertained and make her feel special as well.

Let her do some painting; read aloud to her; get out some of her old toys and play with them together; sing songs or make up a story together; ask her to draw a picture of what she is going to do when she feels better; and, unless she has an infectious illness, let some friends visit her for a brief period during the day. As your child gets better let her play outside, but if she has a fever discourage her from running around too much.

VOMITING
Your child will probably find vomiting a distressing experience and you should try and make her as comfortable as possible. Get her

to sit up in bed and make sure there is a bowl or a bucket within easy reach, so that she doesn't have to run to the toilet. If your child's hair is in the way, tie it back. When she is vomiting hold her head and comfort her. Afterward help your child to clean her teeth, or give her a peppermint candy to suck to take the taste away.

When your child hasn't vomited for a few hours and she's feeling hungry, offer her bland foods, such as mashed potato, but don't encourage her to eat if she doesn't want to. More important than eating is maintaining a constant level of fluids. Give your child lots of water, or use a commercial rehydration solution that you can buy at the pharmacy – be sure to follow the instructions on the package carefully when you make it up. Avoid drinks such as milk, but give fruit juice diluted with water.

TREATING A HIGH TEMPERATURE
The first sign of a high temperature is often a hot forehead, but to check that your child is feverish take her temperature (see p. 515).

Immunization timetable

What is given?	How is it given?	When is it given?
POLIO	Injection	At 2, 4, 6 months and 4–6 years
HIB, DIPHTHERIA, TETANUS, PERTUSSIS,	Injection	At 2, 4, 6, 12–15 months and 4–6 years (no Hib)
VARICELLA	Injection	At 1 year
MEASLES, MUMPS, RUBELLA (MMR)	Injection	At 12 months and 4–6 years
HEPATITIS B	Injection	Usually 1, 2, and 6 months

Call your doctor if the fever is over 102.2°F (39°C), lasts more than 24 hours or if there are accompanying symptoms. Temperatures over 100°F (37.7°C) should be taken very seriously in children under six months.

Try to cool your child down by taking off her clothes and getting her to lie in bed. Cover her with a cotton sheet and take her temperature every hour or so. Changing the sheets on her bed regularly will help keep her comfortable. Try giving her liquid acetaminophen (aspirin is dangerous for children). It's still important for her to drink a lot of fluid since she will be perspiring a lot.

Your child in the hospital

YOU WILL BE DOING YOUR CHILD A GREAT FAVOR IF YOU ENCOURAGE HIM TO THINK ABOUT HOSPITALS AS FRIENDLY PLACES. TRY TO TAKE HIM WITH YOU IF YOU ARE VISITING A FAMILY FRIEND OR RELATIVE – PROVIDED THE PERSON DOES NOT MIND AND VISITING REGULATIONS ALLOW IT.

PREPARING YOUR CHILD
If your child has to go into the hospital, for an operation, for example, and you are given some warning, prepare him by discussing as many aspects of it as possible. Talk about it with the rest of the family as well and get him generally used to the idea.

Answer all his questions honestly. Don't make promises that you can't keep and don't tell lies. If he is having an operation, he will probably ask you if there will be any pain or discomfort after the operation. If you say that nothing is going to hurt and it does, he will simply get a shock and will not trust you in the future. Explain that there will be some discomfort but that it will not last long.

Another good way to prepare him for a hospital stay is to read him a book about someone who goes into hospital. You could also buy him a toy stethoscope and play doctors and nurses with him. Encourage him to be the doctor or nurse and suggest that he makes up a hospital bed for his favorite teddy bear or toy.

IN HOSPITAL
Few children's wards are frightening places. However, hospitals have found that it is very important for parents to be with their children as much as possible while they are in the hospital and, because of this, almost all now allow parents to stay with their child,

particularly if he is very young. Many hospitals have sleeping facilities for parents with children up to the age of six.

When you are there, ask the nurses how you can help with the daily routine. You might be encouraged to bathe and change your child, and to help with his feeding. You can read books and play games with him and any other children in the ward who want to join in. If the ward has a teacher, ask if you can help with your child's schoolwork. If he is well enough and will be in hospital for a while, ask his own teacher to give you the work he would normally be doing at school.

If you cannot be with your child all day, try to arrange a rotation so that someone he knows well is with him all the time.

BACK HOME FROM THE HOSPITAL
It's quite normal for a child to behave a little oddly when he comes out of the hospital. Firstly, your child's sleeping and eating patterns may have changed. Hospital meals, and certainly bedtimes, tend to be earlier than you'd have them at home. Secondly, because your child has been away from his domestic discipline, you may find that he will make a fuss about small things like brushing his teeth. Don't be too hard on him at first, give him time to readjust to being at home before you insist that he fits in with the old routine.

Packing for the hospital

If you can, you and your child should pack his case together a few days before he has to go in.
- Three pairs of pajamas.
- Robe and slippers.
- Three pairs of ankle socks.
- Hair brush and comb.
- Sponge bag with soap, washcloth, toothbrush, toothpaste.
- Bedside clock.
- Portable radio or cassette player with headphones.
- Favorite books and portable games.
- Favorite picture or photograph to put by his bedside.

CONGENITAL CONDITIONS

Congenital conditions are those that are present from birth; they may also be genetic, meaning that they are caused by a defective gene.

Many congenital conditions such as developmental dysplasia of the hip or phimosis are relatively minor, while others, such as some congenital heart defects, are more serious.

The good news is that many congenital conditions are now treatable and children who receive early treatment can expect to lead normal lives.

Cerebral palsy

CEREBRAL PALSY IS THE NAME GIVEN TO DAMAGE TO THE BRAIN THAT OCCURS EARLY IN LIFE AND RESULTS IN A LACK OF FULL CONTROL OF PHYSICAL MOVEMENT.

In most children, the damage occurs in pregnancy though in a few others, during a difficult labor, the baby may suffer from a lack of oxygen. However, it is usually not possible to determine the exact cause of cerebral palsy. It may result if a premature baby has severe breathing problems, with bleeding in the brain and lack of oxygen both contributing to the condition. Noncongenital causes include serious head injury and meningitis.

WHAT ARE THE SYMPTOMS?
Because the more sophisticated voluntary control centers of the brain do not function in the first months of life, cerebral palsy may not be apparent at birth. After a few months it may show itself if the child is slow to sit up, is generally unsteady, or cannot grasp and hold things. Cerebral palsy may affect only one side (for example, the right arm and leg), both legs with the arms hardly affected at all, or all four limbs and the trunk. Walking is delayed but usually possible. If the limbs tend to be stiff and fixed in certain postures the child is technically termed "spastic." If he is prone to frequent, purposeless writhing movements he is said to be "athetoid."

Cerebral palsy is not a progressive disease that gets steadily worse. And it's very common for children with cerebral palsy to have normal intelligence and normal social capabilities.

WHAT IS THE TREATMENT?
The treatment for cerebral palsy consists of trying to develop the child's physical, mental, and social capabilities to the full. Therefore it is important that the child is fully assessed by a specialist and a physical therapist so that he can be given treatment at an early age. Stretching exercises will prevent fixed deformity of the limbs; orthopedic appliances such as calipers, and in some cases surgery, can improve mobility; and treatment, such as speech therapy, can compensate for the physical disability.

When there is no mental handicap, the outlook is extremely good. Children adjust quite well to severe lack of motor function as long as their intellectual capacity is good and they can make themselves understood.

WHAT CAN I DO?
The reaction of the family is of great importance. Parents must guard against feeling sorry for the child. If there are other children in the family the child must be treated as much as possible in the same way as they are, although this may be hard for parents. As with all disabled children the emphasis should be on what the child can do rather than on what he cannot.

Congenital heart disease

CONGENITAL HEART DISEASE MEANS THAT ONE OR MORE DEFECTS OF THE HEART ARE PRESENT AT BIRTH.

WHAT ARE THE SYMPTOMS?
Minor congenital heart defects may not cause symptoms. If symptoms are present, they may include the following things.
■ Shortness of breath, leading to difficulty in feeding.
■ Slow weight gain and growth.
■ Bluish coloration to the tongue and lips, if oxygen levels in the blood are low.
■ Susceptibility to chest infections or infection of the lining of the heart.

WHAT IS THE TREATMENT?
Many heart defects correct themselves or need no treatment. Only about 1 in 3 children requires surgery. Affected children are usually monitored through childhood and if necessary surgery is performed when the child is older and the operation is easier. A heart transplant is now a possibility for children with multiple heart defects. Chest infections need to be treated promptly and if the child has dental treatment or surgery antibiotics are necessary to prevent infection of the lining of the heart. Some children will need drugs such as diuretics to control the symptoms of a heart defect.

WHAT IS THE OUTLOOK?
Septal defects may close naturally or be corrected surgically. Surgical advances over the last 20 years mean that even very severe defects can often be corrected.

Types of congenital heart disease

■ Septal defects (usually a hole in the inner wall that divides the heart, known as the septum; often called a "hole in the heart").
■ Patent ductus arteriosus (failure of a small blood vessel in the heart, known as the ductus arteriosus, to close soon after birth, preventing normal circulation).
■ Valve defects (any abnormality occurring in one or more of the four heart valves).
■ Multiple defects (rarely, several heart defects occur together).

directory children's conditions

Developmental dysplasia of the hip

DEVELOPMENTAL DYSPLASIA OF THE HIP IS A TERM THAT COVERS A WIDE RANGE OF PROBLEMS WITH THE HIP JOINT IN NEWBORN BABIES. THESE PROBLEMS ARE SIX TIMES MORE COMMON IN GIRLS THAN IN BOYS AND SOMETIMES RUN IN FAMILIES, SUGGESTING A GENETIC FACTOR.

In mild cases, the hip joint moves excessively when manipulated; in moderate cases, the head of the femur (thighbone) slips out of the hip socket when manipulated but can be eased back in; in severe cases, the dislocation is permanent with the head of the femur lying outside the hip socket. Simple manipulation of your baby's hips to test for congenital hip dislocation is usually done shortly after birth and by your doctor during routine development checkups.

Hip dislocation occurs more often in the left hip and sometimes affects both hips. In cultures where babies are regularly carried astride their mothers' backs, hip dislocation rarely persists.

WHAT ARE THE SYMPTOMS?

Mild forms of hip dislocation may cause no symptoms. Otherwise, symptoms include:
● asymmetrical creases in the skin on the backs of the baby's legs
● inability to turn the affects leg out fully at the hip
● shorter appearance of the affected leg
● limping when older if the condition is not treated early.

SHOULD I CONSULT THE DOCTOR?

Consult your doctor as soon as possible if you suspect that there is a problem with your baby's hips. If hip dislocation is not corrected early, it may lead to permanent deformity and early onset of osteoarthritis.

WHAT IS THE TREATMENT?

If your doctor suspects developmental dysplasia of the hip, he may arrange for ultrasound scanning to confirm the diagnosis. The less severe forms of the condition often correct themselves during the first 3 weeks of life. If the problem persists, the hip joint may be positioned in a harness for 8–12 weeks to hold the head of the femur in the hip, allowing the hip socket to develop normally. In older babies the hip may have to be held in a cast for up to 6 months to correct the problem. If treatment is unsuccessful surgery may be necessary. If hip dysplasia is treated promptly most babies develop normal hip joints and there is no lasting damage.

Cystic fibrosis

CYSTIC FIBROSIS IS A RARE DISEASE THAT IS PRESENT AT BIRTH AND INHERITED FROM BOTH PARENTS.

If the mother and father are healthy, but each carries one defective gene for cystic fibrosis, each child conceived has a 25 percent chance of inheriting two defective genes and being born with the disease.

Cystic fibrosis causes several glands in the body to be defective, particularly the glands in the lining of the bronchial tubes. Instead of producing the normal thin mucus, the bronchial glands produce a thick, sticky phlegm that creates blockages in the air passages and this in turn leads to lung infections. When small parts of the lungs collapse pneumonia results. This is a common and recurrent infection in cystic fibrosis sufferers.

In cystic fibrosis, the pancreas fails to produce certain enzymes that are vital to digestion. These enzymes break down food so that it can be absorbed easily by the body. When these enzymes are missing food is poorly digested, which leads to diarrhea and foul-smelling stools. Because the body does not absorb many of the nutrients that are essential to good health the child with cystic fibrosis tends to be small, underweight and fails to thrive. Bouts of diarrhea may alternate with constipation that can actually block the intestine.

Parents with an affected child who are planning another pregnancy are offered genetic counseling.

WHAT ARE THE SYMPTOMS?

■ Recurrent chest infections with a cough and some breathing difficulty.
■ Diarrhea, alternating with constipation.
■ Greasy and foul-smelling bowel motions.
■ Failure to thrive.
■ Swollen abdomen and wasted limbs.

WHAT IS THE TREATMENT?

There is no cure for cystic fibrosis, but early detection of the condition lessens the chance of permanent damage to the lungs. Simple tests on the blood or stools of a newborn baby can be carried out, but the definitive test for cystic fibrosis is a sweat test because there is an increased salt level in the sweat of sufferers. This will be done on all brothers and sisters of a child with cystic fibrosis, or if a baby has recurrent bouts of pneumonia or fails to thrive. The tests are carried out when the baby is about three months of age.

Respiratory infections are treated with antibiotics; sometimes a spray form is used for speedy inhalation. Other treatments include inhaling enzymes to help dissolve lung secretions, or a heart-lung transplant.

The gene for cystic fibrosis has been identified and gene therapy will almost certainly be a future option.

WHAT CAN I DO?

A child with cystic fibrosis has to have a special low-fat diet, with vitamin supplements and enzyme replacements, which can be taken orally. Physical therapy and breathing exercises must be done daily to loosen and drain mucus from the lungs. Exposure to moist air and a cold steam vaporizer can also help the lungs.

People with cystic fibrosis need daily chest physical therapy to keep the lungs free of mucus.

Pyloric stenosis

IN CONGENITAL PYLORIC STENOSIS THE RING OF MUSCLE (PYLORUS) THAT LINKS THE STOMACH TO THE DUODENUM THICKENS AND NARROWS, PREVENTING THE STOMACH FROM EMPTYING. THE CAUSE IS NOT KNOWN BUT WHEN THE BABY IS ABOUT ONE MONTH OLD THE SYMPTOMS BEGIN.

Food builds up in the stomach, which contracts powerfully in an attempt to force the food through the thickened pylorus. Because this is impossible milk is vomited up violently after a feeding. This is known as projectile vomiting and the unpleasant smelling milk curds and mucus can be thrown for up to two yards (a meter or two). Projectile vomiting should not be confused with spitting up, in which a baby naturally regurgitates milk after a feeding. Pyloric stenosis is much more common in boys.

Pyloric stenosis is serious. Vomiting eventually leads to dehydration and a failure to thrive.

WHAT ARE THE SYMPTOMS?
■ Projectile vomiting after a feeding, beginning at around four weeks of age.
■ Failure to thrive.
■ Weakness and listlessness.
■ Lack of bowel movements.

SHOULD I SEE THE DOCTOR?
Consult your doctor immediately if your baby vomits violently after every feeding.

WHAT IS THE TREATMENT?
If pyloric stenosis is supected, your doctor will refer your baby to the hospital. A pediatrician will examine your baby's abdomen during a feeding to see if the enlarged pylorus can be felt. Usually an ultrasound and blood tests will be ordered to confirm diagnosis, and a simple surgery is performed, giving a complete cure.

WHAT CAN I DO?
Stay with your baby in the hospital. After the operation you will be advised to feed your baby gradually increasing amounts of milk. 48 hours after the operation, his feeding routine should be back to normal.

Down syndrome

DOWN SYNDROME IS THE MOST COMMON CHROMOSOMAL ABNORMALITY. CHILDREN WITH DOWN SYNDROME HAVE 47 CHROMOSOMES INSTEAD OF THE NORMAL 46 IN EACH CELL. THE EXTRA CHROMOSOME, CHROMOSOME 21, USUALLY COMES FROM THE MOTHER'S EGG.

The incidence of Down syndrome babies rises sharply with maternal age, but various forms of screening in pregnancy can identify the condition in the fetus and a termination can be performed if the parents wish. Chorionic villus sampling or nuchal scanning (scanning of the fetal neck) can be done between 9 and 13 weeks of pregnancy. At around 20 weeks, an amniocentesis test is usually offered to pregnant women of 35 or over. Blood tests (known as the triple test) can also be done at this stage.

A new screening test for Down syndrome can identify more than 90 percent of cases after only 12 weeks of pregnancy. It's done six to eight weeks earlier than the triple test and will detect 30 percent more cases. It works by combining several of the methods to detect Down syndrome described above. The 5 percent of patients deemed most at risk are then offered a definitive diagnosis procedure, such as chorionic villus sampling or amniocentesis.

WHAT ARE THE SYMPTOMS?
■ Small, upward-slanting eyes; nose with a wide bridge; short, broad hands with a deep crease across the palm; gap between the first and second toes.
■ Some degree of learning difficulty.

WHAT IS THE TREATMENT?
The degree of learning difficulty varies widely in children with Down syndrome, and a few may be within the normal intelligence range. Modern theories reject the idea that all children with Down syndrome should be educated in special institutions. The education of a child with Down syndrome must be determined by the specific learning difficulty of the child, but children with Down syndrome are usually educated in mainstream schools. As with all children, the emphasis should be on what the child can do rather than what she cannot.

Almost all children with Down syndrome will learn to walk and talk and some will learn to read and write. They will need extra help to fulfill their potential, but with this help many will go on to lead semi-independent lives.

Muscular dystrophy

MUSCULAR DYSTROPHY IS A GROUP OF GENETIC CONDITIONS IN WHICH
MUSCLES BECOME WEAK AND WASTED.

Hydrocephalus

THE TERM "HYDROCEPHALUS" MEANS WATER ON THE BRAIN, AND THIS CONDITION RESULTS WHEN
THERE IS EXCESSIVE PRESSURE INSIDE THE BRAIN DUE TO A BUILDUP OF CEREBROSPINAL FLUID.

Cerebrospinal fluid, or CSF, carries nutrients to the brain and acts as a protective fluid buffer. If the circulation of CSF is blocked for some reason, or if the fluid is produced in too great a quantity, the buildup of fluid increases pressure inside the brain. The brain tissue becomes thinner and the bones of the skull stretch to accommodate the excess fluid. The pressure on the brain can cause brain damage and if untreated, more than 50 percent of hydrocephalic infants die.

WHAT ARE THE SYMPTOMS?
■ Abnormal head size at birth, or rapid growth of it in the following months.
■ Veins standing out on scalp.
■ Swollen fontanelle.
■ Headache.
■ Vomiting.

The symptoms depend on the age at which hydrocephalus develops in the child. If it is present at birth, the head is abnormally large because the skull bones have been pushed apart by the fluid; in such cases the baby will probably also suffer from spina bifida, a neural tube defect (see below). In milder forms the head may be normal at birth but grow at an excessive rate in the following months.

Hydrocephalus can also develop later in childhood as the result of a tumor or an infection such as meningitis when there may be no appreciable enlargement of the head, although the pressure of the fluid on the brain may cause headaches and vomiting.

WHAT IS THE TREATMENT?
If the condition is present at birth, it will normally be noticed by the doctor at delivery or at regular checkups when your baby's head

is measured to check the size. A careful initial evaluation by a pediatrician is necessary to determine the exact cause of the buildup of fluid. In mild cases drugs may be used to prevent excess production of CSF. Otherwise, provided the hydrocephalus is not too advanced, the condition will be relieved surgically. Under anesthetic, a fine tube with a one-way valve is inserted into the brain through a hole in the skull. The other end is usually inserted into the peritoneal (abdominal) cavity where fluid from the brain drains. After these treatments the baby's head gradually returns to normal; about 40 percent of hydrocephalic infants then go on to develop near normal intelligence. If at some stage after the operation your child becomes irritable and is vomiting, a blockage of the tube will be suspected. The tube will be replaced or the blockage removed.

Neural tube defects

NEURAL TUBE DEFECTS ARE ABNORMALITIES OF THE BRAIN AND SPINAL CORD
AND THEIR PROTECTIVE COVERINGS.

The neural tube, which develops along the back of the embryo by about the third week of pregnancy, later becomes the brain and spinal cord and their coverings. If this tube fails to close completely defects in any of these parts can result. The most common neural tube defect is spina bifida, in which the spinal cord and vertebrae are affected. Effects may vary from a dimple or tuft of hair at the base of the spine and a minor abnormality of the vertebrae to complete exposure of part of the spinal cord. Rarely, the brain and skull are affected. Neural tube defects tend to run in families, suggesting that genetic factors are involved.

Since the discovery in 1992 that folic acid taken before conception and during early pregnancy provides protection against neural tube defects, spina bifida is becoming less common.

WHAT ARE THE SYMPTOMS?
In minor cases, there are no obvious symptoms, and spina bifida may only be diagnosed when a minor condition such as

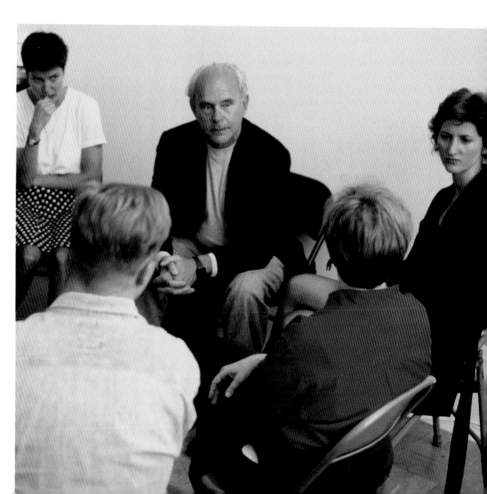

Family support group
*Families of children affected by congenital disorders
such as spina bifida may find it helpful to meet to
offer each other practical and emotional support.*

backache occurs in adult life. Symptoms may become apparent in childhood and mainly affect the lower body, including:
- a dimple or brown, hairy mole at the base of the spine
- paralysis or weakness of the legs
- absence of sensation in the legs
- abnormalities in bladder or bowel function.

Many children with severe spina bifida also have a buildup of fluid in the brain (hydrocephalus).

SHOULD I CONSULT THE DOCTOR?
If you are concerned about your child's ability to move his legs or bladder or bowel functioning, consult your doctor as soon as possible.

WHAT IS THE TREATMENT?
A baby who has a neural tube defect will probably have CT scanning or a MRI of the spine to assess the severity of the defect. If the defect is minor, no treatment is necessary. However, if a baby has a serious defect, he is likely to require surgery in the first few days after birth. Even with surgery, children who are born with severe defects will be permanently disabled and need lifelong care. If no action is taken in such severe cases, the babies usually die peacefully within weeks of birth.

If your child is severely affected, you will need practical and emotional support from a team of specialists including doctors, physical therapists, and special education teachers.

Your family may also find it helpful to join a support group.

WHAT CAN I DO?
You can reduce the risk of your baby having a neural tube defect by taking folic acid supplements (usually 400 micrograms per day) during the first three months of pregnancy, and if possible while you are trying to conceive. Your doctor may suggest a slightly higher dose if you already have an affected child.

See also:
- CT scanning p. 401
- Hydrocephalus p. 524 • MRI p. 409

Hypospadias

HYPOSPADIAS IS A COMMON BIRTH DEFECT IN WHICH THE OPENING OF THE URETHRA (THE PASSAGE THAT CARRIES URINE FROM THE BLADDER TO OUTSIDE THE BODY) DEVELOPS ON THE UNDERSIDE OF THE SHAFT OF THE PENIS INSTEAD OF AT THE TIP.

Most commonly, the opening develops near the end of the penis, but in severe cases it can occur far back toward the scrotum.

Sometimes, part of the foreskin may be missing and the penis curves downward, a condition known as **chordee**. Hypospadias can run in families, suggesting that a genetic factor may be involved. The condition is usually detected during the routine examination following birth.

WHAT IS THE TREATMENT?
Hypospadias is usually treated with surgery before the age of 2. During the operation the foreskin is used to form an extension to the existing urethra so that it reaches the tip of the penis, and it is important that your son is not circumcized if he is born with hypospadias. If chordee is also present, it can be corrected during the same operation. Treatment usually allows urine to be passed normally, and sexual activity and fertility in later life are not affected.

Phimosis

PHIMOSIS IS THE NAME GIVEN TO AN ABNORMAL TIGHTNESS OF THE FORESKIN THAT PREVENTS IT FROM BEING DRAWN BACK OVER THE TIP (GLANS) OF THE PENIS.

Phimosis can result in infections such as balanitis because the penis cannot be properly cleansed; it may also cause problems with urination and pain with erections. If the foreskin fails to loosen naturally, circumcision is usually recommended. Never attempt to force the foreskin back, especially if your child is under five years old.

WHAT ARE THE SYMPTOMS?
- Foreskin cannot be drawn back over the tip of the penis.
- Urine does not come out in a steady stream; it either dribbles out slowly or the foreskin balloons with the pressure of the urine, which sprays out in all directions.

SHOULD I SEE THE DOCTOR?
Consult your doctor if you are concerned about the condition or if the foreskin has not loosened naturally by the time your child is five or six years old. Consult your doctor as soon as possible if the foreskin has been forced back and won't slide forward again.

WHAT IS THE TREATMENT?
- If possible, your doctor will return the foreskin to its normal position if it has been pulled back and won't return.
- Your doctor may refer you to a surgeon for permanent correction of the condition by circumcision. Your child will be admitted to the hospital and the foreskin removed under a general anesthetic. Your child will be discharged from the hospital within 24 hours.

WHAT CAN I DO?
- Try not to worry about the condition if your son is under five years old; it may correct itself in time.
- Make sure your child bathes frequently. A warm bath is the best way to keep an uncircumcized penis clean and to prevent infection. Retraction of the foreskin to clean the penis should not be necessary.
- If your child has just been circumcized, give him baths with a handful of salt in them twice a day to promote healing.
- Let him go around without pants on – anything rubbing on a recently circumcized penis will make it sore.
- Give your newly circumcized child a bowl of warm water to pour over his penis when he urinates. There will be some pain on passing urine for about 48 hours after the operation.

Checking for undescended testicles

When a baby boy is born a pediatrician will examine his testicles to see if they have descended. If not you will be advised of the fact and reassured that they may descend naturally. If your baby's testicles did not descend at birth, feel for them occasionally in the scrotum. If they have descended, they will feel small – each about the size of a pea. Warm your hands before you do this; otherwise the testicles may temporarily retract into the abdomen.

Undescended testicle

THE TESTICLES GROW AND DEVELOP INSIDE THE ABDOMEN NEAR THE KIDNEYS.

Shortly before a boy is born they move down or "descend" into their normal position in the bag of skin called the scrotum. For testicles to develop normally at adolescence and produce sperm they must hang outside the body. This is because sperm production can proceed only at a temperature that is slightly below the body's internal temperature. If the testicles – or more usually one testicle – fail to descend, sperm will not be produced normally but the hormone testosterone (which produces male characteristics, such as a deeper voice and body hair) will be.

SHOULD I SEE A DOCTOR?
Theoretically one descended testicle could be sufficient to produce sperm and male hormones but if your son's testicles have failed

to descend by the age of 2 you should consult your doctor.

WHAT IS THE TREATMENT?
Your doctor will probably take action before your son is five or six years old. If a boy's testicles fail to descend many surgeons recommend operating before the age of 2½ years. An undescended testicle that is producing testosterone can increase the risk of testicular cancer if left untreated.

WHAT CAN I DO?
■ Stay with your child in the hospital when he has the operation to lower his testicles.
■ Keep your son quiet and calm after the operation. If he engages too soon in boisterous play he could damage the scrotum.

Birthmarks

A BIRTHMARK IS A PATCH OF DISCOLORED SKIN CAUSED BY A COLLECTION OF SMALL BLOOD VESSELS OR PIGMENT JUST UNDER THE SURFACE OF THE SKIN. IT IS PRESENT AT BIRTH OR APPEARS SOON AFTERWARD.

There are three types of birthmarks: vascular birthmarks, strawberry birthmarks, and port wine stains.

VASCULAR BIRTHMARKS
These are birthmarks made up of abnormal blood vessels in the skin. The most common is the so-called **salmon patch**, which affects one in every two newborn infants.

Salmon patches are found on the eyelids, the bridge of the nose, the upper lip, and the nape of the neck (where they are called stork bites). They fade during infancy (except perhaps on the nape of the neck) and no treatment is required. More important are the rarer birthmarks, known as strawberry marks and port wine stains. Their features and treatment are discussed below.

WHAT ARE STRAWBERRY MARKS?
Strawberry marks affect 2 percent or more of babies. They are raised red soft lumps on the skin, usually about half an inch or larger, and look like a strawberry. They are also called capillary hemangiomas or cavernous hemangiomas if they are deeper in the skin or appear blue in color. The blood vessels in these birthmarks are increased in size and number.

Strawberry marks are not a sign of ill health, and are not connected with cancer. They can

occur anywhere on the skin but are more important when they affect the face or diaper area. These birthmarks are often not obvious at birth, but grow in the first months of life. Rarely they grow quite large and may bleed or become infected or ulcerated.

WHY DO THEY DEVELOP?
Strawberry marks are more common in premature babies. They seem to arise from "left over" groups of cells in the baby's skin. Many myths have developed about them but no parent should feel responsible for these blemishes.

DO STRAWBERRY MARKS DISAPPEAR?
The birthmark may continue to grow for the first 3 to 6 months and sometimes for longer. Then they slowly shrink. In 30 percent of children the birthmark will fade by the third birthday and by the fifth birthday in 50 percent. By the seventh birthday 70 percent will have faded. Shrinkage is not influenced by the position, the size, or the number of birthmarks. Sometimes the skin over the birthmark remains rather thinned or baggy after the hemangioma has shrunk. Plastic surgery can improve the appearance if there is a problem.

WHAT TREATMENTS ARE AVAILABLE?
Usually no treatment is needed as most hemangiomas will shrink on their own. Children are seldom aware of their blemishes before the age of 3, and by then the birthmark will usually be fading. Large or troublesome strawberry marks in certain places, for instance near the eye, may need treatment to avoid

affecting the vision in that eye. Steroid medicine or injections shrink the blood vessels. Interferon given by injection is used in special cases. Rarely surgery is considered to reduce the size of the birthmark. Laser treatment can be used to speed up healing of ulcerated birthmarks and to stop bleeding but is not used routinely for these birthmarks.

WHAT ARE PORT WINE STAINS?

A port wine stain is a red or purple birthmark that affects 1 out of every 500 babies. Port wine stains are present at birth and grow with the child. They do not improve with time. They can occur on any part of the skin surface but cause most concern when they affect the face. They are also called nevus flammeus.

WHY DO THEY DEVELOP?

Port wine stains develop because the blood vessels in the affected skin lack small nerve fibers that are necessary to narrow them. The result of this is that the affected blood vessels are wide open with increased blood flow through the involved skin. This results in a permanent blush – a port wine stain.

DO THEY CHANGE WITH AGE?

Yes; in babies and children, port wine stains are flat and pink. As people get older the blood vessels in port wine stains may become bigger and blood flows through them more slowly. At this stage, they look more purple than pink. Later, in adult life, port wine stains often develop bumpy areas which can make applying cosmetic camouflage difficult. Occasionally bleeding can occur in the bumpy areas if they are scratched.

ARE THERE ANY ASSOCIATED PROBLEMS?

Facial port wine stains can occasionally affect the eye or other underlying organs and in certain cases further investigation is necessary. If it occurs on an arm or a leg, it is usual to check that the growth of the limb is normal.

PSYCHOLOGICAL PROBLEMS

Port wine stains cause a lot of misery because they occur so often in visible areas important for the body image, such as the face. A lot can be done to reduce the psychological impact including treatments discussed below, camouflage and advice from patient support groups.

IS TREATMENT AVAILABLE AND SUCCESSFUL?

Yes – usually. Treatment with the pulsed dye laser helps most patients although it may not clear the port wine stain completely. It is available in a few specialized centers. Port wine stains in older children can be treated under a local anesthetic, often using an anesthetic cream. Young children and those having very extensive areas treated, especially around the eyes, need to have their laser therapy under a general anesthetic or sedation.

Laser treatment lightens 90 percent or more of port wine stains in children. Depending on the size and site of the birthmark, up to 10 treatment sessions may be required at intervals of eight weeks or so. Port wine stains on limbs respond less well than those on the face.

Cosmetic camouflage

Cosmetic or camouflage creams are often very helpful. Dermatologists can provide advice on where to find these types of products and how to use them. The American Academy of Dermatologists (see Useful addresses, p. 567) also offers information about birthmarks.

Leg and foot problems

MINOR CONGENITAL LEG AND FOOT PROBLEMS INCLUDE IN-TOEING ("PIGEON" TOES), OUT-TOEING, BOWLEGS, KNOCK-KNEES, AND FLAT FEET. DIFFERENT MINOR LEG AND FOOT PROBLEMS IN CHILDREN ARE COMMON AT DIFFERENT AGES.

Minor leg and foot problems rarely interfere with walking or require treatment. Certain of these minor problems can run in families, which suggests that a genetic factor is involved.

In-toeing, in which the toes point inward, is common and occurs at any time from infancy to about age 8. **Out-toeing**, in which the feet point away from each other, is less common but may occur at about 6 months. **Bowlegs**, in which both shinbones curve outward, is normal in a child until about the age of 3. Severe bowing is uncommon and may be a sign of vitamin D deficiency. **Knock-knees**, in which a child's legs curve in at the knees, is common between the ages of 3 and 7.

Most children have **flat feet** until the arch develops between 2 and 3 years of age. Children also have a fat pad beneath the foot that makes the feet look even flatter. Some children, however, have flat feet that persist into adulthood.

SHOULD I CONSULT THE DOCTOR?

Consult your doctor if you are concerned about the appearance of your child's legs or feet or if your child has difficulty walking, has a limp, or complains of pain.

WHAT IS THE TREATMENT?

Most minor leg and foot problems do not require treatment because they are not severe enough to interfere with normal walking; they usually disappear naturally as a child grows up. Out-toeing usually disappears first, often within a year of a child starting to walk. In-toeing and bowlegs usually disappear by age 3–4 and knock-knees by age 11–12. Persistent flat feet usually don't need treatment unless they cause pain.

If your child has difficulty walking or if the shape of his legs is abnormal, your doctor may recommend physical therapy. Rarely, if your child's legs or feet are seriously affected, orthopedic surgery may be necessary.

Clubfoot (talipes)

CLUBFOOT (ALSO CALLED TALIPES) IS A CONDITION IN WHICH A BABY IS
BORN WITH ONE OR BOTH FEET TWISTED OUT OF SHAPE.

Babies are often born with their feet in awkward positions, and there are two types of clubfoot: **positional clubfoot**, in which the twisted foot is flexible and can be manipulated into normal position, and **structural clubfoot**, in which the twisted foot is rigid.

In positional clubfoot, the foot is of normal size but is twisted, possibly due to compression of the baby in the womb. Most cases are mild and correct themselves. Structural clubfoot is a more serious condition in which the foot turns downward and inward and is usually abnormally small in size. In about half of babies with structural clubfoot, both feet are affected. The condition is twice as common in boys and can run in families, which suggests a genetic factor. Both types of clubfoot are usually diagnosed during the routine examination after a baby is born.

WHAT IS THE TREATMENT?

Positional clubfoot may not need treatment. If it does, physical therapy may help straighten the foot, and a cast may be used to move the foot into position. A normal position is usually achieved within three months. Structural clubfoot requires physical therapy and a cast for a long period. In 6 out of 10 cases this treatment is successful. If it is not surgery may be needed between the ages of 6 and 9 months. Surgery is usually successful and enables most children to walk normally.

Cleft lip and palate

A CLEFT LIP AND PALATE ARE SPLITS IN THE UPPER LIP AND THE ROOF OF THE MOUTH THAT ARE
PRESENT FROM BIRTH. THEY MAY OCCUR SINGLY OR TOGETHER AND OCCUR WHEN THE UPPER
LIP OR ROOF OF THE MOUTH DOES NOT FUSE COMPLETELY IN THE FETUS.

In many cases the cause is unknown, but the risk is higher if certain anticonvulsant drugs are taken during pregnancy or if the mother is a heavy drinker. Cleft lip and/or palate sometimes runs in families. Both conditions can be very upsetting for parents, but plastic surgery usually produces excellent results.

If a baby is severely affected, he may find it difficult to feed at first, and if the condition is not treated early, speech may be delayed.

Children with a cleft lip and/or palate are also susceptible to persistent buildup of fluid in the middle ear (glue ear) that impairs hearing and may delay speech.

WHAT IS THE TREATMENT?

A cleft lip is usually repaired surgically by the time a child is three months old, and a cleft palate between the ages of 6 and 15 months. While waiting for surgery, a plate may be fitted into the roof of the mouth if a baby has feeding problems. After surgery, a child may have a hearing test to check for hearing impairment caused by a buildup of fluid in the ear. A child may also need speech therapy when he begins talking. Plastic surgery usually produces excellent results and allows a child's speech to develop normally.

Strabismus (crossed eyes or squint)

IT IS QUITE COMMON FOR THE EYES OF NEWBORN BABIES TO MOVE INDEPENDENTLY
OF EACH OTHER UNTIL THE AGE OF 6 WEEKS. AT ABOUT THIS TIME, THE BABY'S
EYES SHOULD BECOME PERMANENTLY ALIGNED.

If alignment doesn't happen, and one or both eyes wander, it is known as crossed eyes or a squint. This condition is most commonly caused by an imbalance of the eye muscles. It may also be associated with other vision defects such as long or short sight. The brain compensates for the wandering eye by blocking out what it sees.

Your pediatrician will check your child's eyes and vision at the 6-week, 3-month, 2-year, and 3-year development assessments.

WHAT ARE THE SYMPTOMS?

With crossed eyes, the eyes appear to be looking in different directions.

SHOULD I CONSULT THE DOCTOR?

Consult your doctor as soon as possible if the crossed eyes persist after your baby is three months old. Crossed eyes that persist are serious because the child could lose sight from that eye.

WHAT IS THE TREATMENT?

■ Your doctor will treat the condition by blacking out the strong eye with a pad or patch. This forces the muscles of the wandering eye to work and become stronger. The treatment usually corrects the laziness in the eye within four or five months.

■ If your child is older, an eye specialist will teach your child a series of simple eye exercises to help strengthen the eye muscles.

■ If your child's crossed eyes are associated with some vision defect and glasses are required, you will be referred to an optometrist or ophthalmologist.

■ If the crossed eyes persist, surgery may be performed to correct muscular imbalance. This will not be contemplated until your child is at least two years old.

WHAT CAN I DO?

■ Have your child's eyes checked annually.

■ If you are concerned about your child's eyes, ask to be referred to an ophthalmologist for another opinion.

BEHAVIOR AND DEVELOPMENT

In recent years both doctors and the media have paid increasing attention to behavioral disorders in children, especially attention deficit disorder (ADD) and hyperactivity (together called ADHD). More and more children are being diagnosed with behavioral disorders, correctly or not. Diagnosis of autism spectrum disorders also seems to be increasing, probably because the criteria are recognized more than they used to be. Dyslexia and other developmental disorders also concern parents, but much can be done to help.

Attention deficit hyperactivity disorder (ADHD)

FOR WANT OF A LABEL, SOME DIFFICULT BUT COMPLETELY NORMAL CHILDREN ARE SAID TO BE HYPERACTIVE. TO MY MIND THIS IS UNJUSTIFIED.

The word "hyperactive" is the broad term formerly used to describe children who have attention deficit disorder (ADD) and attention deficit hyperactivity disorder (ADHD) – behavioral conditions that include disruptive behavior, poor attention span, sleeplessness, and excitability. Contrary to parental belief, certain food colorings and flavorings have never been proven to contribute to hyperactivity and sympathetic handling by parents can improve the behavior of most children. Only a few degrees of hyperactivity in children are abnormal or serious or need medical treatment.

WHAT ARE THE SYMPTOMS?
- Disruptive behavior.
- Restlessness.
- Short attention span.
- Sleeplessness.
- Foolhardiness and unpredictability.

SHOULD I SEE THE DOCTOR?
Consult your doctor for advice if you find your child difficult to live with, or if his behavior is interfering with his schooling.

WHAT IS THE MEDICAL APPROACH?
It is difficult to find two doctors who agree on the origin, features, or even the fact that there is such a thing as hyperactivity. If minor behavioral problems are combined with any form of learning disability, such as dyslexia, the confusion is compounded. Your doctor may refer your child to a child psychiatrist to establish whether or not the child has ADD/ADHD. If learning difficulties are also present, these are more likely to be detected when your child starts school. Your doctor will not prescribe any drugs unless a definite diagnosis is made.

I, personally, am against the use of drugs such as Ritalin without very careful assessment by several doctors, especially since so many children respond to kinder cognitive and behavioral therapies.

WHAT CAN I DO?
- The essential approach for parents with hyperactive children is sensitive handling and it's best if you both adopt the same approach so that your child gets consistent guidance.
- Learn to live with your child by treating him as an exciting, unpredictable, but nevertheless normal child. While your child is young this will be exceedingly difficult, but by the time he goes to school he should have learned to concentrate.
- You will need to be more vigilant if your child is foolhardy and more inventive at providing games so that he doesn't become bored.

Dyspraxia and DAMP

DYSPRAXIA AND DAMP, WHICH STANDS FOR DEFICIT IN ATTENTION, MOTOR CONTROL, AND PERCEPTION, ARE TWO CLOSELY LINKED CONDITIONS.

Dyspraxia means simply clumsiness but the medical definition would be the partial loss of the ability to perform skilled, coordinated movements in the absence of any defect in motor or sensory functions.

The nervous system is the body's information gathering, storage, and control system and it's organized like a computer that controls a highly complex machine. Disorders of the nervous system may result from damage to, or dysfunction of, its component parts. "Motor" is a term used to describe anything that brings about movement, such as a muscle or nerve. It is usually applied to nerves that

stimulate muscles to contract and thereby produce movement, including muscles which control speech. "Perception" is the interpretation of a sensation. People receive information about the environment through the five senses – taste, smell, hearing, vision, and touch – but the way in which this information is interpreted depends on other factors too.

HELP FOR YOU AND YOUR CHILD
Drug therapy is usually used for those children with dyspraxia who fail to respond to psychotherapy. In long-term therapy drug

treatment should be gradually withdrawn every year to determine if it's still necessary.

It's important to realize that, if your child is experiencing difficulties, he should be praised for what he can excel at, rather than have attention drawn to what he can't do so well. Patient families and teachers can do a lot to make up for a child's lack of skills.

Coping strategies can go a long way to making the situation easier and, with remedial and other help, many children with dyspraxia manage very well in mainstream education.

FOCUS *on* autistic disorders

Autistic children have problems communicating with people and relating to them in a meaningful way and autism spreads over a wide spectrum of conditions. Autism affects about 1 in 500 children. It always develops before the age of 3, but can be detected as early as 18 months old.

Autistic children are not physically disabled in the same way that a child with cerebral palsy may be, and they look like normal children.

THE FACTS
● The whole spectrum of autistic disorders touches the lives of as many as 2 to 6 in 1,000 people in the US.
● Autism cannot be cured, but research has shown that early intervention through specialized education can make a crucial difference to an autistic child's development.
● At the higher-functioning end of the spectrum is a condition called **Asperger syndrome**; people with it are often highly intelligent but are seen as being socially a bit odd.
● At the lower-functioning end of the spectrum are those who compulsively injure themselves, or who never learn to speak or become toilet trained.
● There is no evidence linking the measles, mumps, and rubella (MMR) vaccine to autism.

THE AUTISTIC CHILD
The autistic child is one who is seemingly isolated in his or her own world, who makes no gestures, no eye contact, and doesn't speak; who resists change, doesn't play imaginatively, or show interest in other children, and is locked into inappropriate, repetitive routines. They have no built-in tools of communication. What they all **share** is a way of perceiving the world that is very different from how you or I perceive it.

The various forms of autism can be grouped into autistic spectrum disorder, a lifelong disability. The exact causes are still not known but genetic factors are important, as are certain conditions affecting development of parts of the brain to do with reasoning, social interaction, and communication. Typically, a trio of impairments is seen:
1. Difficulty in communicating and relating to others.
2. Lack of imaginative play.
3. Obsessive and ritualistic behavior.

UNDERSTANDING AUTISM
Autism is four times more likely to occur in boys than girls and knows no racial, ethnic, or social boundaries. Family income, lifestyle, and educational levels don't affect the chances of its happening.

Autism is said to be as common as **1 in 500 children**, but if you include the whole spectrum it may be as common as **1 in 9**.

Within the spectrum of autism are those with severe learning disabilities at one extreme, and those with high ability who become **fully independent** adults at the other.

Early diagnosis is vital and typical behavior can usually be seen between birth and three years old. But because there are many forms, children with autism may not be diagnosed and so cannot benefit from the **specialized education** that could help them later on.

The nature of autism, especially the difficulties with social interaction and relating to others, creates particular pressures for the parents, brothers, and sisters. And because it's not physically visible, it's hard to promote understanding and awareness in the wider community.

THE PARENTS
Being the parent of an autistic child can be hard, leading to frustration and low morale. You may find that professional help isn't always adequate as these statistics show.
● 65 percent of parents see three or more professionals before they get a firm diagnosis, 25 percent see five professionals or more.
● Multiple diagnoses are often given to parents. Over time, the diagnosis often changes from a general and incomplete one to a more specific diagnosis on the autistic spectrum.
● 45 percent of parents state that autism is explained inadequately or not at all at the time of diagnosis; 81 percent state that there's either no assessment of severity or a vague one.
● 45 percent of parents are dissatisfied to some degree with the diagnostic process, with

Daily Life Therapy

Daily Life Therapy was developed in Japan in the 1960s as a way of teaching children with autism in mainstream schools with emphasis on very positive encouragement for all activities and very high praise for all achievement. The overall goal is for children to develop physically, emotionally, and intellectually and therefore achieve social independence and dignity.
Daily Life Therapy has three key objectives:
● to **stabilize** the emotions and build up self-confidence through achievement
● to establish a routine to daily life through physical exercise, which will also build physical strength and control
● to stimulate the intellect with math, language, communication, and social skills.

The approach concentrates on a few basic lessons, so simplifying what's expected from each child. Many activities are group-orientated so that learning isn't only from teacher to child but from child to child as well, often by one child imitating another.
Daily Life Therapy isn't without its critics, who see the group approach as being based on Japanese culture, which might not sit easily in the West. Others are worried about the training element of Daily Life Therapy.

THE UNDERACHIEVING CHILD OFTEN SHOWS CERTAIN CHARACTERISTICS FROM BIRTH, WHICH CAN BE DIFFICULT TO PIN DOWN AT FIRST.

20 percent being very dissatisfied.
- 45 percent of parents report they aren't given any advice about where to go for help/support/counseling after the diagnosis.
- 50 percent of parents say the support they receive at the time of diagnosis is inadequate.

GETTING THE RIGHT HELP
Whatever the age at diagnosis – whether the person is two or 22 years old – the right type of help can make a great difference. Proper assessment can help secure services and support that could improve the quality of life in tangible and practical ways. People with autism and Asperger syndrome need **specialized preschool help and education**, **respite care**, or **support in finding employment** and benefits they have a right to, including **disability benefits**.

THE GOOD NEWS
The earlier that diagnosis of autism is made, the better the chances are of a child receiving the specialized education and support that can really make a difference.
- Autism professionals **worldwide** agree that early intervention is crucial. Therapies such as the intensive behavioral programs pioneered in the US have achieved extraordinary results.
- Staying power is essential. In one study of autistic children under the age of 5, nearly 50 percent of children who received 40 hours a week of therapy over two years achieved normal intellectual and educational skills. In contrast, only 2 percent who received 10 hours a week reached the same standard.

Parents often think they simply have a very good and quiet baby. This can, however, signify an unresponsive baby. If you ever find yourself saying any of the following, you should ask your doctor if all is well.

"She is always a very good and quiet baby and hardly ever cries."

"We hardly know we have him; he never gives us any trouble."

"Sometimes she just lies in her carriage without moving at all, and she sleeps a lot."

"He is as good as gold, a marvelous baby and no trouble, unlike his brother."

"She hardly makes a sound; she seems to live in a world of her own."

"He only just seemed to come alive when he was about eight months old, he never moved much when he was younger than that."

HOW CAN I RECOGNIZE IT?
What distinguishes developmental delay is a slowness that affects **all** the milestones. Lateness in achieving one or two milestones is common and not abnormal. Nearly always the first sign is a lateness in noticing things and in smiling. Occasionally this is so pronounced that even blindness may be suspected. Because the child may appear to take such little notice of what is going on around him both sight and hearing may be questioned.

Sometimes your child may be late in learning to chew, which may lead to difficulty in eating solids or lumpy food. Some of the milestones may last longer than they should. For instance the **grasp reflex** should be lost around 3 to 4 weeks old but may persist beyond three months or hand regard may go on for as long as 20 weeks. Similarly taking all objects to the mouth, **mouthing**, which is quite normal for children between 6 and 12 months, may go on for longer in affected children.

The desire to throw things over the carriage, **edge**, usually stops around 16 months but may go on longer if a baby is mentally slow. And while normal, bright or even exceptionally intelligent children can have attention problems, **lack of concentration** and **interest** may indicate impaired mental ability, as may aimless overactivity. **Pointless overactivity** may not show up for a time and children who were excessive sleepers when they were very young undergo a remarkable transformation and are now unable to concentrate. They may flit from one activity to the other – even flitting physically around the room transiently interested in many tiny things – and this can escalate into almost frenetic activity that is very

difficult to live with. This is particularly true of the autistic child.

WHAT CAN BE DONE?
There is no question that an underachieving child can be helped from a very early age by parental interest, attention, stimulation with songs, chatter, books, games, and educational toys. A generally stimulating environment based on listening, discussion, and questioning will help your child reach his optimum potential.

This is borne out by a meticulous study on infant intervention programs performed by Craig Ramey in North Carolina in the 1980s. Infants who entered the study were those from very poor families whose mothers had low IQs and they were enrolled in special day care programs eight hours a day, five days a week. (This does not mean to say that your child has to have such intensive help and education, it simply shows the effect of an education program.) The children entered the program from 6 to 12 weeks of age until they were five years old when they began kindergarten in an ordinary school.

The program was stimulating and emotionally warm, very much the kind of special family characteristics that help children to develop. At the same time there was a control group from similar backgrounds that did not receive the specially enriched programs but did receive nutritional supplements and medical treatment while being brought up at home.

WHAT THE STUDY SHOWED
The results were unequivocal. At all ages the enriched day care improved IQ scores significantly over the control group who were reared at home before attending school without an enrichment program. Furthermore, the difference between children who had attended a preschool enrichment program remained significant after another eighteen months of regular school.

These results do not mean that impaired mental ability can be cured simply by giving children heavy doses of especially stimulating education in infancy. What they show is that the intellectual power of children who begin life with few advantages can be increased if richer stimulation is provided. To me, the importance of these findings is that parents who have children with slightly less mental power than their peers can only help if they try to provide an **enriching environment** in their own homes from infancy onward.

Dyslexia and learning disabilities

DELAYED SPEECH DEVELOPMENT OFTEN OCCURS BEFORE LEARNING AND READING DISORDERS.
THERE IS SOME EVIDENCE THAT LEARNING DISABILITIES MAY START AS EARLY AS TWO YEARS.

Delayed reading and dyslexia

Delay in learning to read is usually part of a wider spectrum of learning disorders including difficulty in spelling, writing, and learning languages, for example. This compound disorder of language, often called dyslexia, may be defined as a reading age of two years or more below the mental age.

Delayed reading may simply be a variation of normal. However, a child who is mentally slow is more often slow in learning to read than in any other part of school lessons. Common features that go along with late reading are a short attention span, aimless overactivity, defective concentration, impulsiveness, aggressiveness, and clumsiness. Your child's visual perception should also be tested.

The label dyslexia is bandied about very loosely these days, but a child should never be labeled dyslexic unless the diagnosis has been made with the help of expert, psychological advice. Nearly always there is a family history of the same complaint, or at least a learning disorder. Dyslexia is four times more common in boys and nearly

always occurs in both twins. Sometimes there are problems of laterality, which means left- or mixed-handedness, and a tendency to read from right to left or to reverse letters.

Dyslexia is made worse by many factors including young age of the parents, poverty, and unemployment, lack of suitable reading material in infancy, lack of to-and-fro conversation, domestic friction, child abuse, sexual abuse, a one-parent family, or any cause of insecurity. School factors will include poor teaching, lack of motivation, and school absences. Poor teaching or critical teaching may convince a child that he cannot read, and so he stops trying, then teachers are liable to label him as a poor reader and he becomes one so his inability to read turns into a self-fulfilling prophecy.

Dyslexia must have something to do with Western society because it is ten times more common in the West than it is in the East, despite the fact that China has 10,000 "letters" in common use out of a total of about 50,000.

Learning disabilities very often occur along with poor coordination, repetitive movements, poor memory, and the inability to do puzzles and drawing.

WHAT MIGHT BE DONE?

Many children grow out of their dyslexic difficulties without special help though some may have slight spelling difficulties for all of their lives. However, do seek special help. Your child's teacher at school or the principal will put you in touch with a psychologist or a special teacher who is experienced in remedial teaching for dyslexic children. Your child may have to attend special classes in the evening several times a week for several years.

Your support and enthusiasm for your child's special lessons, progress, and achievements is irreplaceable; you must keep in mind that whatever type of remedial teaching is being used, your child cannot help it and is not just being naughty or stupid. Please tell your child that many famous and eminent people who have gone on to achieve much have experienced exactly the same problem as he. Auguste Rodin, one of the greatest sculptors of all time, was described as "the worst pupil in the school." His father said, "I have an idiot for a son" and his uncle said, "He is ineducable." Rodin never mastered spelling throughout the whole of his life but this did not prevent him excelling at his chosen profession.

The Learning Disabilities Association (see Useful addresses, p. 567) will give you support, advice, and information about local schools and support groups where your child's problem and your own difficulties will be treated sympathetically and patiently. It will also provide you with leaflets and books which will help you to understand and care for your child.

Encopresis

IF A CHILD FREQUENTLY PASSES SOLID STOOLS IN HIS PANTS OR IN INAPPROPRIATE PLACES AFTER
HE HAS BOWEL CONTROL, HE IS SUFFERING FROM ENCOPRESIS.

Encopresis that starts in a child who has bowel control should be regarded as a symptom of a problem rather than of slow development. It often starts as the result of some emotional disturbance in the child's life, such as the arrival of a new baby, separation of parents, moving to a new location and losing contact with friends, or divorce. Seen in this way, encopresis should never be punished

or derided. Occasionally, children persist in soiling their pants from infancy onward. This soiling may be a reaction against over-fussy or over-authoritarian toilet training, something that I'm strongly against.

In a child of four or five, a common cause of encopresis is chronic constipation. Holding of the stools, not wanting to pass them, leading to constipation, may also be a feature. This again

can be the result of a parent placing too high a value on a baby or child passing a stool regularly into a potty. Encopresis is not a serious problem. Never blame your child. First, look at yourselves.

SHOULD I CONSULT THE DOCTOR?

Pure constipation is easy to treat so consult your doctor as soon as possible if you think your child has chronic constipation. If you can find no reason for the involuntary soiling, your doctor may be the best person to discover the cause of tension in the family.

WHAT IS THE TREATMENT?

■ If your child is constipated, your doctor may prescribe a mild laxative, specially formulated for babies and children, which is safe for short-term use.

■ Your doctor will advise you on how to reduce the constipation in the future.

■ Where there is some emotional reason for the encopresis, your doctor will assess the situation after discussion with you and your child. If he feels that further counseling is needed, your doctor may refer you and your child to a psychotherapist.

WHAT CAN I DO?

■ NEVER punish your child or show disgust if he soils his pants; this will only make matters worse.

■ Watch for signs of poor school performance.

Your child may become a target of scorn because of the odor if he soils himself at school. Be sympathetic and helpful, he really doesn't want to soil his pants, so provide him with spare underpants and take his teacher into your confidence.

■ Make sure your child has a diet that is rich in dietary fiber and liquids and gets regular exercise.

UPPER AIRWAY CONDITIONS IN BABIES AND CHILDREN

The middle ear, throat, sinuses, nose, and larynx can be thought of as one single and interconnected system in children, because the tubes and passages that connect each component are very short. Given that in certain places only a few millimeters separate one area from another (for example, the throat connects to the middle ear via the Eustachian tube, which in babies is exceedingly short), it follows that bacteria or viruses treat these spaces as one. So a throat infection can spread almost immediately to the middle ear and cause otitis media (infection of the middle ear).

Similarly an infection of the throat will descend very quickly to the lungs and small airways (bronchioles) because, to an invading virus, the throat and the lungs are the same space in a child. And the younger the child the quicker the spread because distances are so tiny.

As children grow, the air passages lengthen and widen and organisms can no longer leapfrog around the upper airways. In adults the spread of infection is rarer because the ear, nose, and throat are anatomically separate. Because of this unifying anatomy in children, there's logic in grouping conditions of the upper airways together, a malfunction of one component nearly always having a chain reaction effect on another.

Colds in children

THE COMMON COLD IS CAUSED BY A VIRUS THAT ENTERS THE BODY THROUGH THE NASAL PASSAGES AND THROAT AND CAUSES INFLAMMATION OF THE MUCOUS MEMBRANES LINING THESE PASSAGES.

The body's defenses take around 10 days to fight off the common cold virus.

A common cold is not serious, but because it lowers the body's resistance, complications such as **bronchitis** and **pneumonia** have been known to arise. A cold should be regarded more seriously in a baby because minor cold symptoms, such as a blocked nose, can cause her to have feeding problems.

WHAT ARE THE SYMPTOMS?

■ Sneezing.
■ Runny or blocked nose.
■ Temperature.
■ Coughing.
■ Sore throat.
■ Aching muscles.
■ Irritability.
■ Mucus.

SHOULD I CONSULT THE DOCTOR?

Consult your doctor immediately if you think your child has developed a secondary infection. If your baby is having trouble sleeping at night or feeding, consult your doctor.

WHAT IS THE TREATMENT?

■ Your doctor will treat any secondary infection to the cold.

■ Your doctor may prescribe nose drops to ease feeding. Use them as directed, since overuse can damage the lining of the nose.

■ Your doctor may prescribe a cough suppressant or an expectorant to ease a bad cough.

WHAT CAN I DO?

■ Ease your baby's breathing by placing a pillow under the crib mattress to raise her head.
■ Give your child plenty to drink.
■ Make nose-blowing easier by blowing one nostril at a time.
■ If possible, create a humid atmosphere in your child's bedroom so that the raw lining of the nose does not become dry.
■ Smear Vaseline on to your child's nose and upper lip if constant blowing has made them sore.
■ Capsules of camphor sprinkled onto clothing and bedding will ease your child's breathing during the night.
■ A hot bedtime drink of freshly squeezed lemon juice and water will ease your child's sore throat and clear her nasal passages.

The flu

IF YOUR CHILD IS OF SCHOOL AGE, THE CHANCES OF ESCAPING AN INFECTION WITH THE COLD
OR FLU VIRUS ARE SLIM. THE FLU IS USUALLY QUITE EASY TO DISTINGUISH FROM A COLD.
IN THE FIRST PLACE, IT'S MORE SERIOUS AND IT STRIKES MORE QUICKLY.

Your six-year-old may be a picture of health one minute and pale, listless, and sweaty the next. Here are a few things to keep in mind.
■ The illness usually lasts around three or four days. Unless there's a secondary infection, treatment of the symptoms is all that's necessary most of the time.
■ The flu virus has the ability to mutate readily to new forms, which means it can spread rapidly around the world in epidemics most winters.

IS IT SERIOUS?

It's rare for serious complications to crop up with the flu in children. However, sometimes secondary infections such as **pneumonia**, **otitis media** (middle ear infection), **bronchitis**, or **sinusitis** may result.

WHAT ARE THE SYMPTOMS?

■ Runny nose.
■ Sore throat.
■ Cough.
■ Temperature above 100.4°F (38°C).
■ Shivering.
■ Aches and pains.
■ Diarrhea, vomiting, and nausea.
■ Weakness and lethargy.

WHAT SHOULD I DO FIRST?

1. Keep children with flu at home. Don't make them stay in bed unless they want to, instead encourage them to play quietly. Strenuous sports should be avoided during viral illnesses. Use cotton sheets – they are much more comfortable for a child with a temperature. Change the sheets regularly, particularly if your child has a fever – clean sheets feel better.

Leave a box of tissues on the bedside table.
2. While your child has a temperature do your best to keep him at an even temperature, even if that means he lies on the sofa downstairs with you.
3. When your child is ill it's the time to relax all the rules, to put a TV in the bedroom and give special treats. Don't forget illness makes your child feel insecure, so read him stories, play games, and give him lots of cuddling.
4. Try to avoid contact with other children outside the family to avoid spreading infection. Avoiding contact with children in the family isn't usually practical.
5. Most children with a fever don't want to eat so, while you should offer food, you should never force your child to eat if he seems unwilling. As long as children are getting plenty of liquid, they can survive perfectly well for two or three days on very little. When the illness is over, your child's appetite will return. As soon as it does, take advantage and let him eat as heartily as he wants to.
6. While you shouldn't worry if your child eats very little for a day or so, make sure that he gets plenty of fluids to drink. School-age children should drink around 80 ounces (two liters) a day when they have a viral infection – this means six to eight glasses of water or other drinks. For toddlers and younger children who still prefer a bottle, you should make sure that they have a bottle of water or other clear fluids always on hand. Feel free to give them their favorite drink, just so that you can be sure they're getting enough fluid.
7. Take your child's temperature twice a day, and when you are worried about how hot he feels. A high body temperature is a natural

defense against viral infection, since viruses can't multiply at high temperature. **For this reason, it isn't recommended any longer to bring a high temperature down with lukewarm sponging, unless it's very high** (over 104°F/40°C).
8. If a rash appears just after the onset of flu symptoms, your child may have measles, so tell your doctor.

SHOULD I CONSULT THE DOCTOR?

Yes, if:
● your child's temperature is consistently higher than 102.2°F (39°C), or your child is unable to manage a good fluid intake. The symptoms of moderate dehydration are a dry cough, highly concentrated (dark yellow) urine or poor output of urine, and general lethargy
● you're concerned that a secondary bacterial infection is developing – a worsening cough, or a cough that produces colored sputum (yellow or green), a puslike discharge from the nose or an earache
● your child isn't starting to improve within 48 hours.

WHAT MIGHT THE DOCTOR DO?

■ If there's a secondary infection, your doctor may prescribe an **antibiotic**.
■ Recently some **new drugs** have been developed that show promise in reducing the duration and symptoms of flu, but their place in the treatment of straightforward cases isn't yet clear. Your doctor may consider using one of these drugs if it's a severe case of flu or if your child has other health problems.

WHAT CAN I DO TO HELP?

■ **Vaccination** can prevent influenza, but it must be repeated each autumn because of the virus's ability to mutate to new forms. An **annual influenza injection** should be considered for children with a serious chronic medical problem such as **asthma**, **diabetes,** or **cystic fibrosis** and for children who are immuno-suppressed, such as transplant recipients or cancer patients. The best time for your child to have a flu shot is between **September and November** to prepare him for the winter. Ask your child's school what plans they have for a vaccination program or speak to your doctor.
■ Let the **school** know that your child has the flu, so that classmates can be diagnosed and treated if necessary.
■ Your child can return to school when the fever and other symptoms have settled down and he's feeling well again.

Croup

CROUP IS THE NAME GIVEN TO THE SOUND MADE WHEN AIR IS BREATHED IN THROUGH
A CONSTRICTED WINDPIPE, PAST INFLAMED VOCAL CORDS.

Croup usually occurs in young children up to the age of about 4, who are susceptible because their air passages (bronchi) are narrow and become blocked with mucus when inflamed – often because of a virus such as a common cold, or an infection such as bronchitis. In rare cases, croup can be caused by an inhaled foreign body. In older children the condition is less serious and is known as laryngitis. The first attack of croup can come on quickly, usually at night, and may last a couple of hours. Your child will have a croaking, barking cough and labored breathing.

If your child has a severe attack of croup, he could develop breathing difficulties. This should be treated as an emergency.

WHAT ARE THE SYMPTOMS?
- Croaking cough.
- Labored breathing when the lower chest caves in at every inhalation.
- Wheezing.
- Face color becoming gray or blue.

SHOULD I CONSULT THE DOCTOR?
Consult your doctor immediately if your child's skin turns gray or blue and he has to fight for breath. Consult your doctor as soon as possible to tell him that your child has had an attack of croup.

WHAT IS THE TREATMENT?
- In a serious attack, your doctor will give your child oxygen and, in some cases, steroids.
- Your doctor may advise inhaling steam.
- Your doctor will give you advice on what to do if your child has another attack.
- If the attack is caused by an inhaled foreign body, your doctor will remove it.

WHAT CAN I DO?
If any other attacks occur, stay with your child and follow your doctor's instructions.

Cough

A COUGH IS EITHER A SYMPTOM OF AN ILLNESS OR THE BODY'S WAY OF REACTING
TO AN IRRITANT IN THE THROAT OR AIR PASSAGES.

A cough may bring up phlegm from the chest and clear mucus from the air passages, for example, during an attack of asthma or whooping cough (this is known as a productive cough).

A dry cough, which produces no phlegm, serves no useful purpose and its cause is not always obvious. The irritation provoking the cough may be mucus from chronically infected sinuses or nasal discharge from a common cold, both of which drip down and tickle the back of the throat. A dry cough may also be the body's way of bringing up a foreign body stuck in the windpipe. Coughing may be caused by "passive smoking." If adults around your child smoke, the smoke may irritate your child's throat and cause a cough. Children may also adopt a cough as an attention seeking device, when it becomes a tic or mannerism.

A cough is not usually serious, although it can be irritating. However, a cough that causes breathing difficulties such that your child turns blue around the lips and gasps for breath is serious and should be treated as an emergency.

SHOULD I CONSULT THE DOCTOR?
Consult your doctor as soon as possible if your child's cough doesn't get better after three or four days, or if your child is not getting any sleep at night, or if you cannot remove a foreign body from your child's throat. Consult your doctor immediately if your baby develops a hacking cough or if your child's coughing is accompanied by rapid, labored, or wheezy breathing. This could be croup or asthma.

WHAT IS THE TREATMENT?
- If your child's cough is part of an infection such as otitis media or tonsillitis, your doctor will prescribe antibiotics to clear up that infection.
- If your child is suffering from a viral infection, your doctor will advise you on how to relieve the symptoms and help your child to cough up the phlegm.
- If the cough is part of an asthmatic condition, your doctor may prescribe bronchodilator drugs that help to widen the air passages.
- Your doctor may prescribe nose drops to administer sparingly to your child before he goes to bed. These drops ease congestion and prevent mucus from dripping down the back of your child's throat.
- Your doctor may prescribe a cough medicine: either a cough suppressant (to reduce irritation and soothe the throat) or an expectorant (to encourage the coughing up of phlegm).

WHAT CAN I DO TO HELP?
- Keep your child quiet and warm to help prevent any minor infection from spreading into the lungs and causing a serious condition such as bronchitis.
- Don't let your child run around too much during the day. Breathlessness can bring on a coughing fit.
- Encourage your child to lie on her stomach or her side at night so that mucus will not drip into her throat.
- Keep the air in your child's room moist by leaving a window open. Don't overheat the room.
- Don't smoke at home and don't take your child into smoky atmospheres.

Tonsillitis

POSITIONED AT THE BACK OF THE THROAT, THE TONSILS ARE THE BODY'S FIRST LINE OF DEFENSE.
THEY TRAP AND KILL BACTERIA, PREVENTING THEM FROM ENTERING THE RESPIRATORY TRACT.

In the process the tonsils can become infected, causing tonsillitis. The adenoids at the back of the nose are usually affected also. Babies under the age of about 1 year rarely suffer from tonsillitis. It occurs mainly among school-age children when the relatively large tonsils and adenoids are exposed to infectious microbes. As resistance to infectious microbes increases, attacks should lessen. Most children do not get tonsillitis after the age of 10. Tonsillitis is not serious unless repeatedly accompanied by infection of the middle ear.

WHAT ARE THE SYMPTOMS?
■ Sore throat, possibly bad enough to cause difficulty in swallowing.
■ Red and enlarged tonsils, possibly covered in yellow spots.
■ A temperature of over 100.4°F (38°C).
■ Swollen glands in the neck.
■ Mouth-breathing, snoring, and a nasal voice.
■ Unpleasant breath.

SHOULD I CONSULT THE DOCTOR?
Consult your doctor as soon as possible if you suspect tonsillitis.

WHAT IS THE TREATMENT?
■ Your doctor may take a throat culture to identify the infection. He may prescribe antibiotics for bacterial tonsillitis.
■ He will examine your child's ears to check for any infection and may prescribe antibiotics.
■ If your child has tonsillitis frequently or if enlarged adenoids cause recurrent middle-ear infections, you may be referred to a specialist.

WHAT CAN I DO?
■ Treat your child as you would for fever.
■ Keep his fluid intake up with regular drinks.
■ Never let your child gargle for a sore throat. It can spread infection from the throat to the middle ear.
■ Offer him foods that slip down easily but don't force him to eat.

Bronchiolitis

BRONCHIOLITIS IS AN INFLAMMATION OF THE SMALLEST AIRWAYS IN THE LUNGS (BRONCHIOLES).
IT IS USUALLY CAUSED BY A VIRUS AND OCCURS IN BABIES UNDER ONE YEAR OLD.
THE CONDITION MAY START AS A COUGH OR COMMON COLD.

The virus causes the lining of the small airways to swell and to fill with mucus. This results in breathing difficulty and the baby will have to struggle for breath. Bronchiolitis is serious because the condition can cause severe breathing difficulties.

WHAT ARE THE SYMPTOMS?
■ Rapid breathing – over 50 breaths per minute.
■ Breathing difficulties.
■ Temperature.
■ Blueness of the lips and tongue.
■ Drowsiness.

SHOULD I CONSULT THE DOCTOR?
Consult your doctor immediately or take your baby to the nearest hospital if he has obvious breathing difficulties or if there is any sign of blueness around his lips and on his tongue. Consult your doctor immediately if you notice any deterioration in your baby's condition following a cold or cough.

WHAT IS THE TREATMENT?
If you doctor is satisfied that your baby's infection is a mild one, he will advise you on procedures that will allow you to care for your baby at home. However, most babies with this condition are usually admitted to the hospital overnight for observation.

WHAT CAN I DO TO HELP?
■ If your baby is admitted to the hospital, stay with him overnight. Your presence will reassure him.
■ Try to keep your baby away from other children and adults who have coughs and colds.

Glue ear

GLUE EAR (SECRETORY OTITIS MEDIA) IS A CONDITION THAT RESULTS WHEN THE EUSTACHIAN TUBE AND MIDDLE EAR ARE FILLED WITH FLUID, OFTEN AS A RESULT OF A THROAT INFECTION.

The Eustachian tube, which runs from the throat to the ear, produces large quantities of fluid as a response to chronic infections such as sinusitis, tonsillitis, or, most commonly, infection of the middle ear. If the tube in either ear is blocked by inflammation, the fluid cannot drain and becomes gluelike, impeding the efficient vibration of sound, causing loss of hearing.

Glue ear should be treated seriously because it can lead to permanent loss of hearing in the affected ear, and can cause problems with speech development and learning.

WHAT ARE THE SYMPTOMS?
■ A feeling of fullness in the ear.
■ Partial loss of hearing or deafness in one or both ears.

SHOULD I CONSULT THE DOCTOR?
Consult your doctor as soon as possible.

WHAT IS THE TREATMENT?
■ Your doctor will examine your child's ears with a special instrument called an otoscope.
■ In mild cases, your doctor will prescribe antibiotics to clear up the infection, and she may also prescribe vasoconstrictor drugs, which promote drainage by reducing swelling in the Eustachian tubes.
■ In severe and recurrent cases, your child will probably be referred to an ear, nose, and throat specialist for a hearing test. He may be admitted to the hospital to have the fluid drained under a general anesthetic and tubes

may be inserted. These tiny plastic tubes allow mucus to drain away. They either fall out after several months when the ears are healthy again, or can be removed by the specialist. If glue ear is a result of repeated infections or enlarged adenoids, the underlying problem will also be treated to prevent recurrences.

WHAT CAN I DO?
■ If your child has had tubes inserted, he should wait until two weeks after the operation to go swimming and should not dive. Some ear, nose, and throat specialists advise against swimming entirely when tubes are in place.
■ Try to keep the ear as dry as possible.

OTHER PROBLEMS IN BABIES AND CHILDREN

A number of conditions that affect babies and children don't fall into a single neat category, and these are included together in the following section.

Some of these conditions, such as cradle cap, diaper rash, teething, intussusception, and colic, only affect young babies and do not usually pose a problem for toddlers or older children. Other conditions included here, such as styes, appendicitis, epilepsy, head lice, and ringworm, can affect adults as well as children, although they are usually seen first or more often in children.

Many of the conditions in this section are minor and easily treatable at home, and where home treatment is a possibility I have included information about what you should do. Other conditions, notably intussusception, appendicitis, and Kawasaki disease, are more dangerous and need urgent medical treatment. If you are ever in doubt about the seriousness of your child's condition, don't hesitate to consult a doctor right away.

In this section you will also find a chart detailing the infectious diseases of childhood, such as measles, chickenpox, and so forth. Many of these can now be prevented by routine immunizations (see box, p. 519), which are very important to safeguarding your child's health and well-being.

Febrile convulsions

A CONVULSION IS A FIT OR SEIZURE THAT OCCURS WHEN THE BRAIN REACTS ABNORMALLY. THE MOST COMMON CAUSE OF CONVULSIONS IN CHILDREN IS A HIGH TEMPERATURE THAT ACCOMPANIES A VIRAL INFECTION SUCH AS THE FLU.

This type of convulsion is known as a febrile convulsion and generally occurs between the ages of 6 months and 6 years.

Any convulsion is frightening but febrile convulsions are harmless and not necessarily a sign of epilepsy. The tendency to suffer from febrile convulsions runs in families. Convulsions may also be caused by **meningitis, encephalitis,** and, rarely, chemical abnormalities of the blood, such as a **low blood sugar level** in diabetics. **Epilepsy** is another cause of convulsions. Sometimes no specific cause is found.

During a febrile convulsion your child loses consciousness, becomes rigid for some seconds while holding his breath, then rhythmically bends and straightens his arms and legs for some minutes. Your child may cry out at the beginning of the seizure. He may urinate and he may defecate. When the convulsion is over your child will be in a confused state and he may want to sleep.

WHAT ARE THE SYMPTOMS?
■ Sudden rise in temperature.
■ Crying out and loss of consciousness.
■ Rigid phase with the breath held.
■ Rhythmic jerking of the limbs.
■ Urination and/or defecation.
■ Confusion and drowsiness.

SHOULD I SEE THE DOCTOR?
If there is someone with you ask him to call the doctor while you stay with your child. Otherwise consult your doctor immediately as soon as the convulsion has passed.

If you can't get to your doctor within 15 minutes, or if the convulsion hasn't passed by then, take your child to the nearest hospital.

Any fit that continues for 20 minutes should be stopped with an anticonvulsant drug.

WHAT IS THE TREATMENT?
■ If the convulsion is continuing your doctor will give your child an anticonvulsant drug, usually administered rectally.
■ If your child is less than two years old when he has his first convulsion your doctor may admit him to the hospital so that tests can be done to exclude any serious cause of convulsions, such as meningitis.
■ With an older child your doctor will refer him to the hospital if the cause of the convulsion is not clear. Tests will be done and the pediatrician will advise whether or not anticonvulsant drug treatment is needed in the event of your child contracting another infectious fever.
■ Your doctor will give you advice on how to avoid a rapid rise in temperature in the future.

WHAT CAN I DO?
■ During the convulsion don't try to hold or touch your child, and move objects away so that he can't harm himself.
■ Once the convulsion is over, if your child is feverish and has a high temperature, remove his clothing and let his skin cool down. Cover him with a light sheet only while he sleeps.
■ Don't give him any over-the-counter medicines without your doctor's advice.
■ Stay calm.

A child with a high temperature should be left to sleep uncovered or covered only with a light sheet.

Epilepsy

I'M DEALING WITH EPILEPSY HERE BECAUSE CHILDHOOD IS WHEN MOST EPILEPSY STARTS. THE SUDDEN ONSET OF EPILEPSY IN ADULTHOOD HAS RATHER DIFFERENT SIGNIFICANCE.

There is the possibility of adult-onset epilepsy being a symptom of a brain tumor, something that is very rare indeed in childhood epilepsy.

WHAT ARE THE CAUSES?

Epilepsy is a disorder that causes periodic seizures, and these occur when the normal electrical impulses in the brain are disturbed. It usually develops in children, sometimes runs in families and is often outgrown. About 3 to 5 percent of children under the age of 6 have an occasional convulsion, but nearly all of these are **harmless** febrile convulsions, when the electrical fault in the brain is caused by a high temperature preceding or during an infectious illness such as the flu.

WHAT ARE THE TYPES?

Epileptic seizures may be **generalized** or **partial**, depending on how much of the brain is affected by abnormal electrical activity. During a generalized seizure, all areas of the brain are affected at the same time, whereas during a partial seizure only one part of the brain is affected. Generalized seizures can be further divided into either **grand mal seizures,** with a fit and sleepiness afterward, or absence seizures, also known as **petit mal seizures**.

WHAT ARE THE SYMPTOMS?

GRAND MAL SEIZURES

■ First there can be a warning of an attack, known as an **aura**, which lasts for a few seconds and may be a feeling of unease, a smell, a taste, a feeling of déjà vu.

■ During the first 30 seconds of a seizure there's stiffening of body and irregular breathing, followed by random movements of the limbs and trunk.

■ There may be involuntary urination.

■ If the muscles of the jaw are involved there may be frothing at the mouth.

After the seizure, consciousness is regained, breathing returns to normal, and muscles relax. Confusion and disorientation may last for a few hours afterward and a headache may develop. There is usually no memory of what has happened.

Status epilepticus is a very rare and serious complication in which a person whose epilepsy is not adequately controlled has repeated grand mal seizures without regaining consciousness in between each seizure. The condition can be life threatening, and medical help is urgent.

ABSENCE SEIZURES

■ There is no real loss of consciousness but loss of touch with surroundings, leading to a daydreamlike state lasting between 5 and 30 seconds from which the child cannot be roused.

■ The eyes may remain open and fixed. Since the seizures are almost never associated with falling down or other abnormal movements, they may not be noticed or may be confused with daydreaming. However, frequent attacks can affect school performance.

SHOULD I CONSULT THE DOCTOR?

Consult your doctor as soon as any convulsion has passed, whether you think it is a grand mal seizure or a febrile convulsion. Consult your doctor as soon as possible if you think your child has absence seizures.

WHAT IS THE TREATMENT?

■ If your child has had a convulsion your doctor will examine him and question you about the attack to help determine what form of seizure your child has experienced.

■ Your doctor may order tests to look for an underlying cause of the seizure. If no cause is found, your doctor may order an EEG to look for abnormal electrical activity in the brain, and if necessary CT scanning or a MRI of the brain.

■ If your child has had recurrent seizures, whether they are grand mal or absence seizures, he will probably be treated with **anticonvulsant drugs**. These are usually prescribed in gradually increasing doses until the seizures are controlled. Occasionally, a

second anticonvulsant may be needed.

■ Your child's condition will be reviewed periodically by your pediatrician or pediatric neurologist. If there are no seizures for 2–3 years drug treatment may be reduced or even stopped. However, any changes in dosage should be carried out only under medical supervision.

■ People who develop status epilepticus need to be admitted to the hospital without delay where intravenous drugs will be given to control the seizures.

WHAT CAN I DO?

■ It can be a shock to realize that your child has epilepsy. Both you and your child will need to get your confidence back. You can do this through your doctor who can advise you how to deal with the seizures, and there are support groups that are very helpful.

■ Make a note of the frequency of your child's absence seizures so that you can tell your doctor.

■ Watch your child carefully and report and mental or personality differences which may be the result of the drugs. It is important that your child's medication is given in the proper amounts so as not to cause any undesirable side effects.

■ Treat your child as normally as possible. Tell his friends and teachers about the condition so that they will not be frightened and shocked if your child has a convulsion in their presence.

■ Have a medic-alert bracelet or medallion with information about your child's epilepsy, in case of an attack when you are not there, and

continued on p. 541

SELF-HELP

Living with epilepsy

If you have recently been diagnosed as having epilepsy, the following points may be helpful:

■ Avoid anything that has previously triggered or may trigger a seizure, such as flashing lights.

■ Learn relaxation exercises to help you cope with stress, which may trigger seizures.

■ Try to eat at regular times.

■ Avoid drinking too much alcohol.

■ Check with your doctor before taking medications that may interact with anticonvulsant drugs.

■ Make sure that you have someone

with you if you are swimming or playing water sports.

■ If you drive, you must stop driving and inform the DMV of your epilepsy. You will have to surrender your licence, but you can reapply for it after one year without a seizure. If you plan to apply for a driver's licence, talk to your doctor first.

■ Consult an adviser before choosing a career because some types of employment may not be suitable.

■ Consult your doctor if you are planning a pregnancy.

FOCUS *on* fever in children

Colds and flu are particularly worrisome in young children because unlike us, they quite often run a frighteningly high temperature which makes them ill and lifeless. It's very scary but less so if you know how to treat a fever and make your child more comfortable.

First of all, what's a fever? Is it serious? And what can you do about it?

WHAT IS A FEVER?

The range of normal body temperature is 96.8°–98.6°F (36°–37°C). Anything over 100°F (37.7°C) is designated a fever, although the height a temperature reaches isn't necessarily an accurate reflection of the seriousness of the illness.

A fever isn't in itself an illness, but rather a symptom of one. Besides any illness, your child's temperature will reflect the time of day and his activity level: after a very strenuous game of soccer, for example, the temperature could be over 100.4°F (38°C) for a short time.

IS IT SERIOUS?

A temperature of over 100°F (37.7°C) is always serious in a baby under six months old. If the temperature remains high there's also a slight risk of a convulsion occurring – not itself a symptom of epilepsy, but the reaction of a child's brain to being too hot. As we grow older we lose that sensitivity.

WHAT SHOULD I DO FIRST?

1. If you suspect that your child has a fever take his temperature then check it again in an hour to see if it has varied. Note each reading.

2. Put your child to bed and remove most of his clothing, even if the room is cool. A child with a fever only needs to be covered in a light sheet.

3. Only if your child's temperature is very high do you need to lower it. A high fever stops a virus from multiplying and so is the body's natural defense. Lower a temperature of over 104°F (40°C) by sponging your child all over with lukewarm water. NOT cold water, lukewarm water. But take his temperature every five minutes and stop lukewarm sponging when the temperature drops to 100.4°F (38°C). The reason for never using cold water is that it causes blood vessels to constrict, preventing heat loss and therefore driving the temperature up, not down.

4. Give liquid **acetaminophen** only if other methods of reducing the fever have failed. Never give aspirin to a child.

5. Encourage your child to drink as much liquid as possible by giving them their favorite drinks, offering small amounts every **half hour**.

SHOULD I CONSULT THE DOCTOR?

● Consult the doctor immediately if your child is under six months old.

● Consult the doctor immediately if your child has a convulsion, if he's had a convulsion in the past, or if febrile convulsions run in the family.

● Consult your doctor as soon as possible if the fever lasts for more than 24 hours.

● Consult your doctor if you're worried about any other symptoms like vomiting, diarrhea, or a rash.

WHAT MIGHT THE DOCTOR DO?

Treatment will depend on what's causing the fever. If the cause is a bacterial infection, antibiotics will probably be prescribed.

If the cause is something like chickenpox or a common cold, then your doctor will probably not prescribe anything, just advise you on how to make your child comfortable.

Likely causes of a fever

Accompanying symptoms	Possible causes
Your child has a cough and a runny nose.	He possibly has a common cold.
Your child has a cough, sore throat, and aches and pains.	He possibly has influenza.
Your child has a rash of itchy, red spots on the trunk.	He may have chickenpox.
Your child urinates frequently and if he's old enough complains of a burning sensation.	He may have a urinary tract infection.
Your child has a runny nose and sore eyes and now has a brownish rash.	He possibly has measles.
The sides of your child's face and the area under his chin are swollen.	He possibly has mumps.
Your child has earache, or if he's too young to tell you, he cries and tugs at his ear.	He possibly has a middle ear infection (**otitis media**).
Your child has diarrhea.	He could have gastroenteritis or food poisoning.
Your baby or child is breathing rapidly and with great difficulty.	CONSULT YOUR DOCTOR IMMEDIATELY. Your child may have bronchitis, **bronchiolitis**, pneumonia, or croup.
Your child cannot bend his neck without pain and turns away from bright light. A purple rash may develop that does not fade when pressed.	CONSULT YOUR DOCTOR IMMEDIATELY Your child may have meningitis.

continued from p. 539
make sure your child wears it all the time.
■ If your child is prescribed anticonvulsant drugs, do not stop them without medical advice. To do so could cause a severe, prolonged convulsion after a few days.
■ Teach your child to recognize the signs of an attack (aura). If your child is old enough to identify these sensations as warning signs, he may be able to avoid having an accident.

WHAT IS THE OUTLOOK?

About 1 in 3 people who have a single seizure will have another one within 2 years. The risk of recurrent seizures is highest during the first few weeks. However, the prognosis for most people with epilepsy is good, and more than 7 in 10 people go into long-term remission within 10 years.

See also:
• Febrile convulsions p. 533
• Relaxation exercises p. 292

Reye syndrome

REYE SYNDROME USUALLY OCCURS A FEW DAYS AFTER A CHILD HAS HAD CHICKENPOX OR FLU, PARTICULARLY WHEN ASPIRIN WAS USED TO RELIEVE SYMPTOMS OR REDUCE TEMPERATURE.

Reye syndrome is a childhood illness in which the child suddenly becomes ill with **vomiting** and **fever**. The body's reaction to the illness causes the **brain to become inflamed**, so your child may also become delirious and even lapse into unconsciousness and then a coma. The cause of Reye syndrome is only now becoming clear: a virus or some other poisonous agent damages cells in various parts of the body. However, only certain children seem susceptible. It is thought that susceptibility may be related to the body's inability to deal with certain chemical substances, especially fats. Reye syndrome is very serious and can result in death if it is not identified quickly. It is, however, rare.

WHAT ARE THE SYMPTOMS?
■ Uncontrollable vomiting.
■ Fever.
■ Delirium.
■ Drowsiness or unconsciousness.

SHOULD I CONSULT THE DOCTOR?
Consult your doctor immediately, or call an

ambulance if there is any delay, if your child has a fever or is becoming drowsy and difficult to rouse.

WHAT IS THE TREATMENT?
■ If your doctor suspects Reye syndrome, he will admit your child to the hospital immediately. Usually many tests are used to confirm the diagnosis, but if there is any doubt, the doctor will remove a tiny piece of liver under local anesthetic, using a hollow catheter (a procedure called a liver biopsy). This sample will then be analyzed for abnormal fat distribution, which characterizes the illness.
■ Your child will be treated in an intensive care unit and given intravenous glucose. Various measures will be taken to control swelling of the brain.

WHAT CAN I DO?
■ Stay with your child in the hospital if possible.
■ Be prepared for a long convalescence. Ask about special precautions that should be taken to avoid a recurrence of the syndrome.

HOW CAN I HELP?
● Change the sheets on your child's bed frequently to make him feel comfortable and cover him with a sheet only.
● Place a cold compress or a wet face cloth on your child's forehead.
● Don't wake your child to take his temperature. Sleep's more important.
● Relax all routines. To my mind, a sick child deserves an easy life. So give them treats to eat, ice cream or yogurt for a sore throat, comforting desserts, favorite games to play on their bed. Put a TV in their room.
● They'll know when they want to get up; don't force the pace.
● As soon as your child is over the worst, lift their spirits by asking their friends over for a gentle play date.

See also:
• Caring for a sick child p. 514

Cradle cap

CRADLE CAP IS A THICK YELLOW ENCRUSTATION ON THE SCALP AND IT'S NOT ABNORMAL.

Cradle cap occurs in young babies, though children up to the age of 3 can have cradle cap. The yellow scales appear in small patches or can cover the entire scalp.

Cradle cap is not due to poor hygiene. Babies who suffer from it probably just have greasier scalps.

Cradle cap is simply due to skin cells being rapidly turned over on a newborn's skin and their collection due to the presence of hair. It

may appear unsightly, but it is quite harmless unless it is accompanied by red, scaly areas elsewhere on your baby's body, in which case your baby may have seborrheic eczema. All babies grow out of cradle cap by 8 or 9 months without treatment.

WHAT ARE THE SYMPTOMS?
■ Thick, yellowish scales over part or all of the scalp.

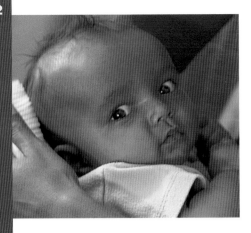

SHOULD I CONSULT THE DOCTOR?
Consult your doctor if you are worried about the condition or if your baby has any red, scaly areas elsewhere.

WHAT IS THE TREATMENT?
NEVER scratch or pick off the scales. Your doctor will prescribe a special shampoo to prevent the scales from forming and give you advice on brushing and other home treatments that help prevent cradle cap.

WHAT CAN I DO?
■ You can prevent scales from building up by brushing through your baby's hair daily, even if there is very little of it, with a soft-bristled brush. Don't scrub at your baby's scalp.
■ Never rub the scalp very hard when washing your child's hair. Shampoos remove dirt within seconds, so you only need to bring the shampoo to a lather and then rinse it off thoroughly.
■ An infallible treatment is to apply baby oil at night and shampoo off the following night when the scales have loosened. Repeat until all scales have gone. If the cradle cap becomes very hard and thick, you may have to continue the baby oil or Vaseline treatment over a 10-day period to loosen all the encrustations.

Head lice

HEAD LICE AFFECT ALL SOCIAL CLASSES AND HAVE ABSOLUTELY NOTHING TO DO WITH PERSONAL HYGIENE. THEY LIKE CLEAN HEADS AS MUCH AS DIRTY ONES AND THERE IS NOTHING SHAMEFUL ABOUT BEING INFESTED.

If you have a child there is a good chance you will come into contact with head lice at some stage.

Head lice live and suck blood from the scalp, leaving tiny red spots that cause intense itching. Adult lice can live for several weeks and the females lay a daily batch of tiny pale eggs (nits) close to the scalp. These hatch out after several days. Lice are spread through direct contact, but it doesn't necessarily have to be head-to-head.

WHAT IS IT?
Infestation of tiny wingless insects on the scalp that may cause intense itching.

WHAT IS THE TREATMENT?
The traditional response to an outbreak of head lice is the application of powerful lotions containing pesticides. The main advantage is that such lotions can penetrate the hard casing of the lice eggs and kill the nits inside.

However, scientists and parents are now beginning to think again because:
● it seems that with repeated use these pesticides are losing their effectiveness. There are reports from some areas that live nits are not being destroyed and it is suggested that some adult lice may also be resistant

● of concern about using powerful chemicals again and again on young children
● of the high cost and unpleasantness of use.
However, there are effective alternatives:
■ The first and most important weapon against head lice is the **small fine-toothed comb** (often called a nit comb because the teeth are so close together it can remove the lice eggs). Plastic combs are recommended rather than metal because they are more flexible and therefore can get closer to the scalp. They are also easier to clean and less likely to pull or snag hair.

Use the nit comb every time you wash your own and your children's hair. But do use plenty of **conditioner** after shampooing. Using conditioner makes the procedures simple and painless (no tangles) and makes it possible to dislodge lice from the slippery strands.

Pay special attention to anyone who has curly hair; it's harder to see the lice or pull the comb through so they may be particularly vulnerable.
■ The use of Quassia chips is an alternative remedy that is also becoming popular with parents. Quassia chips look like pieces of dried wood. They are cheap, natural and don't smell or leave a greasy residue.
To use Quassia chips:
  1. Place 1oz (25g) of Quassia chips in a

saucepan and pour 20oz (560ml) of boiling water over them. This loosens the oil in the chips. Leave overnight and the next day bring to a boil and simmer for 10–15 minutes. Let it cool and transfer to a spray bottle.
  2. Shampoo hair, rinse, and apply conditioner. Comb through with the nit comb. Rinse off the conditioner and towel dry. Spray the Quassia solution all over the hair. Let dry naturally. Spray again when dry.
  3. Spray again the following morning after brushing and repeat over the next couple of days. You can continue to spray as a preventative since the Quassia solution creates a bitter, hostile environment that lice do not like.
■ Natural remedies often blend five essential oils (citronella, geranium, eucalyptus, lavender, and rosemary). They claim to get rid of lice and also act as a repellent.

OVER-THE-COUNTER REMEDIES
Infestations of head lice can be treated with an over-the-counter lotion or shampoo, and the lice can then be removed with a nit comb. Hair conditioner may make it easier for you to comb out the dead lice and eggs, especially if your child's hair is long, thick, or curly. All combs and towels should be washed in very hot water after use to prevent reinfestation.

Ringworm

RINGWORM IS A FUNGAL INFECTION OF THE SKIN AND HAIR THAT SHOWS ITSELF AS BALD PATCHES IN THE HAIR, AND AS ROUND, REDDISH OR GRAY SCALY PATCHES ON THE SKIN.

As the infection spreads, the edges of the ring remain scaly, and the center begins to look

more like normal skin. Ringworm is usually contracted from animals, such as a household pet, or from other infected people.

Although it is not a serious disorder,

ringworm is unattractive and irritating. The infection is also very **contagious** and must therefore be treated promptly.

WHAT ARE THE SYMPTOMS?
■ Red or gray scaly rings on any part of the body, particularly warm, moist areas, and on the scalp, where they produce bald patches.
■ Itchiness in the ringed areas.

SHOULD I CONSULT THE DOCTOR?
Consult your doctor as soon as possible. Ringworm is contagious as well as irritating.

WHAT IS THE TREATMENT?
Your doctor will prescribe an **antifungal cream** for the skin and **oral antifungal pills** or **liquid** for the scalp. The pills will have to be taken for **at least four weeks**.

WHAT CAN I DO?
■ Throw out any brushes, combs, or headgear your child may have used while infected. Disinfectant will not destroy the fungus.
■ Keep your child's washcloth and towel separate from those of the rest of the family

to avoid spreading the infection through the household.
■ Always make sure that you and your child wash your hands thoroughly both before and after touching the affected areas.
■ If you think that your pet is a possible source of ringworm, you should take it to the vet for treatment as soon as possible.
■ Ringworm on the skin clears up quickly, but treatment of the scalp could take a couple of weeks or more. Get your child some kind of cap to hide the bald patches if he is bothered by them.

Erythema infectiosum

ERYTHEMA INFECTIOSUM, ALSO KNOWN AS SLAPPED CHEEK OR FIFTH DISEASE OR SOMETIMES AS PARVOVIRUS INFECTION, IS A VIRAL INFECTION THAT CAUSES A RASH AND OCCASIONALLY INFLAMMATION OF THE JOINTS. IT IS USUALLY MILD IN CHILDREN.

The disease is transmitted by airborne droplets in the coughs and sneezes of infected people and occurs most often in spring. Although it usually causes only a mild illness, the infection briefly halts the production of red blood cells in bone marrow and so can have serious consequences in a child who has anemia.

One attack of erythema infectiosum provides lifelong immunity to further attacks.

WHAT ARE THE SYMPTOMS?
Some children don't develop symptoms. If symptoms appear, they usually do so within

7–14 days of infection and may include:
● bright red rash on the cheeks that may spread to the trunk and limbs
● mild fever
● rarely, mild inflammation of the joints.

SHOULD I CONSULT THE DOCTOR?
Consult your doctor as soon as possible if your child develops a bright red rash on his cheeks, has a fever and if his joints seem stiff or swollen.

WHAT IS THE TREATMENT?
Your doctor may suggest liquid acetaminophen

The infection usually clears up on its own within two weeks. However, if your child is anemic he may need treatment in the hospital.

WHAT CAN I DO?
If your child has erythema infectiosum, care for him as if he had a cold or flu and have him avoid pregnant women since the infection can be dangerous to a developing fetus.

> **See also:**
> ● **Colds in children p. 533**

Stye

A STYE IS A PUS-FILLED SWELLING ON THE MARGIN OF THE EYELID. IT IS CAUSED BY AN INFECTION OF ONE OF THE HAIR FOLLICLES FROM WHICH THE EYELASHES GROW, AND IT ALMOST ALWAYS APPEARS ON THE LOWER EYELID.

A stye usually comes to a head and bursts within four or five days. Styes are encouraged by rubbing and pulling at the eyelashes and may also be associated with a general inflammation of the eyelids known as **blepharitis**. Styes are not highly infectious, but they can be spread from one eye to the other. A stye is usually harmless and can be treated at home.

WHAT ARE THE SYMPTOMS?
■ Swollen, sore red area on the eyelid, which enlarges to become pus-filled.
■ Rubbing and pulling at eyelashes, accompanied by irritation of the eye.

SHOULD I CONSULT THE DOCTOR?
Consult your doctor as soon as possible if home treatment does not improve the stye within 4-5 days, if the eyelid becomes generally swollen, or if the stye is accompanied by blepharitis.

WHAT IS THE TREATMENT?
If there is an infection of the eyelid or the eye itself, your doctor will prescribe an antibiotic ointment or eye drops. If the stye is accompanied by blepharitis, your doctor may prescribe an ointment and warm compresses to clear it up.

WHAT CAN I DO?
■ Keep your child's washcloth and towel separate from those of the rest of the family to avoid spreading any infection.
■ Wash your hands before and after treating the stye and discourage your child from touching the area.

> **See also:**
> ● **Blepharitis p. 471**

Infectious diseases in children

DISEASE	POSSIBLE SYMPTOMS
Chickenpox A less common and mild viral disease.	Red, itchy spots that become fluid-filled blisters and then scabs. Headache and slight fever.
German measles (rubella) A viral infection that is usually mild in children.	Small red spots, first behind the ears, then spreading to the face and all over the body, slight fever, and enlarged lymph nodes at the back of the neck.
Mumps An uncommon viral illness that is seldom serious in children.	Tender, swollen glands below the ears and beneath the skin. Fever, headache, dry mouth, and difficulty chewing and swallowing. Less common symptoms are painful testicles in boys and swollen ovaries in girls.
Measles A highly infectious and potentially serious viral illness.	Brownish-red spots appear behind the ears and then spread to the rest of the body. White spots in the mouth (Koplik's spots) are the diagnostic sign. The child is feverish, has a runny nose, a cough, and a headache. He may have sore eyes and find it hard to tolerate bright lights.
Whooping cough (pertussis) A bacterial infection that clogs the airways with mucus.	A cough with a distinctive "whoop" sound as the child tries to breathe, common cold symptoms (see p. 533), and vomiting. Coughing may stop your child from sleeping.
Hepatitis A viral infection causing inflammation of the liver. There are two common types, A and B. Type A is more common in children than B.	Loss of appetite, jaundice, and flu symptoms. In severe cases, your child may pass dark brown urine and pale stools.
Scarlet fever A bacterial infection whose effects are similar to those of tonsillitis, but accompanied by a rash. It is somewhat common, and rarely serious.	Enlarged tonsils and a sore throat, a high temperature (up to 104°F or 40°C), abdominal pains, vomiting, a rash of small spots that starts on the chest then spreads and merges, but does not affect the mouth area, and a furry tongue with red patches.
Roseola An uncommon viral infection whose symptoms resemble those of scarlet fever.	A fever with a temperature of 102.2–104°F (39–40°C) for about three days. After this, red or pink spots appear on the trunk, limbs, and neck. The rash fades after about 48 hours.
Diphtheria A serious and highly contagious bacterial infection. It is now very rare because of widespread immunization.	The tonsils are enlarged and may be covered by a gray membrane. Your child may have a mild fever, a cough, a sore throat, breathing difficulties, and headaches.
Tuberculosis A highly infectious bacterial infection that most commonly affects the lungs, but can also affect the kidneys, meninges, joints, bones, and pelvis if long-term.	Persistent coughing (with blood and pus in the sputum if the lungs are affected), chest pain, shortness of breath, fever (especially at night), poor appetite, weight loss, and fatigue.
Poliomyelitis A viral infection of the spinal cord and nerves that can cause paralysis.	High temperature, sore throat, headache, vomiting, weakness, paralysis of muscles, usually in the lower limbs or in the chest.
Impetigo A highly contagious bacterial skin infection most often seen around the lips, eyes, and ears.	Tiny blisters around the nose and mouth or ears, which ooze and harden to form crusty, yellow-brown scabs.

TREATMENT	COMPLICATIONS
Apply calamine lotion to the rash, keep your child at home, and discourage scratching. Your doctor may prescribe an anti-infective cream.	In very rare cases chickenpox may lead to encephalitis (inflammation of the brain) and, if aspirin is taken, Reye syndrome (see p. 541), a serious illness whose symptoms are vomiting and fever.
There is no specific medical treatment. You can give your child liquid acetaminophen if he has a fever and you should try and keep him in isolation.	The biggest risk is to pregnant women who come into contact with a child with German measles, since it causes birth defects. There is a slight risk of encephalitis.
There is no specific medical treatment. You should keep your child away from school, give him liquid acetaminophen and plenty of fluids, and liquidize his food.	Occasionally, meningitis, encephalitis, and pancreatitis. Sometimes, one of the testicles is affected and decreases in size. If both testicles are affected, this can lead to infertility, but this occurs very rarely.
Keep your child in bed for the duration of the fever, keep him away from school, and give him liquid acetaminophen and plenty of fluids. Your doctor may prescribe eye drops for sore eyes and antibiotics for secondary infections.	Ear and chest infections, vomiting and diarrhea may occur a couple of days after the appearance of a rash. There is also a slight risk of pneumonia and encephalitis. The lungs and ears may be permanently damaged if antibiotics aren't given.
Your doctor may prescribe antibiotics, and in severe cases your child may need to go to the hospital for oxygen therapy and treatment for dehydration. Encourage your child to bring up phlegm by laying him over your lap and patting his back as he coughs, don't let him exert himself and keep him away from cigarette smoke.	The main danger is dehydration due to persistent vomiting. Sometimes a severe attack of whooping cough can damage the lungs and make your child prone to chest infections. Secondary infections, which are rare, include pneumonia and bronchitis.
Your child should be isolated and rest in bed for at least two weeks. Be meticulous about hygiene – hepatitis is highly contagious – and give him plenty of fluids. If he won't eat, add a spoonful of glucose to his drinks.	Some children suffer post-hepatitis symptoms for up to six months. These may include moodiness and lethargy.
Your doctor may prescribe antibiotics. Home treatment includes giving your child plenty of fluids and liquidizing food to make it easier to eat. Give liquid acetaminophen to lower temperature.	If your child is sensitive to the streptococcus bacterium it may cause complications, including nephritis (inflammation of the kidneys) and rheumatic fever (inflammation of the joints and heart). These are rare.
Keep your child rested and sponge him to reduce his fever if it's very high. Give liquid acetaminophen to lower his temperature.	If your child's temperature is very high, he may have febrile convulsions (see p. 538).
Diphtheria is very serious because of the possibility of breathing difficulties and your child should be hospitalized immediately. He will be given strong antibiotics and may be given a tracheostomy to help him breathe – that is, a small tube will be inserted temporarily into the windpipe to bypass the blockage in the throat.	Without treatment diphtheria can cause other serious complications: pneumonia and heart failure.
Tuberculosis is a serious disease if left untreated but is rare nowadays. The disease can usually be treated at home. Your doctor will prescribe antibiotics.	The main complications of tuberculosis of the lungs are pleural effusion, in which fluid collects between the lung and chest wall, and pneumothorax, in which air is present between the lung and chest wall.
Quiet and bed rest are important; physical therapy may be necessary. Polio has become rare in recent times due to immunization.	If the disease progresses it can cause paralysis, particularly in the muscles of the lower limbs and chest.
Your doctor will prescribe an antibiotic cream or oral antibiotics.	Impetigo rarely has serious side effects, but because it is highly contagious it should be treated immediately.

Teething

TEETHING IS THE TERM USED TO DESCRIBE THE SYMPTOMS THAT MAY ACCOMPANY THE ERUPTION OF A BABY'S FIRST TEETH. TEETHING USUALLY BEGINS AT ABOUT THE AGE OF 6 OR 7 MONTHS, WITH MOST OF THE FIRST TEETH BREAKING THROUGH BEFORE YOUR BABY IS 18 MONTHS OLD.

Your baby will produce more saliva than usual and will drool; he will try to cram his fingers into his mouth and chew on his fingers or any other object that he can get hold of. He may be clingy and irritable, have difficulty sleeping, and he may cry and fret more than usual. Most of these symptoms occur just before the teeth erupt. It is important to realize that the symptoms of teething do not include bronchitis, diaper rash, vomiting, diarrhea, or loss of appetite. These are symptoms of an underlying illness, not teething. Teething itself and the symptoms associated with it are never serious. No serious symptoms, for example earache, should ever be explained away as teething.

WHAT ARE THE SYMPTOMS?
- Increased saliva and drooling.
- Desire to bite on any hard object.
- Irritability and increased clinginess.
- Sleeplessness.
- Swollen red area where the tooth is being cut.

SHOULD I CONSULT THE DOCTOR?
You don't have to consult a doctor unless your child's symptoms cannot be attributed to teething.

WHAT IS THE TREATMENT?
Your doctor will give you advice on how to cope with the symptoms of teething and may prescribe a mild analgesic to relieve the pain.

WHAT CAN I DO?
- Nurse your baby often. A teething baby needs comfort and closeness. The arrival of teeth doesn't mean a necessary speeding up of the weaning process. Babies with teeth can still be breast-fed, with no discomfort to the mother.
- Distract your child with a chilled teething ring (never freeze it or your baby may get frostbite) or a piece of carrot – something with a firm texture. Never leave him alone with food, in case he chokes.
- Try not to resort to giving your baby acetaminophen. Over the course of the teething process, doses of such pain relievers could become too large. Only use pain relief on your doctor's advice.
- Rub the swollen gum with your finger. Try to avoid teething jellies that contain local anesthetics since they have only a temporary effect and can sometimes cause allergy.
- If your child refuses food, encourage him to eat by giving him cold, smooth foods such as yogurt, ice cream, or jello.

Intussusception

INTUSSUSCEPTION IS A CONDITION THAT OCCURS WHEN PART OF THE SMALL INTESTINE TELESCOPES INSIDE THE INTESTINE AHEAD OF IT, SOMEWHAT LIKE A FINGER OF A GLOVE BEING TURNED INSIDE OUT. THE FOLDED INTESTINE SWELLS AND THIS CAUSES A BLOCKAGE.

In an effort to overcome this blockage, the affected intestine goes into spasm, causing pain and vomiting. There is no known cause for intussusception but it mostly affects baby boys under 12 months of age who have previously been in excellent health. The baby may suddenly cry out as the muscular spasms begin and may vomit and be pale and feverish. In between spasms he may appear quite normal and have normal bowel movements for the first few hours. However, as the attacks continue the bowel movements characteristically look like dark red jello because they consist mostly of blood and mucus.

Though rare, intussusception is a serious condition. Never leave it untreated.

WHAT ARE THE SYMPTOMS?
- Severe abdominal pain, possibly accompanied by screaming.
- Vomiting.
- Paleness.
- Slight fever.
- Bowel motions containing blood and mucus that resemble redcurrant jelly.

SHOULD I CONSULT THE DOCTOR?
Consult your doctor immediately if your baby has a number of attacks or abdominal cramps, or if you notice any blood or mucus in your baby's bowel movements.

WHAT IS THE TREATMENT?
Your doctor will refer your baby to hospital and he will possibly have a barium enema to confirm the diagnosis of intussusception. This is a painless investigation in which fluid is pumped into the intestines through your baby's rectum; the condition of the intestines can then be seen on X-ray. The barium enema sometimes causes the condition to right itself; if it does not, your baby will have an operation in which the intestine will be maneuvered back into its normal position.

See also:
• Contrast X-rays p. 353

Colic

COLIC, AS APPLIED TO A BABY UNDER FOUR MONTHS OF AGE, DESCRIBES A CRYING SPELL, DURING WHICH THE BABY'S FACE BECOMES VERY RED AND BOTH LEGS ARE DRAWN UP TO HIS STOMACH AS IF HE IS IN GREAT PAIN.

This crying spell usually comes in the early evening; during the rest of the day the baby is generally contented. The crying can reach screaming pitch and last from one to three hours. It doesn't usually respond to soothing techniques that work at other times. Colic is so common that it is regarded by pediatricians as normal, but for parents it can be difficult to endure. The cause of the apparent spasmodic crying is not known. It is often at its worst at three months of age but disappears by four months. Recent research has failed to confirm that colic is caused by pain, even though it looks like your baby is in pain.

The fact that your baby is contented during the rest of the day means that this crying bout is not related to a serious physical problem. Colicky babies are usually healthy and thriving.

WHAT ARE THE SYMPTOMS?
■ Your baby cannot settle in the early evening and cries no matter what you do to calm him.
■ He becomes red-faced and draws his legs up into his stomach as if in pain.
■ He may wake from a short sleep with a startled cry.

SHOULD I CONSULT THE DOCTOR?
Consult your doctor as soon as possible if you find you cannot cope with the nightly crying sessions.

WHAT IS THE TREATMENT?
Colic rarely requires treatment with drugs. Your doctor will reassure you that your baby is healthy and that he will grow out of the colic eventually.

WHAT CAN I DO TO HELP?
■ Make sure you take care of yourself. You will be better able to cope if you get as much sleep as you possibly can during the day while your baby sleeps.
■ Invite good friends in to share that time of the evening with you; a relaxed atmosphere may calm both you and your baby.
■ Talk to other parents who have had colicky babies. Once you realize that colic attacks do pass you may find them easier to handle.
■ Consult your doctor for valuable advice and support.

Appendicitis

THE APPENDIX IS A SHORT BLIND TUBE STICKING OUT FROM THE JUNCTION OF THE SMALL AND LARGE BOWELS. APPENDICITIS OCCURS WHEN THE APPENDIX BECOMES PARTLY OR WHOLLY BLOCKED AND A BUILDUP OF BACTERIA CAUSES AN INFECTION.

The appendix then becomes inflamed and swollen and may need to be removed surgically. An appendectomy is a common emergency operation among children. However, appendicitis in babies under the age of 12 months is rare.

If appendicitis is diagnosed early it is not a serious condition. However, if treatment is delayed for any reason the buildup of pus in the blocked appendix can cause it to burst. This condition is known as **peritonitis** and requires immediate attention.

WHAT ARE THE SYMPTOMS?
■ Abdominal pain, starting around the navel, then moving down to the lower right abdomen.
■ Mild temperature, rarely over 100.4°F (38°C).
■ Loss of appetite.
■ Vomiting, diarrhea, or constipation.

SHOULD I CONSULT THE DOCTOR?
If you suspect that your child has appendicitis consult your doctor immediately. If the appendix has burst any delay could allow the infection to spread to the rest of the intestines.

WHAT IS THE TREATMENT?
Your doctor will examine your child's abdomen and ask you to describe the symptoms. He will probably arrange for your child to be admitted to the hospital to confirm the diagnosis and for surgical removal of the appendix, if this is considered necessary.

WHAT CAN I DO TO HELP?
■ Arrange to stay with your child at the hospital overnight.
■ Encourage your child to rest and eat normally when he returns home from hospital, usually about five days after the operation. Your child should recover fully after two to three weeks.

Balanitis

BALANITIS IS THE INFLAMMATION OF THE TIP (GLANS) OF THE PENIS. IT MAY BE CAUSED BY DIAPER RASH, BY AN ALLERGIC REACTION TO THE LAUNDRY DETERGENT IN WHICH YOUR CHILD'S CLOTHES ARE WASHED, OR BY A TIGHT FORESKIN (PHIMOSIS) IN BOYS AGED 3 TO 5 YEARS.

Up to the age of 5 or 6 years, the foreskin is normally tight.

WHAT ARE THE SYMPTOMS?
- Red, swollen tip to the penis.
- Discharge of pus from the tip.
- A foreskin that cannot be drawn back.
- If your child is still in diapers, a general inflammation around the buttocks and genital region.

SHOULD I SEE THE DOCTOR?
Consult your doctor as soon as possible if your child complains of pain, if you cannot retract the foreskin in a child over the age of 5, or if home treatment fails to relieve the swelling in 48 hours.

WHAT IS THE TREATMENT?
Your doctor may prescribe an antibiotic cream to relieve the inflammation.

If the foreskin is tight, your doctor will keep a regular check on it. If the foreskin has failed to stretch by the time your son is six years old, the condition may need to be corrected surgically with circumcision. Your doctor will refer you to a pediatric urologist who will assess your child to see if he needs to be circumcised.

WHAT CAN I DO?
- Always change your child's diapers frequently to help prevent the recurrence of diaper rash.
- Teach your child good personal hygiene from an early age. Up until the age of 5, regular bathing will keep the penis adequately cleaned. After this age, encourage your child to draw back the foreskin and wash the area every day.
- If an allergic reaction has caused balanitis, try changing your laundry detergent, and make sure that your child's clothing is thoroughly rinsed.

Diaper rash

DIAPER RASH IS A SKIN CONDITION THAT AFFECTS THE AREA NORMALLY COVERED BY A BABY'S DIAPER, AND CAN OCCUR WHETHER THE DIAPERS USED ARE CLOTH OR DISPOSABLE.

There are several causes of diaper rash, but it is most commonly caused by urine and stools being left in contact with the skin for too long. Bottle-fed babies are more likely to suffer from this form of diaper rash than breast-fed ones. Diaper rash can also be caused by inadequate drying after bathing your baby. In such cases the diaper rash is usually confined to the skin creases at the top of the thighs. If the rash covers most of the diaper area and you use cloth diapers, it may be due to an allergic reaction to chemicals in the laundry detergent used to wash them, or to fabric softener. This reaction is an early sign of a form of eczema known as atopic eczema. Diaper rash is not serious and is easily prevented and treated.

A rash that starts around the anus and moves over the buttocks and on to the thighs may not be diaper rash but a candida infection (yeast).

WHAT ARE THE SYMPTOMS?
- Redness over the diaper area.
- Redness that starts around the genitals and is accompanied by a strong smell of ammonia.
- Tight, papery skin with inflamed spots that have pus-filled centers.
- Redness that starts around the anus and moves over the buttocks and on to the thighs.

WHAT IS THE TREATMENT?
- If the diaper rash has become infected, your doctor may prescribe antibiotics.
- If your baby has signs of eczema, he may advise you to change your brand of laundry detergent or softener. He may prescribe a cortisone ointment to be used sparingly.
- If the diaper rash is caused by yeast, your doctor will prescribe an antifungal cream.

WHAT CAN I DO?
- When you notice redness on your baby's bottom, wash it with warm water and dry thoroughly. Apply a small amount of emollient cream to prevent skin irritation.
- Change diapers and wash your baby's bottom at least every two to three hours and as soon as he's had a bowel movement.
- Check inside your baby's mouth. If there are white patches, try to wipe them off. If they leave raw, red patches, your baby has oral thrush (yeast), which may have caused the diaper rash. Consult your doctor as soon as possible.
- Don't use talcum powder, it irritates the skin.

See also:
- Eczema in babies and children p. 313
- Candidiasis p. 450

Worms

THERE ARE A NUMBER OF WORMS THAT CAN LIVE IN THE HUMAN BODY BUT THE MOST COMMON IN TEMPERATE CLIMATES IS THE PINWORM. ROUNDWORMS ARE ALSO SOMETIMES SEEN.

Pinworms usually enter the body as eggs in contaminated food, which then hatch in the intestine and develop into adults in 15 to 28 days. The female worms then lay more eggs around the anus, which causes itching, especially at night. If your child scratches himself, he can easily pick up the eggs on his fingers and under his fingernails and by putting them into his mouth start the whole cycle again. Pinworms, which are $\frac{1}{16}$-$\frac{1}{2}$in (2-13mm) long, are harmless but they can produce unpleasant symptoms. The worms are highly infectious and all the family should be treated simultaneously.

WHAT ARE THE SYMPTOMS?
PINWORMS
- Itching around the anus, usually at night.
- White threadlike worms in the stools.
- Sleeplessness that is caused by intense itching.

ROUNDWORMS
- Failure to gain weight appropriately.
- White worms in the stools.

SHOULD I CONSULT THE DOCTOR?
See your doctor as soon as possible if you find any worms. See your doctor as soon as possible if you've been in an area where roundworm is common and your child is not gaining weight.

WHAT IS THE TREATMENT?
- Your doctor will prescribe a simple treatment, usually in the form of a pleasant tasting, soluble powder to be taken by the whole family.
- If your child has a roundworm, your doctor will prescribe a drug taken by mouth that will paralyze the worm. He may also prescribe a

laxative so that your child can pass the worm easily in his stools.

WHAT CAN I DO?
- Follow the instructions for the medication carefully. The bowel movements may be loose for 12 hours afterward, so you may be advised to give the medication early in the morning.
- Repeating the dosage may be necessary depending on the type of worm and on the medication taken.
- Be meticulous about hygiene. The eggs can be picked up under the fingernails and reingested.
- Make sure your child wears pajamas or pants at night so that when he scratches, his hands don't come into direct contact with the anus.

Roundworms

Roundworms are rare but are most likely to infect children in areas where sanitary conditions are poor; they are more common in tropical climates. These worms are long – 6–14in (15–35cm) – and resemble a white earthworm. The eggs are swallowed with contaminated food and drink and, after hatching in the intestine, the worms lay eggs that are sometimes excreted in the stools. Your child will appear undernourished and he will fail to thrive.

Crib death (SIDS)

CRIB DEATH, ALSO KNOWN AS SUDDEN INFANT DEATH SYNDROME (SIDS), IS THE SUDDEN
AND OFTEN UNEXPLAINED DEATH OF A SEEMINGLY HEALTHY BABY.

There is no single known cause of crib death, although research has shown that some deaths can be the result of an abnormality in the breathing and heart rate. There are several current areas of research, including the development of a baby's temperature control mechanism and respiratory system in the first six months, and the recent discovery that an inherited enzyme deficiency may be responsible for around 1 percent of cases. Studies connecting SIDS with flame-retardant chemicals in crib mattresses have, so far, proven inconclusive.

The death of an infant from SIDS is a particularly distressing experience. Severe grief can be compounded by intense feelings of guilt and misplaced blame, and family relationships can sometimes suffer as a result. Parents of crib death infants may have to discuss the incident with the police and be prepared for postmortem examination of the baby. Your pediatrician should be able to provide valuable support and counseling in this situation, and talking to other parents who have also experienced a crib death, or to a professional organization, can also provide great comfort (see Useful addresses, p. 567).

WHAT ARE THE SYMPTOMS?
- Common coldlike symptom of stuffy nose.
- Inexplicable weight loss.

WHAT CAN I DO?
While the causes of crib death are not clear, there are ways in which you can significantly reduce the risks.
- Always put your baby to sleep ON HIS BACK, NEVER ON HIS FRONT. Babies who sleep on their backs are at less risk of crib death. This position also helps control your baby's body temperature (see below).
- Don't wrap him in too many night-clothes or bed linens, especially during winter, or put him to bed in a room that is too warm. Use a thermostatically controlled heater in his room so that temperatures do not rise too high or drop too low. Make sure he has enough blankets – a sheet and three blankets is sufficient in a room temperature of 64°F (18°C). Use fewer if the temperature is higher – no more than one sheet and blanket on a warm night of 75°F (24°C).
- Avoid smoking during pregnancy and after your child is born.
- Ban smokers from the house.
- Be careful not to swaddle or tuck your baby in. Don't use comforters, sheepskins, or crib bumpers since they all prevent heat loss.
- Whenever possible, breast-feed rather than bottle-feed your baby.
- Avoid taking unnecessary drugs during pregnancy.
- If you think your baby is unwell, contact your doctor. If he has a fever, don't increase

the wrapping – reduce it so he can lose heat. After a minor illness, keep a closer eye than usual on him for several days until the symptoms disappear.

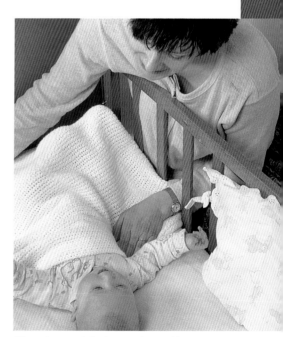

Always put your baby down to sleep on his back with his feet at the foot of the crib ("feet to foot") to prevent him from slipping under the bed linens.

Kawasaki disease

KAWASAKI DISEASE IS A PROLONGED FEVER DURING WHICH THE HEART AND BLOOD VESSELS
MAY BE DAMAGED. IT IS MORE COMMON IN CHILDREN UNDER AGE 5, IN BOYS
AND IN PEOPLE OF ASIAN, AFRICAN, OR CARIBBEAN DESCENT.

First observed in Japan in the 1960s, Kawasaki disease is now being diagnosed more often in Western countries. Heart damage occurs in about 1 in 5 of all cases of the disorder. Early diagnosis is important because Kawasaki disease can be life threatening.

WHAT ARE THE SYMPTOMS?
Symptoms develop over about two weeks and include:
● prolonged, constant fever lasting more than five days
● sore or itchy, watery eyes
● cracked, swollen, and painful lips
● sore throat
● swollen glands in the neck, under the arms, and in the groin.
   After about a week of fever the following symptoms may develop:
● reddening of palms of hands and soles of feet, with peeling skin on tips of fingers and toes
● blotchy pink rash over the entire body.

SHOULD I CONSULT THE DOCTOR?
Consult your doctor immediately if your child develops a fever that cannot be lowered by taking liquid acetaminophen.

WHAT IS THE TREATMENT?
■ If your doctor suspects Kawasaki disease your child will be admitted immediately to the hospital because treatment is most effective if started within 10 days of the onset of the disease.
■ Your child will probably have blood tests to look for evidence of Kawasaki disease.
■ Echocardiography may be done to look for damage to the heart and blood vessels.
■ Intravenous immunoglobulin may be given to fight the infection and reduce the risk of inflammation of the heart muscle (myocarditis).

■ High doses of aspirin may be given until the fever subsides, with lower doses following for a period of several weeks.
   Most children with Kawasaki disease recover completely within three weeks but need regular follow-up visits to the doctor, and sometimes echocardiography, for a few months. Any inflammation of the heart muscle usually disappears after several months. Children who have had Kawasaki disease have a slightly increased risk of developing coronary artery disease later in life.

WHAT CAN I DO?
Care for your child as you would for a child who has just come home from hospital.

See also:
● **Your child in hospital p. 519**

Juvenile rheumatoid arthritis

JUVENILE RHEUMATOID ARTHRITIS (JRA) IS PERSISTENT INFLAMMATION OF ONE OR MORE
JOINTS THAT OCCURS ONLY IN CHILDHOOD.

Juvenile rheumatoid arthritis is the result of an abnormal response of the immune system, leading to inflammation, swelling, and pain in the lining of one or several joints. Although the cause is not understood, juvenile rheumatoid arthritis sometimes runs in families, suggesting a genetic factor may be involved. In mild cases, mobility is rarely affected. In severe cases, there may be reduced mobility and eventually joint deformities.
   Juvenile rheumatoid arthritis is divided into three types according to the number of joints affected by the disease and the specific symptoms involved.

WHAT ARE THE TYPES AND THEIR SYMPTOMS?
SEVERAL JOINTS ARE AFFECTED
This type affects more girls than boys and occurs at any age. Symptoms include inflammation, stiffness, and pain in five or more joints. Those joints commonly affected include the wrists, fingers, knees, and ankles.

FEW JOINTS AND SOMETIMES OTHER PARTS OF THE BODY ARE AFFECTED
This type affects both sexes equally and usually occurs during early childhood. Symptoms

include inflammation, stiffness, and pain in four or fewer joints, and girls are at high risk of an eye condition known as **uveitis**. The joints commonly involved include those in the **knees, ankles,** and **wrists.**

THE JUVENILE FORM OF ADULT RHEUMATOID ARTHRITIS
This type is also known as Still's disease and affects boys and girls equally at any age during childhood. Any number of joints may be affected, but, although they are painful, they do not become swollen. The other symptoms of the disease include **fever, swollen glands,** and a **nonitchy rash.** Some children recover totally.

SHOULD I CONSULT THE DOCTOR?
Consult your doctor as soon as possible if your child complains of pain in his joints, if his joints are swollen or if you otherwise suspect that your child may have JRA.

WHAT IS THE TREATMENT?
If the doctor suspects that your child has a type of juvenile rheumatoid arthritis, he may arrange for X-rays of the affected joints and blood tests to look for particular antibodies associated with the condition.

The goal of treatment for JRA is to reduce inflammation, minimize joint damage, and relieve pain. If your child is mildly affected, he or she may only need to take **nonsteroidal anti-inflammatory drugs** (NSAIDs) to reduce inflammation and relieve pain. In more severe cases your child may be prescribed **oral steroids,** or she may be treated with locally acting steroids **injected into the affected joints.** Sometimes, inflammation can be reduced by using **antirheumatic drugs,** such as gold-based drugs or penicillamine.
   Other treatments may include **physical therapy** to maintain joint mobility and sometimes, **occupational therapy. Splints** may be used for support and to help prevent deformity. **Special devices** are also available and may help with daily activities such as dressing. If damage to the joints is severe and has caused deformity, **joint replacement** may be necessary.

WHAT IS THE OUTLOOK?
Juvenile rheumatoid arthritis usually clears up in a few years. Severely affected children may be left with deformed joints, and some may develop rheumatoid arthritis in adult life.

Moles

MOLES ARE CAUSED BY AN OVERPRODUCTION OF PIGMENTED SKIN CELLS CALLED MELANOCYTES.
THEY CAN FORM ANYWHERE ON THE SKIN, AND THERE ARE SEVERAL TYPES.

WHAT ARE THEY?

Moles are flat or raised growths on the skin, which are rough or smooth and vary in color from light to dark brown. Freckles, by contrast, are multiple, small, brown-colored spots on the skin that are usually harmless.

Moles may exist from birth, or appear during childhood and early adolescence; nearly all adults have about 10–20 moles by the age of 30. Most moles are noncancerous, but in rare cases a mole may undergo changes that make it cancerous.

Alterations in the shape, color, or size of moles are not always a sign of cancer, and changes during puberty or pregnancy are usually normal. However, any change in moles should always be evaluated by a doctor.

WHAT MIGHT BE DONE?

You should consult a doctor immediately if you have a mole that is more than ⅜in (1cm) in diameter and is growing rapidly. A mole that changes shape or color, becomes itchy or inflamed, or starts bleeding should also be investigated by a doctor.

If your doctor suspects that a mole is cancerous, he or she may recommend that you have it removed and examined for cancerous cells (a biopsy). Noncancerous moles can also be removed either for cosmetic reasons or if they are being chafed by clothing.

> **See also:**
> • **Tissue tests p. 259**

Children's teeth

DENTISTS HATE TAKING OUT TEETH, EVEN BABY ONES, BUT OCCASIONALLY
AN ORTHODONTIST WILL DECIDE TO TAKE OUT A PRIMARY TOOTH TO PREVENT
OVERCROWDING WHILE THE PERMANENT TEETH EMERGE.

Most orthodontists feel that they have to "educate" parents as well as treating the children, because parents often demand corrective treatment for malpositioned teeth long before it should be given. There is no point considering cosmetic dentistry for a child until she is eight years old, since she will not have the requisite number of teeth on which to attach a brace or wire. Most dentists would prefer to wait until a child is about 12 years old before undertaking orthodontic treatment because if this is given too early other faults may occur. In addition, many problems improve naturally if left to the correcting effects of chewing and the position of the tongue, cheeks, and lips.

Reference 5

FIRST AID

In an emergency situation you need to assess what has happened and what you need to do, and you must stay as calm and be as methodical as possible while you do so. You need to consider:

• Risks to yourself.

Do not put yourself at risk. If you are injured too, you will not be able to help anyone. Be aware of your limitations; do only as much as you feel able to do.

• Risks to the person.

If you can't eliminate a hazard, try to move it away. Move the person only as a last resort.

• Risks to bystanders.

• What help you need.

• Resources you can use to help.

The recovery position

The recovery position prevents an unconscious person's tongue from falling back and blocking the throat and allows liquids to drain from the mouth, making it less likely that the person will inhale vomit. Do not use the recovery position if you suspect a spinal injury, and only use the log roll (see p. 562) if you have help.

FOR A BABY UNDER ONE YEAR
If a baby is unconscious but is breathing and has signs of circulation (see below), cradle him in your arms with his head tilted downwards. This will prevent him from choking on his tongue or inhaling vomit.

The leg is bent to prevent the person from rolling forward

The hand supports the head, allowing drainage from the mouth

The ABC of resuscitation

Once you have determined that it's safe, you can quickly assess the state of the person and give emergency aid if necessary. Determine whether or not he is conscious by asking what has happened and gently shaking his shoulders.

You must also assess whether he:

• has an open **airway**

• is **breathing**

• has signs of **circulation**.

A good way to remember what to do is the ABC of resuscitation (see below).

A = airway
Open the airway by gently tilting the person's head back and lifting the chin.

B = breathing
Check to see if he's breathing by looking at the chest to see if it's rising and falling, listening for sounds of breathing, and feeling for breath on your cheek. Do this for up to 10 seconds before you decide that breathing is absent.

If the person is **not breathing**, you can keep his blood supply oxygenated by giving **rescue breaths** (see p. 555)

Place a person who is **breathing** but unconscious in the **recovery position** (see above) to ensure that his airway remains open.

NEVER delay in getting help that you need.

C = circulation
Spend up to 10 seconds looking for evidence of circulation, such as breathing, movement, coughing, and a healthy color of the skin. If **circulation is absent**, you can use **chest compressions** to keep the blood circulating around the body (see p. 555). You need to do these along with rescue breaths to keep the blood oxygenated.

If the person is **not breathing**, you can keep his blood supply oxygenated by giving **rescue breaths** (see p. 555)

Rescue breathing
Body tissues, and especially tissues in the brain, need oxygen to keep their cells alive. Although the air that you breathe out contains only about 16 percent oxygen, it's still enough to maintain life if it's blown into the lungs of someone who has stopped breathing due to illness or injury. If there are no signs of circulation (see above), you need to perform chest compressions (see p. 555) also; together the two are known as cardiopulmonary resuscitation or CPR.

Mouth-to-mouth rescue breaths

1. With the person lying flat on his back, open the airway by placing one hand on the person's forehead and gently tilting the head back.

2. Remove any obvious obstruction from the mouth and lift the chin.

3. Pinch shut the nostrils of the person (inset). Take a full breath; place your lips around his mouth to provide a good seal.

4. Blow into the person's mouth until you see his chest rise. It will take about two seconds for full inflation.

5. Remove your mouth from his and let the chest fall completely – this will take about four seconds. Repeat the procedure once more and then check for signs of circulation (see p. 554).

■ **If there are no signs of recovery,** such as return of skin color or any movement, begin CPR (see below) immediately.

■ **If there are signs of recovery,** but no breathing, give 10 breaths per minute and check for signs of circulation every 10 breaths.

■ **If spontaneous breathing returns,** put the person in the recovery position (see p. 554).

RESCUE BREATHING FOR A BABY UNDER ONE YEAR

1. Seal your mouth tightly around the baby's mouth and nose and breathe out into his lungs.

2. Give two breaths, that raise the chest, trying to provide 20 breaths every minute. Look for signs of recovery, such as breathing, coughing or return of color to the skin.

RESCUE BREATHING FOR A CHILD AGED 1–7

1. Pinch the nostrils closed. Seal your lips around his mouth and breathe out into the lungs until the chest rises.

2. Give two breaths, trying to give 15 breaths every minute. Look for signs of recovery, such as breathing, return of skin color, or movement.

Cardiopulmonary resuscitation (CPR)

■ **If there are no signs of circulation** (see p. 554), you need to keep the blood circulating around the person's body using artificial circulation, which you can provide by chest compressions. You must combine these with rescue breaths to keep the blood oxygenated (see above). Together these are known as cardiopulmonary resuscitation (CPR). Two people can perform CPR together.

1. Kneel beside the person, who should be on his back on a flat surface.

2. Find one of the lowermost ribs using the first two fingers of the hand that is closest to the person's legs. Slide your fingers along the rib to the point where the lowermost ribs meet the breastbone. Place your middle finger here (inset) and your index finger above it on the lower breastbone.

3. Put the heel of your other hand on the breastbone. This is where you should apply pressure to compress the chest.

4. Put the heel of your first hand on

top of the other hand; interlock your fingers (inset).

5. Leaning right over the person, keep your arms straight and press down vertically to depress the breastbone up to one-third of the depth of the chest (about 1½–2in/4–5cm for an average adult). Remove the pressure but leave your hands in position.

6. Compress the chest 15 times, trying to do so at a rate of 100 compressions per minute. Then give two breaths (see above) before calling for an ambulance. Continue this procedure, alternating 15 compressions with two breaths until help arrives, the person recovers or you become exhausted.

CPR FOR A BABY UNDER ONE YEAR

1. With the baby on his back on a flat surface, put the tips of your first two fingers on the midbreastbone between the nipples. Press down at this point to a third of the depth of the baby's chest. Do this five times, going for a rate of 100 compressions per minute.

2. Give one full rescue breath into the baby's nose and mouth (see above).

3. Alternate five chest compressions with one breath for one minute before calling an ambulance. Continue giving CPR alternating five compressions with one breath while you are waiting for help to arrive.

CPR FOR CHILDREN AGED 1–7

1. Place your hand on the child's chest as you would for an adult (see left), but use the heel of one hand only to compress the chest to a third of its depth. Do this five times going for a rate of 100 compressions per minute.

2. Give one full rescue breath.

3. Alternate five chest compressions with one breath for one minute before calling an ambulance. Continue giving CPR alternating five compressions with one breath while you are waiting for help to arrive.

Choking

Choking happens when an object or piece of food gets stuck at the back of the throat, blocking it or causing the throat muscles to go into spasm. Young children and babies are prone to choking since they often put things in their mouths. Choking always requires prompt action. Be prepared to resuscitate if the person stops breathing.

Choking in a conscious adult

1. Assess the severity of his breathing difficulty. Encourage coughing, which may help him dislodge the obstruction.

2. If he starts to become weaker or stops coughing, position yourself close behind him and put your arms under his arms, encircling his torso.

3. With one hand, make a fist. Place the thumb side of the fist on his upper abdomen, slightly above the navel and well below the tip of the breastbone. Grasp your fist with your other hand.

4. Give up to five abdominal thrusts. Pull

your fist sharply inward and upward against his abdomen. Each thrust should be a quick, separate movement. The thrusts should force air out of the lungs. The pressure may dislodge the obstruction. Look in the mouth, and remove visible obstructions. Continue thrusts until the blockage is cleared or he becomes unconscious.

Choking in a conscious baby of up to one year

■ **If at any point the object clears** or the baby becomes unconscious, open the airway and check breathing (see p. 554).

1. Lay the baby facedown against your forearm, supporting the back and chin. Give up to five sharp slaps on his back.

2. Check the baby's mouth and remove any obvious obstruction with a finger. NEVER feel around in the throat.

3. If this fails, turn the baby face up on your arm or lap. Give up to five sharp thrusts into the chest at the nipple line with your fingertips. NEVER use abdominal thrusts on a baby. Check the baby's mouth.

4. If the object has not cleared, repeat steps 1–4 three times and then take the baby with you to phone for an ambulance. Repeat steps 1–4 until help arrives.

■ **If the baby loses consciousness at any time,** follow the steps below.

Choking in a conscious child aged 1–7

1. Assess the severity of the child's breathing difficulty. Encourage the child to cough, which should help dislodge the obstruction.

2. If the child stops coughing, without dislodging the obstruction, or if he becomes weaker, prepare to give him abdominal thrusts. Position yourself close behind her and put your arms under her arms, encircling her torso. If she is small, kneel behind her.

3. With one hand, make a fist Place the thumb side of the fist against the child's upper abdomen; position it slightly above the navel and well below the tip of the breastbone. Grasp your fist with your other hand.

4 Perform up to five abdominal thrusts. To do this, pull your fist sharply inward and upward against the child's abdomen. Each abdominal thrust should be a quick, separate movement. These thrusts should be sufficient to force air out of the child's lungs. The sudden pressure of the air may dislodge the obstruction from his airway.

5 Continue giving the child abdominal thrusts until the obstruction is cleared or he loses consciousness. If the child becomes unconscious, see Choking in an unconscious child (below).

Choking in an unconscious adult, child, or baby

FOR ADULTS AND CHILDREN AGED 8 AND OVER

1. Open the airway and check breathing (see p. 554). If there is no breathing, give rescue breaths (see p. 555). Make five attempts to do two effective breaths.

2. If the person's chest rises during these attempts, continue rescue breaths. If the chest does not rise, do 15 chest compressions and alternate these with two attempted rescue breaths.

3. After each set of 15 chest compressions, check the mouth to see if the obstruction has cleared using one finger to remove any obvious obstruction.

■ **Follow this procedure for one minute** and then, if it has not already been done, phone for an ambulance.

■ **If at any stage the person begins to breathe normally,** you should put him in the recovery position (see p. 554). Phone for an ambulance.

FOR BABIES AND CHILDREN AGED 1–7

1. Open the airway by gently tilting the head back. Pick any obvious obstruction out of the mouth and lift the chin.

2. If there is no breathing, give two rescue breaths (see p. 555). Check circulation and if there is no circulation, alternate five chest compressions (see p. 555) with one rescue breath. Do this for one minute before taking the baby with you to phone for an ambulance.

Asthma attacks

In an asthma attack the muscles of the air passages go into spasm and the linings of the airways swell. This makes the airways narrow and breathing becomes difficult. Sometimes there is a "trigger," such as an allergy or a cold, for an attack; other times there is no obvious reason for an attack coming on.

People who have been diagnosed with asthma usually carry "reliever" inhalers, which are used to relieve an attack and usually have blue caps. Sometimes they also carry "preventer" inhalers, which are used regularly to help prevent attacks and usually have brown or white caps. Plastic "spacers" are sometimes attached to inhalers to help people breathe in the medication correctly.

If you are with someone who is having an asthma attack, do the following:

1. Keep calm and be as reassuring as you can. Ask the person to use their reliever inhaler and help them to do so if necessary; you may need to fit a spacer to the inhaler. Remember that, although asthma can be

frightening, a reliever inhaler usually has an effect within a few minutes.

2. Let the person get into the position they feel is most comfortable; this is often sitting down. DO NOT make the person lie down. Encourage the person to breathe slowly and deeply.

3. If the attack is a mild one and eases within 5 or 10 minutes, ask the person to take another dose from his reliever inhaler. Immediate medical help is not vital, but he should tell his doctor about the attack soon.

4. If this is a person's first attack or if it is a severe attack and the inhaler has no effect after 5 or 10 minutes, the person is getting

worse and breathlessness makes talking difficult, phone for an ambulance. Help him use his inhaler every 5 or 10 minutes, and monitor and record his breathing and pulse regularly.

5. If the person stops breathing or loses consciousness, open his airway and check breathing and circulation (see p. 554). Call EMS.

> **DO NOT use a preventer inhaler during an asthma attack.**

Croup

Croup is an attack of breathing difficulty in a baby or a child that is caused by inflammation in the larynx and windpipe. The child may make a barking noise when he coughs and make noise when trying to breathe. It can be frightening but an attack usually passes without any lasting harm. Croup often occurs at night.

If an attack of croup does not clear or is severe or there is noise with breathing, phone for an ambulance immediately.

If you are with a child who is having an attack of croup, do the following:

1. Sit the child up and reassure him. Make sure his back is supported against something. NEVER stick your fingers into the child's throat, and do not panic, since you will only

frighten the child and worsen the attack.

2. Either create a steamy atmosphere by using a humidifier or boiling a kettle in the child's room or move the child into the bathroom and run the hot faucet or the shower. Sit him down and encourage him to relax and breathe in the steam. Be sure you keep the child well away from the hot water.

3. If that doesn't work, take the child

outside in the cold air.

4. When the child is put back to bed, create a humid atmosphere in the bedroom by using a humidifier, boiling a kettle, or hanging a wet towel over a radiator. The humidity may prevent an attack from recurring.

5. Call your doctor or call EMS if the steam doesn't bring relief or if the attack is severe.

Anaphylactic shock

Anaphylactic shock (anaphylaxis) occurs when the body has a serious, general allergic reaction to something. Medical attention is urgently required and first aid is limited to helping breathing and minimizing shock until medical help arrives.

A person who develops anaphylactic shock may have widespread red blotches on the skin, obvious difficulty breathing, and swelling in the face and neck. An injection of epinephrine (adrenaline) eases the symptoms, and people with severe allergies usually carry injectable epinephrine (an Epi-Pen) with

them. If an affected person has an Epi-Pen, help her to use it as soon as signs of anaphylactic shock become apparent.

1. Call EMS immediately. Say that you suspect anaphylactic shock.

2. If the person is conscious, help her sit up in a position that helps breathing the most.

3. If the person is unconscious, put her in the recovery position and monitor her breathing, pulse and level of response regularly. Be prepared to resuscitate if necessary.

Seizures

A seizure (also known as a convulsion or fit) occurs when disturbance in the function of the brain causes involuntary contraction of muscles in the body. There are many causes of seizures, including head injury, certain diseases or conditions that affect the brain (such as epilepsy), or shortage of oxygen to the brain.

In babies and young children, high fever may cause seizures (see Febrile convulsions, below). Seizures usually cause consciousness to be lost or impaired, and in any seizure in which consciousness is lost, follow the treatment rules for unconsciousness (see below).

Epileptic seizures

There are two basic types of epileptic seizures: petit mal and grand mal. Petit mal seizures are also known as absence seizures, because people who experience them do not lose consciousness completely but enter into a state like daydreaming. Grand mal seizures involve unconsciousness and uncontrollable twitching or jerking of the limbs.

PETIT MAL (ABSENCE) SEIZURES

1. Help the person experiencing the seizure to sit down; remove any sharp objects or hot drinks from the nearby area.

2. Talk to her calmly but don't ask her unnecessary questions. Stay with her until the seizure has passed and she is behaving like her normal self again.

■ **If the person is unaware of her absence seizures,** suggest to her that she see her doctor soon.

GRAND MAL SEIZURES

1 If the person is falling, try to ease his fall if you can. Clear the space around him and ask any bystanders to stand back.

2 Loosen clothing around the neck and put something soft under his head if possible.

3 Once the seizures have stopped, put him in the recovery position (see p. 554). Check his breathing, pulse and level of response, and stay with him until he is fully recovered.

■ **If a person is unconscious** for more than 10 minutes or the convulsions last for more than 5 minutes, phone for an ambulance. You should note the time the seizure occurred and its duration.

Febrile convulsions

Babies and small children are prone to seizures when their core body temperature rises very high, as in a fever. Febrile convulsions are frightening but are not usually dangerous or indicative of epilepsy.

1. Put pillows or other soft objects around the child so that she won't harm herself. Undress her down to underwear.

2. Sponge her with lukewarm (not cold) water (cold water makes blood vessels constrict and drives body temperature up).

Start at her head and work down the body.

3. Ensure that her airway is open and put her in the recovery position once the seizure stops.

4. Phone for an ambulance.

> **DO NOT** lift or move a person having a convulsion unless he is in danger.
>
> **DO NOT** put anything into his mouth or attempt to restrain him in any way.

Unconsciousness

Unconsciousness occurs when the brain's normal electrical activity is interrupted, for whatever reason. A number of different conditions and accidents can cause unconsciousness, including fainting due to low blood sugar or low blood pressure, epilepsy, and head injury. If a person is unconscious, follow these rules:

1. Open airway, check breathing and be ready to resuscitate (see p. 555). Place him in the recovery position.

2. Examine the person for injuries, but in doing so you should not move him unnecessarily.

3. Check his response level regularly. In doing so you should consider whether he can open his eyes, can obey commands,

The recovery postition

or respond to a pinch, and answer sensibly a simple question such as "what is your name?".

■ **Even if the person regains full consciousness** and remains well, he should see his doctor as soon as possible. If he does not recover or his condition deteriorates, phone for an ambulance and continue monitoring the person's response level until help arrives.

Concussion

Concussion occurs when the brain is shaken a little in a fall or a violent blow. Although there may be a brief or partial loss of consciousness, it is followed by complete recovery. Concussion can only be safely diagnosed by medical personnel after the person has made a complete recovery.

You should keep in mind that all head injuries are potentially serious and should be assessed by a doctor.

1. If the person is unconscious following a head injury, assume there may be a neck or back injury (p. 562). Watch her closely; while you are doing this you should also remember

to monitor and record her breathing, pulse and response level regularly. If the person remains unconscious, phone for an ambulance.

2. If the person regains consciousness, you should continue to watch her carefully, looking for any change in her level of

response, even if she has apparently made a full recovery.

3. Advise the person to see her doctor, even if she appears to have made a full recovery. It is particularly important for her to see a doctor if she experiences headache, sickness, or fatigue afterward.

Bleeding

Minor bleeding can be distressing but is not usually cause for alarm; it can usually be controlled or stopped by applying direct pressure to the wound and does not need medical attention. More severe bleeding needs prompt action to control blood loss and requires immediate medical attention.

Minor bleeding

First aid for minor injuries that break the skin helps to minimize the risk of infection developing and aids healing. However, you should always seek medical advice if:
● a foreign object, such as a piece of wood, glass, or gravel, is embedded in a wound
● the wound is a puncture wound or a bite
● a previous wound shows signs of becoming infected, for example if it becomes red and sore or if there is pus in it.

TO TREAT MINOR EXTERNAL BLEEDING:
1. Wash your hands well in soap and water before you treat the wound. Put on disposable gloves if available.

2. If there is dirt on the wound, rinse it under running water; alternatively, use an antiseptic wipe. Pat the wound dry with clean gauze. Cover the wound with clean gauze.

3. Elevate the part of the body that has been wounded above the level of the heart. Don't touch the wound directly and support the elevated part with one hand.

4. Clean the area around the wound with soap and water. Pat dry and remove the gauze. Apply an adhesive dressing.

Severe bleeding

Severe bleeding is very upsetting and frightening, but keep in mind that blood loss is rarely so great that the heart stops beating. It is, however, likely that the injured person will be in shock and may lose consciousness. Try to remain calm.

TO CONTROL SEVERE BLEEDING, DO THE FOLLOWING:
1. Put on disposable gloves if available. Remove clothing from the area of the wound, cutting it off if necessary.

2. Apply direct pressure on the wound with your fingers or palm. Use a clean dressing if one is at hand, but don't waste time looking for one. If an object is embedded in the wound, apply pressure firmly on either side of it.

3. Carefully raise the injured area so that it is above the level of the person's heart. Lay her down to reduce blood flow to the wound.

4. Apply a sterile dressing, but leave any original dressing in place. Make the bandage tight, but not so tight that it prevents circulation. Apply another bandage on top if blood is seeping through.

5. Phone for an ambulance and treat the injured person for shock (see p. 560). Make sure that the bandages you have applied do not impede circulation.

> **NEVER apply a tourniquet; it can actually worsen bleeding and can cause tissue damage.**

A foreign object in a minor wound

1. Do not try to remove objects embedded in a wound. Small pieces of glass, wood, or gravel may be picked off the surface of a small wound, but if you try to remove objects more deeply embedded you may damage the tissue further and make bleeding worse.

2. Control bleeding by applying pressure to the wound on either side of the object using a piece of clean gauze. Elevate the injured part if possible.

3. Cover the wound with clean gauze and put pads made of gauze or cotton padding around the object so that you are able to put a bandage over it without pressing directly on the object. If you can't build the pads high enough, put the bandage around the object instead.

4. Arrange for the person to go to the hospital as soon as possible.

Nosebleeds

Nosebleeds happen when blood vessels inside the nose get broken. A nosebleed can be alarming, but it is only dangerous if a great deal of blood is lost. However, if the fluid that comes out of the nose appears thin and watery following a head injury, this is a serious condition that may indicate that cerebrospinal fluid is leaking from the area surrounding the brain.

1. Ask the person to sit down and put his head forward. NEVER put the head back during a nosebleed since the blood running down the throat can cause vomiting.

2. Ask the person to breathe through his mouth and pinch his nose below the bridge. Help him if he cannot do this himself. Ask him not to speak or try to clear his nose, since these things can interfere with blood clotting. Give him a tissue or handkerchief to hold against his nose to mop up any blood.

A young child can lean over a bowl and spit into it if this helps.

3. Ask the person to stop pinching his nose after 10 minutes. If the bleeding continues, repeat the procedure for another 10 minutes and check again. If after 30 minutes the person's nose is still bleeding, take the person to an emergency department with his head in the forward position.

4. When the bleeding has stopped, ask the person to stay leaning forward; gently clean the area around the nose. The person should rest for a few hours and should not blow his nose, which could cause bleeding to start again.

Shock

Shock occurs if the supply of blood to the body's vital organs is reduced. This may occur for a variety of reasons: if the heart doesn't pump blood normally (as in a heart attack); if blood vessels dilate, reducing blood pressure (as in anaphylactic shock); or if blood or other bodily fluids are lost through injury, burns, diarrhea, or vomiting.

The type of shock a person experiences in stressful situations where there is no physical injury is called psychogenic shock or fainting and is a separate condition needing different treatment.

SIGNS OF SHOCK
- Rapid pulse.
- Pale, sometimes bluish skin.
- Sweating and cold skin.

IF SHOCK DEVELOPS FURTHER
- Weakness and dizziness.
- Nausea and possible vomiting.
- Thirstiness.
- Rapid and shallow breathing.
- A weak pulse.

IF SHOCK CONTINUES
- Restlessness and possible aggressiveness.
- Yawning and gasping for air.
- Unconsciousness.
- Failure of the heart to beat.

TREATING SHOCK
1. Lay the person down (on a coat or a blanket if outdoors or on a cold surface), and keep her head low. Talk to her reassuringly.

2. Raise the person's legs; this will help the blood supply to the vital organs.

3. Loosen any tight clothing; the person may be wearing, such as a tie, a tight collar, cuffs, or a belt.

4. Keep the person warm by covering her with coats or blankets. DO NOT put any direct source of heat near the person or use an electric blanket or hot water bottle. Phone for an ambulance. Record the person's breathing, pulse, and response level and be prepared to resuscitate if necessary (see p. 555).

A person in shock should not smoke, eat, drink, or move around unnecessarily. Don't leave a person in shock alone. If she become unconscious, refer to p. 558.

Eye injury

All eye injuries should be considered potentially serious. They require prompt medical attention to minimize the risk of infection or scarring of eye tissues, which may lead to permanently impaired vision. The injured eye may appear bloodshot or may bleed or leak clear fluid.

1. Lay the injured person on his back, keeping his head still.

2. Tell the person not to move his eyes, since movement of the uninjured eye will also cause movement of the injured one.

3. Ask the person to hold a sterile dressing over the injured eye, which will help keep him from moving it and will help prevent infection.

Support his head so that it is straight

4. Take the person to a hospital emergency department immediately.

> **DO NOT touch an injured eye or attempt to remove any object embedded in it.**

Foreign objects in the eye

While a speck of dust or a contact lens that is floating on the surface of the eye may be easily removed, anything that is actually stuck to the eye or embedded in it should not be touched. Take the person to a doctor or an emergency department.

1. Ask the person not to touch or rub her eye. Ask her to sit down and face a light source. Then gently pull back the upper and lower eyelids and look carefully at the eye.

2. If there is a foreign object floating on the surface of the eye, wash it out by pouring clean water over it from nose side outward, or by using an eyebath filled with clean water.

3. If this doesn't work, you can try to lift it out with a moist cotton swab, or a dampened corner of a tissue or clean cloth. DO NOT try to do this if the object is stuck in place.

4. If the object is under the upper eyelid, ask the person to pull the upper eyelid over the lower one. This often dislodges the object.

Foreign objects in the nose

Young children are especially prone to this situation. They may put small objects up their noses, which can cause injury, infection or blockage. Do not try to remove an object from the nose yourself, since you may cause further injury or push the object farther in. Instead keep the person calm and quiet, encourage him to breathe through his mouth, and take him to a hospital emergency department immediately.

Foreign objects in the ear

An object in the ear may cause temporary deafness or may injure the eardrum. Do not try to remove any object in the ear yourself, since you may worsen the injury. However, if an insect has flown or crawled into the ear, you can try rinsing it out using the following method.

1. Ask the person to sit down and stay calm.

2. Gently pour a glass of clean, lukewarm water into the ear, which may wash the insect out.

3. If this doesn't work, take the person to a hospital emergency department.

Broken bones and soft tissue injuries

If a person is unable to move an injured part of the body, or if the injured area is misshapen or very painful, you should suspect a bone fracture. Soft tissue injuries, such as injuries to joints, ligaments, tendons, and muscles, may also cause severe pain and swelling and may sometimes be difficult to distinguish from fractures.

Bone fractures

There are two basic types of bone fracture: open fractures, in which the skin is broken and the bone is exposed, and closed fractures, in which the skin near the bone is not broken and bone doesn't protrude from the skin. An open fracture is more likely to become infected than a closed fracture, because the bone is exposed to bacteria in the air. A closed fracture will often have extensive bruising and swelling on the skin covering, and near the site of, the break.

TO TREAT AN OPEN FRACTURE:

If possible, get a helper to steady and support the injured area while you work.

1. Cover the wound with a clean dressing and apply pressure to control bleeding,

if necessary. However, you should NOT press down directly on a protruding bone.

2. Put some clean padding over the dressing and around it. Do not touch the wound with your fingers.

3. Keep placing padding around the wound until it is possible to put a bandage over the pads without pressing directly on the bone.

4. Fasten the dressing and padding firmly, but do not make it so tight that circulation might be impaired. Immobilize the injured part by taping or tying it gently but firmly to an adjoining part of the body (i.e. an arm against the trunk of the body, a leg against the other leg).

5. Phone for an ambulance. Check the circulation beyond the bandage regularly, and observe the injured person for shock (see p. 560).

TO TREAT A CLOSED FRACTURE OR A DISLOCATED BONE:

1. Ask the injured person to stay still, and gently immobilize the injured part by taping or tying it firmly to an adjoining part of the body (i.e. an arm against the trunk of the body, a leg against the other leg).

2. Phone for an ambulance. Look for signs of shock and check the circulation beyond the injured area regularly.

Muscle strains and tears

Remember "RICE" (Rest, Ice, Compression, and Elevation) when treating soft tissue injuries, such as muscle strains or sprains. If the injury isn't better in 24 hours, consult a doctor.

1. Apply an ice pack (ice cubes in a plastic bag, or a bag of frozen peas wrapped in a cloth) to lessen swelling and relieve pain.

2. Wrap the injured area firmly but not too tightly using a layer of thick, soft material (such as cotton balls or padding) on the inside and an elastic bandage on the outside.

3. Raise the injured area to reduce blood flow to it.

4. If the injured person is still in pain, go to the emergency department at the nearest hospital. Otherwise, he should continue resting the injured area and see a doctor if the injury seems no better after 24 hours.

> **DO NOT** try to put a dislocated bone back into its socket.

Neck or back injury

The main danger in any neck or back injury is damage to the spinal cord. If the spinal cord is damaged, paralysis or loss of sensation may occur below the damaged area. So any neck or back injury must be treated very carefully.

If you suspect a neck or back injury, DO NOT move the affected person unless she is in danger or she is unconscious and her airway is not open. If you must move the person, use the following procedure for "log roll":

1 Keep the person's head, trunk, neck, and toes in a straight line throughout the procedure.

2 While one person supports the head and neck, get helpers to straighten her limbs and roll her, as if she were a log, onto a stretcher on her back. Get five people to help if you can. Generally, this should be done after EMS arrives.

Slings

A sling is used to support an injured arm. You can improvise a sling with a shirt or jacket if necessary.

1. Hold the injured arm so that the hand is above the elbow, if this is possible. (If it is not possible, don't force the arm into this position.) Put one end of the sling through at the elbow and pull it around to the person's opposite shoulder. Open the bandage so that its bottom is level with the person's little fingernail on the hand of the injured arm.

2. Bring the lower end of the sling over the person's forearm so that it meets the other end at the shoulder of the injured arm.

3. Tie a knot and tuck the ends in under it to act as padding.

4. Fold the point of the sling (by the injured elbow) forward and tuck it into the sling. Pin it in place with a safety pin. If you don't have a safety pin, twist the point and tuck into the back of the sling.

5. Check the circulation in the person's fingers regularly. If they seem cold or numb, undo the sling and loosen any bandages.

Crepe roller bandages

Roller bandages can be used to hold dressings in place or to provide compression for soft tissue injuries. The method of application is slightly different for each of these purposes.

To hold a dressing in place:

1. Put the end of the bandage below the injured area and, working outward, make two straight overlapping turns to anchor it.

2. Wind the bandage from the inside to the outside of the limb in spiraling turns, working up the limb and over any dressings.

3. Use one straight overlapping turn to finish, and fasten the end of the bandage using clips, safety pins, or adhesive tape.

To compress a soft tissue injury to a joint:

1. Hold the injured limb in a comfortable position. Flex the joint if possible.

2. Place the end of the bandage on the inside of the joint. Fix the bandage by winding it around the joint one and a half times.

3. Wind the bandage once around the limb just above the joint. Make a diagonal turn and wrap the bandage down just below the joint.

4. Continue wrapping in this manner, above and below, overlapping the bandage in a figure of 8 so that it extends a short way up and down the limb.

5. Use two straight turns to finish, and fasten the end of the bandage using clips, safety pins, or adhesive tape.

6. Check circulation by pressing on a finger or toenail (color should return right away) every 10 minutes. If the bandage is too tight, undo it and wait until circulation is normal before reapplying it more loosely.

Burns

Before you treat a burn, you must try to determine its depth and extent. Deep and/or extensive burns are likely to cause shock (see p. 560) because they cause the body to lose tissue fluids. They also destroy the skin, which is the body's natural barrier to bacteria in the environment, and so infection is also a risk.

There are three types of burn: superficial, partial-thickness, and full-thickness.

1. A superficial burn involves the outermost layer of skin only; the skin looks red, swollen, and tender. Medical help is needed if the burn covers more than 5 percent of the body surface.

2. A partial-thickness burn affects the underlying layer of skin, the dermis, and looks raw and blistered. Medical attention is needed.

3. A full-thickness burn affects all layers of skin and possibly nerves, fat tissue, and muscle. The skin looks yellow, pale, or charred. Urgent medical attention is essential.

Blisters

Blisters form on skin damaged by heat or friction. The "bubble" appearance of a blister is due to tissue fluid, called serum, entering the area just below the skin's surface. If left alone the serum is reabsorbed by the tissue, new skin forms, and the outer layer of dead skin falls off.

Blisters usually need no treatment. Do NOT burst them, because this interrupts the healing process and could cause infection. If a blister breaks on its own, cover the area with a sterile dressing and leave it until the area has healed.

Minor burns

These are superficial burns that will heal naturally after first-aid treatment. (You should always seek medical advice if you are not sure how serious an injury is.)

1. Run the burned area under cold water for at least 10 minutes. If there is no water available, any cold, harmless liquid such as canned drinks will work just as well.

2. Cover the area with a sterile dressing or a piece of clean material that is not linty or fluffy. Bandage it loosely in place.

3. If blisters appear, DO NOT break them. This could introduce infection into the wound.

> **DO NOT apply lotions, butter, or other fats to the wound. This could cause infection and further tissue damage.**

Severe burns

Your main goal in treating a severe burn is to cool the burn. You must also make sure that the person affected is able to breathe and you must get emergency help.

1. Make sure the person is lying down. Cool the burned area by pouring cold liquid on it for 10 minutes or until emergency help arrives.

2. Gently remove any clothing or jewelry from the injured area, cutting it off if necessary, unless it is sticking to the burn.

3. Cover the injured area with a clean, lint-free dressing (if a dressing isn't available you can improvise with a piece of a clean sheet or plastic kitchen towel).

4. Call EMS. Reassure the injured person while you wait for help to arrive.

Heatstroke

In heatstroke the body's ability to control its own temperature fails and the body becomes dangerously overheated. It can occur rapidly, within a matter of minutes, and may cause unconsciousness. A person affected by heatstroke may be dizzy and have a headache, and may seem restless or confused. Her skin may be dry but hot and flushed, and she may have a rapid pulse.

1. Make sure the affected person is in a cool place. Indoors is best, but at least move her into the shade. Take off as much outer clothing as possible. Call EMS.

2. Cover the person in a cold, wet sheet and keep wetting it. Take her temperature frequently and continue this procedure until her temperature has fallen to 100.4°F (38°C).

3. When her temperature has fallen to this level, remove the wet sheet and cover her with a dry one. Reassure her until help arrives.

Sunburn

Sunburn is usually a mild burn caused by over-exposure to sunlight, although it can be severe, in which case the skin will be very red and blistered and heatstroke (see left) may be present. Sunburn can happen even on overcast days and may be due to the reflection of the sun's rays from snow or sand.

1. Cover the affected skin with a light towel or with light clothing. Take the affected person indoors or at least into the shade.

2. Cool the skin by pouring cool water over it or sponging carefully with cold water. If there is blistering, seek medical advice.

3. Give the affected person cool water to drink. Calamine lotion or after-sun cream may soothe the affected area if the burning isn't severe.

Bites and stings

Insect bites and stings may be painful but are relatively harmless compared to animal and human bites, which must always receive medical treatment. However, certain snakes and spiders may be highly poisonous and if you are in doubt as to the seriousness of a bite, you should seek medical attention.

Insect bites and stings

1. To remove a sting such as a wasp or bee sting, gently scrape the affected area with a blunt-edged knife or a credit card until it comes out. Do not use tweezers to remove the sting since this can squeeze the poison sack and inject more of it into the skin.

2. Apply a cold cloth to the area. If swelling becomes worse or persists, call a doctor.

■ **If someone is stung in the mouth,** let the person suck on an ice cube or something cold and call EMS.

■ **To remove a tick,** grasp the tick as close to the person's skin as possible using fine tweezers. Using a slight rocking action, gently dislodge the tick from the skin. Keep the tick in a container and take it to a doctor for analysis, since ticks can carry diseases, such as Lyme disease (see p. 354).

Snake bites

There are many poisonous snakes that are native to the US. Some people keep exotic snakes as pets and their bites may be severe. If a snakebite occurs, try to put the snake in a secure container or make a note of what it looks like; this may help identify the snake so that the correct antivenom may be given. If the snake has escaped, tell the police.

1. Ask the injured person to lie down. Try to keep him as calm and still as possible to help prevent the venom from spreading.

2. Wash the wound gently and pat it dry.

3. Compress the area above the wound lightly with a bandage and immobilize the injured area as you would for a broken bone (see p. 561).

DO NOT put a tourniquet above the wound, cut the wound open with a knife, or try to suck out the venom.

Animal and human bites

Puncture wounds caused by an animal's teeth can carry germs deep into the flesh. Human bites can introduce infection if they break the skin and can also cause crush injuries. Any contact between teeth and skin that breaks the skin must receive prompt first aid and then medical attention.

1. If there is serious bleeding, control it by putting direct pressure on the wound and raising the injured part above the level of the heart, if possible.

2. If the bite is not bleeding seriously, wash the wounded area with soap and water and pat it dry.

3. Cover the wound with a sterile bandage.

4. Take the person to an emergency department and tell the staff what type of animal caused the bite.

Poisoning

Most homes contain everyday substances that are potentially poisonous, such as detergents, bleach, and paint solvents. Medicine cabinets also may contain over-the-counter and prescription drugs and remedies that are poisonous if taken in excessive doses. Gardens may contain poisonous plants.

Children are especially at risk of poisoning, and hazardous substances should be locked away or, at the very least, kept well out of their reach. NEVER store hazardous substances in anything but their original containers, particularly old soft drink bottles which could mislead a child.

Household poisons

If a household poison, such as bleach or detergent, has been swallowed, NEVER attempt to induce vomiting.

1. If the person is unconscious, check that his airway is open and that he is breathing. Be prepared to resuscitate if necessary (see p. 555).

2. Call EMS. Say what substance has been swallowed, if you can. If the person is conscious and his lips have been burned by a corrosive substance, give him sips of cold water or milk.

Drug poisoning

If you suspect a drug overdose, whether accidental or deliberate, DO NOT attempt to induce vomiting, which rarely helps and may make things worse.

1. If the person is unconscious, check that his airway is open and that he is breathing. Be prepared to resuscitate if necessary (see p. 555).

2. Call EMS. If the person has vomited, keep a sample of the vomit to help identify the drug. Look for empty drug containers and if you find one, send it to hospital with the person.

Poisoning from plants

Children are most at risk from poisonous plants, since they may be attracted by their berries or seeds and may eat them. Teach your children from an early age never to eat anything they find outside unless an adult says that it's safe.

If you suspect that someone has swallowed a poisonous plant DO NOT induce vomiting, which rarely helps and may make matters worse.

1. If the person is unconscious, check that his airway is open and that he is breathing. Be prepared to resuscitate if necessary (see p. 555).

2. Phone for EMS or call a poison center (1-800-222-1222).

3. Try to find out which plant has been swallowed, and if possible what part of it was eaten. Keep pieces of the plant and a sample of any vomit to give to the paramedic or doctor.

Plants that cause poisoning if swallowed

Death cap mushroom

Foxglove

Brown roll rim mushroom

Spotted fly agaric

Wild arum

Your first-aid kit

Every household should keep a well-stocked first-aid kit on hand at all times. In addition, it's a good idea to keep a first-aid kit in your car. Keep the kit in an easily accessible location with everything clearly marked.

YOUR KIT SHOULD INCLUDE:
- 20 adhesive dressings in assorted sizes
- 6 medium sterile dressings
- 2 large sterile dressings
- 2 extra-large sterile dressings
- 2 sterile pads
- 6 triangular bandages
- 2 crepe or elasticated roller bandages
- 6 safety pins
- disposable gloves
- scissors
- tweezers
- cotton balls or rolls
- nonalcoholic cleansing wipes
- notepad, pencil, writable tags
- plastic face shield.

Adhesive dressings

Sterile dressings in three sizes

Sterile pads

Triangular bandage

Roller bandage and clip

Cotton rolls

cleansing wipes

Safety pins, scissors, and tweezers

Disposable gloves

Notepad and pencil

Face shield

Travel health

Travel is part of most people's lives these days – whether for business or pleasure – and it's easy to forget that, even with routine immunizations, risks to health during travel are still very real. On top of that, obtaining health care in other countries can be much more complicated than it is in the US, and can end up being extremely expensive if you travel without the proper level of insurance.

There are however many ways you can minimize your risk of getting ill and/or facing large medical bills when you travel. Be sure to take the following precautions:

● **International health insurance**
Injuries and illness can be frightening when traveling abroad. If a US citizen becomes seriously ill or is injured abroad, a US consular officer can assist in locating appropriate medical services and informing family or friends. A consular officer can also assist in the transfer of funds from the US. However, since payment of hospital costs and other medical expenses are the responsibility of the traveler, travel health insurance can be a real lifesaver. Before you travel, find out if you are covered by your regular health insurance policy. Some health insurance companies will pay "customary and reasonable" hospital costs abroad but few will pay for medical evacuation to the US, which can cost more than $10,000 depending on the location and medical condition. Supplemental policies that cover emergency evacuations are available.

● **Check with your doctor** about whether you and your family will need immunizations for the countries you plan to visit. You should do this at least two months before you travel since some immunizations need time to take effect. You should still check with your doctor if you need to travel suddenly, since some protection may be better than none at all. Many state and local health departments provide travel immunizations. If your area does not have a travel clinic, your state health department can usually

provide information on who in the area provides travel immunizations. Check with the US Centers for Disease Control's travel health department for a list of which immunizations are needed for where you are traveling.

● **Be very careful in the sun.** Over-exposure to the sun can cause sunburn and heatstroke, and children are especially at risk. Don't go out in the sun at midday, stay in the shade when you can, and use a high-factor sunscreen at all times. Make sure your children wear a high-factor sunscreen and headgear that also protects the back of the neck. Drink plenty of fluids, but make sure they're safe – canned and bottled drinks are usually best.

● **Be on guard against insect and animal bites.** Even in areas where malaria is not a problem, ticks can be a carrier of disease. If you go walking in areas of high grass or woodland, wear long trousers and socks, and keep your arms covered too. Make sure that your children are also adequately dressed. Use insect repellents. If you've been prescribed antimalarial medicine, make sure you take it regularly.

Bites from animals can cause very serious, and sometimes fatal, illness if they are not promptly treated. Be extremely cautious of all animals, even those that appear to be tame, and teach your children to be cautious too. If someone does get bitten by an animal, seek medical advice immediately.

● **If the water at your destination may not be safe to drink**, drink only

bottled or canned drinks. Use disinfectant tablets if you need to use the water to wash food or brush your teeth. Don't ask for ice in your drinks or use ice to keep food cool.

● **Make sure hot food is piping hot** and cooked all the way through. Avoid uncooked food such as raw fruits or vegetables; if you must eat them, peel them yourself. Avoid eating shellfish, especially any shellfish that is eaten raw, such as oysters. Do not drink unpasteurized milk.

● **Never swim alone**, and always make sure that children are supervised by an adult who is a good swimmer. Don't leave children alone near any water – a young child can drown in a wading pool or even a large puddle.

● **Be extra vigilant** when driving, walking, or bicycling on foreign roads. Make sure you know which direction the traffic is traveling, especially when crossing roads – most countries drive on the right instead of the left. Be aware of local traffic laws.

● **If you are taking a long-haul flight**, get up and walk around at least once an hour or so to keep your blood circulating freely – this reduces the risk of developing deep vein thrombosis (see p. 235).

● **If you haven't been to the dentist recently**, have a dental checkup before you travel. Dental care can be difficult to find and very expensive in some countries.

Useful addresses

AIDS

CDC National HIV/AIDS Hotline
Tel: (800) 342-2437
Website: www.cdc.gov

AIDS Action Council
1875 Connecticut Avenue NW
Washington, DC 20009
Tel: (202) 986-1300
Email: aidsaction@aidsaction.org
Website: www.aidsaction.org

Alopecia

National Alopecia Areata Foundation
P.O. Box 150760
San Rafael, CA 94915-0760
Tel: (415) 472-3780
Website: www.alopeciaareata.com

Alzheimer's disease

Alzheimer's Association
919 North Michigan Avenue
Chicago, IL 60611-1676
Tel: (800) 272-3900
Tel: (312) 335-8700
Email: info@alz.org
Website: www.alz.org

Arthritis

Arthritis Foundation and American Juvenile Arthritis Organization
1330 West Peachtree Street
Atlanta, GA 30309
Tel: (800) 283-7800
Tel: (404) 872-7100
Email: help@arthritis.org
Website: www.arthritis.org

Asthma

Asthma and Allergy Foundation of America
1125 15th Street NW
Washington, DC 20005
Tel: (800) 7-ASTHMA
Tel: (202) 466-7643
Email: info@aafa.org
Website: www.aafa.org

American Lung Association
1740 Broadway
New York, NY 10019
Tel: (800) 586-4872
Tel: (212) 315-8700
Email: info@lungusa.org

Website: www.lungusa.org

Attention deficit disorder (ADD)/Attention deficit hyperactivity disorder (ADHD)

Attention Deficit Disorder Association
9930 Johnnycake Ridge Road
Mentor, OH 44060
Tel: (440) 350-9595
Email: natladda@aol.com
Website: www.add.org

Autism

Autism Society of America
7910 Woodmont Avenue
Bethesda, MD 20814-3015
Tel: (800) 328-8476
Website: www.autism-society.org

Birthmarks

American Academy of Dermatology
930 N. Meacham Road
Schaumburg, IL 60173-4965
Tel: (888) 462-3370
Tel: (847) 330-0230
Website: www.aad.org

Blindness

American Foundation for the Blind
11 Penn Plaza
New York, NY 10001
Tel: (800) 232-5463
Tel: (212) 502-7662 (TTY)
Email: afbinfo@afb.org
Website: www.afb.org

Cerebral palsy

UCP Association
1660 L Street NW, Suite 700
Washington, DC
Tel: (202) 776-0406
Website: www.ucpa.org

Cancer

American Cancer Society
1599 Clifton Road NE
Atlanta, GA 30329-4251
Tel: (800) 586-4872
Tel: (404) 320-3333
Website: www.cancer.org

National Cancer Institute Information Service

9000 Rockville Pike
Bethesda, MD 20892
Tel: (800) 442-6237
Tel: (301) 435-3848
Tel: (800) 332-8615 (TTY)
Website: www.nci.nih.gov

Crib death

Pregnancy and Infant Loss Center
1421 East Wayzata Boulevard
Wayzata, MN 55391
Tel: (612) 473-9372

SIDS Alliance
1314 Bedford Avenue, Suite 210
Baltimore, MD 21208
Tel: (410) 653-8226
Website: www.sidsalliance.org

Counseling

American Counseling Association
5999 Stevenson Avenue
Alexandria, VA 22304-3300
Tel: (800) 347-6647
Tel: (703) 823-9800
Tel: (703) 823-6862 (TTY)
Website: www.counseling.org

Cystic fibrosis

National Cystic Fibrosis Foundation New York Chapter
60 East 42nd Street
New York, NY 10165
Tel: (212) 986-8783
Website: www.cff.org

Deafness

Alexander Graham Bell Association for the Deaf
3417 Volta Place, NW
Washington, DC 20007-2778
Tel: (202) 337-5220
Email: Bellchaps@aol.com
Website: www.agbell.org

Depressive illness

National Mental Health Association
11021 Prince Street
Alexandria, VA 22314-2971
Tel: (800) 969-6642
Tel: (703) 684-7722
Website: www.nmha.org/index.cfm

**National Institute of Mental Health
NIMH Public Inquiries**
6001 Executive Boulevard
Bethesda, MD 20892-9663
Tel: (301) 443-4536
Tel: (888) 8-ANXIETY
Tel: (800) 421-4211
Website: www.nimh.com

The Samaritans of USA
9 Wild Harbour Road North
Falmouth, MA 02256
Tel: call directory assistance for local chapter
Website: www.befrienders.org

Diabetes

American Diabetes Association
149 Madison Avenue
New York, NY 10016
Tel: (800) 342-2383
Email: customerservice@diabetes.org
Website: www.diabetes.org.

Down syndrome

**Association for Children with Down
Syndrome**
2616 Martin Avenue
Bellmore, NY 11710
Tel: (516) 221-4700
Email: info@acds.org
Website: www.ACDS.org

Drugs and alcohol

Alcoholics Anonymous
Grand Central Station
P.O. Box 459
New York, NY 10163
Website: www.alcoholics-anonymous.org

**National Drug Information Treatment
and Referral Hotline/Center for
Substance Abuse**
Tel: (800) 662-4357

Partnership for a Drug Free America
405 Lexington Avenue
New York, NY 10174
Tel: (212) 922-1560
Website: www.drughelp.org

Dyslexia

Learning Disabilities Association
4156 Library Road
Pittsburgh, PA 15234-1349

Tel: (412) 341-1515
Email: ldanatl@usaor.net
Website: www.ldanatl.org

Eating disorders

**The American Anorexia/Bulimia
Association, Inc.**
165 West 46th Street
New York, NY 10036
Tel: (212) 575-6200
Website: www.aabainc.org

**National Association of Anorexia
Nervosa and Associated Disorders.**
P.O. Box 7
Highland Park, IL 60035
Tel: (847) 831-3438
Email: anad20@aol.com
Website:
www.members.aol.com/anad20/index.html

Eczema

National Eczema Association
1221 Southwest Yamill
Portland, OR 97205
Tel: (800) 818-SKIN
Email: nease@teleport.com

Epilepsy

American Epilepsy Society
638 Prospect Avenue
Hartford, CT 06105
Tel: (860) 586-7505
Email: infor@aesnet.org
Website: www.aesnet.org

Epilepsy Foundation of America
4351 Garden City Drive
Landover, MD 20785
Tel: (800) 332-1000
Tel: (800) 332-2070 (TTY)
Email: postmaster@efa.org
Website: www.efa.org

Family planning

Planned Parenthood
810 Seventh Avenue
New York, NY 10019
Tel: (800) 230-PLAN
Tel: (212) 541-7800
Website: www.plannedparenthood.org

Food allergies

National Institute of Allergy and

Infectious Disease
31 Center Drive MSC 2520
Bethesda, MD 20892-2520
Tel: (301) 496-5717
Website: www.niaid.nih.gov

Heart disease

**American Heart Association National
Center**
7272 Greenville Avenue
Dallas, TX 75231
Tel: (800) 242-8721
Website: www.americanheart.org

Herpes infection

National STD Hotline of the Centers for Disease
Control and Prevention
P.O. Box 13827
RTP, NC 27709
Tel: (800) 227-8922
Website: www.ashastd.org

Impotence

Men's Health Network
P.O. Box 770
Washington, DC 20044-0770
Tel: (202) 543-MHN1
Email: theia@btinternet.com
Website: www.menshealthnetwork.org

Infertility

Resolve, Inc.
1310 Broadway
Somerville, MA 02144-1779
Tel: (617) 623-1156
Tel: (617) 623-0744
Email: resolveinc@aol.com
Website: www.resolve.org

Ferre Institute
1258 Genesse Street
Utica, NY 13502
Tel: (315) 724-4348
Website: members.aol.com/ferrinf/ferre.html

Irritable bowel syndrome (IBS)

Digestive Disease National Coalition
507 Capitol Court NW
Washington, DC 20002
Tel: (202) 544-7497

**National Institute of Diabetes and
Digestive and Kidney Diseases**
2 Information Way

Bethesda, MD 20892-3570
Tel: (301) 654-3810
Website: www.niddk.nih.gov

Lupus
Lupus Foundation of America
1300 Piccard Drive
Rockville, MD 20850-4303
Tel: (800) 558-0121
Tel: (301) 670-9292
Essex RM1 3NH
Email: lupusinfo@aol.com
Website: www.lupus.org

Miscarriage
MEND (Mommies Enduring Neonatal Death)
P.O. Box 1007
Coppell, TX 7519
Tel: (888) 695-MEND
Website: www.mend.org

Pregnancy and Infant Loss Center
1421 Wayzata Boulevard
Wayzata, MN 55391
Tel: (612) 473-9372

Multiple sclerosis
Multiple Sclerosis Society
30 West 36th Street
New York, NY 10010
Tel: (800) 344-4867
Email: info@nmss.org

Muscular dystrophy
Muscular Dystrophy Association
Website: www.mdausa.org

Osteoporosis
National Osteoporosis Foundation
1150 17th Street NW
Washington, DC 20036-4603
Tel: (800) 223-9994
Tel: (202) 223-2226
Email: nofmail@nof.org
Website: www.nof.org

Polycystic ovary syndrome
Polycystic Ovarian Syndrome Association
P.O. Box 80517
Portland, OR 97280
Tel: (877) 775-PCOS

Website: www.pcosupport.org/

Prostate problems
The American Foundation for Urologic Disease
300 West Pratt Street
Baltimore, MD 21201
Tel: (800) 242-2383

The Prostatitis Foundation
1063 30th Street, Box 8
Smithshire, IL 61478
Tel: (888) 891-4200
Website: www.prostate.org

Psoriasis
National Psoriasis Foundation
6600 SW 92 Avenue
Portland, OR 97223
Tel: (800) 723-9166
Email: getinfo@npf.usa.org
Website: www.psoriasis.org

Rape
Rape, Abuse, and Incest National Network Hotline
Tel: (800) 656-HOPE

Restless legs syndrome
NIH Neurological Institute
P.O. Box 5801
Bethesda, MD 20824
Tel: (800) 352-9424
Tel: (301) 468-5981 (TTY)
Website: www.ninds.nih.gov

Sexual problems
Sexuality Information and Education Council of the United States
130 West 42nd Street
New York, NY 10036
Tel: (212) 819-9770
Email: siecus@siecus.org
Website: www.siecus.org

Sexuality
The Gay and Lesbian National Hotline
Tel: (888) 843-4564

Spina bifida and hydrocephalus
Spina Bifida Association of America

4590 MacArthur Boulevard NW
Washington, DC 20007-4226
Tel: (800) 621-3141
Tel: (202) 944-3285
Email: ir@sbaa.org
Website: www.sbaa.org

Hydrocephalus Association
870 Market Street
San Francisco, CA 94102
Tel: (415) 732-7040
Email: hydroassoc@aol.com
Website: www.hydroassoc.org

Stroke
American Stroke Association
7272 Greenville Avenue
Dallas, TX 75231
Tel: (800) 553-6321
Website: www.americanstroke.org

Testicular cancer
National Cancer Institute
616 Executive Boulevard, Suite 3036A
Bethesda, MD 20892-8322
Tel: (800) 4-CANCER
Website: www.cancer.gov/cancer

Tinnitus
America Tinnitus Association
P.O. Box 5
Portland, OR 97207
Tel: (503) 248-9985
Email: tinnitus@ata.org
Website: www.ata.org

Travel health
CDC Travel Information Hotline
Tel: (404) 332-4559
Website: www.cdc.gov/travel

International Association for Medical Assistance to Travelers
417 Center Street
Lewiston, NY 14092
Tel: (716) 754-4883
Website: www.sentex.net/~iamat

Women's health issues
National Women's Resource Center
5255 Loughboro Road NW
Washington, DC 20016
Tel: (202) 537-4015
Website: www.healthywomen.org

Australian useful addresses

AIDS

Australian Federation of AIDS Organisations (AFAO)
PO Box 876
Darlinghurst NSW 1300
Tel: 02 9281 1999
Website: www.afao.org.au

National Association of People Living With HIV/AIDS
Tel: 02 9281 2511
www.napwa.org.au

Alopecia

Alopecia Areata Support Association of Victoria Inc.
PO Box 89
Camberwell VIC 3124
Tel: 03 9513 8580

Alzheimer's disease

Alzheimer's Association National Dementia Behaviour Advisory Service
Tel: 1800 639 331
Email: www.alzheimers.org.au

Arthritis

Arthritis Foundation of Australia
Tel: 1800 011 041
Website: www.arthritisfoundation.com.au

Asthma

Asthma Foundation
Tel: 1800 645 130
Website: www.asthma.org.au

Attention deficit disorder (ADD)

VIC Vic Active Inc.
Tel: 03 9650 2570

ACT ADD Support Group
Tel: 02 6290 1984

NSW Hyperactivity and Attention Deficit Association
Tel: 02 9411 2186

QLD ADD Information and Support Services
Tel: 07 3817 2429

SA ADD Information Service
Tel: 08 8221 5166

Autism

Autism Council of Australia
VIC Tel: 03 9885 0533

Cerebral palsy

Cerebral Palsy Support Network
Tel: 03 9348 2677
Website: www.cpsn.info

Cancer

The Cancer Council Australia
Level 4, 70 William Street, East Sydney NSW 2011
Tel: 02 9380 9022
Website: www.cancer.org.au

Cancer Helpline & Information Service
Tel: 13 11 20
Website: www.accv.org.au

Continence

Continence Foundation of Australia
National Continence Helpline
Tel: 1800 330 066
Website: www.contfound.org.au/

Cot death

SIDS (Sudden Infant Death Syndrome)
Tel: 1300 308 307

Counselling

National Association for Loss and Grief
VIC Tel: 03 9351 0358
NSW Tel: 02 9976 2803
ACT Tel: 02 6259 3940
WA Tel: 08 9385 4748
Website: www.grieflink.asn.au

Lifeline
Tel: 02 6282 6511

Relationships Australia
Tel: 1300 364 277

Coeliac disease

Coeliac Society of Australia
Tel: 02 9411 4100

Cystic fibrosis

Cystic Fibrosis Australia Inc.
51 Wicks Road, NSW 2113
TeL: 02 9878 5250
Website: www.cysticfibrosisaustralia.org.au

Dementia

Dementia Helpline
Tel: 1800 639 331
Website: www.alzheimers.org.au

Depressive illness

Lifeline
Tel: 13 11 14, 03 9662 9030, 02 6282 6511

SANE Australia
Tel: 1800 688 382
Website: www.sane.org

Diabetes

Diabetes Australia
Tel: 1800 640 862
Website: www.diabetesaustralia.com.au or www.dav.org.au

Down's syndrome

Down Syndrome Association
ACT Tel: 02 6290 0656
NSW Tel: 02 9683 4333
NT Tel: 08 8985 6222
QLD Tel: 07 3356 6655
SA Tel: 08 8365 3510
TAS Tel: 03 6244 0490
VIC Tel: 03 9486 2377
WA Tel: 08 9358 3544
Website: www.dsav.asn.au

Emphysema and lung support

Quality of Life Through Patient Support
Tel: 1800 654 301
Website: www.lungnet.org.au

Epilepsy

National Epilepsy Association of Australia
PO Box 879
Epping NSW 1710
Tel: 02 9856 7075, 1300 36 6162
Website: www.epilepsy.org.au

Hearing problems

The Western Australian Deaf Society Inc
16 Brentham Street
Leederville WA 6007
Tel: 08 9441 2677
Website: www.wadeaf.org.au

Haemophilia

Haemophilia Foundation Australia Inc (HFA)
213 Waverley Road
East Malvern VIC 3145
Tel: 03 9572 5533
Website: www.haemophilia.org.au

Head injury organizations

Head Injury Council of Australia Inc
Tel: 1800 626 370, 02 6290 2253
Website: www.headinjurycouncil.org.au

Heart disease

Heart Foundation of Australia
Cnr. Denison Street and Geils Court Deakin
ACT 2600
Tel: 1300 36 27 87
Website: www.heartfoundation.com.au

Hepatitis C infection

Hepatitis C Helpline
Tel: 1800 032 665

Herpes infection

Australian Herpes Management Forum
P O Box N159
Grosvenor Place NSW 2000
Tel: 02 9291 3358
Website: www.herpes.on.net

Kidney disease

Kidney Foundation, Australia
GPO Box 9993 (in your capital city)
Tel: 08 8334 7555, 1800 682 531
Website: www.kidney.org.au

Miscarriage

Stillbirth and Neonatal Death Support (SANDS)
Suite 208/901 Whitehorse Road, Box Hill
Tel: 03 9899 0218

Multiple sclerosis

Multiple Sclerosis Australia
Tel: 02 9955 0700
Website: www.msaustralia.org.au

Muscular dystrophy

Muscular Dystrophy Australia
Tel: 1800 656 632
Website: www.mda.org.au/

Osteoporosis

Osteoporosis Australia
Level 1, 52 Paramatta Road
Forest Lodge, NSW 2037
Tel: 02 9518 8140, 1800 011 041
Website: www.osteoporosis.org.au

Palliative care

Palliative Care Australia
Tel: 02 6232 4433
Website: www.pallcare.org.au/

Parkinson's disease

Parkinson's Australia
Tel: 1800 644 189
Website: www.parkinsons.org.au

Prostate problems

Cancer Council of Australia
Level 4, 70 William Street, East Sydney
NSW 2011
Tel: 02 9380 9022
Website: www.cancer.org.au

Spina bifida and hydrocephalus

Spina Bifida information line
Tel: 1800 819 775

Spinal cord injury

Australian Quadriplegic Association (AQA)
Tel: 03 9489 0777
Website: www.aqa.org.au

Paraplegic and Quadriplegic Association of Victoria
Tel: 1800 805 384
Website: www.paraquad.asn.au

Stroke

Stroke Recovery
National Stroke Foundation
Tel: 1800 787 653
Website: www.strokefoundation.com.au

Testicular cancer

Anti-Cancer Council of Victoria
Tel: 13 11 20
Website: www.accv.org.au

Cancer Council of Australia
Level 4, 70 William Street
East Sydney, NSW 2011
Tel: 02 9380 9022
Website: www.cancer.org.au

Thalassaemia

Thalassaemia Society
VIC   Tel: 03 9888 2211

Tinnitus

Australian Tinnitus Assoc (NSW) Ltd
9 Ice Street
Darlinghurst NSW
Tel: 02 8382 3331
Website: www.tinnitus.asn.au

Tinnitus Association of Victoria
Better Hearing Advisory Centre
5 High Street, Prahran, Vic 3181
Tel: 03 9510 1577

Index

441
see also arthritis
joint replacement 420, *428*
joints 420, *421*, 427
JRA (juvenile rheumatoid arthritis) **550**
junk foods & candy 85

K

Kaposi's sarcoma 339, 340, 455
Kawasaki disease **550**
kegel exercises 166, **169**, 373, **375**
keratin 445, 461
keratoconjunctivitis sicca (dry eye) **473**
ketamine 30
ketoacidosis 504
keyhole (endoscopic/minimally invasive) surgery *358*
kidney & bladder conditions
  acute, chronic, & end-stage kidney failure **380–1**
  bladder tumors 380
  cystitis **378–9**
  glomerulonephritis **377**
  infection of the kidneys (pyelonephritis) **376**
  kidney stones **377**
  urinary hesitancy & obstruction 266
  urinary incontinence, stress incontinence, & irritable bladder 373, **375**
kidneys *242, 374*
kissing disease (infectious mononucleosis) **342**
knee joint replacement *428*
knock-knees 527
kyphosis (curvature of the spine) 423, 425, 431

L

labia *242*
labor **132–3**
labyrinthitis 418, **478**
lactose intolerance 361, 364, **366**
language, speech, & talking, babies & children **54–5, 74–5**
laparoscopy 250, *250*, 276
large cell carcinoma 394
large loop excision of the

transformation zones (LLETZ) 259
larynx (voice box) *384*, 476
  cancer of the larynx **482**
  laryngitis (sore throat) **482**, 535
laser treatment *254*
  for birthmarks 527
  for cervical precancer & cancer 258, 259
  for genital warts 282
  for hair removal *460*
  laser-assisted in-situ keratomileusis (LASIK) *470*
  laser-assisted uvuloplasty (LAUP) 480
  laser iridotomy, for acute glaucoma *466*
  laser trabeculoplasty, for chronic glaucoma 467
  for prostate conditions 267
LASIK (laser-assisted in-situ keratomileusis) *470*
LAUP (laser-assisted uvuloplasty) 480
lavender (essential oil) 32, 33, *290*, 361, 453, 542
LDL (low-density lipoproteins) 222, *223*
learning difficulties *see* behavior & development conditions; Down syndrome
learning spurts, children 59
left-handedness 65
left-sided heart failure 232
leg conditions
  congenital leg & foot problems **527–8**
  deep vein thrombosis (DVT) **235–6**, 395, 566
  restless legs 297, **437–8**
  sciatica 435, 437
  varicose veins **235**, 264
Legionnaires' disease 392
lenses
  contact lenses & glasses 463, *469*, 470
  lens of the eye *463, 464*
lentigo maligna 455
letter-matching test *468*
leukemia (bone marrow cancer) **239**, 359, 422
levodopa 415
libido *see* sex & sexuality
lice *332, 453*, 542
life stages
  0–1 years **36–57**
  1–4 years **58–79**
  4–11 years **80–101**
  11–18 years **102–28**

18–40 years **134–55**
40–60 years **160–81**
60+ years **182–203**
see also babies; children; pregnancy & birth; teenagers
lifestyle changes *see* specific conditions for which changes are required (e.g. high blood pressure)
lifting objects correctly *436*
lindane 453
lip augmentation *156*
lipids 223, *223*
  cholesterol **222**
  cholesterol levels & tests 222, 223, *223*, 505
  lipid-lowering drugs 225, 230
liposculpture 142
liposuction **157**
lips, cleft lip, & palate **528**
liquid crystal thermometers 515, *515*
listeriosis 339, **346**
lithium 448
lithotripsy 377
liver *349*, 355
liver biopsy 541
liver conditions
  alcohol-related liver disease 355, **356**
  cirrhosis 356, **357**
  fatty liver 356
  hepatitis **341–2**, 357, *544–55*
  jaundice 341, **355–6**
  liver cancer 355, **359**
  liver failure 341
living will (advance directive) **202–3**
LLETZ (large loop excision of the transformation zones) 259
lone parents 150, 151
loneliness **192**
longevity 183
loperamide 363, 364
Losec 351
loss of appetite *212, 515*
low back pain *210*, **434–6**
low blood pressure (hypotension) **234**
low blood sugar 294
low-density lipoproteins (LDL) 222, *223*
lower back stretch *435*
LSD (acid) 30
lukewarm sponging 534, 540
lumbar puncture 413
lumbar spondylosis 432
lumpectomy 241, 245–6, **262**
lumps
  breast lumps **244–6**

lump in scrotum, symptom guide 215
lung cancer 24, **394–5**
lung conditions *see* chest & airway conditions
lung function tests *391*
lung volume reduction surgery 391
lung volume test *391*
lungs *384*
lupus (systemic lupus erythematosis/SLE) **324–5**, 393
lying & truth, children 70, 71, 98
Lyme disease **344**, 417
lymph & lymphatic system 327
lymph nodes
  breast cancer spread 246, 262, 327
  enlarged lymph nodes (swollen glands/lymphadenopathy) **327**
lymphangitis **328**
lymphatic drainage 328
lymphocytes *311*, 323, 339
lymphoedema **328**
lymphoma **328–9**, 340, 359
lysozyme 463, 471

M

macula *463, 464*
macular degeneration 473
magnesium *410, 499*
magnetic resonance imaging (MRI) 250, *409, 412*
makeup & cosmetics 170–1
malabsorption 360, **365**, 366
malaria **343**, 566
male conditions *see* men's conditions
male menopause **172–3**
male-pattern baldness 140, 459
male reproductive & urinary systems *242, 374*
male sterilization (vasectomy) **269**
malignant melanoma **455, 458**
malocclusion (poor bite) 494, **489.492**
malpositioned teeth 490, 491
mammograms 159, *245*
manganese *499*
manners, children's 93
marijuana 30

see also bone conditions; joint
conditions; muscle & tendon
conditions
MUSE (medicated urethral
system for erection) 274
mutual masturbation 115
myalgic encephalopathy
(ME/chronic fatigue
syndrome/CFS) **410–11**
myelin *399*, 412
myocardial infarction (heart
attack) 165, 220, **230**
myopia (nearsightedness) 468,
469
myxedema (hypothyroidism) **507**

N

nails 444, *445*, **461**
named patient prescribing 27,
438
naproxen 247
nasal polypectomy 480
nasal polyps **479**
natural methods, contraception
118
nausea & vomiting
antihistamines for 418, 477,
479
in children 514, 518–19, 522
morning sickness 129
naxtrexone 27
nearsightedness (myopia) 468,
469
near-vision test *468*
nedocromil sodium *387*
nephrons *374*
nerves, structure *399*
nervous system *399*
nervous system conditions *see*
brain & nervous system
conditions
nettle rash (urticaria) 41, **322**
neural tube defects **524–5**
neuralgia
postherpetic neuralgia 335,
408
trigeminal neuralgia **408**
neuroblastomas 409
neuroma, acoustic neuroma 417,
418
neurotransmitters 168, 298, 415
nevus flammeus (port wine
stains) 527
newborn babies **40–1**, 73
adjusting to parenthood
148–51
NHL (non-Hodgkin's

lymphoma) 328, 340
nickel allergy 314
nicotine 23–4
night sweats 498, 503
nightmares & night terrors 77
nipple conditions 244, **246**
nitrate drugs 224
nits & nit combs 453, 542
no-bleed HRT 502–3
noncyclical breast pain *215*,
243–4
non-Hodgkin's lymphoma
(NHL) 328, 340
nonsteroidal anti-inflammatory
drugs *see* NSAIDs
nose *384*, *476*
nose & throat conditions
cancer of the larynx 482
choking, first aid **556**
common cold **333**, 385, **533**
foreign object in nose *561*
laryngitis (sore throat) **482**,
535
nasal polyps **479**
nosebleed **479**, **481**, **560**
sinusitis **481–2**
snoring 475, **480–1**
tonsillitis **536**
nose drops *517*
nosebleed **479**, **481**, **560**
NSAIDs (nonsteroidal anti-
inflammatory drugs) **431**
causing peptic ulcer 353, 354,
431
trigger for asthma *386*, 387
see also specific conditions
requiring NSAID treatment
for pain & inflammation
(e.g. arthritis)
nuchal scanning 522
nudity 72, 95
numbers & counting
(numeracy) 97
nursing children at home
518–19, 534
nuts 19

O

OA (osteoarthritis) 186, 420,
427, **428–9**
spondylosis 427, **432**
oblique (spiral) fracture *422*
obsessive-compulsive disorder
(OCD) 285, **293**
occult blood, fecal tests 369
occupational asthma *386*
occupational dermatitis 314

OCD (obsessive-compulsive
disorder) 285, **293**
oily fish 17, 139, 186
older people
60+ years, life stages **182–203**
caring for eldery relatives 178
mental fitness 183, 192–3
see also specific topics related
to older people (e.g.
retirement)
on-off phenomenon, Parkinson's
disease 415
open-angle (chronic) glaucoma
467
open biopsy 245–6
open (compound) fractures 422,
561
optic nerve *463*, *464*
optical migraine 470
optimism 183
oral sex 115
organ transplants *see* transplants
orgasm 31, 115
failure to orgasm, women *141*
premature ejaculation *143*
orthodontic treatment *492*, 551
ossicles *476*
osteoarthritis (OA) 186, 420,
427, **428–9**
spondylosis 427, **432**
osteophytes *428*, 432
osteoporosis 420, **423–5**, 503
see also fractures
otitis media (middle ear
infection) 475, 533, 537
otoplasty *156*
otosclerosis **478**
out-toeing 527
oval window *476*
ovaries *242*, 496
ovary conditions *see* uterus &
ovary conditions
overbite (overjet) *492*
oxaliplatin 369
oxygen therapy 391, *393*

P

pacemakers, cardiac pacemakers
231
pacifiers 43
pads & tampons 89, 147
pain
abdominal pain, symptom
guide *211*
angina **224–5**, 230
back pain, symptom guide *210*
breast pain (mastalgia) *215*,

243–4, 500–1
chest pain, symptom guide
207
chronic pelvic pain **250–1**
dysmenorrhea (period pain)
107, **247–8**
earache, symptom guide *215*
fibromyalgia 438, **440**
frozen shoulder 420, **441–2**
headache *215*, **403**
joint pain, symptom guide
208–9
labor pains & pain relief **132–3**
low back pain *210*, **434–6**
migraine **403**, 407, 470
muscle cramp **438**
painful intercourse in women
(dyspareunia) **271**
pleurisy 392, *393*
polymyalgia rheumatica **440**
postherpetic neuralgia 335,
408
sciatica 435, 437
symptom guides *207–11*, *215*
trigeminal neuralgia **408**
see also other conditions
causing pain (e.g. arthritis)
palate, cleft lip & palate **528**
palpitations **231**
palsy, facial palsy **417**
pancreas *349*, *355*, *496*
pancreas conditions
acute pancreatitis 355, 358,
359–60
diabetes mellitus 273, 323, 365,
504–6
pancreatic cancer 355, **360**
see also cystic fibrosis
pancreas transplant 505–6
panic attacks **287**, 293
Pap (cervical) smears 119, 138,
258, 259, 281, 282
parathyroid gland *496*
paratyphoid & typhoid **343**
parenthood, adjusting to **148–51**
Parkinson's disease &
parkinsonism 168, **415**
paroxetine (Seroxat) 293, 295,
303
see also SSRIs
partial seizures 539
partial-thickness burns 563
partnership & marriage
problems 151, **152–3**, **177**,
197, 200
parvovirus infection (erythema
infectiosum/slapped
cheek/fifth disease) **543**
patch testing 318, *318*
patent ductus arteriosus 520
pathological fractures 422

Acknowledgments

DK would like to thank the following people for their contribution to the book:

CONSULTANTS
Directory: Professor M.W. Adler, Dr. Robert Allan, Dr. Robin Blair, Professor Charles Brook, Dr. Christopher Davidson, Mr. J.M. Dixon, Professor Andrew Doble, Dr. Tony Frew, Mr. Michael Gillmer, Professor Terry Hamblin, Dr. Paresh Jobanputra, Professor P. Kendall-Taylor, Dr. David Kerr, Professor P.T. Khaw, Professor Leslie Klenerman, Professor David Mabey, Dr. Hadi Manji, Dr. Martin Partridge, Professor Robert Peveler, Dr. J.A. Savin, Professor Martin H. Thornhill
Dietary information: Lyndel Costain **First aid:** Dr. Vivien Armstrong

Thanks also to: Laboratory Spa and Health Club in London, Corinne Asghar, Angela Baynham, Sue Bosanko, Peter Byrne, Ellie King, Alyson Lacewing, Mary Lyndsay, Ruth Midgley, Michelle Pickering, Esther Ripley, Lucas Mansell, and Sally Smallwood for additional photography

The publisher would like to thank the following for their kind permission to reproduce their photographs: (Abbreviations key: t=top, b=bottom, r=right, l=left, c=center)

Britesmile 491 (bc, br); Corbis Stock Market 486; Corbis Stock Market/Ariel Skelley 425 (c); Corbis Stock Market/Darama 104 (br), 127 (br); Corbis Stock Market/David Raymer 184 (bc), 198 (bl); Corbis Stock Market/David Woods 327; Corbis Stock Market/DiMaggio/Kalish 185 (bl), 199 (tr); Corbis Stock Market/Ed Bock 163 (cr), 179 (bl); Corbis Stock Market/George Disario 77 (bl); Corbis Stock Market/George Shelley 191 (b); Corbis Stock Market/John Henley 175 (bl); Corbis Stock Market/Jon Feingersh 530-531; Corbis Stock Market/Jose Luis Pelaez Inc. 45 (tl), 92 (tr), 197 (b), 342 (c) ; Corbis Stock Market/Jules Perrier 63(bl); Corbis Stock Market/Michael Keller 136 (tl), 138 (tr); Corbis Stock Market/Norbert Schäfer 82 (b, c), 99 (bl), 100 (tl); Corbis Stock Market/Tom & DeeAnn McCarthy 105 (br), 124 (tr); Corbis Stock Market/Tom Stewart 93 (bl); Corbis/Martin Hughes 162 (tl), 168 (tl); Eyewire 157 (cla, ca), 226 (bl), 285, 345 (b), 537 ; ImageState 114 (tr), 162 (cr), 176 (tr); ImageState/AGE Fotostock 7 (cb), 85 (tl); ImageState/Stock Image 171 (br), 500 (t); Masterfile UK 164 (tr), 166 (tl); Masterfile UK/Brian Kuhlmann 42 (tl), 47 (tcr); Masterfile UK/Dan Lim 39 (bc), 57 (cl); Matt Meadows 401 (br); Meningitis Research Foundation 405 (tr, cl); Photodisc 157 (tl), 294, 310, 329 (t), 417; Photonica/Neo Vision 411; Powerstock Photolibrary 144 (tr), 163 (t, c), 169 (cr), 301 (tr); Rex Features 156 (cb, b, c); Science & Society

Picture Library/Science Museum 473 (b); Scott Camazine 412 (b, cl); SPL 353 (bc, br), 392 (b); 541 (tl); SPL/Alfred Pasieka 474, 495; SPL/Antonia Reeve 406; SPL/Biophoto Associates 397; SPL/BSIP 319 (tl); SPL/BSIP VEM 372; SPL/BSIP, Laurent 344 (b); SPL/BSIP, LA/Filin.Herrera 442 (t); SPL/BSIP, Sercomi 219; SPL/Chris Priest 146 (br), 245 (cr), 549 (br); SPL/CNRI 382; SPL/Conor Caffrey 334 (b); SPL/David Parker 243 (br), 263; SPL/Department of Clinical Radiology, Salisbury District Hospital 412 (bl); SPL/Dr Linda Stannard UCT 330; SPL/Dr. P. Marazzi 337 (b); SPL/Faye Norman 376 (bl); SPL/Gaillard, Jerrican 466 (t); SPL/Geoff Tompkinson 331 (b), 401 (tr); SPL/Gusto 387 (tr), 482 (cr); SPL/Hattie Young 493 (b, c); SPL/J. C. Revy 423 (cl, c, cr); SPL/James King-Holmes 391 (c); SPL/John Greim 431; SPL/John Radcliffe Hospital 318 (t, c), 405 (tl); SPL/Lauren Shear 513 (br); SPL/Mark Clarke 315 (b, c), 317 (r); SPL/Martin Dohrn 462; SPL/Matthew Munro 383; SPL/Mauro Fermariello 521 (br); SPL/Mehau Kulyk 218 (b, c), 231 (cr), 240; SPL/NIBSC 510-511; SPL/Oscar Burriel 308; SPL/Peter Menzel 395 (tr); SPL/Philippe Plailly/Eurolios 225 (br); SPL/Prof. P. Motta/Dept of Anatomy/University "La Sapienza", Rome 419, 424; SPL/Quest 8 (cl), 309, 347, 443; SPL/Robin Laurance 522 (b); SPL/Samuel Ashfield 277; SPL/Saturn Stills 23 (bl), 506 (cl); SPL/Sheila Terry 535 (br) ; SPL/Simon Fraser 224 (b); SPL/Tim Beddow 284; SPL/Tissuepix 483; SPL/Will & Deni McIntyre 409; SPL/Y. Beaulieu, Publiphoto Diffusion 381(c); Stone/Getty Images 3, 6: (tr, c), 7 (tc), 8 (bl), 14-15, 17 (tr), 20, 21 (tr), 22 (tr), 25 (tl), 26 (bl), 27 (bl), 29 (tr), 32 (b), 34-35, 38 (tr, cr), 44 (br), 46 (bcl), 48 (tr), 51 (br), 53 (tr), 70 (bl), 80, 83 (cl,

b, c), 90 (tr), 91 (br), 98 (tr), 101 (tr, bl), 102, 105 (cl), 115 (tr), 117 (t), 120 (bl), 126 (tl), 129 (t), 133 (t), 136 (tc, br), 137 (b, c), 141 (bl), 143 (bl), 153 (bl), 154 (bl), 155 (br), 157 (tc, tr), 158 (tr), 160, 167 (br), 184 (br), 187 (b), 195 (bl), 198 (tr), 200 (tl, br), 201 (b), 204-205, 216-217, 220 (b), 228, 254, 286 (b), 290 (tl), 418, 427 (b), 444, 475, 478, 479 (c), 491 (tl), 501, 524 (b), 527 (br), 547 (br), 552-553; TCL/Getty Images 6 (cl, br), 16, 19 (tr), 28, 36, 38 (tl), 39 (cl, br), 41 (b), 47 (bcl), 50 (c), 52 (br), 53 (c), 55 (cr, bl), 57 (br), 58, 72 (bl), 75 (t), 111 (tr), 119 (tr), 131, 136 (tr, c), 139 (br), 149 (b), 178 (tl), 179 (t, c), 182, 184 (tl, bl, cl), 190 (tl), 192 (bl), 196 (br), 203, 229 (tr), 266, 289, 292 (b), 297 (tr), 315 (tr), 325 (tr), 356 (cl), 373 (b), 433 (bl), 455 (br), 534 (tl); Telegraph Colour Library 74; The Image Bank/Getty Images 33 (tr), 38 (cl), 39 (tc), 49 (c), 54 (tl), 66 (br), 86 (tl, br), 97 (br), 104 (cr), 116 (tl), 118 (tl), 121 (b), 125 (t), 134, 158 (tl), 159, 162 (tc, cl, bl), 163 (tl), 167 (br), 172 (tr), 173 (bl), 176 (bl), 180 (tl), 188 (tl), 194 (tr), 202 (tr), 291, 302 (br), 420, 440 (t), 484, 551; The Photographers' Library 502 (tr); The Wellcome Institute Library, London 324, 526 (br)
Back jacket
Corbis Stock Market/Jon Feingersh (cl); ImageState/Blackdog Productions (tr); SPL/Hank Morgan (clb)

All other images © Dorling Kindersley.

For further information see:
www.dkimages.com